p. 493-501
516-530

THE BIOMECHANICS OF HUMAN MOVEMENT

MARLENE J. ADRIAN, D.P.E.
Professor of Kinesiology, Rehabilitation, Bioengineering
Director of Biomechanics Research Laboratory
University of Illinois at Urbana-Champaign

JOHN M. COOPER, Ed.D.
Professor Emeritus of Physical Education
Indiana University

Benchmark Press, Inc.
Indianapolis, Indiana

Library of Congress Cataloging in Publication Data:
ADRIAN, MARLENE 1933-
COOPER, JOHN 1912-
THE BIOMECHANICS OF HUMAN MOVEMENT

Cover Design: Gary Schmitt
Copy Editor: Alicia Rasley
Illustrations: Craig Gosling
              Ellyn Traub
              John Nixon

Manufactured By: Edwards Brothers
                Ann Arbor, MI

Library of Congress Catalog Card number: 86-71388

ISBN: 0-936157-06-2

Printed in the United States of America
10 9 8 7 6 5 4 3 2 1

The Publisher and Author disclaim responsibility for any adverse effects or consequences from the misapplication or injudicious use of the information contained within this text.

Contents

The essentials of human movement, human anatomy,
   environment, movement system, communication system,
   and posture

iii

CONTENTS

CONTENTS   **v**

CONTENTS   **ix**

CONTENTS   **xi**

Dedication

TO:

The curious, inquiring students who are not satisfied with known knowledge but are striving to gain new understandings and insights, who will be the future explorers and scientists probing into the mysteries of human action.

EACH AUTHOR'S SPECIAL TRIBUTE:

To Anne, my inspiration; and Michael, my first artist.

Marlene J. Adrian

To my family: Charlianna, my wife; Carolyn, Jack, and Joanna, my children, for their support and forbearance while I searched, examined, and wrote about the field of movement through 40 years.

John M. Cooper

Foreword

"Citius, Altius, Fortius"—Swifter, Higher, Stronger—the motto of the Olympics. Striving for excellence is the goal of every Olympic athlete. To achieve that goal, the athlete must be able to move in the most effective and efficient manner possible. The goal of the Olympian is not unlike the goal of everyone who performs the tasks of daily living or who engages in leisurely activities. The joy and satisfaction of movement occurs when it is done correctly, effortlessly, and safely.

The study of biomechanics allows one to scientifically analyze the techniques involved in the performance of human movement skills. The meaning of biomechanics in the current text is described as an integrated study of forces produced by and acting on the human body. Further, it is the study of the consequences of those forces in producing motion and tissue deformation. This implies that the study of biomechanics encompasses the whole of body movement, both internally and externally.

The responsibility for teaching effective human movement through a knowledge of biomechanics rests with the physical educator/biomechanist. He or she must have an understanding of and must be able to communicate the principles underlying movement patterns. To this end, Adrian Cooper's *Biomechanics* provides the vehicle by which this can be accomplished. The text is a comprehensive undertaking. Writing something new and innovative in a competitive market is a challenge. The authors have more than met the challenge. *The Biomechanics of Human Movement* explores biomechanics from every aspect involving the moving living body. In their attempt to use the holistic approach, Adrian and Cooper have included discussions on developmental biomechanics, occupational biomechanics, rehabilitative biomechanics, exercise biomechanics, and biomechanics in the arts. The traditional topics of kinematics, kinetics, and musculoskeletal system biomechanics also are included.

To the beginning student in biomechanics, this text provides a blend of theory and practice. There are mini-labs to assist in learning concepts, numerous illustrations to clarify points, and a summary discussion of principles after each concept has been introduced and discussed. These should serve as motivational tools for learning.

Adrian and Cooper long have been recognized as pioneers and leaders in the field of biomechanics. They will take their place in history along with the others who have so ably promoted the study of human movement. Their enthusiasm is contagious and their dedication to the field second to none.

Carole J. Zebas, P.E.D.
Professor of Physical Education
University of Kansas
Kinesiology Academy Chair-Elect
CS-ACSM President

Preface

We acknowledge the influences of all those who have worked and written with us, especially Larry Morehouse and Ruth B. Glassow. We wish to recognize the pioneering work of Ruth Glassow in the synthesis of theory and application of human movement.

Though this is our second collaboration, we truly believe this is essentially a first, written from a different and fresh viewpoint. We have written a biomechanics of human movement text in which the application of the concepts of biomechanics is made to a wide spectrum of environments. In addition, we kept in mind teaching and coaching situations. We consider this to be a unique and comprehensive approach representing a frontier of knowledge approach with some topics, heretofore, never included in a biomechanics book.

We have continued the tradition of presenting the pertinent concepts and newest research findings, both domestic and foreign, have followed the current guidelines for content and experiences in biomechanics and have been futuristic in our approach. The contents of this book have been designed to challenge the reader's thirst for the latest on movement information, to take the reader beyond what exists into what can be. Additionally, we have incorporated the international system of units of measure, injury aspects of participation, handicapped mobility problems and improvement of human movement based on a holistic and individualized approach. Quantitative measurement of human movement is reported when available, as the authors believe that without the quantitative, there cannot be adequate assessment and understanding of human movement.

The Mini-Lab Learning Experiences have been retained, and in many instances, enlarged. Teachers have stated that these exercises have aided in providing learning experiences that reinforced concepts and strengthened the ability to apply knowledge. In addition, new movement activities have been included to expand knowledge and extend applications.

Two very unusual features are included in this book. One, each section, large or small with one or two exceptions, is so constituted that it is an entity within itself, and the information can be extracted from the book and used separately. Two, a number of quest authors have either reviewed and brought material up-to-date, or have written on specific topics in which they are experts. Many of them are not only biomechanists, but are also teachers and coaches of human movement. We are pleased and excited about their contributions.

PART I encompasses the general background required to study

the biomechanics of human movement and posture. This part consists of an introduction, effect of gravitational environment, human structure, movement systems, communication system and motion mechanics. All of these are related to the human being in motion.

PART II is a detailed summary of methodology for human movement analysis. Tools, guidelines for improvement and predictions, and qualitative and quantitative techniques are discussed.

PART III includes occupational biomechanics, rehabilitational biomechanics, developmental biomechanics, the arts and biomechanics, and exercise biomechanics. This features some new and exciting concepts.

PART IV consists of concepts for teaching, coaching, injury prevention, enhanced performance and training in sports. Individual and team sports and specific movements related to sports, some of which occur in unusual environments, are described.

PART V is the future. New ideas and projected theories and applications of biomechanics are described. A challenge is given to the reader concerning the use of biomechanics in the future.

The Appendices include basic trigonometry and metric-English system tables, procedures for calculations of characteristics of projectiles, muscle-joint charts, anthropometric chart and moments of force chart.

Marlene J. Adrian
John M. Cooper

Contributors

Marlene J. Adrian, D.P.E., F.S.M.
Professor of Bioengineering
Director, Biomechanics Research Laboratory
University of Illinois at Urbana-Champaign
Urbana, IL

John M. Cooper, Ed.D., F.S.M.
Professor Emeritus
Former Director of Biomechanics Laboratory
Indiana University
Bloomington, IN

Connie Bothwell-Myers, Ph.D.
University of New Brunswick
Fredericton, N.B. Canada
Chapter 17, Curling

Carol Brink, Ph.D.
St. Cloud State University
Minneapolis, MN
Chapter 13, Biomechanics in the Arts

Joy Hendrick, Ph.D.
State University College at Cortland
Cortland, NY
Chapters 3, 4, & 6, Human Structure,
Movement and Communication Systems

Phillip Henson, Ph.D.
Indiana University
Bloomington, IN
Chapters 15, 16, & 17, Track and Field Runs,
Jumps and Throws

Lois Klatt, P.E.D.
Concordia Teachers College
River Forest, IL
Chapter 19, Field Hockey

Anne Klinger, Ph.D.
Clatsop Community College
Astoria, OR
Chapter 20, Combatives

Sharol Laczkowski, M.S.
Indiana University
Bloomington, IN
Chapter 21B, Power Skating

Dawn L. Orman, B.S.
University of Indianapolis
Indianapolis, IN
Chapter 18, Badminton

Lynda E. Randall, Ph.D.
Florida State University
Tallahassee, FL
Chapter 9, Clinical Diagnosis

James Richards, Ph.D.
University of Delaware
Newark, DE
Chapter 21B, Bobsled and Luge

Mary Ridgway, Ph.D.
University of Texas at Arlington
Arlington, TX
Chapter 19, Volleyball

Lela June Stoner, Ph.D.
University of Minnesota
Minneapolis, MN
Chapter 13, Biomechanics in the Arts

Tonya Toole, Ph.D.
Florida State University
Tallahassee, FL
Chapter 9, Aging

John Wasilak, P.E.D.
California State University, Los Angeles
Los Angeles, CA
Chapter 21A, Swimming

Jerry Yeagley, M.S.
Indiana University
Bloomington, IN
Chapter 18, Soccer

Part I General Biomechanical Concepts

The essentials of human movement, human anatomy, environment, movement system, communication system, and posture

1

Introduction to Human Movement

Welcome to the exciting and diversified world of biomechanics! When you elect to explore this world, you will be embarking on an immense journey which has fascinated human-kind since time's beginning. The human body contains more mysteries than the cosmos or the deep, and studying it and how it thinks, dreams, imagines, feels, and moves is more fascinating than the best novel or greatest movie.

Through biomechanical studies, engineers, mathematicians, zoologists, biologists, computer scientists, and others strive to measure, model, explain, equate, categorize, and catalog the movement patterns of all sorts of living creatures. There are persons who exclusively study one of the following: snake biomechanics, amoeba biomechanics, equine biomechanics, animal biomechanics, and human biomechanics.

Some human biomechanists also study selected body parts and tissues, rather than the body as a whole. (Thus, a person might be interested in bone biomechanics, muscle biomechanics, lung biomechanics, or blood biomechanics.) The study of specific parts of the body usually has had clinical objectives. Two of the very prominent areas of study with clinical applications are orthopedic and podiatric biomechanics. If you were interested in orthopedic biomechanics you would investigate movement patterns and forces acting at the joints and on the bones of individuals prior to surgery or treatment and after surgery. Podiatric biomechanics is probably less than twenty years old. The concern of the latter is how and why the feet and legs function or malfunction. Interest in this area has been influenced by improved technology, the "fitness running revolution," and its concomitant high numbers of injuries. Others might be interested in the third category, that of biomechanics of movement of the living body as a whole.

This latter area has been conveniently categorized into sports,

3

occupational, activities of daily living (ADL), rehabilitative, and exercise biomechanics. In addition, special populations have often become the subject for these areas of study. The athlete is most often studied in sports biomechanics. The disabled and the elderly are studied utilizing knowledge from ADL biomechanics.

All these areas of application will be discussed in this book, to provide a more holistic and broader perspective to the reader. Although some persons may apply biomechanical knowledge solely in one sub-area, such as sports biomechanics, some people may not wish to channel themselves so narrowly. Since the approaches, tools, basic foundation of knowledge and ultimate goals are similar, one biomechanist may learn and teach another biomechanist. For example, what is learned in the study of joint biomechanics in pigs quite often has some direct value to the person studying gait (i.e., walking and running) patterns of human beings.

All of the above examples have been applied to biomechanics areas of study. The biomechanist is interested in improving performance, preventing injury, correcting a dysfunction or weakness, and identifying ways to alter the movement patterns of human beings. When a scientific method is used to investigate phenomena, this is termed research. Research with application as a goal is termed applied research. Research that has no immediate application is termed basic research. The latter research in the biomechanics area would consist of investigations of underlying mechanisms and formulation of theories as to the why of the action. It is improbable that much biomechanics research would be pure (basic) research in the sense that an application would not be "in the back of the researcher's head," if not in the forefront of the investigation. Yet, some biomechanists may devote most of their energies in basic research. Most likely, some of their findings will eventually be applied by others.

The explosion of knowledge within any field of almost every discipline has been enormous in the last twenty years, and the sub-discipline of biomechanics is no exception. The study of this specialty requires comprehension of certain aspects of several sciences which form the foundation for investigative procedures. They may be augmented by information from social sciences and humanities, but the main supportive parts are the biological sciences. The utilization of these knowledges are essential to thoughtful inquiry. This is true especially in biomechanical inquiry involving human movement. Also, an open mind is necessary to a scientific approach.

Yet, whatever the focus or area of study, biomechanists will fail miserably unless they remember that they are studying the most complete and challenging organism ever to evolve—the human being. When one grasps this point and holds it fast, the philosophy of the biomechanist emerges. Human motion must be analyzed and studied as a means to an end, not as an end in itself. We move not only to live, but also to express our joys and sorrows, our struggles and our triumphs, and the incredible experience of being a living, thinking being. It is to persons of this orientation that the material in this book will be most meaningful.

MOVEMENT AND LIFE

Movement is basic to life. There can be no life without movement, whether that movement is extrinsic or intrinsic to the organism. To survive, one must move: move to eat, to breathe, to reproduce, to defecate, to develop bone and muscle, and to continue all the life processes. Movement allows human beings, birds, fish, quadrupeds, and other life forms to achieve a degree of independent living. Through the acquisition of skilled movement patterns, human beings are able to work and to play more effectively and more efficiently. The thrill of being able to tie one's shoes, saw wood, hit a baseball, kick a soccer ball, swing an axe, ride a horse, shovel snow, peel and slice potatoes, hoe a garden, sing a song, play a piano, swim or walk a mile, play a game of racquetball, or jump from an airplane and form a free-fall skydiving pattern is part of the joy of life. These overt movement patterns, however, do not arise spontaneously at birth. Overt movement patterns must be learned, although some movements are more reflex based and therefore are easier to learn than others. Nevertheless, there is always some trial and error involved in every attempt at locomotion, manipulation, or a combination of these and other types of movements.

One of the underlying goals of any human being, then, might well be to learn to perform skilled movement patterns with the least amount of frustration, failure, and danger. Another important goal may be that of helping others, human beings or animals, to develop effective, efficient, and safe movement skills. Additionally, one might be merely curious about movement: how it occurs and how it can be changed. All these goals are best accomplished by receiving instruction from persons who have conducted a scientific study of movement. This scientific study of movement, in the past, was termed "kinesiology," which literally means the science of motion.

In its purest form, kinesiology is synonymous with the term biomechanics. In the therapy world, kinesiology often is synonymous with applied (functional) anatomy. The meaning of kinesiology as used by the therapist, however, has been expanded to include all of the sciences related to human movement: sociological, psychological, physiological, anatomical, cultural, pedagogical, and biomechanical.

Currently, however, biomechanics is considered to be the physics of human or other living being's motion, an integrated study of forces produced by the human body and forces acting on the human body and the consequences of motion and tissue deformation.

Studying biomechanics includes studying the temporal and spatial characteristics of motion, which are referred to as the "kinematics" of motion. The spatial characteristics of motion include (1) the direction of the motion with respect to the three-dimensional world in which all things move, and (2) the path of the motion. Temporal characteristics include the time span needed to execute the motion or selected phases of the motion. These characteristics can be described in qualitative or quantitative terms. Thus, some of the words and phrases used to denote the kinematics of motion are as follows: fast, slow, right, left, forward, diagonally, in a straight line, in a circle, 30 m/sec, 200 rad/sec, 4 kmph, 6 m, 180 degrees/sec, and 5 m at a 60-degree angle with the horizontal. Biomechanics also includes the study of the "kinetics" of motion, which refers to the forces causing, modifying, or otherwise facilitating or inhibiting motion. Force, work, kinetic and potential energy, momentum, and power are some of the terms used to describe the force aspects of motion. Examples of the units of measurement are Newtons, pounds, joules, and watts.

An expanded definition that can be used by the student of biomechanics is as follows: Biomechanics is that branch of science concerned with the understanding of the interrelationships of structure and function of living beings with respect to the kinematics and kinetics of motion. Thus, concepts from anatomy, physics, and mathematics are used to determine and measure the quantities of motion— time, space, and force—and to fully understand movements of living things.

Historically, kinesiology often did not include the investigation of deformation and stresses to the human and animal body or their parts. This limitation, however, may have been a result of four factors: (1) inadequate instrumentation, (2) a primary interest in the analysis of movement patterns, (3) a movement-effects approach toward the analysis of muscle force, and (4) limited knowledge about movement; qualitative analysis had to come first. Steindler (1955), however, more than three decades ago included discussion of pressures within the hip joint and structural deformities of bones in his treatment of kinesiology. Therefore, in this book no differentiation will be made between "kinesiology" and "biomechanics." For persons who wish to pursue this topic further, Atwater (1980) provides an informative discussion of various meanings of kinesiology and of biomechanics.

THE AGE OF BIOMECHANICS

The field of biomechanics is new, yet very old. It is relatively new in that the big surge in biomechanical research and subsequent publications began in earnest in the 1960's. Prior to 1950, many research studies were often conducted with only a few subjects or only one subject. Valid results were obtained with crude instrumentation, but to apply the findings to a specific population was often difficult. Nevertheless, that was done because additional data were not available. Perhaps one of the reasons for the surge was that technology was advanced sufficiently to enable investigators to process data rapidly from large numbers of subjects. The present generation owes a huge debt to those of the past. Some few examples will be mentioned here.

In prehistoric times, parents taught the skills of survival to their children, usually on a one-to-one basis. To hunt, fight, work, and/or escape successfully was based on skills handed down from one generation to another. The correct mechanics as known were presented until new methods were developed, mostly on a trial and error basis.

The ancient history of human beings is depicted on cave walls, showing the mechanics of performance. The ancient Egyptians (5000–3000 B.C.) built the pyramids without the use of power tools. They were also familiar with many games and contests and how to perform certain skills, such as what is now called Greco-Roman style of wrestling, the crawl stroke in swimming, and the correct positions in running. These are shown by drawings on some of the tomb walls.

The Greek Aristotle (384–322 B.C.) must have had the eye of an eagle (without the use of any instruments) to make his comments about runners, jumpers, and throwers regarding body position and the center of gravity (Cooper). Aristotle gave the world, including coaches, therapists, physical educators, physicians, and even industrial workers, the idea of using detailed observations. Hart (1925) said, "From the point of view of mechanics, we may regard Aristotle's work as the starting point in the evolution of the subject up to the days of Leonardo da Vinci." In fact, some historians believe many of da Vinci's ideas were gleaned from and enlarged upon from the thoughts found in Aristotle's writings.

Archimedes (287–212 B.C.), a Greek mathematician, proposed principles of flotation which are the basis of modern swimming concepts. Also, his comments on the lever system and compound pulley are classics, and of practical use today. His insights must have been phenomenal, taking into account the mathematical knowledge of the period. Leonardo da Vinci (1452–1519 A.D.), a Roman citizen, never has been equalled in talents. He was a biologist, an artist, and an engineer of a high quality. His knowledge of anatomy and mechanics make him one of the forerunners of biomechanical thought. He had the ability to draw the action of muscles when the human body was performing a dynamic act. This was of great value to medical students and to future biomechanists. Also, da Vinci's intelligence and versatility are exemplified in his description in his treatise on the "Flight of the Birds." Pilots of modern planes use the method of lowering a wing in righting a plane in flight that he mentioned concerning birds.

Galileo (1452–1519 A.D.), Newton (1642–1727 A.D.), and Borelli (1608–1679 A.D.) gave the biomechanists much information on the mechanical aspects of human motion. Galileo's contributions were many in the field of mechanics, including identifying the rate of acceleration of falling objects. Newton, an Englishman, proposed three laws of motion which are used today to understand human movement.

Borelli, a pupil of Galileo, applied Galileo's mathematical concepts to movements. Steindler (1955) believed that Borelli should be considered the Father of Modern Biomechanics. He supported this contention by saying that "the essential feature of kinesiology (nee biomechanics) is that it treats all motor functions, normal and abnormal, as mechanical events."

Finally, Amar, a Frenchman, made great contributions to biomechanics in the area of efficiency and body mechanics. He wrote *The Human Motor* which is considered by many as one of the outstanding publications on mechanics of performance in industrial work and sports. Each generation has investigators who diligently study human motion. Their instrumentation, techniques, and findings often can be improved upon by the next generation of investigators and practitioners.

WHAT IS MOVEMENT?

Based on the spatial characteristics of motion described previously, movement patterns can be categorized as planar or non-planar. A planar movement occurs in one plane; that is, if the movement occurs in a vertical plane, there will be no horizontal deviation. One might liken planar movement to movement on a sheet of paper (one plane). One might then tilt the paper to produce a new plane, and, in fact, a multitude of planes. The inclined planes are termed diagonal planes of motion.

Visualization of the basic orthogonal planes of motion can be achieved via a cube, representing a piece of cheese being sliced. (Fig. 1-1). The top and bottom are horizontal planes. If the cheese is sliced, parallel to the top surface, the cutter moves in a horizontal plane. The front and back of the cube are vertical slices in the frontal plane. The two sides are parallel to each other and vertical. The slices would be achieved by movements in the sagittal plane. The planes as slices through the center of gravity of the human being are depicted in Fig. 1-2.

Although locomotion tends to be in a vertical plane known as the sagittal, or anteroposterior (AP) plane, the anatomy of the body is such that some horizontal motion occurs as the body alternates between right-leg support and left-leg support. Only during imposed conditions and during limited single-limb movements used in exercising is pure planar motion likely to occur. Human movement usually occurs in two or more planes and is referred to as non-planar or three-dimensional.

If movement is primarily in one plane and movement in a second plane is negligible, the movement may be analyzed as a planar movement for ease of analysis. For example, many movements of human beings and quadrupeds are sagittal-plane movements primarily, since anatomically the flexor and extensor muscle groups are the principal locomotor muscles. Birds use their wings in the frontal plane, a vertical plane with movements right and left of body center. Fish move their tails in a horizontal plane. Thus, these three planes (sagittal, frontal, and horizontal) are considered to be the basic planes of motion in our three-dimensional world. Logan and McKinney (1977) have defined several diagonal planes of motion because many human arm motions occur in diagonal planes. Two of these diagonal planes are (1) right high to left low and (2) right low to left high. Additional planes of motion have been identified in human-factors engineering and in aerospace research. The complexity of describing spatial motion increases as the need increases for more precision in locating the path of movement. It is through knowledge of the planes of movement that the movement analyst can determine the probable muscles involved in producing the movement (Fig. 1-3).

The three types of motion that occur within a plane or through several planes may be described as follows. "Translatory motion" is motion of a body from one plane to another, with each part of the body moving an equal distance. The movement may be linear, that is, occur in a straight line, as in the movement of a child being carried. Another example of translatory movement would be gliding on ice skates (see Fig. 1-4). Because we live in a gravitational field, many of the observed translations of objects are curvilinear, or parabolic, such as the flight of a ball.

Contrast translation with the second type of motion, "rotary motion." This type of motion differs from translation in that the body or body segment rotates about an axis, causing each part of the body to

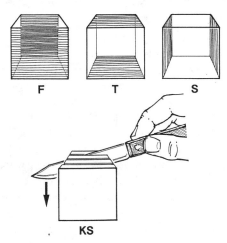

Fig. 1-1. *Three-dimensional space can be visualized as a cube, rectangle, or a room in a house. The surfaces of the structure represent the planes of the body: F, the front and back surfaces of the cube lie in the frontal (medial-lateral) plane; T, the top and bottom surfaces lie in the transverse (horizontal) plane; and S, the side surfaces lie in the sagittal (anteroposterior) plane. The movement involved in slicing the cube occurs in the plane of the surface being sliced: KS, the movement of the knife occurs in the frontal plane since the slices are separated front-to-back. Describe the movements of the knife to cut in the sagittal, transverse and oblique planes.*

INTRODUCTION TO HUMAN MOVEMENT **9**

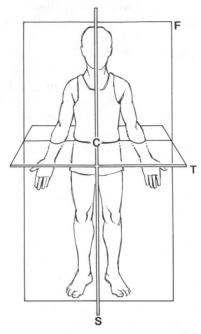

Fig. 1-2. *The center of gravity (center of mass) of the human body is at the intersect (C) of the three cardinal planes: transverse (T), sagittal (S), and frontal (F) (coronal). In this case the body is divided into top and bottom halves (cephalic-caudal halves), right and left halves, and front and back halves (anterior-posterior halves). The human body is depicted in a position known as "the anatomical position."*

move a distance proportional to its position from the axis. For example, a person performing a giant swing on the high bar (Fig. 1-5) will experience only a slight movement of the wrists, whereas the hips will move a distance equal to $2\pi r$, with r equal to the length of the body from hands to hips. Logically the feet travel the greatest distance of all the body parts, a total of $2\pi r$, with r now being the length of the body from hands to feet ($\pi = 3.1416$).

Many limb-segment exercises utilize pure rotation; however, human and animal movements tend to be complex, and a third type of motion, a "combination of translation and rotation" (general motion) is the more common type of motion produced voluntarily. The human anatomy consists of a number of body parts attached by means of joints, which act as axes of rotation. Locomotion occurs, and the body translates as a result of rotations of two or more body segments. Therefore, one or more of the axes of rotation translate, and only one axis is stationary, or fixed. The complexity of locomotion is illustrated again when one notes that the same axis does not remain fixed during locomotion. At one point, the fixed axis is the intersection of the heel of one foot with the ground; next, the fixed axis occurs at the intersection of the metatarsal-phalangeal joint and the ground. Later the

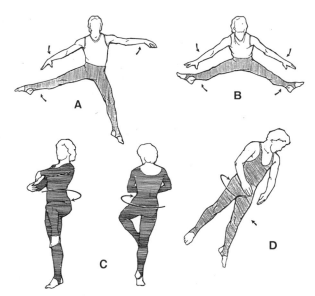

Fig. 1-3. *Recognition of the planes of movement and general spatial orientation of body parts is a primary part of movement analysis. Identify the planes of movement of the depicted figures prior to reading the rest of this paragraph. A: Arms and legs have moved in the frontal plane. B: Arms and legs move across the sagittal and frontal planes as the trunk moves in the sagittal plane. C: Total body twisting (turning) movements have occurred in the transverse plane. D: The body moves in the oblique plane as the leap is taken and the body moves in the transverse plane as the twist is executed. Test your ability to describe the planes of movement depicted in the many figures in this book.*

fixed axis transfers to the opposite limb. Thus, the human body has been referred to as a kinematic link system. Movement of one segment of the body creates movement and a repositioning of another body segment (Fig. 1-6). One can readily see what happens to the position of the forearm and hand when the following movements are executed:

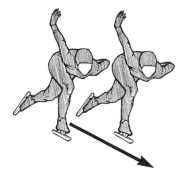

Fig. 1-4. *At this instant during ice skating, translation occurs since the total body of the skater glides along the ice. There is no rotation of any body segment.*

INTRODUCTION TO HUMAN MOVEMENT **11**

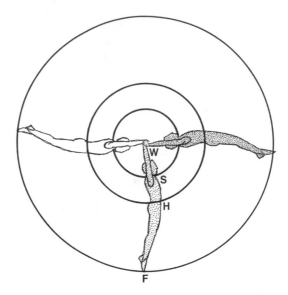

Fig. 1-5. *This giant swing on the gymnastics high bar is an example of rotary motion. The bar is a fixed axis of rotation. The wrist (W) travels a circumferential distance of 2πr, where r represents the radius of rotation. Note the circumferential distances increase as the body part (S, shoulder; H, hip; and F, foot) is farther from the axis of rotation. The shoulder travels approximately one-fourth the distance the foot travels. The actual distances can be calculated by measuring the figure and multiplying the values by 60 (the figure is 60 times smaller than the actual human being). What is the approximate distance the hip will travel?*

1. Starting in the anatomic position, with the arm vertical at the side of the body, flex the arm at the elbow to an angle of 90 degrees.
2. Abduct the arm at the shoulder and note that position of the forearm and hand.
3. Medially rotate the arm at the shoulder and note the position of the forearm and hand.
4. Extend and flex the forearm from the position described in movement 3.
5. Simultaneously extend the forearm while adducting the arm.

The difficulty of the last movement illustrates the interrelationships of the movements of the limb segments. Adduction at the shoulder also adducts the forearm, which, in this situation, is an opposite movement to that of the extension at the elbow.

With respect to the giant swing depicted in Fig. 1-5, the body may not maintain its rigid extended length throughout the swing. A common action is flexion at the hip to assure that a complete revolution can be achieved. Thus the movement now will consist of two axes of

THE BIOMECHANICS OF HUMAN MOVEMENT

rotation, one fixed and one stationary. A rotation takes place about another rotation without any translation.

Axes of rotation are represented by the joints of the body, by axles of wheels and other inanimate objects, and by imaginary lines within the body or between the living body and another body, living or inanimate (Fig. 1-7). For example, a person pivots (rotates) about an invisible axis at the intersection of the hands with the ground when doing a cartwheel.

Each anatomic axis and each axis external to the living body (external axis) may be described with respect to space. The axis may be represented as a line passing through the plane of motion and at a right angle to that plane. Therefore, any rotary motion in a horizontal plane will occur about a vertical axis (Y). When rotary motion occurs within one of the two vertical planes of motion, the axis of rotation will be one of the two horizontal axes. The sagittal plane of motion occurs about the horizontal-frontal axis (Z), and the frontal plane of motion occurs about the horizontal-sagittal axis (X). Rotary motion occurring in diagonal planes will have diagonal axes.

This description of motion provides the underlying basis for the analysis of motion. From this basis, a determination of the sources or forces producing motion can be made, in particular, the mathematic evaluation of motion in terms of linear displacement or angular displacement. It must be kept in mind, however, that aspects of both types of motion almost always occur during a movement pattern.

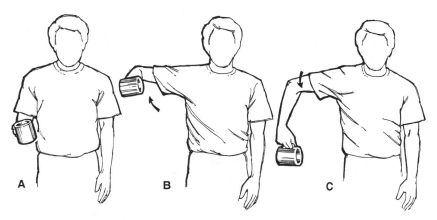

Fig. 1-6. *The human body is a kinematic link system with movement of one body segment influencing another body segment. In these examples, movements of proximal body segments reorient the distal body segments. A: Abduction of the arm causes the palm to change from a palm up position to a palm down position. Fluid would spill from a cup held in the palm. B: Medial rotation of the arm causes the forearm to assume a vertical position. Experiment with other movements: for example, starting in the anatomical position, flex, then horizontally extend, and then adduct the arm. Repeat as many times as possible. What is the limiting factor?*

INTRODUCTION TO HUMAN MOVEMENT   **13**

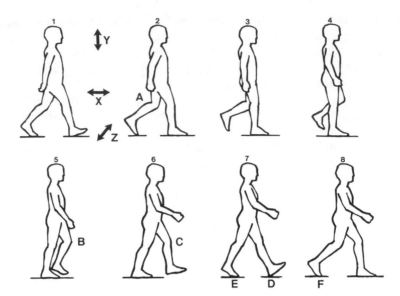

Fig. 1-7. *Using nomenclature of the Cartesian Coordinate Reference System, the common rotary movements are depicted with each major axis of rotation.: vertical axis (Y), lateral-horizontal axis (X) and frontal-horizontal axis (Z). Prior to reading the following sentences identify the axis or axes of rotation in each figure and determine the plane of movement of the body parts rotating about the identified axes. During this walking sequence there are six axes present with respect to the movements of the leg. A: The leg rotates in the sagittal plane (flexes) about the frontal-horizontal hip axis; B: the shank rotates in the sagittal plane (extends) about the frontal-horizontal axis at the knee; and C: next, both hip and knee axes are present as the thigh flexes and the shank extends. D: As heel contact is made, the axis of rotation becomes the intersect of the heel with the floor (again a frontal-horizontal axis) as the total body rotates about the axis; E: next, the body rotates about the metatarsal joints; and F: lastly, during the toeoff position the axis of rotation becomes the toe-floor intersect. Select the figures in chapter 21B to identify axes and planes of movement for airborne activities.*

MINI-LAB LEARNING EXPERIENCES

1. Observe a variety of movements: locomotion, manipulation, and single-limb movements. Identify planes and axes of motion.
2. Ask two persons to rise from a chair. Does each utilize the same body segments, axes and planes? How do they differ and why do you think the difference occurred?

CLASSIFICATIONS OF MOVEMENT

In addition to the planar-3 dimensional translatory descriptions of motion, there are several classification systems of movement patterns that may be used by the movement analyst. One classification consists of work, activities of daily living (ADL), and leisure. The kinesiologist, biomechanics specialist, or human engineer interested in greater work productivity might well be concerned only with movement patterns related to the work situation. The physical therapist might be concerned with ADL and the restoration of independent living for the physically disabled. The physical educator and coach might be concerned only with leisure activities of sports and dance. This broad classification system is not always effective, however, since many movement patterns do not exist solely in only one of each of these categories. For example, walking is an activity of daily living and is also used in the work situation, in folk and disco dancing, and in several sports, including golf.

One might also group movement patterns according to the amount of learning involved, for example (1) new movements to be learned or to be relearned if rehabilitation is the goal, (2) movements learned in a wrong or unusable manner that need to be unlearned and then learned correctly, (3) movements to be refined that are partially learned, and (4) movements that are automatic, requiring no learning but needing reinforcement. This method of classification does not lend itself to a scientific study of movement, since what is a new skill for one person may not be a new skill for another person. Therefore, more definitive classifications of movement that are more useful for the purpose of biomechanical analysis have been developed.

Higgins (1977) has grouped movement patterns into three categories: locomotion, manipulation, and a combination of the two. Although these categories are useful, many biomechanists have preferred to further subdivide movement patterns into more specific, yet rather broad categories, such as locomotion on land, locomotion in the water, locomotion in the air, projecting oneself into the air, returning to earth, swinging and suspending one's body, projecting external objects, receiving external objects, and manipulating objects. Manipulation has been divided into gross motor skills such as using long-handled instruments, and into fine motor skills such as piano playing, using a fork and spoon, and typing.

Movement may also be described as being effective or ineffective, efficient or inefficient, and safe or unsafe. If a movement is effective, it may not necessarily be the most efficient movement.

Efficiency may be determined physiologically, that is, by evaluating the metabolic cost of the movement with respect to the amount of work performed. The relationship of work of the movement or energy input and work or energy output determines the efficiency. When the mechanical work performed by the human body on some object is only slightly less than the mechanical work performed to produce the respective movement of the human body, the movement is considered to be efficient. The formula for the percentage of efficiency from the biomechanists' point of view is as follows:

Efficiency (%) = (work out/work in) × 100.

Rarely does the human body accomplish more than 25% efficiency with respect to a movement task. There are times when efficiency is not as important as effectiveness. For example, in sprinting, the expenditure of energy is of little concern. Being effective over a short time is the goal. Utilization of a high rate of energy is expected, and the most efficient pattern may not be the fastest. Long-distance running, on the other hand, requires more efficient movements if the person desires to complete the race.

There are many ways to perform a task effectively. Very young persons and animals usually perform movements using excessive muscle forces and extraneous motions. "Wasted" effort goes unnoticed. To be effective day after day or during movements lasting hours in duration, efficient movements need to be developed. The more efficient a person is in executing a basketball jump shot during the first minutes of a game, the more that person is likely to be able to execute the movement effectively during the last minutes of a strenuous game. On the other hand, a basketball player may be so tense early in the game that unnecesary muscles will be used to perform the task of shooting. As the game progresses and relaxation occurs, the movement becomes more efficient and more effective. The differences between efficiency and effectiveness must be remembered when analyzing movement. They are not the same. Effectiveness is easy to measure; efficiency is not.

Finally, movement may be safe or unsafe. Great concern has arisen concerning the type of movements and the velocities at which these movements are being performed by young athletes. The challenge, the prize, and the glamour of being the best have caused many performers to practice long hours, to exert great forces by the body and on the body, and consequently to reach the pinnacle of human tolerance. If biomechanical analysis is undertaken, we will SEE the difference in performance outcome:

S   for safety
E   for effectiveness
E   for efficiency

Whatever the method selected for categorizing movements, the ultimate purpose is to be able to define general principles of biomechanics for ease in analyzing many movement patterns. The cross-country runner, recreational jogger, racehorse, and domestic dog all utilize similar principles in their execution of locomotor patterns.

Categorizing movements enables one to see similarities but may obscure differences. For example, throwing movements that require high accelerations, greater use of muscles, and near-maximal efforts are described analytically in a different manner from throwing movements requiring accuracy but not great speed. Broad categories in the classification of movement patterns do, however, provide the basis for reducing the varieties of possible movements into a workable whole.

Specialists may then benefit from knowledge gained in other fields of study. For example, the clinical kinesiologist has provided information related to walking patterns that has proved helpful to the sports biomechanist investigating the forces produced by and imparted to the jogger and sprinter.

WHAT IS THIS THING CALLED THE HUMAN BEING?

What are some of the feats that human beings have accomplished? Some remarkable feats are as follows:

1. Many persons have been able to swim the rough and stormy English Channel. It has taken 20 or more hours of continuous swimming to perform this feat. A few years ago, James Counsilman (former U.S. Olympic swimming coach), at age 58, was able to perform this arduous task.
2. Some persons, after becoming quadruple amputees, have been able to participate in many physical activities, including sports.
3. A few people have fallen to the earth from great heights and lived to tell about it, without permanent injury.
4. One man walked around the world (wherever there were land masses) in four years. Other feats have included marathon dancing, running, sailing, cardio-pulmonary resuscitation performed for record-setting numbers of hours and days.
5. Human beings have the ability to pace themselves over a long-distance run. Indians, often in relay fashion, were able to run down a deer.
6. A blind person can play a game of golf. With the aid of an assistant for posture placement, a blind man has obtained a score of 85 on a typical 18-hole course.
7. Human beings have obtained running speeds of 45 kmph (27 mph); some say only 22 depending upon calculation procedures. When it is realized that the human being has only two legs with which to propel a body designed as a cylinder offering maximum wind resistance, this is truly remarkable.

The fastest and strongest movements tend to be seen in the sports arena. Baseballs are thrown overarm at 167 kmph, and softballs are pitched underarm at a slightly faster speed. The volleyball overarm serves attain speeds of 117 kmph, which must be dissipated by the receiver. Tennis balls are projected at 257 kmph, badminton smashes travel at 400 kmph, and the slap shot in ice hockey has been recorded at 197 kmph. Although locomotor speeds are not as fast, human beings ride skateboards at 100 kmph and enter flight at 110 kmph from a ski jump. Contrast these speeds with such ADL movements as walking at 5 to 8 kmph and mopping a floor at 6 to 9 kmph.

Persons do become injured during movements and wonder how to determine the safe limits of movement. This question is of concern to investigators in the animal world as well. The safe limits of animal, and sometimes human, movement in the rodeo events of calf and steer roping and wrestling, bronco and brahma bull riding, and barrel racing are yet unassessed quantitatively. What are the limits to which horses and dogs may be taken in preparation for and during races? The same question could be, and should be, asked about human racing.

Comparison of Human Beings and Animals Regarding Running, Jumping, and Swimming

Another approach to an understanding of the movement potential of human beings is to compare their feats with animals in running, jumping, and swimming. The same could be done for several other skills.

It is noted (see Table 1-1) that in speed running on land the human male is below the average (22 plus miles per hour for the selected animals); the slowest is the tortoise (not even one mile per hour) and the swiftest, the cheetah (70 miles per hour but lacks endurance). The latter's long stride and spine flexibility enables it to attain great speed. On the other hand, the gazelle with its short body and long legs can outrun the cheetah over a long distance. It can be seen that the human being is among the slower runners.

With respect to jumping, the most powerful jumper for its size is the flea, which can jump 200 times the length of its body. It can jump 6 in. vertically and 12 in. horizontally. The human male is able to jump horizontally 29 ft. $2^1/_2$ in., while the impala can jump 40 ft. The kangaroo is able to jump 9 ft. vertically, and the dolphin 14 ft.

In swimming, the tuna and sailfish are the fastest, with the sailfish attaining a speed of 40 miles per hour. The human male swimmer attains a speed of 8 miles per hour.

Incidentally, flying is not a skill human beings have attained unless they use artificial means. Flight in the air by the peregrine falcon and Indian swift is up to speeds of 100 miles per hour. Birds have a light skeletal framework, hollow bones, and warm internal temperature system (105 degrees Fahrenheit). On a dive, the falcon can reach a speed of 200 miles per hour. Human beings have flown across the English Channel by means of powered wings.

It is obvious that the human being is not capable of equaling or surpassing many of the large animals in speed races and in height and length of jumps. The human body is not designed for great speed, agility, or even strength (which is not compared here). (However, with a great deal of training and systematic study from a mechanical viewpoint, the human beings might reduce to a degree this superiority of other animals.)

The human being consists of:

1. More than 200 major muscles supplying energy (out of a total of over 600 muscles).

Table 1-1. *Comparison of performances of human beings and animals with respect to land speed, jumping distances and water speed. How would we fare if we had an Olympic sports competition open to all species?*

ON LAND	SPEED (miles per hour)	
Tortoise	1	
Elephant	12	
Human male	25	
Racing camel	27	
Horse	40	
Gazelle	60	
Cheetah	70	

JUMPING DISTANCE (feet and inches)		
	Horizontal	Vertical
Flea	12″	6″
Frog	15″	9″
Grasshopper	30″	15″
Hare	22′ 4″	15″
Human male	29′ 2$^1/_2$″	7′10″
Deer	30′	8′
Puma	38′	12′
Horse	39′	8′ 6″
Kangaroo	27′	9′
Impala	40′	8′

IN WATER	SPEED (miles per hour)	
Beaver	4	
Human male	8	
Trout	19	
Flying fish	22	
Tarpon	25	
Tuna	30	
Sailfish	40	

*Information taken from various sources, including, where possible, world records. Some of the above has been estimated.

2. More than 206 bones providing the framework for movement.
3. 43 major joints of the appendages (126 bones involved), about which body parts rotate.
4. Several miles of nerves transmitting messages.

Levers and the insertion points of muscles have an effect on performance. The angle of the bony lever that is assumed in action likewise influences the action. Usually, the arms are placed at approximately 90 degrees and the legs at 115 degrees in order to sustain great weight or exert great force. It has been mentioned that it takes 30–40 times more energy to carry messages along the nervous system than to move muscles. The fastest moving muscles are those that are fast twitch or white muscles; the slow twitch or red are slow sustaining muscles. For example, the track sprinter usually has 60%–70% or more fast twitch muscles in the legs than a distance runner who has percentage-wise higher slow twitch muscles. It may be as high as 70%–80%.

The human body often has been compared to a machine, a product of human ingenuity. The human motor is probably best described as an "electro-capillary" engine in which nervous excitation modifies the tension of the muscles and produces contraction (Amar).

The efficiency of the human machine as compared with the steam engine is high. Steam engines require about double the fuel consumption. Walking is one of the most efficient movements, varying from 25% to 30%, based on caloric intake and work output. The ability to develop power of a sustained nature is less than one horsepower (contrast that with the horsepower developed in the automobile engine). The human being can, however, develop 6 HP for a fraction of a second during activities, such as shot putting.

The human body and how it performs must not be thought of as a machine, but a living and changing entity. Many factors can affect human performance. Coordination of muscles, health, and general condition of the person, level and type of techniques, readiness for action, previous experience, temperature, fatigue, anxiety, motivation, cultural setting, social expectations, gender, and age of participant all enter into determining movement performance achievements.

Men and women perform skills in much the same manner. The anatomical and physiological differences are evident but only to a degree. Since strength is a function of the cross-sectional area of muscle, and men have greater musculature, the strength factor favors the male. This difference in strength, however, is evident only on an absolute basis because when strength is equated with lean body weight pound-for-pound, there is no difference in strength between males and females. The ability, however, to move quickly in a small space favors the female. Top women athletes now are performing certain skills, especially in swimming and track and field events, as well as Olympic male athletes did only a few years ago.

There may be a systematic order to human motor movement that can be vertical and lateral in nature, ergo, a developmental sequence. Development proceeds from head-to-toe (cephalo-caudal) and from trunk-to-limbs (proximal-distal). With respect to gross locomotor movements, many children may be observed to follow this progressive order: swimming, crawling, climbing, walking, running, jumping, throwing and on to complex movements involving part or all of the above. The one action that must be developed and understood is walking (at least, a step), which is a part of almost all gross body movements.

Movement has a definite rhythm. Frequently, performers remark about their rhythm in performing a motor task. If the sports performer or worker is out-of-synch (synchronization) with the action and one's own body rhythm, then completion of the act at a high level is not apt to occur.

Most workers and sports performers are often unaware of the exact details of performing a movement; a type of automatic pilot takes over. Performers rarely can verbalize about the action but prefer to "show" how it is done. Usually, this is a good idea since cerebrating (thinking) about an action is contra-indicated while performing, because once movements are learned, they become seemingly automatic and thinking about the details of a movement while performing causes interference. What performers believe they do, however, may not be what they actually do.

RELATED AREAS

There are areas and ideas, some including new fields of study, related to biomechanics in which new concepts about motion can be learned. The field of "kinanthropometry" is a relatively new scientific discipline that has emerged to focus solely on the measurement of size, shape, proportion, composition, maturation, and gross function as related to such concerns as growth, exercise, performance and nutrition. Because of the physical (anatomic) characteristics of human beings, it is known that researchers, teachers, coaches, physical therapists, and all those associated with education in and improvement of human movement have attempted to relate anatomic characteristics to movement achievement. An understanding of this discipline's concepts offers a great opportunity to gain new insights. It is closely aligned with ergometry, the measurement of the work of muscles.

Morphology, another field of measurement, is a branch of biology encompassing the form and structure of plants and animals. The form of an organism, such as a human being is considered apart from function.

One of the methods more commonly used to study proportionality characteristics is the body typing method called "somatotyping" (Sheldon et al., 1954). Since persons tend to observe the total body in rather general terms such as skinny, fat, or muscular, the somatotype has been very popular. The ectomorph is the linear or lean person, the endomorph is the person with excess adipose tissue, and the mesomorph is the person with a high proportion of muscle. Few persons exhibit only one of these attributes; most have a combination of all three. On a 7-point scale, the average person would be rated 4, 4, 4 (endo-, meso-, ecto-). Athletes tend to be more mesomorphic, except for the ectomorphs found in events such as long-distance running. Athletes also are usually taller than the normal population. In addition, numerous researchers, more recently those using the Carter anthropometric somatotyping method, have shown that athletes in certain sports cluster in unique places on the somatotype chart (Fig. 1-8). One consequence of these findings is that preselection and training of young children for national and international sports competition has been conducted solely on the basis of the child's anatomic characteristics. Unfortunately, we do not know whether athletes develop their body characteristics because of the sport or choose the sport because of their body characteristics.

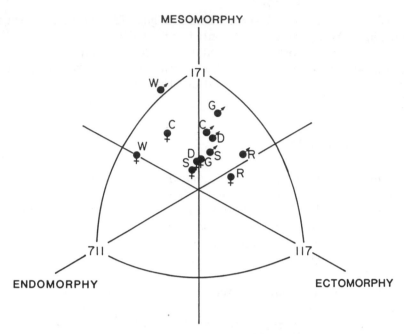

Fig. 1-8. *Mean somatotypes of sports groups participating in Mexico Olympic Games. ♂, male; ♀, female; W, weight throwers; C, canoeists; G, gymnasts; S, swimmers; D, divers; R, middle-distance runners. (Based on data presented by de Garay, A. L., Levine, L., and Carter, J. E. L.:* Genetic and anthropological studies of Olympic athletes, *New York, 1974, Academic Press, Inc.)*

Widths, lengths, girths, and other single anthropometric measurements do not correlate highly with any known skill. Ratios, indexes, and comparisons of one measurement with another have shown higher correlations with performance than did single measurements, but even these parameters do not provide more than a group predictability. A more complete approach is the use of a unisex phantom, or representation of a bilaterally symmetric average human body. When the unisex phantom model (Ross et al., 1978) was applied to data collected by Eiben on 125 women athletes participating in the European Track and Field Championships, 1966, the following significant differences among long jumpers, shot-putters, discus throwers, and the phantom were found:

1. Long jumpers had smaller arm breadth and girth measurements than that of the phantom.
2. Long jumpers had longer tibial heights than shot-putters.
3. The shot-putters and discus throwers had much greater chest depth and bitrochanteric width than did the phantom.
4. Long jumpers' thigh circumference and body weight were equal to the phantom; the discus throwers' were greater than the phantom, and shot-putters' measurements were greater than discus throwers.

22   *THE BIOMECHANICS OF HUMAN MOVEMENT*

More than 100 measurements are taken on a person to construct an anthropometric profile of that person. The profile can then be compared with profiles at various times with respect to age, sports participation, nutrition, and other factors, as well as with profiles of other persons, including champion performers.

From a biomechanical perspective, the athlete who is successful in projecting the body into space must be proportionally different from the one who projects objects. Just as Murpurgo found exercise to change the body, one cannot be sure how much the body is changed through participation and how much is inherited, and which proportion of each is vital to success in a motor skill. High correlations merely show relationships, that is, the one item is likely to occur with another item related positively to it. One must be cautious, however, not to confuse relationships with cause and effect. It has been shown that both bone and muscle hypertrophy with use. Tennis players, bowlers, baseball pitchers, and other unilateral sports performers have heavier and larger limbs on one side of the body than on the other.

In the succeeding chapters, anatomic characteristics that enhance and inhibit certain movement performances will be described. In some cases, the interaction and interdependency of factors prevent a complete identification of the pertinent anatomic characteristics.

Open-minded readers must be aware that there are numerous movement specialists who have developed procedures and instrumentation to further the understanding of human movement and analyze the action of participants. Among these specialists are:

Psychometrists noted that people can best learn information about an object by just holding and moving it. This technique is employed by workers in industry and by specialists in sports, such as basketball players, pitchers in baseball, and passers in football. The greater use of psychometry might not only add credence to the concept, but also be applicable to human movement analysis.

Dianeticists subscribe to a system that involves the analysis, control, and development of human thought. This method helps provide techniques for increasing ability. It embodies "mind over matter." Many who deal with human performance at a high level believe that the mental aspect of performance is 4 times as important as the physical. The dianetics concepts expressed by Hubbard (1975) can be adapted and utilized in biomechanics in some instances.

Physical therapists are professional medical people who spend a great deal of time with rehabilitating the movement of permanently or temporarily disabled persons. The application of some of their ideas to the field of biomechanics is enlightening and worthwhile.

Psychologists who study the application of psychological knowledge to sports have many concepts the biomechanist may utilize. For example, the relationship of anxiety of muscle tension, speed of movement and coordination is within the psychological domain. The psychological orientation toward movement is different but worthy of consideration by the biomechanists.

Physiologists' investigations overlap and sometimes augment that of the biomechanists. The internal body system is their main area of study.

Anatomists deal with the structure, the framework including muscles, bones and nerves of the body. Information from this field undergirds that of the biomechanists. It is the basis for the "bio" part of biomechanics.

REFERENCES

Amar, J. (1920). *The Human Motor,* E.P. Dutton & Co., Inc.: New York.

Aristotle (1945). *Parts of Animals, Movements of Animals and Progression of Animals:* Loeb Classical Library, Harvard University Press: Cambridge, MA.

Atwater, A. E. (1980). Kinesiology/Biomechanics: Perspectives and Trends, *Research Quarterly, Exercise Sport,* 51:193–218.

Braun, G. L. (1941). "Kinesiology": From Aristotle to the Twentieth Century, *Research Quarterly* 12:163.

Cooper, J. (1979). Biomechanical Research in Sport: Past, Present, and Future, In *Science in Athletics,* Terauds, J. and Dales, G. (eds.) Academic Publishers: Del Mar, CA, pp. 3–15.

Hart, I. (1897). *The Works of Archimedes,* University of Cambridge Press: London.

Higgins, J. R. (1977). *Human Movement: An Integrated Approach,* the C. V. Mosby Co.: St. Louis, MO.

Hubbard, L. R. (1975). *Dianetics,* Bridge Publications, Inc.: Los Angeles.

Locke, L. F. (1965). Kinesiology and the Profession, *JOPHER* 36:69.

Logan, G. and McKinney, W. C. (1977). *Anatomic Kinesiology* (2nd ed.), Wm. C. Brown Co.: Dubuque, IA.

O'Malley, C. D. and Saunders, J. B., de C. M. Leonardo da Vinci (1952). *On the Human Body,* Henry Schuman, Inc.: New York, p. 174.

Ross, W., Eiben, O., Ward, R., Martin, A., Drinkwater, D. and Clarys, J. (1984). Alternatives for the Conventional Methods of Human Body Composition and Physique Assessment. In *Perspectives in Kinanthropometry,* J. Day (ed.), Human Kinetics: Champaign, IL, pp. 203–220.

Sheldon, W. H., Dupertuis, C. W. and McDermott, E. (1954). *Atlas of Men,* Harper: New York.

Steindler, A. (1955). *Kinesiology of the Human Body Under Normal and Pathological Conditions,* Charles C. Thomas: Springfield, IL.

2
Human Gravitational Environment

Imagine the anatomic changes that would occur, particularly in muscle development, should human beings be compelled to move in another environment than on earth. At the sun, for example, body weight would be more than 30 times that on earth. Without some major change in muscle morphology, human beings would weigh two and one-half times their earth body weight if they lived on Jupiter. Contrast this with a weight of approximately 40% on Mars and 17% on the earth's moon. The astronauts had a great deal of difficulty walking on the surface of the moon. Since their bodies kept rising upward, they had to use a short-step pattern with very low accelerations of the body parts. Atrophy of muscles, particularly those identified as antigravity muscles, would result from living on the moon.

Plants, animals, and human beings respond according to their unique structure, and each structure can be and is modified by the environment in which it exists. Within the earth's environment, bodies are attracted to the earth at an acceleration rate of approximately 9.8 m/sec^2. This rate varies with respect to the distance of the body from the center of the earth, but any attempt to move the body upward requires muscular force in opposition to this attraction known as gravity. The required force is directly proportional to body mass, which is the quantity of matter the body possesses. The product of mass and acceleration of gravity is equal to body weight. The effectiveness and efficiency of upward movement is therefore determined to a major degree by the relationship of body weight to the force that the muscles of the body can produce, as well as to the speed of this force production.

According to physicists, although gravity is one of the minor forces in nature, gravity is one of the major forces with respect to movement. Every movement of a body part upward or downward is influenced by gravitational force—facilitating the downward movement and inhibiting or indirectly causing an upward movement. Since every volitional movement of body parts is rotary, there will always exist a vertical component for every movement. Furthermore, since the force of gravity is a vertical vector (an arrow having a vector quantity, or magnitude of force, acting toward the center of the earth), it influences the efficiency of every posture or stance, as well as every movement. When muscle force is required to maintain a posture, the amount of force required is directly proportional to the efficiency of that posture. To determine whether or not muscles will need to contract, thereby exerting a counterforce to the gravitational force, one must resolve the gravitational force vectors acting on every particle of the body either into one force vector or into one force vector per body segment.

This single force vector acting on the body is called the gravitational line. This line passes through a point known variously as the balance point, center of weight, center of gravity, or center of mass. The position of the center of mass of a body is important in determining equilibrium and dynamic control. In this chapter we will investigate the erect posture and the relationship of the gravitational line to muscle force and body structure and then will present techniques for determining the position of the center of mass in a stationary body and in a moving body.

STANDING UPRIGHT

Human beings are bipeds whose upright posture makes them distinct from all other animals. Using "man" and "his" as neutral gender, Morton and Fuller say that "in his body form, in his completely erect bipedism and mental development, Man possesses characteristics that separate him undeniably from all other living creatures." They are of the opinion that the physical differences that distinguish the human being from other, closely related animal forms developed as a result of reaction to the force of gravity. (See Fig. 2-1.) To maintain an erect position, human beings had to undergo certain skeletal and muscular changes. The human foot became the sole weight-bearing organ. Concerning the human foot arrangement, Morton and Fuller (1952) state:

(1) It permits the body center to occupy its central position over the area of ground contact so that the margin of postural security is equal forward and backward;
(2) It places the direction of structural unbalance toward the front so that the muscular tension needed to maintain our erect posture is imposed entirely upon the large and powerful calf muscles;

(3) The weaker anterior group of muscles is released from any active counterbalancing tension.

In addition, they stress the value of an anteriorly unbalanced position of the body center in aiding the initiation of forward movement.

Human lower limbs are more extended than are those of partially bipedal animals and are extended in line with the body. The human gluteus maximus as an extensor of the hip is unusually large and is counterbalanced by the large quadriceps femoris in front. The latter arrangement helps prevent the leg from flexing, which would cause a person to fall in moving forward as the foot strikes the ground.

The use of the arms and hand to support the body weight in the hanging position and to move is called brachiation. Species using this form of locomotion, brachiators, are considered ancestors of homosapiens and had to develop morphological changes in the arms and hands that produced free mobility in the shoulder girdle and wide movement in all directions in the shoulder joint. The upper limbs were lengthened and strengthened, and the movements of supination and pronation were developed in the forearms. The hand, including the digits and thumb, is common to certain related animal forms, but the human hand is the most flexible and dexterous.

To provide better balance, human beings developed one unique skeletal part, the human foot. Bony segments above the foot were altered, and among these was the pelvis, which gradually took a vertical, rather than a horizontal, position to support the weight of the torso better. To meet this function, the pelvic bones shortened, thickened, and broadened. (For a detailed description of this evolutionary change, see Napier.) Again using "man" and "his" as neuter terms, Howell (1944) says:

> Man is a biped with a unique pelvis, and although neither cursorial (running) nor saltatorial (jumping) in a strict sense, his

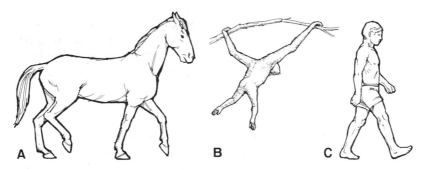

A   B   C

Fig. 2-1. *Anatomical structure is the foundation for functional movement. Quadrupeds, brachiating animals and human beings have unique structures that favor walking on four legs (A), locomotion by swinging from the arms (B), and walking on two legs (C). Study the skeletal structure of the horse and human being and postulate what the structure of this brachiating animal would be.*

adaptations should receive some attention. His pelvis has been shortened (craniocaudally) and broadened. The ilium has expanded not only ventrally but dorsally (thereby accentuating the greater sciatic notch). The position of the thigh in the upright posture has tended to reduce to zero the angle of the leverage of the hamstring muscles—a quandary that the ischium has met by migrating dorsally.

Since human lower limbs perform the functions of both weight bearing and locomotion, structural differences exist between the human being and the lower animals. Essentially the human being is less well equipped to run, jump, or even stand than are other animals. However, the upper limbs are free for manipulation. Structural differences from the feet to the pelvis provide for the weight-bearing and locomotor functions. Likewise, differences, especially the lumbar curve, are present in the spinal column and torso to adjust to the upright position. The C-shaped curve of the spine in an infant develops into the anterior, posterior, or lateral S curve of the adult. During the period of creeping and progress into walking, the spine undergoes changes, especially in the lumbar region, to enable the child to become an upright creature. The lumbar curve is seen only in the human species.

Medawar (1958) states:

> The . . .vertebral column. . . is not a column at all, but is more like a cantilever having the four legs as piers. The vertebral column of a human being is no longer a simple uninflected arc; it bends slightly forwards in the neck, slightly backwards in the thoracic cage, forwards again in the lumbar region, the small of the back, and backwards in the fused vertebrae that form the sacrum. That is the mature pattern; in development, the neck flexture appears somewhat before birth, and the lumbar flexure between the ninth and eighteenth months of age.

The center of gravity of the human body is elevated to a position high above and to the outer borders of the feet, the supporting parts. This unstable and potentially mobile structure must be held in a standing position by continuous muscular action because it is a high vertical structure with a small base.

Above the midline, any body portion that is moved to the rear or front to any great extent makes the maintenance of balance more difficult. A person whose body is unusual, such as large or tall, or who has a specific body part that is unusually large or long, may find that these conditions affect the ability to maintain an upright position. For example, a male with a heavy, tall body and small feet will experience some difficulty in standing and walking comfortably. His base is not large enough to allow him to withstand as great a displacement of force as he should. However, Morton and Fuller believe that this instability of normal individuals is an aid in the initiation of forward movement. Joseph (1960) has said:

> One may therefore conclude that in the posture of standing at ease (military position) in most subjects, stability at the ankle joints is maintained by the calf muscles, mainly the soleus, at the knee and hip joints by the appropriate ligaments and at the vertebral joints by only some parts of the sacrospinalis muscles. There are no apparent differences between the sexes with regard to the leg and thigh muscles. Movements such as swaying at the ankle joints or flexion at the knee or hip joints or flexion of the vertebral column result in activity in the appropriate muscles, usually the extensors, which resist the force of gravity.

In other words, not all muscles are used to maintain the standing position, as would be more likely in a vigorous movement such as running. The specific muscles used are rightly called "postural muscles."

Hellebrandt has said that standing is really movement on a stationary base and that swaying is inseparable from the upright stance. Hellebrandt and others have shown that considerable sway occurs in forward, backward, and sideward directions. Cooper has had his students measure the amount of sway that occurs during 5- and 10-minute periods of standing erect without moving (other than swaying) and with the feet placed close together. It was found that the longer the individual stands, the greater is the amplitude of sway. Usually after 15 minutes, the individual will tend to faint and fall to the floor. One individual in a special experiment was able to stand erect for 25 minutes with his feet in a bucket of ice water. At the end of 25 minutes, he fell to the floor and had to be revived. In speaking of a study of standing, Hellebrandt and Franseen (1943) state:

> Weiner (1938) in South Africa combined the factors of exercise and a hot, humid environment in studying the ability to stand. He found that most of his adult male Bantu subjects could tolerate an hour of quiet standing after shoveling gravel for an equal period of time. When, in a controlled experiment, the standing was undertaken in a cool room, no cases of collapse occurred.

The muscles act as "little hearts" in helping push the blood back through the veins to the heart. When this action is lacking, the blood pools in the feet and the individual faints from lack of blood in the brain. Feet have increased in size as much as one and one-half shoe sizes after prolonged standing. A walk of one-half mile reduced the feet to normal size.

Concerning sway, Hellebrandt and Franseen (1943) have said:

> There is general agreement that stance is steadied when the eyes are open and focused on a fixed point and least stable with the eyes closed. Distraction reduces sway. When the feet are to-

gether, the stance is unsettled. Turning the toes out to an angle of 45 degrees or separating the feet so as to equalize the coronal and sagittal planes of support steadies the stance. Sway is much greater in the anteroposterior vertical orientation plane than in the transverse plane. Height and weight correlate poorly with stability. Thus, the body may compensate in other ways for mechanically disadvantageous factors in physical build. When carefully measured, postural sway patterns are characteristic for each person and highly reproducible. There is lack of agreement chiefly as to whether stance training reduces postural instability or not, and whether fatigue is reflected as readily, as is often implied in an augmentation of sway.

Postural sway patterns obtained recently are indicative of the validity of Hellebrandt and Franseen's conclusions of more than four decades ago.

Joseph (1960) also investigated sway. He showed that activity in the muscles of the calves of the legs was greater when subjects wore high-heeled shoes ($2^1/_2$ inches) than when they were barefoot. The increased muscular activity was necessary to counteract the otherwise unstable position created by the high-heeled shoes. Activity in the gastrocnemius muscle was increased the most. Researchers now are interested in evaluating postural sway as related to neurological disease, aging, incidences of falling, and shooting (pistol, rifle, or an arrow in archery).

The term "posture" has many meanings, depending on the person who is defining the term, as illustrated in the following discussion. In 1889 Braune and Fischer described a posture in which a vertical line erected from the ankle intersected the axis of the knee joint, the axis of the hip joint, the axis of the shoulder joint, and the ear. This linear alignment of the body is an erect position representing a convenient posture from which to measure deviations, since all reference points fall along the same line. This posture, in which no part deviates from the vertical line, was named the "normal-stellung," or "normal standing posture." Other postures, such as the relaxed and military, were also described, and deviations from normal posture were discussed. Normal posture does not correspond with the usual position of the body and can be maintained only momentarily. The usual position of the body is a more relaxed posture. Although no attempt was made by Braune and Fischer to depict the normal standing as the ideal posture, such an interpretation became wide-spread. Many logical reasons have been given to support the contention that the normal posture of Braune and Fischer is the ideal one. Most of the reasons were based on the relationship of this posture to the healthy function of the internal organs. Posters showing this normal posture are displayed even today on some schoolroom walls to depict a perfect standing position. Modifications are also seen in posture charts showing a similar "normal" sitting position—a non-natural but "ideal" position.

The statistical interpretation of normality is in terms of the frequency distribution of a population. In a healthy population, the normal posture would be that assumed by the majority. Observations of people standing in line before ticket windows or on street corners reveal that practically no one is using the "normal-stellung." Instead, people shift from one position to another while standing or sitting. An investigator attempting to measure the usual postures of a population would be confronted with the task of erecting a frequency distribution of postures assumed by each person from day to day in various conditions of heat and cold, sickness and health, and sadness and joy. For women, as well as for men, a researcher would face the additional problem of fashion changes. After the model posture of each person has been determined, the frequency distribution for this population could then be projected. This statistical expression of normality of posture derived by the frequency of occurrence of one posture among others would necessarily include the range of differences and the amounts of deviations from the normal that could be expected from time to time. Thus, the statistical normal posture cannot be a fixed value.

The physiological concept of normality is that condition in which the organs and systems of the body function efficiently. Body postures affect physiologic functions. For one thing, the energy requirements of different postures vary considerably. The rigid military posture requires about 20% more energy than the easy standing position. An extremely relaxed standing position requires about 10% less energy than an easy standing position. If one stands so as to be practically hanging on the ligaments (completely relaxed as much as possible), little more energy is used than in sitting or reclining. Hellebrandt and co-workers determined that the energy cost of standing is relatively small and that oxygen consumption during graded degrees of gravitational stress deviates insignificantly from the normal variations characteristic of recumbency.

Blood pressure rises when a person assumes a rigid, erect posture because of the muscular effort involved. The respiratory efficiency is difficult to assess in the resting state, since only a small part of the available lung tissues would provide ample area for the small requirement of gaseous exchange. Because of this excessive respiratory tissue, the small gain in maximal diaphragmatic excursion and vital capacity resulting from changes in posture is inconsequential. Thus, from the point of view of physiologic efficiency, the rigid, erect posture is not the normal, since the efficiency of metabolic and circulatory systems is reduced.

Extreme curvature of the spine and poor alignment produce physiological changes and are considered to be pathologic. Just how much deviation is possible without causing impairment of health and inefficient function of vital organs is a subject of discussion by several authors. Minor deviations do not appear to greatly affect the health and efficient function of the internal organs.

Erect posture is commonly associated with attitudes of readiness, self-confidence, and assurance. A relaxed or slouched posture may generally denote laziness and incompetence. For this reason, the erect posture is the one to which we most often aspire and is considered to be normal. We should not think, however, that a standing posture is a rigid set of aligned anatomic landmarks—lobe of ear, tip of acromion process, middle of trochanter, and head of fibula. Certainly the erect posture gives a better appearance, since clothes fit better, the physique is shown to better advantage, and the face is held up so that attentiveness is indicated. Clothing models, stage and screen performers, and beauty contestants assume erect and stately postures to appear to the best advantage before an audience. However, exceptions have occurred in successful individuals. Superior intelligence and tremendous energy are sometimes housed in a body that is habitually slouched. Some great athletes assume a habitual posture of extreme relaxation.

Normal posture, then, is that which best suits one's own condition and the conditions of the environment. During attention to a stimulating situation, the normal posture will be erect. In a condition of distress because of sad circumstances, normal posture will be characterized by a general sagging of all body parts. In extreme fatigue, the normal posture will be that which conserves energy. The normal posture of physical attractiveness is one that displays the special qualities of the physique to the best advantage.

Metheny (1952) stated her concept of posture as follows:

> There is no single best posture for all individuals. Each person must take the body he (she) has and make the best of it. For each person the best posture is that in which the body segments are balanced in the position of least strain and maximum support. This is an individual matter.

Based upon anatomical differences, gravitational stress patterns are highly individual. Furthermore, body alignment measured repeatedly during uninterrupted standing is variable. The criterion for posture must not be determined by aesthetic ideals, but must be based upon biomechanical and physiological concepts.

CULTURAL DIFFERENCES IN POSTURE

Individuals, as well as family groups, various cultures, and age groups within cultures, show differences in standing and sitting postures. Although individual differences may be linked to many causes, including attitudes and emotional states, the cultures and subcultures appear to develop postures distinct to their groups. The reasons probably are many but certainly include nutrition, climate, and training. Over 1000 different postures ranging from standing, squatting, kneeling, and sitting have been identified by Hewes (1957). Although not common to the United States, at least a fourth of the population of the world habitually crouch in a low squat, both to rest and to work. In certain parts of Africa, India, Australia, and South America the "Nilotic stance" is a common resting position. This stance is a stork-like posture in which the sole of the one foot is planted against the support leg near the knee. Warm climate, bare feet, and unkown cultural reasons are likely reasons for adoption of this stance, as well as occupation or habit of carrying a long staff. Clothing affects styles of sitting for both men and women. However, clothing alone does not explain all posture differences.

MINI-LAB LEARNING EXPERIENCES

1. Observe the postures depicted in Fig. 2-2 and determine which ones might indicate a characteristically rigid posture, which would tend to produce kyphosis (increased convex curvature of upper back), which would tend to produce lordosis (increased concavity of lumbar region), and which would tend to produce scoliosis (lateral curvature of the spine).
2. Identify the muscles that would contract against gravity for each of the postures.

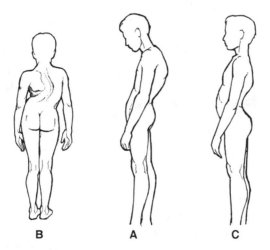

B   A   C

Fig. 2-2. *Standing postures with various spinal column deformities. Match the following to the appropriate posture: scoliosis (lateral curvature of the spine), kyphosis (exaggerated posterior thoracic convexity), and lordosis (exaggerated posterior lumbar concavity). The matching is B, A, C.*

INDIVIDUAL DIFFERENCES IN STANCE

Among the various body types, obese persons are likely to have the most erect posture as a result of the effort required to support excessive fatty tissues. Fat persons twist as they walk, and to reduce the amount of this turning they stiffen and take short steps. Persons with large abdomens often lean slightly backward to balance the weight in front. Some short, stocky people stand erect to make themselves appear taller and slimmer. Extremely thin individuals often lack the muscular strength needed to hold themselves erect. During the teen-age years, many tall girls voluntarily slouch to appear more nearly the size of their shorter boy companions. Specialization in certain forms of hard work or strenuous athletic activity results in adaptations of posture. A coal miner carries the head and shoulders forward and the arms slightly bent in the position of work. The side-horse specialist in gymnastics tends to become overly round shouldered and kyphotic if this activity is not balanced with others that exercise contralateral musculature. Posture adaptations to specialized events may also be counteracted by a conscious effort to improve the carriage at all times when the person is not bent to the task.

Structural deformities cause postural compensations. A short leg produces scoliosis. This may be corrected by elevating the heel to lengthen the short leg. Pronated feet result in an anteriorly tilted pelvis and lordosis, which are corrected when the pronation is remedied.

Effect of Pregnancy

The later weeks of pregnancy are marked by a large forward displacement of the center of gravity because of the combined weight of the embryo, its surrounding amniotic fluid, and the massive uterus. The resulting postural compensation is a light backward lean and backward shift of weight in the lumbar region. More weight is borne by the heels. The backward lean (although the center of gravity stays over the base) becomes more exaggerated as the pregnancy progresses. This adaptation occasionally corrects a customary slouch but usually causes increased lumbar stress.

Effect of Shoe Heel Height

Julius Ceasar is thought to have been the first to discover the advantage of elevating the heels. He observed that when heels were added to the sandals of his legions, the soldiers were able to march farther with less fatigue. When the calcaneus is elevated about 1.27 cm (0.5 inches) above the level of the base of the ball of the foot, its shaft is brought to a tangent with the Achilles tendon, and thus the gastrocnemius and soleus muscles are able to exert a greater force in plantar flexion. If shoes without heels or with higher heels are worn after an individual has become accustomed to wearing heels of a certain height, the legs and feet become fatigued more quickly.

The ability of the human body to adjust to heel heights of 7.5 cm or greater is attested to by the skilled movements of women jitterbug dancers of the 1940's and disco dancers of the 1970's. Cowboy boots are worn by both women and men without mishap. High-heeled pumps, however, appear to be the cause of numerous falling accidents. The high heel combined with the high sole may have caused a reduction in perceptual awareness of the position of the foot and delayed the kinesthetic and tactile responses to loss of balance, in addition to elevating the center of gravity of the body about 9 cm. The changes in line of gravity and position of the center of gravity with different heel heights appear in Fig. 2-3. Note that similar alignment of body parts, as well as knee angle and trunk position, can be achieved with any of these heel heights.

Standing at Work

Continued standing may result in a pooling of blood and of other fluids in the feet, as well as lowering of the arches to such an extent that the foot may increase in size as much as one or two shoe sizes. Thus, clerks, dentists, ticket takers, and barbers commonly wear shoes at work that are lacerated at the toe, ball, and top to allow for the expansion to take place. Probably in such work two pairs of shoes should be worn, one pair in the morning and a larger pair in the afternoon. A compromise in the form of loose-fitting shoes is sometimes made; however, this solution is poor because when no support is given,

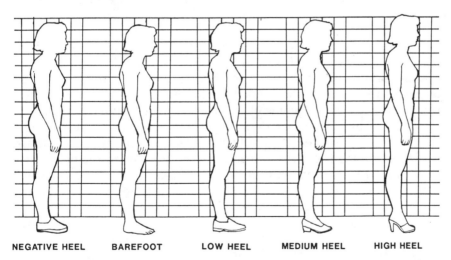

NEGATIVE HEEL   BAREFOOT   LOW HEEL   MEDIUM HEEL   HIGH HEEL

Fig. 2-3. *Effects of changes in elevation of heels on standing posture and forefoot weightbearing. Hip joint and background grid may be used to estimate gravitational line and center of gravity of the body. Note the decrease in forefoot surface area (reproductions of pedographs) and change in weighting of toes and fifth metatarsals as the height of heel increases. What implications do these changes have?*

pronation occurs. A well-designed shoe for standing is constructed so that most of the weight is borne on the outside of the foot, since this part of the foot is supported by strong ligaments, whereas the inside of the foot is supported by long, thin muscles that are easily fatigued.

Posture of Readiness

The standing posture is affected by a person's anticipation of forthcoming action. If no action is anticipated and the conditions of the external environment are unexciting, the response will be a relaxed posture. This is so well-known that athletes can simulate a relaxed posture to deceive their opponents. In a game of basketball a player about to receive a pass can often deceive the defender by assuming a relaxed posture and passive countenance.

The posture of readiness when a rapid or strong movement is about to be performed is an alert one. The peak of attention is reached between 1 and 2 seconds after concentration is directed to the situation. The posture adapts to the condition; after the peak of attention is past, the posture either is relaxed or becomes unstable because of extreme tremor, resulting possibly from accommodation of the coordinating centers of the nervous system.

The position assumed during a state of readiness is in accord with the immediate tasks to be accomplished (Fig. 2-4). If the direction of movement is not known, the weight should be distributed over the surface of both feet. When the direction is known, the center of gravity should be shifted toward the anticipated direction. A slight flexion may occur at the ankle, causing the equilibrium of the body to be unstable and thus facilitating movement. The head, arm, and leg positions are also adjusted to the action to follow. The infielder in baseball leans forward and rises on the toes as the ball is pitched. The base runner taking a one-stride lead off the base will lean toward the next base and rise on the toes as the ball is pitched. In each instance, the mechanical equilibrium of the body is disturbed and movement is commenced. The football quarterback crouches with the arms forward and heels of the hands close together in a position of readiness to catch the ball. Such postures of readiness should not be held motionless for an extended length of time, since proprioceptro sensations, which govern the senses of position and relationship of the body parts to objects in view, will be diminished and have to be reestablished before accurate movement can be accomplished. For this reason, the golfer waggles the club near the ball while adjusting the stance position in readiness for the swing. While poised for the pitch, the batter in baseball does the same thing to heighten the sensation of the position of the bat in relation to the body and to the path of the ball.

The causes of poor posture and the defects associated with pathologic handicaps should be the topic of discussion in books on adapted and corrective physical education. The discussion here has been centered only on the standing position of all human beings, normal and handicapped.

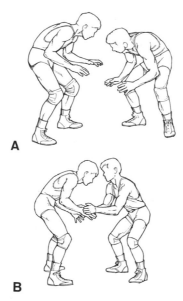

A

B

Fig. 2-4. *Postures of readiness. A, Wrestlers are using staggered stances, which are best for moving rapidly forward or backward. B, Wrestlers are using parallel stances, which are best for moving right or left. Modifications of these two stances are also used in preparation for certain actions and against certain opponents. (From Boring, W. J.:* Science and skills of wrestling, *1975, St. Louis: The C. V. Mosby Co.)*

BALANCING ON HANDS

To keep the base of support wide when the handstand is being executed, the athlete spreads the fingers as wide as possible. The hands are turned slightly outward so that the fingers will be able to help counteract movements to the outside, and the thumbs are turned inward to maintain balance. A plumb line dropped through the center of gravity should fall at the base of the fingers to provide a supporting area from the heel of the hand to the tips of the fingers and thumb, through which the gravity plane can move without the performer's losing balance. This is especially true in the execution of the one-armed handstand. It is also important, in the performance of this move, to hold the parts of the body (arms, torso, and legs) in a relatively stationary position so that control is centered at the shoulder area, where the large muscles (deltoideus, triceps, pectoralis major, and latissimus dorsi) are able to exert their force.

CARRYING OBJECTS

Carrying an object increases the weight that must be supported by the feet and affects the position of the gravity planes with reference to the body. If the carrier is to remain upright, these planes must be kept within the area of the supporting foot; segmental adjustments must be made. This is usually done by altering the trunk position. If the object is held in front of the body, the trunk will be inclined backward; if it is held to the side, the trunk will be inclined to the opposite side. The amount of inclination will be related to the weight, size, and distribution of weight of the object and to the height at which the object is carried. Note in Fig. 2-5 the differences in body position when carrying an identical weight, well distributed and not well distributed with respect to symmetry of the body.

When loads are carried on the head, there is no inclination of the trunk. Visitors to regions in which carying objects on the head, especially among women, is common frequently comment on the excellent carriage of these persons. Undoubtedly the additional weight high above the feet requires careful alignment of body segments.

Walking with heavy load alters the stepping pattern. The center of gravity is not allowed to fall as far forward as it does in normal walking. With the load the step will be shortened, and the center of gravity will be held over the supporting foot for a longer time. It is interesting to note that when bulky packs of produce are loaded onto the backs of Mexican Indian men by fellow workers, the carrier cannot sit down during the 16-km (10 mile) trip from the fields to market, because once the load is lowered, he cannot lift it again without assistance.

PRINCIPLES OF EQUILIBRIUM

With respect to the various postures of static positions that have been presented, the following principles may be stated:

1. To maintain balance, humans beings, as with all living beings, as well as with inanimate objects, must keep the center of gravity in an area within and directly above the supporting base.
2. The larger the base, the greater the range in which the center of gravity can be moved without the body's falling.
3. The closer the center of gravity to the base of support, the greater will be the angle of tilt necessary to move the center of gravity outside the base area. Thus, the stability of the body is often said to be increased as the center of gravity is lowered.
4. The human body can use many body segments as a base—the feet, one foot, the hands, one finger (in the case of acrobats), the head, the thighs, or the entire body.
5. The segments above the base can be adjusted to bring them into various positions. No general balance pattern exists, but whatever the base and the positions of the segments above it, the center of gravity must be kept over the base area if balance is to be maintained.

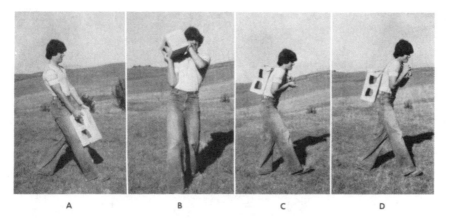

Fig. 2-5. *Variations in body segment alignment as a result of carrying the same load in four positions. A, functional lordosis; B, functional scoliosis; C and D, trunk flexion with possible functional kyphosis.*

It is evident that each object a person carries is added to the weight of the human body in determining the center of gravity of the human-object system. In essence, the object becomes part of the human body, affecting the body's balance point and determining the position of the gravitational vector.

The principles stated above are applicable in situations in which movement does not exist. These principles may or may not be valid for the dynamic situation, since movement itself introduces another force: ma, or $I\alpha$. The mass (m) of the body represents its resistance (inertia) to translation, which is multiplied by acceleration (a) to depict the force of a translating body. The "I" is the moment of inertia, or the resistance to rotation of a body. This resistance is multiplied by rotary, or angular acceleration (α) to depict the moment of force of a rotating body. Therefore, the moving human body may be in "dynamic balance", that is, may not fall during instances in which the line of gravity falls outside the base of support. Note the lean of the bodies depicted in Fig. 2-6 during surfboarding and snow skiing. A further explanation of this phenomenon and of situations in which other forces are present will be considered in Chapter 6.

DETERMINATION OF CENTER OF GRAVITY

The techniques presented in this section use the human being as the subject for the determination of the center of gravity of a body. Some modifications may be made in size of equipment, but the concepts are valid for all applications to living and inanimate objects. In activities such as horseback riding, the investigation of the center of gravity of the horse, the rider, and the horse-rider system may prove useful in determining the positions of the rider that either interfere with the progress of the horse or enhance it. A review of the concepts

HUMAN GRAVITATIONAL ENVIRONMENT   **39**

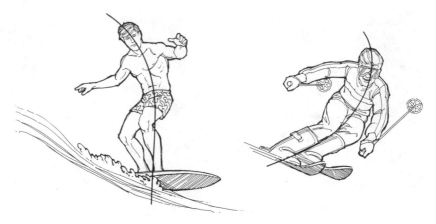

Fig. 2-6. *Typical body leans and curvatures during snow skiing and surfboarding. Can you list other activities that produce similar curvatures?*

involved in the center of gravity is presented first, and then the determination of its location will be discussed.

All masses that are within the gravitational field of the earth are constantly subjected to a pull toward the earth's center; the greater the mass, the stronger will be the force of that pull. The force of gravitational attraction that the earth exerts on a body is called its "weight." Gravitational force pulls downward on each point of a given body. The distribution of these points determines the position of the center of gravity of the body. If a board is suspended on a support as in playground teeterboards, a downward pull is exerted on each side of the support. If the board mass on each side is equal in size and in distance from the support, the board will balance. If a child sits on one side of the balanced board, that side will be pushed downward, and the opposite side will move upward. In such unbalanced situations, gravitational force, interestingly, is responsible for the upward as well as the downward movement. This upward movement caused by gravitational force will be shown later to be used by the body in many forms of locomotion. On the teeterboard, a second child can take a position on the opposite side of the board, and if the distance from the board is adjusted, the board and the two children can be balanced. Within every mass is a point about which the gravitational forces on one side will equal those on the other. This balance point, determined in three planes of the mass, is the center of gravity.

Center of Gravity in the Transverse Body Plane

The point of balance in the human body has long interested investigators. The earliest of these employed the teeterboard to locate the transverse plane of that point. An Italian physicist, Borelli (1608–1679), placed a nude subject on a board in the prone position and then moved the board back and forth as it rested on a knife-edged support until the total mass balanced. He reported the balance plane to be one that cut the body "between the genitals and pubis." Somewhere within this plane would lie the subject's center of gravity. Two German brothers, the Webers, in 1836 improved Borelli's method by first balancing the board and then sliding the subject back and forth until balance was obtained. They found the transverse plane of the center of gravity to be 56.8% of the height above the heel.

Half a century later (1889), the two Germans Braune and Fischer reported that the center-of-gravity plane was 54.8% of the height measured from the soles. Their conclusion was based on finding the point of balance in four fresh "normally built" cadavers that were frozen solid. The cadavers were first balanced on a knife-edge, and then a steel rod was driven into the cadaver at the determined plane. Each cadaver was suspended by the steel rod, and gravitational force moved the mass into a balanced position. When the body attained equilibrium, a plumb line was dropped from the point of suspension to locate the transverse plane of the center of gravity. Since fluid volume and tissue weight varies between live and dead bodies, other methods for determination of centers of gravity of bodies and body segments were sought. Hay (1973) has summarized common methods and data with respect to segmental and body weights, centers of gravity and moments of inertia.

The most convenient early method of locating the plane of the center of gravity was that proposed by the two Americans Reynolds and Lovett (1909). (See Fig. 2-7.) A board of a known length is supported at either end of a knife-edge. The knife-edges are placed on scales that can be adjusted to eliminate the weight of the board. The subject lies on the board, and the plane of the center of gravity is determined mathematically. It will be at a point on the board that can be determined by multiplying the weight on one scale by the distance from that knife-edge to the plane of the center of gravity. This product will equal that obtained by multiplying the weight on the second scale by the distance between the second knife-edge and the plane of the center of gravity: $w_1d_1 = w_2d_2$, where w_1 equals the weight on scale 1, d_1 equals the distance from the line of gravity to w_1, w_2 equals the weight on scale 2, and d_2 equals the distance from the line of gravity to w_2. This equation can be reduced to one unknown by redefining d_2 as the distance between the knife-edge minus d_1. The use of this equation will be shown in the solution of the following problem:

> *Problem:* A subject weighing 660 N lies on a board, with the top of the head in line with the knife-edge on scale 1. The distance between the knife-edges is 1.50 m. The scale reading on the head scale 1 is 320 N; the other scale 2 reads 340 N. These values are placed appropriately into the previously presented equation, which in essence is the determination of the moments of force about the line of gravity.

Solution: $320 \text{ N} \times d_1 = 340 \text{ N} (1.50 \text{ m} - d_1)$

$320 \text{ N} \times d_1 = 510 \text{ Nm} - 340 \text{ N} \times d_1$

$660 \text{ N} \times d_1 = 510 \text{ Nm}$

$d_1 = 0.773 \text{ m}$

$N = \text{newton}$

$Nm = \text{newton-meter}$

One newton (unit of force) is that force which gives a mass of 1 kg an acceleration of 1 m/sec.

Since the head was even with the knife-edge, the distance from the top of the head to the transverse plane of the center of gravity is 77.3 cm. If the subject is 171 cm in height, the plane line of gravity is 45% of the height measured from the top of the head, and 55% of the height measured from the soles of the feet.

This procedure can be used when only one scale is available, since the reading on the second scale will always be the total weight minus the reading on the single scale (Fig. 2-7).

Using the scale method, other investigators have reported findings on the location of the transverse plane of the human center of gravity. Croskey and associates reported in 1922 that this plane is slightly higher in men than in women. The average height of the plane in men was 56.18% measured from the soles; the range of percentages was 55% to 58%. For women, the average was 55.44%; the range was 54% to 58%. Additional observations were made by Hellebrandt and co-workers, who found that in 357 college women the transverse plane averaged 55.17% of the height; the lowest observed was 53%, and the highest was 59%.

The most extensive early study is that reported by Palmer (1944), who located the transverse plane of the center of gravity in 1172 subjects—596 boys and 576 girls from birth to 20 years of age—and in 18 fetal cadavers. Palmer concluded that regardless of age or sex, the plane can be estimated as follows:

0.557 height plus 1.4 cm (0.551 in.) from soles of feet

Since body segments differ in proportion to total height from birth to maturity, the plane of the center of gravity will lie in a different section of the body as age increases, but the proportion of height will be constant (Figs. 2-8 and 2-9).

Obviously, a change in position of the limbs with reference to the prone torso will change the position of the center of gravity. If the arms are raised overhead or the hips flexed, the plane will move toward the head. Loss of body parts will also alter the position. Amputation of any part of the lower limb will raise the plane, and the height of the center of gravity will increase with the amount of body mass lost. The addition of a prosthetic appliance to replace the amputated limb will lower the center of gravity toward the normal position (Fig. 2-10).

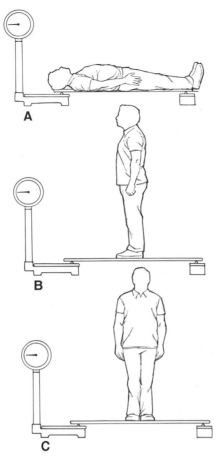

Fig. 2-7. *One method used for determining position of the line of gravity and the center of gravity of the body. The known weight of the human body and the recorded weight acting on the scale are used to mathematically calculate the position of the vertical force vector acting through the center of gravity of the body (line of gravity): A, line of gravity (balance point) top and bottom halves of body; B, balance point of front and rear halves of body; C, balance point of right and left halves of body. The intersect of the position of three calculated force vectors is the site of the center of gravity of the body.*

Center of Gravity in Frontal and Sagittal Body Planes

In the preceding discussion, the transverse plane of the center of gravity was located at a distance from the top of the head or from the soles of the feet. In balance and locomotor activities, it is important to locate the gravity plane in the frontal and sagittal planes. If the Reynolds-Lovett method is used, the body must be stationary on the board, and some body point must be located with reference to the knife-edges; if the frontal gravity plane is to be located while the subject is standing, some part of the foot will be taken as the reference point, and the distance of this part from one of the knife-edges must be known.

HUMAN GRAVITATIONAL ENVIRONMENT **43**

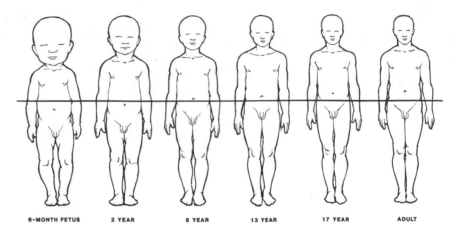

6-MONTH FETUS   2 YEAR   5 YEAR   13 YEAR   17 YEAR   ADULT

Fig. 2-8. *Contourograms of ventral aspects of body at pre-birth and various ages after birth. Body lengths are scaled to reduce all figures to the same height. The transverse plane at the level of the center of gravity of each body is represented by the transverse line. (From Palmer, C. E.: Child Dev. 15:99, 1944.) Is it any wonder that infants have locomotor problems and head control problems?*

Since it is more convenient to stand near the middle of the board rather than near one end of it, a line on the board halfway between the knife-edges is convenient for measuring distance.

The same mathematical procedure described in the preceding section, with respect to the center of gravity in the transverse body plane can be used to determine both the frontal gravity plane and the sagittal gravity plane (Fig. 2-7). Often it is desirable to locate the frontal

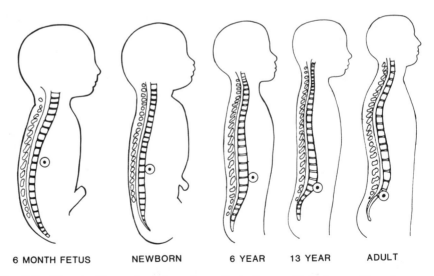

6 MONTH FETUS   NEWBORN   6 YEAR   13 YEAR   ADULT

Fig. 2-9. *The positions of center of gravity in the sagittal plane with reference to the spine are depicted as ⊙. Note how the C-curve changes to a 4-curve as the center of gravity drops and the head weight is reduced. (Modified from Palmer, C. E. Child Dev. 15:99, 1944.)*

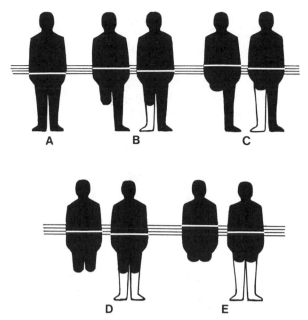

Fig. 2-10. *Diagrammatic representation of influence of amputation of lower extremities on height of center of gravity and compensatory effect of prosthetic limb. The white transverse line represents the plane at the level of the center of gravity. A, able-bodied person; B, below-knee single leg amputee without and with below-knee prosthesis; C, above-knee single leg amputee without and with above-knee prosthesis; D, double leg below-knee amputee without and with prosthesis; E, double leg above-knee amputee without and with prosthesis. (From Hellebrandt, F. A.:JAMA, 142:1353, 1950.)*

plane with reference to the ankle joint. In this case, if the ankle joint is 15 cm from the tip of the toes, the frontal plane is 4.5 cm in front of that joint. A perpendicular line passing through the foot at this point is often called the gravity line; in postural measures, certain body landmarks are described in terms of deviation from this line.

When a person stands erect, the frontal gravity plane lies in front of the ankle joint and in back of the metatarsophalangeal joints. The location between these points differs with individuals and may differ from time to time in the same individual. This location between the ankles and the proximal end of the toes has been so frequently observed that it can be accepted as a human characteristic. Among the published reports are those of Cureton and Wickens, Hellebrandt, Fox and Young, and Brown. Over the years, hundreds of students in our kinesiology classes have observed this phenomenon in themselves and in their classmates. Not only have they observed the location, but they have also seen that this plane is rarely stationary; it usually fluctuates, and the degree of fluctuation varies with the individual and the movement.

As the subject stands on the board for gravity-plane determination, the observer finds it difficult to make an exact scale reading because the dial needle fluctuates rapidly. The range of the needle varies with individuals, but rarely exceeds 20 N. If one reading is desired, the best one to take is that about which the needle hovers; however, the extremes will also provide interesting information. The reason for the changes in scale readings is understood when one remembers that the body must balance on the small base provided by the upper surface of the talus at the ankle joint. Since the center of gravity of the body is ahead of the ankle joint, the body is unbalanced on this small surface. Gravitational force would tilt the body forward if no counterforce were present. The ankle extensors provide this force; the tension in these muscles must be sufficient to withstand gravitational pull if the erect position is to be maintained. Any slight change in any body part (solid, liquid, or gas) will change the distribution of weight; this will change the force of gravitational pull and consequently change the demand on the ankle extensors. The tension in the muscles may change also. Whatever the cause, the frontal plane is constantly shifting; yet it remains within the limits described. Class observations in which students are asked to lean forward as far as possible without raising the heels and then backward as far as possible without lifting the toes (and without falling) rarely find that the gravity plane has moved back of the ankle or ahead of the proximal end of the toes. It does not move beyond the normal limits for the individual.

Segmental alignment above the ankle is not a universal characteristic. Individuals differ in degree of pelvic tilt, in depth of lumbar, dorsal, and cervical curves, and in shoulder girdle and head position. All these factors will affect the distribution of weight. Yet when an individual stands in a habitual position, the frontal plane of the center of gravity will fall between the ankle and the metatarsophalangeal joints.

For location of the sagittal gravity plane, the subject stands on the board, with the right side toward one knife-edge and the left side toward the other. This plane has frequently been located to determine whether the subject is likely to carry more of the weight on one foot than on the other.

An arrangement for simultaneously determining the frontal and sagittal planes of the center of gravity has been presented by Waterland and Shambes. The subject takes a position on a base supported by three dial scales. Two photographs, a side and a front view, are taken by a synchronized shutter arrangement. The three scale readings shown in the photographs will equal the total weight of the subject. With these readings the positions of gravity lines in the frontal and sagittal planes can be calculated. These investigators have shown fluctuations of the gravity line in a "static" standing position. By placing on the supported board a paper on which the footprints of the subject were traced, they located the gravity line with reference to the feet (Fig. 2-11).

The triangular platform shown in Fig. 2-11 was used by Has-

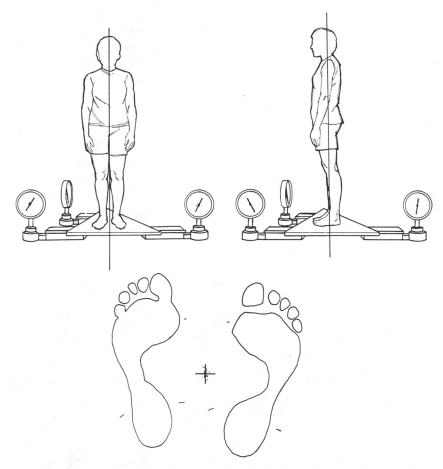

Fig. 2-11. *Two methods for obtaining line of gravity during standing. A: Equipment used to determine mean gravity line in sagittal and frontal planes. Front and side view photographs are taken simultaneously; each view presents two of three dial scales. Gravity lines added to photographs after calculations represent mean of 30 determinations; each dot between feet represents one determination; center point of crossed lines represents mean of 30 determinations. (From Waterland, J. C. and Shambes, G. M.:Biplane center of gravity procedures, Percept. Mot. Skills 30:511, 1970.) B: Pattern of sway automatically collected using an AMTI Force Platform System.*

selkus to compare the postural sway of 10 women 21 to 30 years of age, with 10 others 73 to 80 years of age. Greater sway was thought to be a possible indication of aging of the neuromuscular system. Each subject stood on the platform for three 18-second periods, during which cameras recorded the scale readings every second. The area enclosed in the outer borders of the 54 calculated positions of gravity lines (such as plus in Fig. 2-11) was expressed as a percentage of the functional base of support, a quadrilateral area enclosed in lines drawn along the lateral borders of the feet and across the back of the heels and connecting the heads of the first metatarsals. The older women's sway area covered an average of 43%, and the younger women's, an average 23%. For all subjects, the position of the gravity line tended to be to left and posterior of the geometric center of the functional base. Today, computerized force platform systems automatically display the magnitude, direction, and pattern of sway.

Center of Gravity in a Moving Body

Two methods, the scale (or whole body) and the segmental (or indirect or parts), have been used to determine the center of gravity in the moving body. Both methods require that the investigator "freeze" the moving body into static positions. This is done by selecting still photographs, frames of movie film, or posed positions determined by the observer and used to represent the sequencing of the movement. It is important to attempt to duplicate exactly the position of all body parts at each of the imposed stationary images of the movement. The position of the center of gravity in two planes can be found from each image.

Scale Method. Triangular and rectangular boards utilizing two-four scales have been used in much the same way as the one-two scale method for determining the line of gravity in one plane. Davis (1973) devised a center-of-gravity board with three accompanying scales (Fig. 2-12). After the subjects had assumed various performer-position combinations, he determined (1) the center of gravity in the transverse and sagittal planes for the pike and stride positions and (2) the center of gravity in the transverse and frontal planes for the normal position. Davis also photographed these performer-position combinations and utilized the segmental method.

Segmental Method. Another method of determining the location of the center of gravity in the moving body is the segmental method suggested by Dawson (1935). This method is used when the performer is not present; only a photograph or movie film of the performance is available. Estimations of the weight of each body segment and the estimation of its center of gravity are utilized on the segmental method. Since the position of the center of gravity of the body is changed each time a body segment moves to assume a new position, the effect of this new position must be ascertained. In 1955, Cleaveland using 11 college men, determined these data on live subjects by means of water-submersion technique.

Marks on the body indicated the limits of each segment, and the body was lowered into a tank of water to each mark in succession. The weight of each segment was calculated by the weight lost and the amount of water displaced at each stage of submersion. The center of gravity of each segment was located at the point at which half the amount of weight was lost.

Kjeldsen and Morse (1977) have described significant differences in anthropometric measurements, including percentages of body segment weights, among women gymnasts, women non-gymnasts, and

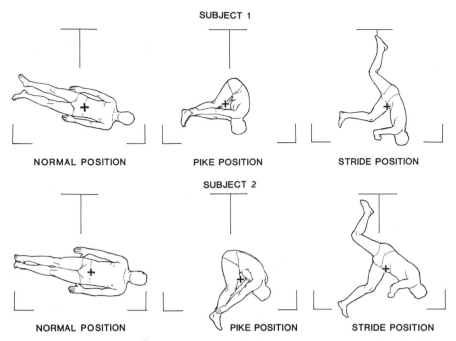

Fig. 2-12. *Performer-position combinations assumed by two performers on center-of-gravity board. Position of center of gravity in each of the six positions is at the cross (+). Note the differences between subject 1 and subject 2. The center of gravity lies outside the body in the pike positions, and in all conditions, is in the vicinity of the pelvis. (From Davis, M.: Quality of data collected by the segmental analysis technique, unpublished doctoral dissertation. Indiana University, Sept., 1973.)*

men. To further clarify differences, Hay presents an excellent compilation and discussion of the extensive data on segmental body weights and segmental centers of gravity. Partial listings of these differences are given in Tables 2-1 to 2-4. Note the similarities as well as the differences.

Limitations. Care must be taken when using the segmental method. The precision of the estimation of the center of gravity is significantly affected by the type of segmental data applied. Segmental data collected on men should not be used when analyzing the movements of women and children.

Furthermore, data from older persons, and physically disabled persons need to be acquired for a better understanding of the anatomic differences among people. Therefore, it might be misleading to analyze the position of the center of gravity of a person based on the data from a small sample of cadavers or live subjects.

Davis found the reliability and validity of the segmental method acceptable for use in his kinematic analyses. Pike and Adrian (unpublished) used three sets of data to determine forces acting at the knee joint during kicking. Although two sets of data varied less than the third, the third set was significantly different from the other two.

Table 2-1. *Weights of body segments expressed in percentages relative to total body weight for women as cited by various authors.*

Segment	Bernstein	Plagenhoef	Kjeldsen
Trunk		55.00	60.20
Upper arm	2.63	2.90	2.74
Forearm	1.82	1.55	1.61
Hand	0.64	0.50	0.51
Thigh	12.48	11.50	8.26
Calf (lower leg)	4.73	5.25	5.49
Foot	1.31	1.20	1.24

Thus, kinetic data, based upon cadaver or other values in data bases, will not be true value.

The segmental method is best used with data from the actual performer, at least submersing the limbs and estimating only the trunk weight to determine center of gravity location. The segmental method, by means of the computer and without the errors of the scale method, allows the calculation of centers of gravity for many positions. Remember that the scale method requires that the person exactly duplicate the position of the movement.

Simplified Version. A simplified version of the segmental method will be used to illustrate the basic theory underlying the method. Think of three children seated on a teeterboard, with each child representing a part of one human body. For example, child 1 would be the legs, child 2 would be the head and trunk, and child 3 would be the arms of a single human body. One child weighs 240 N and is seated on the board 1.0 m from the fulcrum. Another child seated on the same side weighs 200 N and is 0.6 m from the fulcrum. The third child is seated on the opposite side, weighs 360 N, and is 0.8 m from the fulcrum.

Table 2-2. *Weights of body segments expressed in percentages relative to total body weight for men as cited by various authors.*

Segment	Braune and Fischer	Cleaveland	Williams and Lissner	Dempster
Head and neck	7.06	7.03	7.9	
Trunk	42.70	48.30	51.1	49.4
Upper arm (2)	6.72	6.25	5.4	7.0
Forearm (2)	6.24	4.33	4.4	3.2
Hand (2)	(With forearm)	(With forearm)	(With forearm)	1.0
Thigh (2)	23.16	22.52	19.4	27.4
Calf (lower leg) (2)	14.12	11.52	12.0	9.4
Foot (2)	(With calf)	(With calf)	(With calf)	2.6

Values for upper forearm, hand, thigh, calf, and foot are for both segments in each case.

Table 2-3. *Locations of centers of gravity of body segments expressed as percentage of total segment length as measured from proximal end for women as cited by two authors.*

Segment	Matsui	Bernstein
Head and neck	63	
Trunk	52	
Upper arm	46	48.40
Forearm	42	41.74
Hand	50	
Thigh	42	38.88
Calf	42	42.26
Foot	50	

Since these body weights act as rotating forces, the effect of each force, multiplied by the distance from the fulcrum, is known as a moment of force. On the side where the heaviest child is seated, the moment will equal 360 N × 0.8 m, which is 288 Nm; on the side where the two lighter children are seated, it will be 240 N × 1.0 m plus 200 N × 0.6 m, which equals 360 Nm.

The board will not be balanced with this arrangement. The board can be balanced by using one of two possible methods. First, the positions of the children may be changed. The child weighing 360 N might be moved to a position 1.0 m from the fulcrum, and the moment on that side of the board would equal the 360 Nm moment of the opposite side. The second possibility would be to move the fulcrum. To determine the distance that the fulcrum should be moved, one would use the percentage weight of each child in relationship to the total weight of the three children to determine the force of each side:

240 N: 0.30 × 1.0 m = 0.30 m
200 N: 0.25 × 0.6 m = 0.15 m
      Total 0.45 m

360 N: 0.45 × 0.8 m = 0.36
      Total 100%

Table 2-4. *Locations of centers of gravity of body segments expressed as percentage of total segment length as measured from proximal end for men as cited by various authors.*

Segment	Cleaveland	Dempster	Matsui
Head and neck		(With trunk)	65
Trunk	53	60.4	52
Upper arm	42	43.6	46
Forearm	28	43.0	41
Hand	(With forearm)	50.6	50
Thigh	36	43.3	42
Calf	42	43.3	41
Foot	(With calf)	42.9	50

The difference between 0.45 and 0.36 (0.09), is the distance (in meters) that the fulcrum should be moved. The board is balanced by increasing the distance between the heaviest child and the fulcrum by 0.09 m; that between the fulcrum and each of the lighter children should be decreased 0.09 m. With these distances and the percentage weights, the moment values are as follows:

$$0.30 \times 0.91 \text{ m} = 0.273 \text{ m}$$
$$0.25 \times 0.51 \text{ m} = 0.128 \text{ m}$$
$$\text{Total } 0.401 \text{ m}$$

$$0.45 \times 0.89 \text{ m} = 0.401 \text{ m}$$
$$\text{Total } 100\%$$

This proves that the center of gravity of the body (actually, only the line of gravity in one plane) is 0.09 m toward the head, which is represented by the lighter children. Thus, what we did was consider one line of gravity, as represented by the fulcrum of the teeterboard, and reject it as not being the true balance point, or line of gravity, of the system. To find the position of the center of gravity of the total body, one may arbitrarily choose any line (which may or may not pass through some part of the body) as the line from which the position of the segmental centers of gravity will be measured. Moment of force values for each segment can be calculated (by use of percentage weights). The difference between the sums of the values on each side of the line will show the distance that the line should be moved to pass through the total-body center of gravity.

In using the segmental method for determining the location of the center of gravity of the body traced from a film of a boy throwing a ball (Fig. 2-13), the investigator must have the following information:

1. The percentage of total body weight of each segment (Tables 2-1 and 2-2).
2. The location of the center of gravity in each segment, usually reported as a percentage of the total segment length as measured from the proximal end of the segment (Tables 2-3 and 2-4).
3. The horizontal and vertical distance of each body segment center of gravity from a vertical and horizonatl axis in the form of an x- and y- coordinate system as depicted in Fig. 2-13.

The steps to follow in calculating the total-body center of gravity from a projected film image are as follows:

1. Project the image onto a piece of graph paper and trace the performer.
2. Establish a coordinate system on the graph paper in such a way that the origin is in the lower left-hand corner (Fig. 2-

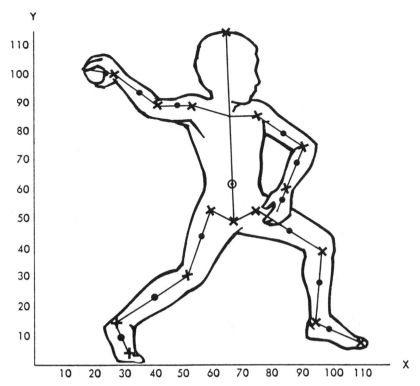

Fig. 2-13. *Tracing from film of young child throwing a ball. The center of gravity (⊙) has been determined using the segmental method. Tabulations are listed in Table 2-5.* **X**, *end points of segments;* ●, *segmental centers of gravity.*

13). This confines all the data to the upper right quadrant, where all x- and y-coordinate values will be positive.

3. From the picture, select two reference points (stationary objects) that can be viewed in all the frames to be analyzed for a given performance, for example, the center of the dial on a wall clock or an electric wall socket.

4. Record the x- and y-coordinate values of the two reference points from the graph paper. In analysis of future frames of this same performance, these reference coordinate values must be exactly the same.

5. Record the x- and y-coordinate values of each of the following segmental end points:
   a. Tragus of the ear (cartilage anterior of ear opening)
   b. Sternal notch
   c. Crotch
   d. Right shoulder
   e. Right elbow
   f. Right fingertips (distal point of right fingertips)
   g. Left shoulder
   h. Left elbow

i. Left wrist
j. Left fingertips (distal point of left fingertips)
k. Right hip
l. Right knee
m. Right ankle
n. Right toe
o. Left hip
p. Left knee
q. Left ankle
r. Left toe (distal point of left toes)

These points are marked on Fig. 2-13.

6. Connect the segmental end points to form a stick figure.
7. Locate the center of gravity for each segment by the following procedure:
   a. Measure the segment lengths
   b. Multiply this value by the appropriate percentage from Table 2-3 or 2-4.
   c. Measure this amount from the proximal end of the segment. Mark this spot as the center of gravity for the segment; that is, if the trunk and head measure 10 cm, then the center of gravity for this segment would be 0.604 × 10 = 6.04, or 6.04 cm from the crotch (using Dempster data on men, Table 2-2).
   d. Repeat the procedure for all segments
8. Record all the x- and y-coordinate values for each segment's center of gravity.
9. Multiply the x values for each segment's center of gravity by the percentage of the total body weight contributed by that segment (Table 2-3). Sum these values. This sum represents the location of the center of gravity of the total body in the x, or horizontal, plane.
10. Repeat step 9, using the y values for each segment's center of gravity.
11. The x- and y-coordinate total-body center of gravity can be located on the graph paper. Table 2-5 contains sample coordinate values on the image in Fig. 2-13.

Graphing the Center of Gravity. These measures and calculations illustrate a method by which the path of the body's center of gravity can be depicted in any skill. Such a procedure was used by Sparks, as seen in Fig. 2-14. To do so, there must be a vertical and a horizontal reference line, neither of which has to pass through some part of the body, as did the lines in the illustration. The number of film frames necessary to determine the path will depend on whether the body is in flight or whether segments are changing position while the body is supported on a stationary base.

Table 2-5. *Segmental center of gravity locations determined for position of body and coordinate reference frame in figure 2-13. Weighted values used in this determination were averages from data listed in previous tables. These weighted values were multiplied by the appropriate coordinate values of each segmental center of gravity to obtain the X value weighted and Y value weighted.*

Segment	% of body weight	X-coordinate	X value weighted	Y-coordinate	Y value weighted
Head and neck		(With trunk)		(With trunk)	
Trunk	51.4	65.0	33.41	76.0	39.01
Upper arm (left)	3.0	81.5	2.45	81.0	2.43
Forearm (left)	1.6	88.0	1.41	69.5	1.11
Hand (left)	0.17	83.5	0.50	57.0	0.34
Thigh (left)	12.8	83.5	10.77	48.0	6.19
Calf (left)	4.7	95.5	4.58	30.0	1.44
Foot (left)	1.5	99.0	1.49	13.0	0.20
Upper arm (right)	3.0	48.0	1.44	89.0	2.67
Forearm (right)	1.6	35.0	0.56	93.0	1.49
Hand (right)	.50	23.5	0.14	101.0	0.61
Thigh (right)	12.9	55.5	7.16	44.5	5.74
Calf (right)	4.8	41.0	1.97	24.0	1.15
Foot (right)	1.5	29.0	0.44	10.0	0.15
Total body			66.32		62.53

Once the contact with the supporting surface has been broken and the body is in flight, the path of the center of gravity is determined by the velocity and direction imparted to it at takeoff and by gravitational pull. It is now a projectile and can be treated as such. The line of flight can be found by the method described in Appendix D. Once the body is in flight, no segmental movement will affect the path of the center of gravity. Therefore, it is necessary to locate the position of the center of gravity at only two points (and the corresponding times). One point must always be the first frame in which contact has been broken—in which the body has just begun its flight. The second can be any frame before landing, but it is well to select a frame that is as far as possible from the first. The frame selected will depend on the number of frames included in the film. The choice of the second frame is as far as possible from the first because there are always likely to be measurement errors; the longer the time and the distance that are measured, the smaller the percentage of error. Since the in-flight path of the center of gravity will be a parabolic curve, the equation for that curve can be calculated from any two points on the curve. In this text, when direction and velocity of body projections are reported, they have been determined by this method.

When the path of the center of gravity is depicted while the base is stationary and segments are moving, its position should be found

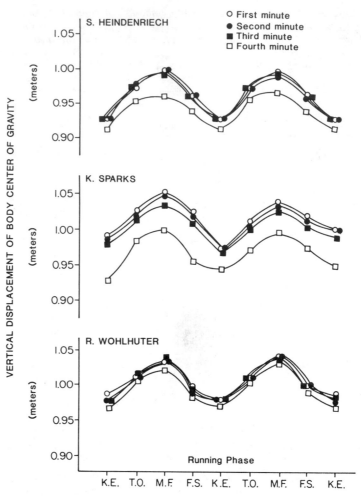

Fig. 2-14. *Vertical displacement (measured from the ground) of body center of gravity of runners was calculated by the segmental method for four positions during each of two cycles each minute in a four-minute-mile run. Only during the fourth minute did the runners show effect of fatigue. The reduced vertical displacement differed among the runners and was due to greater flexion at the knees and general alteration of running style. K.E., knees even; T.O., toe off; M.F., midflight; F.S., foot strike. (From Sparks, K.E.: Physiological and mechanical alterations due to fatigue while running a four-minute mile on treadmill, unpublished doctoral dissertation, Indiana University, May, 1975.)*

in every film frame. In such situations, the center of gravity is not a projectile, and movement of a segment will affect its path. To determine the path of the center of gravity in the takeoff phase of a standing long jump, Johnson (1958) drew the vertical references line through the metatarsophalangeal joints and the horizontal line along the bottom of the toes. At the time the heels left the floor, she found the center of gravity to be 72.6 cm (28.6 in.) above the floor and 7.6 cm (3 in.) ahead of the metatarsal joints. As the flexion occurred at knees and hips and the arms moved downward from the height of the backswing, the center of gravity moved downward and forward to a position 55.6 cm (21.9 in.) above the floor and 26.4 cm (10.4 in.) ahead of the metatarsophalangeal joints.

At takeoff, the center of gravity was 74.4 cm (29.3 in.) above the floor and 57.9 cm (22.8 in.) ahead of the metatarsophalangeal joints. Note that interestingly, the center of gravity was ahead of the toes at the time the heels were raised—a further indication that gravitational pull, not muscle action, tilts the body (raising the heels). As the muscles act and move body segments, the position of the center of gravity is changed, so that it is outside the base of support, and the body falls forward, a fall that is controlled by the ankle extensors.

Calculations to determine the center of gravity by this method involve a relatively long and involved process, yet understanding of the effect of segmental positions will be furthered by a limited number of determinations. If films are not available, various positions can be taken on the gravity board. For example, the subject either may stand on the board in a stride position with feet separated at a measured distance and trunk flexed at a measured angle or may lie on the board with upper and lower limbs held at measured angles to the trunk. Segmental calculations can then be compared with scale determinations.

For more extensive studies, work can be reduced by means of recently developed techniques. Motion analyzers and digitizers used in conjunction with computers (on-line or separate) can greatly increase the number of frames that may be feasibly analyzed in a given time.

Because of the diversity of physical (anatomic) characteristics of human beings, it is no wonder that researchers, teachers, coaches, physical therapists, and others concerned with education in and improvement of human movement have attempted to relate anatomic characteristics to movement-performance achievements. A new scientific discipline has emerged to focus solely on the measurement of size, shape, proportion, composition, maturation, and gross function as related to such concerns as growth, exercise, performance, and nutrition. This discipline, as mentioned in Chapter 1, has been termed *kinanthropometry* and is closely aligned with *ergometry,* the measurement of work of muscles.

Some practical comments on the use of knowledge about the center of gravity in the movement environment are:

1. Stability and mobility factors have to do with the height of the center of gravity. If center of gravity is lower, the position is more stable; if higher, the position is more mobile. If the size of the base of support is wider, then the body is more stable. Increased stability is accomplished by flexing at the knees and moving the feet farther apart. Size of feet affect mobility and stability; if they are large, there is more stability and less mobility. Positioning the body so that its center is near the

edge of the base, but still within the gravitational lines, gives some stability and some instability for fast action.

2. The center of gravity is at times outside the body, such as is demonstrated by the position a sprinter takes to get quick movement off the blocks. A high jumper drapes the body around the bar to clear it.

3. It must be kept in mind that movement of the limbs up or down changes the position of the center of gravity, affecting the stability and mobility.

4. In flight, the path of the center of gravity is parabolic and cannot be changed unless acted upon by an outside force. The type of force to change the center of gravity when the performer is in contact with the floor or ground is an eccentric force.

MINI-LAB LEARNING EXPERIENCES

1. On graph paper, trace the outline (contourgram) of a performer from one frame of a movie film, mark the joints, and draw line segments between the joints. Using the segmental method described in this chapter, determine the center of gravity in two planes of the performer, as traced.

2. Using the scale method described in this chapter, determine the center of gravity in three planes of two human beings:
   a. In the anatomic position
   b. In a track starting position
   c. In a posture of your choice.

REFERENCES

Braune, W. and Fischer, O. (1889): Ueber den Schwerpunkt des menchlichen Korpers mit Ruchsicht auf die Austtustrung des deutschen Infanteristerm, Abh. D. K. Sachs Ges. Wiss. 15:2.

Carter, J. E. L. (1970): The Somatotypes of Athletes: a Review, *Hum. Biol.* 42:535–569.

Cleaveland, H.G. (1955): The Determination of Center of Gravity in Segments of the Human Body, Thesis, University of California at Los Angeles.

Croskey, M. L. et al. (1922): The Height of the Center of Gravity in Man, *Am. J. Physiol.* 61:171.

Davis, M. (1973): Quality of Data Collected by the Segmental Analysis Technique, Unpublished Doctoral Dissertation, Bloomington, IN, Indiana University.

Dawson, P. M. (1935): *The Physiology of Physical Education.* Williams and Wilkins Co.: Baltimore.

Garrett, R. E., Widule, C. J. and Garrett, G. E. (1968): Computer-aided Analysis of Human Motion, *Kinesiology Review,* p. 1.

Hay, J. G. (1973): The Center of Gravity of the Human Body, *Kinesiology,* Vol. III, AAHPER.

Hay, J. G. (1974): Moment of Inertia of the Human Body, *Kinesiology IV,* AAHPER, Washington, DC, pp. 43–52.

Hellebrandt, F. A., Brogdon, E. and Tepper, R. H. (1940): Posture and Its Cost, *Am. J. Physiol.* 129:773.

Hewes, G. W. (1957): The Anthropology of Posture, *Sci. Am.* 196:122–128, February.

Howell, A. B. (1944): *Speed in Animals,* The University of Chicago Press: Chicago.

Johnson, B. P. (1958): An Analysis of the Mechanics of the Takeoff in the Standing Broad Jump, Thesis, University of Wisconsin.

Joseph, J. (1960): *Man's Posture-Electromyographic Studies.* Charles C. Thomas Publishers: Springfield, IL.

Kjeldsen, K. and Morse, C. (1977): *Research reports,* Vol. 3 (Adrian, M. and Braume, J., editors), Washington, DC: AAHPER.

Medawar, P. (1958): *The Uniqueness of the Individual.* Basic Books Inc. Publishers: New York.

Methany, E. (1952): *Body Dynamics.* McGraw-Hill Book Co.: New York.

Morton, D. J. and Fuller, D. (1952): *Human Locomotion and Body Form.* The Williams and Wilkins Co.: Baltimore.

Napier, J. (1967): The Antiquity of Human Walking, *Sci. Am.* 216:56, April.

Palmer, C. E. (1944): Studies of the Center of Gravity in the Human Body, *Child Dev.* 15:99.

Pike, N. and Adrian, M. (1985): Effect of Body Segment Parameter Data Upon Generated Kinetic Parameters. *Abstracts of Research Papers* (Haymes, E., editor), AAHPERD: Reston, VA, p. 46.

Plagenhoef, S. (1971): *Patterns of Human Motion.* Englewood Cliffs, NJ: Prentice-Hall, Inc.

Waterland, J. C., and Shambes, G. M. (1970): Biplane center of gravity procedures, *Percept. Mot. Skills* 30:511.

3

The Human Structural System

Human beings, animals, fish, and birds do not choose their structure; each structure is inherited. Within limits, structure can be modified by environment, exercise, and nutrition. Since movements are dependent on structure, they also often become modified. Furthermore, movements have inherent limitations imposed by the structure of bone, muscle, joints, and nerve innervations. Thus structure influences function, and function influences structure. For example, the tall, thin high jumper and the small monkey in a zoo have inherited different structures and also modified these structures to be able to perform what they best like to do. The high jumper will most likely have a longer and stronger takeoff leg (right) than left leg. The monkey will have a bilaterally developed strong shoulder girdle and arm muscles. It is important to understand this interrelationship because movements are produced by forces, and forces act on body structures. In this chapter, we will discuss the structure of bones, joints, and muscles to provide a basis for the understanding of the foundation of movement: the muscle-bone lever systems. See Appendix for anatomical charts. In addition, the effect of forces on bone will be presented to describe how this particular structure can be, or is, modified.

THE SKELETON

Skeletons of modern terrestrial forms have many similarities. Differences exist in the number of bones and in the types of articulations between the bones that limit the types of locomotion and manipulation possible by any given species. The human skeleton has more than 200 bones, 126 forming the appendicular skeleton comprising the bones of the upper and lower extremities. The appendicular skeletons of hoofed quadrupeds, however, have fewer bones; therefore,

61

quadrupeds lack versatility in manipulation skills. On the other hand, the lack of a clavicle in the cat allows it to leap farther than would be possible with a clavicle limiting the flexion of its forelimbs.

Joints

Bones articulate with other bones to produce joints. They are important to the kinesiologist since they are the locations of movement. Arthrology, the study of joints, often begins with the classification of the six major types of joints (Fig. 3-1) that are important to movement analysis:

1. The gliding joint (arthrodia), in which either the bones glide over one another or one or more bones glide over another bone, is best illustrated by the articulating surfaces of the vertebrae and the tarsal and carpal bones. Most of the movement between any two surfaces is extremely small, but may be large with respect to the entire segment, such as the whole foot. Each

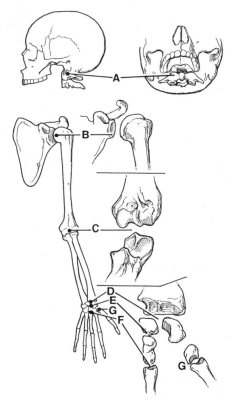

Fig. 3-1. *Major types of diarthrodial joints with respect to articulating surfaces are depicted for the upper extremity and head-neck joint. A: pivot (atlantoxial), B: ball-and-socket (shoulder, also termed humero-scapular), C: hinge (elbow, also termed humero-ulner), D: condyloid (radiocarpal), E: gliding (intercarpal), F: condyloid (metacarpophalangeal), G: saddle (thumb). Referring to the appendix, identify the types of diarthrodial joints in the lower extremities.*

THE BIOMECHANICS OF HUMAN MOVEMENT

small movement is added to the movement from adjacent joints to achieve a wide range of movement.

2. The hinge joint (ginglymus), in which one surface is round, with a knoblike end that fits into another concave surface, usually provides for movement in only one plane about a single axis. This hingelike movement is exemplified by the elbow joint as it moves in flexion and extension in the sagittal plane.

3. The ball-and-socket joint (enarthrosis) has the capacity to move in many planes and many axes. The spherical head of one bone fits into the hollowed concave surface of the other bone, like the head of the femur fits into the acetabulum of the hip. This tri-axial joint has many actions, such as extension, flexion, abduction, adduction, circumduction (the combined movement of the preceding four movements), horizontal flexion and extension (also termed horizontal adduction and abduction), and rotation.

4. The condyloid joint (ovoid or ellipsoid joint) has movement similar to the ball-and-socket joint, but occurring in only two planes, sagittal and frontal (no rotation is allowed). In this joint, a more oval-shaped head (condyloid) fits into a concave surface. The articulations between the carpal bones of the wrist and the metacarpals of the fingers are examples of this joint.

5. The saddle joint (sellar joint), which may be thought of as a modification of the condyloid joint with a greater freedom of movement, is shaped much like a western saddle, with the ends of a concave surface tipped up to form a convex surface in the other direction. This surface fits over an opposite concave-convex surface which allows for flexion, extension, abduction, adduction, and circumduction. This joint is found only in the carpal-metacarpal joint of the thumb.

6. The pivot joint (trochoid joint) permits only rotary movement about the longitudinal axis of the bone. An example of such uniaxial movement is the radius, rotating about its superior (proximal) articulation with the ulna.

The joints listed above are diarthrodial joints: they possess an articular cavity and have a ligamentous capsule that encases the joint and the synovial fluid, which lubricates the joint and regulates the pressure within the capsule. The articular surfaces of these joints are smooth and covered with cartilage. Two other types of joints, synarthrodial and amphiarthrodial, are not discussed here because they allow negligible or no movement.

Although the types of movements are predetermined by the structure of the joint, the range of motion (ROM) is determined not only by the structure of the joint, but by such factors as use, disease, injury, extensibility of muscles, tendons, and ligaments, and by the size of more distal body parts involved in the change of angle at the joint.

The arrangement and number of muscles, ligaments, and tendons

THE HUMAN STRUCTURAL SYSTEM   **63**

surrounding a joint influence range of motion (ROM) at that joint. These tissues are lengthened through use, and ROM increases with respect to the direction of lengthening. Thus, if movement is practiced in the flexion mode, but never in the extension mode, ROM of flexion will increase, whereas ROM of extension will show a decrease. Likewise, an injury that separates (tears) the medial collateral ligament at the knee will show an increased abduction capability, but no change in adduction.

Very young persons appear to be more flexible (have a greater ROM) than any other age group, and females appear to be more flexible than males. Specific flexibilities, however, may be due to specific adaptations to such factors as exercise routines. Thus differences that appear as a result of comparisons of age or sex groups can be attributed to primary causes, such as physical activity patterns, participation in specific sports, and habitual postures of work. For example, gymnasts have greater hyperextension at the elbow; baseball pitchers have greater ROM at the wrist; and hurdlers have greater flexion at the hip than do members of an average population. Conversely, persons whose occupations involve constant sitting usually show a decrease in horizontal extension at the shoulder. The ROM at the elbow also may be reduced after participation in a weight training program designed to cause hypertrophy of the biceps brachii. In the case of extreme development of the biceps brachii, the ROM may be limited to 90 degrees of flexion at the elbow, whereas the norm shows 120 degrees of flexion before the tissues of the upper arm and forearm contact each other and prevent further change in the angle at the joint. Often it is lack of stretching of the other muscles crossing the joint that limits the range of motion rather than the hypertrophy of the biceps brachii.

Tendinitis, bursitis, calcium deposits in the muscle, osteoarthritis, and other disorders produce pain and resistance to movement at a joint. Therefore the ROM will be decreased, or it may be normal, but executed at a slower-than-normal speed. The contralateral (opposite) limb can be used as a comparison of ROM that has been lost as a result of one of these disorders. This comparison, however, may not be totally valid since asymmetry exists in most people.

Two types of ROM are often determined. Active ROM is that ROM possible by voluntary muscle contraction. Passive ROM is ROM resulting from an application of some external force. Another person is often the applicator of this force, pushing the joint beyond its normal active limits. As one would expect, passive ROM should always be greater than active ROM. Examples are shown in Figure 3-2.

Active ROM can be thought of as the range through which one can apply muscular force. The greater time a person can apply a force, the greater will be the resulting impulse. Therefore, as one's active ROM increases, for example shoulder flexibility of the baseball pitcher, the resulting impulse will also increase.

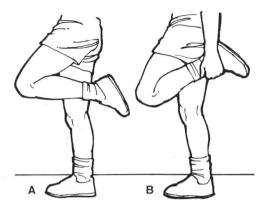

Fig. 3-2. *Range of motion is specific to body parts, orientation to gravity, and other factors. In this figure, active movement (A) is less than passive movement (B). Under which circumstances would active movement at this joint be equal to, or greater than, passive movement?*

The stability of a joint is important from a safety perspective. Some joints are inherently more stable than others, particularly as one compares the number of dislocated shoulders with that of dislocated hips. The type of joint and the bony articulations of the joint will affect stability, usually in one plane more than the others. The arrangement of the surrounding ligaments and muscles can also add stability, particularly in the knee, ankle and shoulder joints. Atmospheric pressure, creating a vacuum in the acetabulum of the hip, also adds stability. It is important to understand that flexibility and stability are not inversely related. For example, gymnasts desire great flexibility to perform the various routines, however, stability is also important; for example, to absorb the forces of landing and rebounding off the floor.

MINI-LAB LEARNING EXPERIENCES

1. Do we become shorter during the day? Measure the height of the arch of the foot with a ruler while standing immediately after rising in the morning. Repeat the measurement in the evening. What is the difference? Why?
2. Does the rear view mirror of the driver become elevated during a day's drive? Measure the sitting height in the morning and in the evening. Are there any differences? Explain.

Study figs. 3-3, 3-4, and 3-5 to better understand normal ranges of motion.

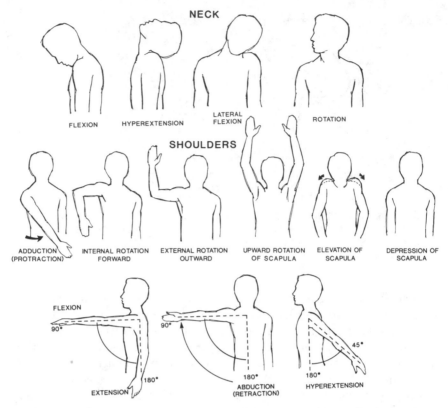

Fig. 3-3. *Basic movements and normal ranges of motion of skeleton: of the neck, and at the shoulders. The depicted body segment movements are those of the head, arm, and scapula.*

Bones

Bones constitute the rigid structure of the body that must withstand the forces of all the muscles, tendons, and ligaments, as well as the force of gravity and external forces resulting from blows, falls, or other types of collisions. Bones are classified by their sizes and shapes into four groups. The long bones, those most directly involved with movement, have a long shaft with broad knobby ends. Those classified as long bones include the humerus, radius, ulna, metacarpals, phalanges, clavicle, femur, tibia, fibula, and metatarsals. Short bones, characterized by their short, chunky shape, include the carpals and tarsals. The flat bones have a large flat area used to attach muscles. Most flat bones (with the exception of the scapulae) enclose various bony cavities. Flat bones include the ribs, sternum and several cranial bones. The remaining bones are called the irregular bones, due to their irregular shape. these include the vertebrae, sacrum, coccyx and several facial bones.

Each bone has an outer, compact layer and an inner, cancellous (spongy) layer. The compact layer (cortex) usually is thicker in the

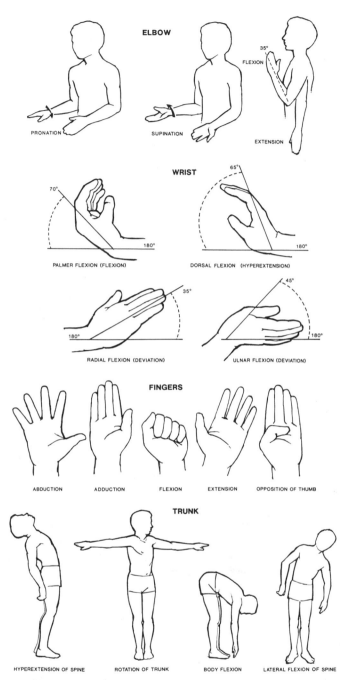

ELBOW

PRONATION · SUPINATION · FLEXION 35° · EXTENSION

WRIST

PALMER FLEXION (FLEXION) 70° 180° · DORSAL FLEXION (HYPEREXTENSION) 65° 180°

RADIAL FLEXION (DEVIATION) 35° 180° · ULNAR FLEXION (DEVIATION) 45° 180°

FINGERS

ABDUCTION · ADDUCTION · FLEXION · EXTENSION · OPPOSITION OF THUMB

TRUNK

HYPEREXTENSION OF SPINE · ROTATION OF TRUNK · BODY FLEXION · LATERAL FLEXION OF SPINE

Fig. 3-4. *Basic movements and normal ranges of motion of skeleton: at the elbow, wrist, metacarpal and interphalangeal joints and spine. The depicted body segment movements are those of the hands, fingers, including the thumb, and trunk.*

THE HUMAN STRUCTURAL SYSTEM **67**

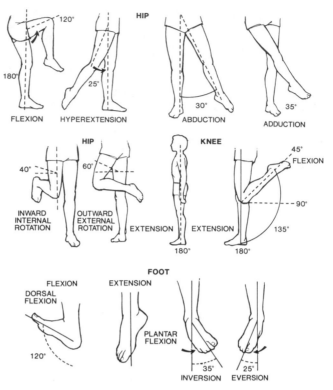

Fig. 3-5. *Basic movements and normal ranges of motion of skeleton: at the hip, knee and ankle. The depicted body segment movements are those of the thigh, shank, and foot.*

cylindrical or long bones forming the appendages than in flat bones, which tend to have large muscle masses attached to them. The cancellous layer consists of a network of trabeculae (Fig. 3-6) enclosing spaces filled with blood vessels and marrow. Bone in general, and the long bones in particular (since long bones have a central cavity) acquire maximal rigidity with minimal weight of material. Bones are approximately 32 times stronger than muscles.

There are two major forces acting on bones: gravity and muscles. Gravity is always present and acting on bone. In addition, muscles contract, forces are exerted on bones. The forces produce stress, which is the force per unit area. The bone reacts with an equal internal resistance to the force. There are two stresses that act axially (along the longitudinal axis), tending to elongate or to compress a bone. Elongation can be produced by a force that acts to pull the bone apart; this type of stress is termed tension. The bone also would become narrower as it elongates. The tensile deformation of bone is minuscule. The opposite deformation would occur with compression, which is the type of stress produced by a force that tends to shorten and widen the bone. Pure compression and pure tension occur only if the force, also

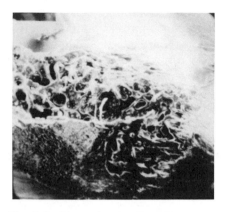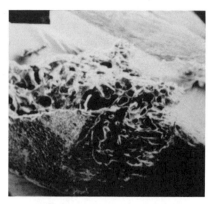

Fig. 3-6. *Example of trabecular structure of bone. Note the various orientations within the network as a result of stresses being applied from different directions.*

called a load, acts directly along the long axis; otherwise a bending moment occurs, causing tension in some portions of the bone and compression in other portions. In addition, some portions may have no stress placed on them. When a material is stressed in a fashion that causes one part to slide over another because of a blow, this stress is termed shear. Examples of various kinds of stress are given in Fig. 3-7, bone being the stressed material.

A person in the upright position will experience compression on

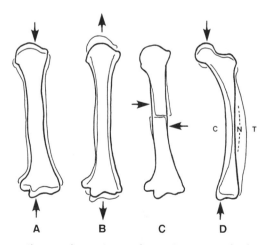

Fig. 3-7. *Forces acting on bone to produce stress are depicted by the arrows (vectors). A, compressive stress with potential to shorten and widen the bone; D, tensile stress with potential to lengthen and narrow the bone; C, shearing stress with potential to severe the bone; D, bending moment with both tension (T) and compression (C), the mid-portion experiencing no stress (N).*

THE HUMAN STRUCTURAL SYSTEM   **69**

the skeletal system because of gravity. For example, the weight of the upper body rests on the knee, producing compression at the joint. The alignment of the bones, however, is such that true compression does not exist. Note in Figure 3-7D how the weight of the upper body on the hip does not act through the long axis of the femur, but produces a bending moment. The placement of the feet also will determine how the line of gravity acts through the bones. Muscle forces act to produce stresses in bone, in addition to causing them to rotate. Usually a bending moment that produces both compression on the concave side of the bone and tension on the convex side of the bone is the result of muscle action.

MINI-LAB LEARNING EXPERIENCES

1. Using a goniometer, measure the range of motion of right and left joints of selected individuals. Identify possible reasons for these differences by asking questions concerning such factors as sports training, job, and previous injury.
2. Measure both passive and active range of motions at various joints. Which joints tend to have the greatest margins between the two measurements? What factor(s) could be limiting the range of motions at each joint?

The interplay of muscles acting on a single bone is complex and interesting as one studies the effect of muscle force on bone. Comparison of the shape of the humerus and that of the femur, for example, can be made by drawing the muscle force vectors and gravitational line vector representing the bone weight. The potential for a curved femur, as compared with a straight humerus can clearly be identified in Fig. 3-8.

Many materials of the body have a linearly elastic characteristic; that is, they deform at a measurable rate for each increment of stress up to or approaching the breaking point of the material. The result of forces acting on materials is deformation. If the deformation tolerances of the material are exceeded, breakage will occur. The deformation per unit length is termed strain. Fractures of bone, even the large femur, have occurred simply due to excessive strain caused by muscular force applied at such an angle to overcome the tolerances of the bone.

Bones are strongest in compression, next strongest in tension, and least strongest in shear. When a bending moment occurs, the fracture occurs on the tensile side. Take a piece of wood (pencil, ruler, or stick), hold it at each end, and bend it. Notice where the stress fracture appears initially. The same phenomenon is true for ligaments, tendons, and muscles. Although figures are not available on human tolerances

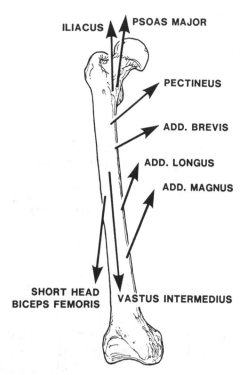

ILIACUS PSOAS MAJOR

PECTINEUS

ADD. BREVIS

ADD. LONGUS

ADD. MAGNUS

SHORT HEAD
BICEPS FEMORIS VASTUS INTERMEDIUS

Fig. 3-8. *Muscle forces depicted as vectors capable of deforming and bending the femur. The deformation is influenced by such factors as amount of collagen in bone, amount of potential tensile force in each muscle, frequency and duration of muscular force production, and angle of pull of muscle.*

in life, the limits of bone strength (ability to withstand stress) have been estimated from cadavers. For example, in a femur, the limits are as follows: compression, 1406 to 2109 N/cm^2 (20,000 to 30,000 psi); tension, 703 to 1406 N/cm^2; 10,000 to 20,000 psi); and shear, 281 N/cm^2 (4000 psi). Naturally these values differ for each bone and each person. Physical exercise can increase the strength of bones; disease often decreases the strength of bone.

The hardness, compressive strength, and rigidity of bone are due to its mineral content. The tensile strength and elasticity of bone— that is, its ability to revert to original form after deformation—are due to the presence of collagen. Young bone is mainly collagenous. With age, the collagen content is reduced and bone mineral is increased to constitute 60% to 70% of adult bone. The main minerals are calcium and phosphate. Water, primarily in a bound state, constitutes 25% to 30% of adult bone. During old age, the mineral content of bone is reduced, and breaking strength decreases as a result of further loss of collagen, causing the bone to become brittle. The changes in this deformation-strength relationship with age are depicted in Fig. 3-9.

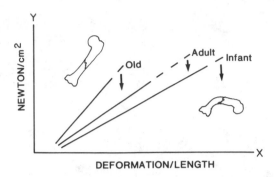

Fig. 3-9. *Changes in stress and strain characteristics of bone with age. Stress is measured on Y-axis, and strain on x-axis. Fracture is depicted with vertical vector, and shape of bone at fracture point is depicted for the old and the young.*

Normal Growth of Bones in Children

The bones of infants are mostly cartilaginous and deform readily. Breakage is rare, and the bones are considered to be very elastic. As the upright position is achieved, the spinal column, which is C-shaped at birth, begins to acquire the characteristic S-shaped appearance seen in the adult. The weight of the head, the position of the ribs anteriorly to the spinal column, and the movement of the arms and tilting of the pelvis to a functional sitting position—all produce forces that re-model the shape of the spinal column. One might state that no two spinal columns are alike; that is, heredity, nutrition, and specific pos-tures that cause forces to act along certain lines with respect to the spinal column, result in differing degrees of curvature in the cervical, thoracic, lumbar, and sacral regions.

Once the child begins to walk, a bowlegged appearance is noted. Since the bones of the legs also tend to deform with body weight, the amount and permanency of bowleggedness will depend on the calcium content in the bones, the laying down of new bone in response to the bending moment caused by the upright posture, and other factors. Permanent bowleggedness and other bone deformities will affect movement patterns and the ability to perform certain types of move-ments.

An extreme remodeling of the fibula has been reported in a boy born without a tibia. The fibula (which is not a weight-bearing bone) was made to bear the body weight. After the boy learned to walk, a second x-ray film revealed that the fibula had taken on the shape of a tibia similar to any tibia shown in any anatomy book.

Ridges, tuberosities, and other protuberances existing at the site of muscle or tendon attachments on the bone are a direct response to the tensile stress at the site. The size of these bony landmarks might well be an indication of early muscle use and strength. The strength of the bone can be exceeded, and sports injuries to young children have included bone pieces being separated from the rest of the bone.

Such an injury, called avulsion, occurs at the site of a muscle (or tendon) attachment when the muscles have become too strong too early in relation to the bone strength.

A common site of injury to the long bones is the epiphyseal plate. This plate is a cartilage ring separating the long shaft of the bone from the bulbous end. Until this cartilage ossifies (is replaced by bone), it represents a weakness in the otherwise ossified bone and is a probable site for dislocation during instances of trauma to the bone. This cartilage normally ossifies after puberty, usually before the age of 21 years, but may vary with respect to the specific bones (Fig. 3-10).

The primary center for ossification in long bones is in the center of the shaft, the diaphysis. As the bone ossifies the center enlarges, spreading towards the ends of the bone where it will eventually meet with the secondary centers, the epiphyses, which are also expanding.

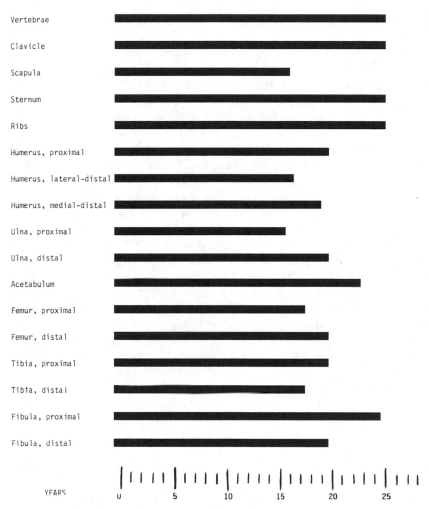

Fig. 3-10. *Approximate ages of Epiphyseal closures.*

THE HUMAN STRUCTURAL SYSTEM
73

The epiphyseal plate separates these centers until ossification is complete leaving an epiphyseal line on the surface of the bone.

The bones are weakest at the growth plate before ossification. Thus contact sports offer one of the greatest risks of bone fractures to children. Large children are often placed in positions of high injury risk due to their size. A sizable body does not mean that the young bones are mature (ossified). Having large children assume the position of the base of pyramid, for example, may be very dangerous to their bones.

Bones of Elderly Persons. The later decades of life are high-risk decades with respect to bone fractures. If osteoporosis, or loss of bone minerals, occurs, fractures may occur as a result of forces no greater than those experienced during normal activities of daily living. Since bones serve to protect body organs, act as part of the movement system, and support body weight of terrestrial species, damage to the bones because of their inability to cope with the forces acting on them is a vital concern to all kinesiologists and students of movement.

Bone Responses to Treatment, Immobilization, and Changes in Environment. When slight tensile stress is placed on a fractured bone, the bone heals faster and becomes stronger than it does without this stress. Conversely, a bone that is immobilized begins to atrophy, bone cells are resorbed, and the bone loses strength. The influence of gravity as a stressor was recognized when the astronauts returned from trips to outer space, where the strong gravitational force of the earth was not present. The loss in mineral content—that is, the strength substances of bone—was measurable. This destruction of bone is of major concern to the kinesiologist because, increasingly, possibilities of living or traveling other than on the earth and within its atmosphere have become realities.

Effects of Sports and Physical Work on Bones. Persons participating in unilateral sports such as tennis, bowling, baseball (especially a baseball pitcher), and racquetball typically show asymmetric development of bones. The tennis arm shows hypertrophied bones as well as muscles. The bones and muscles of the jumping leg of high jumpers also are hypertrophied. A male high jumper, whose performance caliber was in the 2 m (7 ft) range, was able to execute a standing vertical jump twice as high with the left leg as with the right leg. Indirect measurements of bone and muscle were made by measuring the girth of the thigh and the diameter of the shank and knee. Differences between these anthropometric measurements of the legs corresponded to the differences between the jumping performances.

Thus bones may be strong or weak, depending on the stresses placed on them. Muscles pulling against weak bones have been the cause of bone fractures, especially in baseball pitching, javelin throwing and the throwing of hand grenades. These fractures are due to torsion on the bone. Torsion involves a twisting or turning of the bone with one end fixed and constitutes primarily a shearing stress on the bone.

Although data concerning ethnic or racial influences on bone density are not conclusive, blacks have been found to have denser and therefore stronger bones than whites. Men, both whites and blacks, have denser bones than women. The effect of exercise cannot be ruled out as a factor in these differences, since many of the population samples consisted of active, low-income blacks and more affluent, sedentary whites. One study in South Africa indicated that the diet was an important influence on bone density. Affluent blacks floated in water as easily as did whites, whereas the less affluent blacks showed the generally accepted characteristics of low fat, dense bones, and decreased ability to float. Caution is advised when attempting to link a cause and effect to bone strength and ethnic groups.

Muscles

Muscles, ligaments, and tendons produce their own forces and, in turn, may be stressed as a result of collisions to the body, shearing forces to the bone, and tensile forces greater than the tolerances of the muscles. The muscles of the body produce stresses on many body parts other than bone, such as skin, organs, and connective tissue. When muscles allow the inhalation and exhalation of air, the airflow produces stresses on the walls of the airways. Similarly, the cardiac muscle initiates the blood flow, which causes arterial, capillary, and venous wall stress.

Ligaments primarily contract to restrict movement at the joint, and tendons transmit the forces of the muscle to the bone. Since muscles are the prime producers of movement, the remainder of this chapter will be devoted to a description of the muscles, the nature of muscle tension development, and the roles muscles play in the scheme of movement.

Approximately 435 voluntary muscles are found in the human body. Schottelius and Schottelius (1978) state that the importance of the body musculature is readily appreciated when one learns that muscles constitute 43% of the body weight, contain more than one-third of all the body proteins, and represent approximately one-half of the metabolic activity of the resting body. Simple and complex activities are involved when the muscles are activated against the bones to which they are attached, causing the bony levers to move. Coordination and organization of these muscles are necessary when movement takes place. This often involves not only individual muscles or a group of muscles, but also constituent parts of muscles. To completely understand muscle function, it is important to learn the basic physics, chemistry, and anatomy of muscles.

Types of Muscle. The three kinds of muscles—cardiac, smooth, and skeletal (striated)—vary in accordance with their function. Cardiac and smooth muscles have similar functions, and both surround hollow organs. Cardiac muscle is that of the heart. It has some characteristics in common with skeletal muscles and is classified as striated. However, single muscle fibers such as those noted in skeletal and smooth muscle are not obvious in cardiac muscle. Smooth muscle is found in blood vessels, the digestive tract, and certain other organs of the viscera. Cardiac and smooth muscles contract slowly, rhythmically, and involuntarily. Skeletal muscles are different. They are activated voluntarily as well as reflexively and their fibers contract with great rapidity. Huxley has stated that striated muscles can shorten at speeds of up to 10 times their resting length in a second. Skeletal muscles are usually attached to bone and cartilage. Under an ordinary light microscope, these muscles are seen to be crossed by striations, whereas the smooth muscles have none.

Characteristics of Fibers of Skeletal Muscle. Skeletal (striated) muscle fibers are so named because they are found principally in the muscles moving the skeletal framework. Skeletal muscle is also attached to cartilage and is characterized by the cross-straited arrangement within the fibers. Functional characteristics of striated muscle are rapidity and volitional control. Whereas the contraction of cardiac and smooth muscle is mainly reflexive, the striated muscles can also be contracted by voluntarily initiated motor nerve impulses.

The individual unit of the skeletal muscle is the long, slender muscle fiber; depending on arrangement within the muscle, it will vary from 1 mm to 30 cm in length. The biceps muscle has some 600,000 fibers. Elftman (1940) has estimated that 250 million muscle fibers are present in the human body. Each fiber has an elastic connective tissue covering with slender extensions attached to bones. The muscle fiber sizes in infants are approximately 10 micron meters and increase six times prior to age 17 years. We can expect another two-fold increase during adulthood.

A muscle consists of many thousands of fibers arranged parallel to each other (Fig. 3-11). These single muscle cells are covered with a connective tissue, or membrane, called endomysium. These fibers are arranged together in bundles, 20 to 1000 in number, called primary bundles. These bundles are often called fasciculi and are grouped by connective tissue called perimysium. Several bundles wrapped together with perimysium form secondary bundles, and several of these bound together form tertiary bundles. The entire muscle is covered with connective tissue called epimysium, which holds the bundles together as a unit. The connective tissue makes up the framework of the muscle and becomes the area of attachment either by a tendon or by itself directly to the bone. The blood is housed in the capillary beds, which are single-celled, layered structures embedded in the endomysium.

Each muscle fiber is cylindrical in shape and tapers toward the ends. Its component parts, myofibrils, sarcoplasm, and sarcolemma are defined as follows:

The myofibrils, also called fibrils or sarcostyles, are arranged in

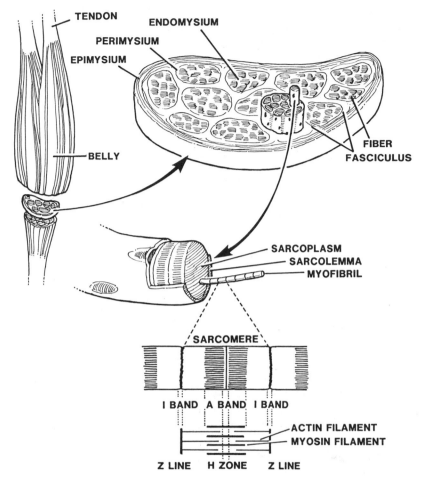

Fig. 3-11. *Details of muscle structure from the gross morphology to the microscopic.*

columns of several hundred to several thousand in each muscle fiber. These are the contractile units of the muscle.

The sarcoplasm comprises about half the muscle fiber and is the fluid within which the contractile part of the muscle moves.

The sarcolemma is the membrane that conducts the action potential through the fiber. The endomysium is the covering on the outside of the sarcolemma. Technically, the endomysium acts as the insulator, whereas the sarcolemma functions as a vehicle through which the action potential is carried to all sarcomeres. The sarcolemma also acts to hold the sarcoplasm in place.

The myofibril is the contractile structure of the muscle and is composed of long, thin elements. Myofibrils are arranged longitudinally parallel and are cross striated. The repeated variations in density, that is, the amount of proteins and the type of protein along the myofibrils, cause this appearance. A myofibril is 0.5 to 1 mm in diameter. Each myofibril is composed of 400 to 2000 tiny filaments arranged parallel to the length of the myofibril, and each consists of light and dark bands. Mautner has stated:

> A more lucid picture of these structures is obtained by observation in polarized light, where only substances that have the property of anisotropism, or birefringence, may be seen to glow. Skeletal muscle possesses this quality. The dark or dense band glows in polarized light, and therefore is called the anisotropic or A band. In the polarized light, the light band becomes the dark band and is called the I or isotropic band.

When a muscle contracts, its attachments are normally drawn toward each other. This contraction exerts a tension on whatever is attached to the ends of the muscle. If the muscle fibers are pulling against the tendons or ligaments attached to bones, the muscle will tend to draw the bones closer together. The proximal end of skeletal muscle is usually attached to a heavier bone than is the distal end. Therefore, when the muscle contracts, the distal bone is the one more likely to move. The effect of the contraction on the lever depends on the position of the attachment and also on the length of the muscle fibers and their arrangement within the muscle.

Although, as previously stated, a contracting muscle usually moves the lighter of the bones to which it is attached, when the feet (or the hands) are fixed and supporting the body weight, the proximal (heavier) segment is moved. This is called reversed action. When the foot is on the ground in running and jumping, contraction of the ankle extensors moves the leg, not the foot; contraction of the knee extensors moves the thigh, not the leg (Fig. 3-12). When the hands are supporting the body weight in a hanging position, contraction of the elbow flexors moves the upper arm, rather than the forearm.

Fiber Arrangements. There are two main types of arrangement of muscle fibers: fusiform and penniform. In the fusiform arrangement the muscle fibers are distributed in longitudinal fashion in the muscle, allowing for maximal range of contraction. The sartorius is an example of a fusiform muscle. Its long, slender fibers are stretched between two heavy tendons. It is the longest muscle in the body and has the greatest range of contraction. The sartorius in an average size man will shorten approximately 20 cm (8 in.) during the full action of flexion at the hip and knee joints and when turning the thigh outward. Since the muscle fibers are arranged longitudinally, there are fewer fibers in this type of arrangement than in others. With fewer fibers, muscular force is reduced. The large range of contraction is thus achieved at the sacrifice of strength. In addition, the parallel arrangement of muscle fibers permits such muscles to move body parts with great speed with a small amount of muscle shortening.

The penniform arrangement of muscle fibers is similar to that of the barbs of a feather. A tendon is the position of the quill of a feather.

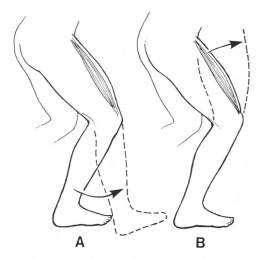

Fig. 3-12. *The function of the rectus femoris: A, the muscle moves the lower leg (shank) during a swinging action; B, the muscle moves the thigh during the initial phase of jumping since the foot is planted on the ground, not free to move. This action in B is termed reverse muscle action.*

Variations in the penniform arrangement include demipennate, unipennate, bipennate, multipennate, and circumpennate. Some of these arrangements are illustrated in Fig. 3-13. In the demipennate muscles, such as the adductor magnus, the fibers are arranged diagonally between two tendons and look like a feather cut in two along the quill. Unipennate muscles, like the semimembranosus and the extensor digitorum longus, have the muscle fibers located to one side of the tendon. Pennate muscles possess a feather-shaped fiber arrangement and include the flexor digitorum longus, peroneus tertius, and flexor pollicus longus. Fibers of bipennate muscles are double feather shaped, as in the vasti medialis and lateralis. Multipennate arrangements of muscle fibers are found in the broad muscles, such as the deltoideus and the pectoralis major.

The diagonal pulling position of the penniform muscles allows a greater number of fibers to act in a given mass, but there is a loss in the range of contraction because these fibers are shorter. As a rule, a long sheath of tendon extends nearly the entire length of penniform muscles. In the peroneus longus, the tendinous sheath is 46 cm (18 in) long, whereas the longest muscle fibers measure only 2.5 cm (1 in). The great number of fibers available for action in the penniform muscles allows only a limited shortening of the muscle, but provides great strength.

Muscle fibers always contract in a straight line; thus a three-part muscle may actually have discrete and different actions because of the manner in which its fibers are laid. This is evident in large muscles, such as the deltoideus. However, those muscles with tendinous extensions, such as those to the hand and foot, as they cross the wrist

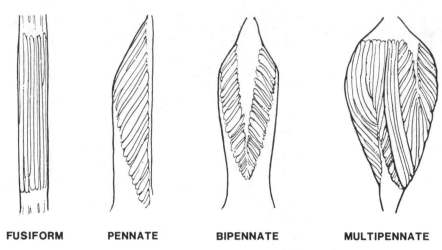

FUSIFORM   **PENNATE**   **BIPENNATE**   **MULTIPENNATE**

Fig. 3-13. *Fiber arrangement in skeletal muscle. Measure the cross-sectional area orthogonal to the fiber orientation to estimate the amount of force that can be developed in each muscle.*

and ankle to connect with each finger phalange or toe phalanx, are able to pull at a changed angle to contract in a straight line. Furthermore, in fusiform as compared to multipennate arrangement, the muscle has the advantage of long fibers, but has a narrow origin and insertion. The reverse is true in the multipennate muscle—with broad origin and insertion, there are muscle fibers running parallel to the contracting ones. Depiction of force vectors (direction of muscle tension) for three muscles is shown in Fig. 3-14.

Stimulation of Muscle Fiber. The conduction of an electrochemical impulse along the sarcolemma of a muscle fiber causes sufficient shift of ions within the fiber to bring about the formation of an actomyosin complex. With the change in the membrane potential, a reaction of the contractile proteins in the muscle results. Dudel (1978) refers to this as electromechanical coupling. Mautner has commented on the importance of the elastic properties of the sarcolemma and its collagenous fibrils in muscle contraction. He contends that the stretching of elastic fibers constitutes a creation of mechanical energy by the chemical process of contraction. He continues, "Implications of these springlike structures are that a bouncing or recoil effect upon reversal of motion exists, making the reversal smoother and faster." Recent work by Komi and Bosco attribute much of the benefits of a counter movement in vertical jumping to the potential energy generated by the elastic component in the muscle.

In the stimulation of a nerve, an action potential either travels over the entire neuron or does not travel at all. This is known as the all-or-none law. However, the force of contraction of a muscle fiber may vary in accordance with its contractile state, appropriate nutrients present, fibers not fatigued, and other such conditions. As to

80   *THE BIOMECHANICS OF HUMAN MOVEMENT*

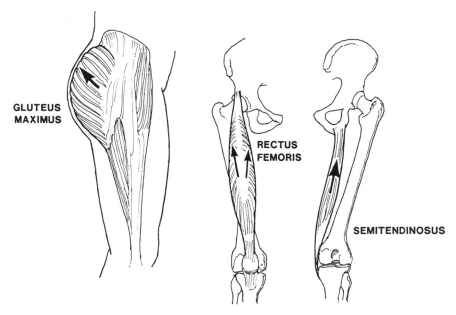

Fig. 3-14. *Force vectors representing lines of contractile forces in three muscles.*

the compliance of muscle fibers to the all-or-none law, one should note that "all" must be recognized as subject to a quantitative variation in interpretation. A muscle fiber may also obey the all-or-none response, but a muscle may not, since it is graded in its response. According to Dudel, the membrane of the muscle fiber, with a sufficient stimulus, evokes an action potential. The contraction, however, does not obey the all-or-none response. The contractile force increases approximately proportional to the amount of depolarization up to a limit where no further change occurs. This graduation of contraction resulting from gradations in depolarization does not occur in skeletal muscle. Muscles may not have a refractory period. This could be called an all-or-something response, since the force of contraction may vary. Not only does an entire muscle display a graded response, but the same phenomenon can also be exhibited by individual fibers. Therefore, the contractile force of an individual muscle fiber can be controlled by the frequency of excitation.

One might ask the following questions: (1) Do muscle fibers always obey the all-or-none law? The variation comes in what all means. If the stimulus is insufficient, it will be nothing, not something. (2) Can a muscle fire a second time without a refractory period? Yes, it may be reliably stated that such is the case. (3) Does myelination really come in degrees of thickness? The measure of thickness of myelin sheath has been given as 180 A. The sheath is described as lamellar, and it is suggested that there may be about 100 layers in a mature sheath.

Some muscles give the appearance of being redder in color than others because in some fibers the sarcoplasm contains relatively more myoglobin than in others. Myoglobin, which is a pigment in muscle similar to hemoglobin, has a greater affinity for oxygen and also dissociates oxygen five times faster than does hemoglobin. The redder muscles are supplied with a red pigment that may serve to store oxygen. They are therefore more suited for performing long, sustained, slow (static) pulls. These muscle fibers are referred to as Type I or slow-twitch muscle fibers. Thus, it is not surprising to find that postural muscles are a darker red than are many other muscles. Whiter muscles tend to tire more quickly when subjected to sustained loads over a prolonged time. These are referred to as Type II or fast-twitch muscle fibers. They are, however, peculiarly adapted to performing fast contractions. Fast-twitch fibers are suited for bursts of activity in which large power outputs with high velocities are generated.

A comparison of the muscles of domestic fowl with those of wild fowl illustrates this point. Muscles in the wings and breast, as well as in the legs of a wild fowl, are usually composed of many red fibers, whereas a domestic bird has more pale fibers in the muscles of the breast and wings from lack of use. In the human body, the soleus, as well as most extensor muscles (antigravity muscles), has a higher percentage of red pigment than do the gastrocnemius and most flexor muscles. The gastrocnemius is fast acting and initiates an action quickly; the soleus moves to sustain the action. The extensor muscles have the task of maintaining posture, whereas the flexors initiate action. In human muscle, however, the distinction between red and white fibers is not as clear as in muscle of fowl and domesticated birds.

Muscle stimulation is also influenced by the ratio of muscle fiber to motor neuron. Weiner (1953) explains the difference between the finely coordinated function of the central portion of the eye, particularly its concentration on visual information, and the function of the periphery of the eye. In the central portion, there is often a one-to-one relationship between a motor neuron and the muscle fibers (one-to-one relationship between the rods and cones and the fibers of the optic nerve). On the periphery of the eye, the relationship is one optic nerve fiber to ten or more end organs of muscle fibers. Thus, the middle of the eye is used to discriminate movement details, and the peripheral fibers are used as pickup mechanisms for centering and focusing, which are necessary in determining the details of an action. A somewhat similar arrangement exists betweeen a motor neuron and the muscle fibers of the fingers as compared to those of postural muscle. In the finger muscles, the ratio of muscle fibers to each motor neuron is less than in postural muscles. Thus finger muscles can perform more finely coordinated movements.

Muscle Tension. The approximately 150 muscles that are directly involved in moving the levers to maintain posture or in activating movement of all or a part of the body are capable of performing a great amount of mechanical work. Schottelius and Schottelius (1978) commented on the work of muscle by saying that the amount of mechanical work done by a muscle is determined by multiplying the newtons of the load lifted by the height to which the load is lifted as measured in millimeters (or meters); the result expresses the work in newton-meters. It is possible for a muscle to contract when no mechanical work is involved. If a load is too heavy and is not lifted, the muscle has then accomplished no mechanical work; all the expended energy appears as heat and would have to be measured by the amount of oxygen consumed. The optimum load for a muscle to lift is one in which maximum work can be accomplished each time the muscle contracts. On the other hand, if the muscle can barely lift the load and develops the maximal tension that it can generate in doing so, it lifts the maximal load. It has been stated that no muscle can do sustained work when the load that it lifts is greater than one-third to one-half of its total capacity. It is generally believed that a given muscle's strength is directly proportional to its physiological cross section. This means that the cross section is measured in such a way that the section is perpendicular to all the fibers of the muscle and not at an angle, as is often the case in an anatomic cross-section measurement. Thus penniform muscles are deemed to be stronger than quadrilateral muscles. Evans, however, states, "The force which a muscle can exert when it contracts depends upon the number, length, and arrangement of its fibers, the geometric relations of the muscle fibers to the tendon, the angle of insertion of the tendon on the bone, and the distance the tendon inserts from the joint axis about which movements occur." Therefore, the determination of potential strength of a muscle is a complex task.

The tension that can be exerted by a muscle becomes less as the muscle shortens. It has been postulated by some writers that this decrease results from internal friction. Since a muscle does not liberate more heat as it rapidly shortens, however, this does not appear to be the case. Huxley has said:

> When the muscle shortens, it exerts less tension: the tension decreases as the speed of shortening increases. One might suspect that the decrease of tension is due to the internal viscosity or friction in the muscle, but it is not. If it were, a muscle shortening rapidly would liberate more heat than one shortening slowly over the same distance, and this effect is not observed.

Hill (1965) has shown that a muscle while shortening does liberate more heat, but only in proportion to the distance that it shortens and not to the speed. When a muscle is stretched between two bones in such a fashion that it is elongated, this elongation gives the muscle an advantage, in that the range of contraction is large before tension is significantly reduced. The techniques of thermography have been used to measure changes in heat within tissues of the body. In the sports world, heat liberated by muscles during a discus throw was measured by researchers in the USSR.

Power is defined as the rate of work, that is, how much work can be performed in a given unit of time. Maximum power is the maximum work a muscle can perform in a unit time. This is dependent upon the maximum rate of cross-bridge cycling at the level of actin and myosin. This bridging is a function of the total cross-sectional area of a muscle that can be activated. Power can be altered by training although it is not a linear function of total change in cross-sectional area. The angle of pull of muscle fibers may change as muscle hypertrophies (gets larger), and, thus, power and tension potential change.

Huxley has further stated that striated muscles can shorten at speeds that are equal to 10 times their resting length in a second. They can also relax in a fraction of a second. This is because each fiber of a muscle is surrounded by an electrically polarized membrane that has one-tenth of a negative volt. When an impulse travels down a nerve to the motor endplate, which is in contact with the muscle fiber, it depolarizes the membrane, and a substance (probably calcium) is released throughout the fiber. Then the process of liberation of energy takes place as mentioned previously, and the fiber contracts.

Changes in muscle length and tension can be visualized in Fig. 3-15. The amplitude of a muscle is the range from maximum contraction to maximum stretch. A muscle works through a range somewhat less than its total amplitude, and its created contractile power is in the elongated phase.

A muscle that shortens (when contracting) to a greater extent than another has the advantage of contracting through a great distance, but lacks strength in lifting a limb. The classic long-fiber muscle is the sartorius, which is reported to be able to contract a maximum of 57% of its resting length. Normally muscles with short fibers contract considerably less than this—some even less than one-third their length.

Graduation of Contraction. Since an electrically polarized membrane surrounds each muscle fiber, if the fiber is depolarized, contraction results. An electrical impulse is sent to the muscle via the alpha motor neuron and is transmitted to the muscle over the motor endplate. This results in a depolarization (action potential) that spreads throughout the muscle fiber resulting in a single muscle twitch. The smallest unit of muscular movement is therefore the twitch. A weak contraction is one in which only a few fibers are involved. During postural tonus a few fibers are asynchronously contracting all the time at frequencies up to 5 per second. As the volleys of impulses to the muscle through the motor nerve fibers are increased, new fibers are stimulated and thus brought into contraction. The extent of the effort is determined by the number of fibers sent into contraction.

Measurement of the increase in the number of active muscle fi-

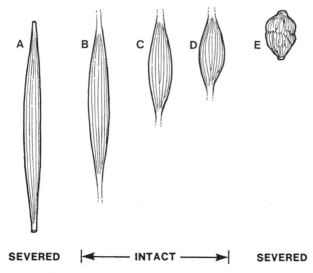

SEVERED |◄──── INTACT ────►| SEVERED

Fig. 3-15. *Length of skeletal muscle in five different conditions. A, maximum resting length after distal end has been severed; B, maximum length of intact muscle when elongated by pull of muscles on opposite side (according to Weber-Fick law, twice the length of condition D); C, natural length of noninnervated muscle; D, maximum shortening of intact muscle in extreme flexion (usually half the length of condition B); E, length of maximally stimulated muscle after distal end has been severed (one fourth to one sixth the length of condition B).*

bers is only one way in which contraction may be graded in strength. The interval between repeated stimuli and the frequency of the responses account for changes in tension. As the interval is shortened and responses become more frequent, the muscle tension is increased. This is referred to as summation (Fig. 3-16).

A muscle fiber that receives a second stimulus while still responding to the first contracts to a greater degree than if it is responding to a single stimulation. If the interval between the first and second stimulus is as brief as 25 to 50 ms, the resulting summation of contraction may triple the tension of a single twitch.

A continuous series of rapidly repeated stimuli at frequencies of about 50 per second sent to a muscle evokes a prolonged contraction, or tentanus, with tension as much as four times as great as that of a simple twitch. The stimuli may arrive in such rapid succession that the muscle remains in a contraction as long as the stimulation continues or until the muscle becomes fatigued.

Force Development in the Muscle. The time of development of muscular force is much greater than the time of the action potential. According to Dudel (1978), contraction in an isometric muscle twitch begins around 2 ms after the rising phase of the action potential (this period is know as the latent period) and does not reach its maximum force until around 100 ms. About halfway through this rising phase, the elastic tension that has been developing in the muscle begins to

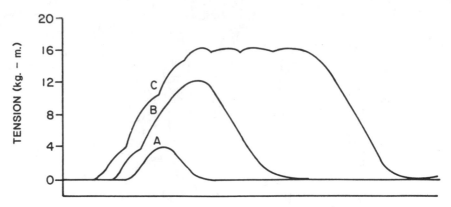

Fig. 3-16. *Response of skeletal muscle to successive excitations. A, single twitch; B, summation; C, tetanus.*

slow the rate of tension development. Gowitzke and Milner noted that at peak tension the contractile tension is equal to the elastic tension elements. The developed tension than becomes less than the elastic tension and the muscle relaxes.

The amount of force development depends on the length of an isolated muscle (Fig. 3-17). In the isolated muscle, maximum developed tension occurs with the muscle slightly longer than resting length. As resting length increases, so does the series elastic component, thus reducing the developed tension in the muscle. If the muscle length is shorter than its resting length, the total tension decreases (even though the elastic tension is almost nonexistent). Below 50% of resting length the muscle is unable to develop contractile force. Our movements are often modified to take advantage of this tension-length relationship. The person performing lower leg extensions on a universal machine leans backward (extending at the hip) as fatigue sets in, so that the length of the rectus femoris muscle is increased and consequently its force will increase. Two-joint muscles have the advantage of being able to position one joint so that the muscle can be made more productive at the other joint.

Beyond these general applications, however, the isolated muscle experiments on which the length-tension curves are based may not have too much practical value when investigating muscle torque and power in a live human being. The biophysics of maximal power output was investigated by Perrine using an isokinetic device (velocity-controlled resistance producing machine). The torque curves were ascending and descending curves, but not of the same type found by Hill. These data were collected from 15 subjects performing extensions of the lower leg (shank) at different rotational speeds. Peak power was achieved at a speed of 240 degrees per second, whereas peak torques occurred at a much lower speed, i.e., 96 degrees per second. Thus the tension-velocity curve differs at the two velocities. According to Kulig and Hay (1984), these two curves and a parabolic curve are common in strength curves. The parabolic curve is typical of flexion at the elbow. There is an interaction between the changes in the muscle moment arm and the changes in length as the angle of the joint changes. Therefore, it is difficult to predict the exact angle at which the body will be able to produce the greatest force. This is compounded further by the fact that more than one muscle usually is contracting to produce a movement.

Types of Muscle Contraction. Muscle contraction can be classified generally in three types: concentric, eccentric, and static. Concentric contraction occurs when a muscle develops sufficient tension to overcome a resistance and shortens. A body lever is moved in opposition to a given resistance. When an individual picks up an object, such as a book, some of the muscles of the arm, such as the biceps brachii, contract and shorten as the book is lifted. Eccentric contraction occurs when the resistance is not overcome, but the muscle develops tension and lengthens during the action. Eccentric contractions may occur when muscles are used to oppose a movement, but not to stop it, as in the action of the biceps brachii in lowering the arm gradually, whether the weight is greater than can be lifted or is a light object being slowly placed on the floor. The main characteristic is that the muscle lengthens during the action and this action is usually in the same direction as the force (for example, in line with gravity). Both concentric and eccentric contractions are called isotonic because the muscle changes length due to its own contraction during a movement with a load (Fig. 3-18).

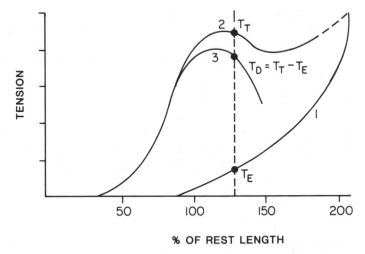

% OF REST LENGTH

Fig. 3-17. *Tension-length curves for isolated muscle. Curve 1, passive elastic tension Te in a muscle passively stretched to increasing length; curve 2, total tension T_T exerted by muscle contracting actively from increasingly greater initial lengths; curve 3, developed tension calculated by subtracting elastic tension values on curve 1 from total tension values at equivalent lengths on curve 2, i.e. Td = Tr − Tg. (From Gowitzke, B. A. and Milner, M. Understanding the scientific bases of human movement. Baltimore, Williams and Wilkins, 1980.)*

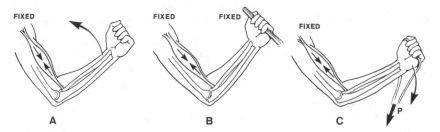

Fig. 3-18. *Concentric, isometric and eccentric contractions of the biceps brachii muscle. A, concentric contraction to produce movement of distal segment, muscle shortens; B, isometric contraction with no movement of body segments since they are restrained from responding to muscular contraction, there is no external manifestation of the minute muscle shortening; C, eccentric contraction with movement caused by external force (P) acting in opposition to muscular contraction, muscle lengthens despite its attempt to shorten.*

MINI-LAB LEARNING EXPERIENCES

1. Palpate the muscles of the arm and back while a person performs an isometric contraction against resistance to flexion at the elbow. Describe your findings and explain them with respect to muscle function.
2. Ask this same person to lift a heavy weight, using flexion at the elbow. Palpate the muscles and compare your findings with those in step 1.
3. Have a person perform a half or full squat, first with the trunk in an erect position and then with the trunk in a flexed position. Palpate the thigh muscles during the descending and ascending movements under these two conditions. Discuss your findings with respect to muscle function and stress to joints, including the spine.

A static contraction occurs when a muscle that develops tension is unable to move the load and does not change length. The effort exerted by the muscle is insufficient to move when the load is too heavy or when opposing muscles contract in opposition to each other, thus preventing movement. This fixation of a muscle's action into a static contraction is termed isometric because the muscle develops tension without changing appreciable length.

Preceding a concentric contraction phase with an eccentric phase is referred to as a stretch-shortening cycle. As noted by Viitasalo, Komi, and Bosco (1984), putting the muscle under stretch in the eccentric phase enables the muscle to store potential (elastic) energy. Work by Komi and Bosco demonstrated the effect of this stretch-shortening cycle in vertical jumps performed with and without a counter movement. Jumps utilizing the counter movement produced higher vertical jump height, average force and power output than without the counter movement. Furthermore, factors such as fiber composition (fast-twitch and slow-twitch fibers), length of prestretch, velocity of the stretch, and coupling time between the eccentric and concentric contractions affected the amount of potential energy. It was found that:

> Subjects rich in FT fibers in the vastus lateralis muscle benefit more from the stretching phase performed with high speed and short angular displacement [at the knee]. The slow type muscle, on the other hand, may be able to retain the cross-bridge attachment longer and therefore also utilize elastic energy better in a slow type ballistic motion.

The authors also noted that training was another important characteristic in force-time characteristics.

Weight Training Effects. Resistance training at a high percentage of one's maximal strength results in numerous morphological changes in skeletal muscle. Gains in muscular strength are usually accompanied by an increase in the size of the muscle fibers, known as hypertrophy. This change in size is mainly due to fiber size increase, but may also be due to muscle fiber splitting. The greater the resistance, the greater will be the hypertrophy. Isotonic training (10-20 repetitions) has resulted in greater increases in muscle size than isometric training since in the former condition the load is usually applied for a greater period of time. Explosive-type, low-resistance training, on the other hand, produces little or no hypertrophy. An acceptable theory to explain the hypertrophic changes is based upon the fact that such changes are due in part to the mechanical stress of contraction. Damage occurs as a result of the contractions and the muscle repairs itself. Thus heavy weight-training sessions should probably be no less than three days apart.

Classification of Muscles According to Function. For action to take place, the muscles of the body develop teamwork through training and practice. However, individually they can do only two things—develop tension to various degrees or relax in various manners.

Since a muscle either develops increased tension within itself or relaxes (in varying degrees), it performs various roles as action of the skeletal levers takes place. The shape, arrangement, size, and location, including whether it is one- or two-joint muscle, the length and nature of the tendons at the insertions, the type and mechanical advantage(s) of the bone(s) to which it is attached, and the insertion's angle with and distance from the fulcrum of the action bones are all factors in determining how the muscle functions in moving its bony lever. Some method of classifying and naming these roles and functions of muscles is needed by the student of kinesiology. Muscles are normally classified with regard to their direction of pull on the joint and subsequent skeletal movement. Such actions as extension, flexion, adduction, abduction, and lateral and medial rotation are classified according to the direction of the movement produced in the limb. If the proximal and distal insertions of a muscle lie in a single plane, only one of the previously defined actions can be carried out by that muscle. Muscles that cross one of the cardinal planes usually produce more than one action, a primary one and a secondary one. In the following pages, descriptive terms are used to define and describe these roles and functions.

It has been mentioned previously that muscles seldom operate singly; rather, they act in cooperation with one or more other muscles or as members of a team (sometimes involving most of the major muscles of the body) in a variety of combinations and patterns. Muscles do not always contract for the purpose of causing lever movement. Muscles may contract to help steady or support the lever, to stabilize a body part, to neutralize a body part, or even to neutralize the undesired action of some other muscles. Primarily, then, muscles are movers, stabilizers, and neutralizers.

Mover, or Agonist. A muscle that is known to be the principal mover or one of the principal movers of a lever is called a mover or agonist. This muscle, which contracts concentrically, may be directly responsible, along with one or more other muscles, for movement of a lever. The muscle is known as a prime mover when it has or shares primary responsibility for a joint action. When a muscle aids the prime mover in its action, it is known as an assistant mover. The biceps brachii is known as a prime mover of both the forearm in flexion and forearm in supination. In addition, because of the position of its two-headed origin on the scapula, this muscle aids in action at the shoulder joint, thereby acting as an assistant abductor. For example, the long head of the biceps brachii, although not often involved in shoulder abduction, becomes involved under certain circumstances. Brunnstrom claims that patients have been taught by therapists to use this muscle to abduct the shoulder when the deltoideus and supraspinatus have been paralyzed.

Antagonist. A muscle that acts as an antagonist is one that in contraction tends to produce movement opposite to that of the mover. In extension, the extensors are the movers and the flexors are the antagonists. After studies of muscle action, Elftman concluded that antagonists play a strong role in walking and running. In such actions when the limbs are about to complete a movement, the pull of the antagonists contract eccentrically in the deceleration of the limb. During a maximum effort by the agonists, the antagonists must relax so that they do not hinder the movement.

Stabilizer, Fixator, or Supporter. A muscle that steadies, fixes, or anchors a bone or body part against contracting muscles is known as a fixator, stabilizer or supporter. The stabilizer may also be used to combat the pull of gravity and the effects of momentum and interaction. For action to take place, one end of a muscle must be free to move and the other end firmly anchored.

A stabilizing muscle is rarely in static contraction, because the part being stabilized is in motion. Actually the anchoring part may be gradually moved to direct or guide the moving part as it performs its task.

The hip flexors stabilize when the rectus abdominis and other muscles flex the thoracic and lumbar spine (from the supine position). On the other hand, the abdominal muscles and lumbar spine extensors stabilize when the thigh is being extended by the gluteus maximus, hamstrings, and adductor magnus (especially when the knee is extended and the thigh is flexed beyond a 45-degree angle). However, when the foot is fixed and supports the weight, knee action extends the thigh (reversed muscle action). The parallel pull along the long axis of the bone that is accomplished by certain muscles makes them better suited for stabilizing a joint than others. This arrangement is convenient because the slower, stronger muscles help support the limbs, whereas the weaker, faster ones produce the limb movement.

Neutralizer, or Synergist. A muscle that acts to prevent an undesired secondary action of another muscle is called a neutralizer. Rasch and Burke use this term to avoid the difficulty with the term synergist. Authors have presented many different meanings of the term synergist. Morris has stated that writers in this field show little agreement, but the term continues to be used. Some call a muscle that functions as a neutralizer a synergist, and others use this term to mean a muscle that aids and abets the action of other muscles.

If a muscle both extends and adducts, but the performer wishes to extend only, the abductors are activated to prevent adduction. They are neutralizers and prevent the undesired action of the agonist. Wright classifies synergists as true synergists and helping synergists. The true synergist is a muscle that acts to prevent an undesired action of an agonist, but has no effect on its desired action. A true synergist often contracts statically to prevent undesired action of two-joint muscles. For example, in clenching a fist, the wrist extensors must contract statically to prevent flexion of the wrist. The helping synergist is one that helps another muscle to move a lever in a desired way and at the same time prevents an undesired action. A helping synergist then acts like a neutralizer.

Another Classification of Muscles. Muscles are also classified based on the ratio of the stabilizing component to the rotary component of their force. All muscles vary with respect to the magnitude of these components based on their angle of pull related to the position of the limbs. However, this variation is also dependent on the location of the muscle attachment with respect to the moving joint. A shunt muscle has a greater distance to the distal attachment than to the proximal attachment. Thus, the primary force of a shunt muscle acts along the line of the moving bone, producing a large stabilizing component and preventing the joint from being pulled apart. Shunt muscles come into play during quick movements to counteract the centrifugal force acting on the joint. The brachioradialis, when flexing the forearm, is a shunt muscle. A spurt muscle, with a longer distance from the joint to the proximal attachment than to the distal attachment has a large rotary component giving motion to the joint. The biceps brachii flexing the forearm is a spurt muscle (Fig. 3-19). When muscles act in reverse muscle action, their classification also reverses. For example, during a pull up with the hands grasping a bar, the forearm remains stationary and the upper arm flexes. In this instance, the biceps brachii has a shunt role and the brachioradialis a spurt role.

Classification of Movement Type with Respect to Muscle Contraction. Based upon studies of the electrical activity and the changes in tension in the various muscles involved in a voluntary movement, we know that a close cooperation exists between anatomically antagonistic muscles. The adjustment of the time relations and the magnitude of the responses to degrees of resistance and velocity of movement are infinitely variable. Nevertheless, rather fixed patterns of responses to different movements have been the basis for another system of classification of movement. Some of these systems have been reviewed and summarized by Hill. One classification along these lines is as follows: (1) slow tension movements, (2) rapid tension movements, and (3) rapid ballistic movements. In addition, there are oscillating (repetitive) movements.

Slow Tension Movements. Slow movements of body parts and objects that offer great resistance are phasic in character. A phasic movement is indicated by moderate to strong co-contraction of antagonists. The co-contraction serves to fix the joints involved in the action and to aid in accurate positioning of the body part or object being moved.

In the slow, controlled forms of movement, the antagonistic muscle groups are continuously contracted against each other, giving rise to tension. Tremors occur when antagonistic muscles are in contraction and balanced against each other in fixation.

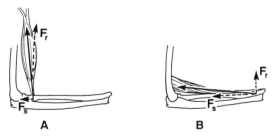

Fig. 3-19. *Examples of spurt (A, biceps brachii) and shunt (B, brachioradialis) muscles. Fr = rotary or movement force (perpendicular to longitudinal axis of forearm), Fs = stabilizing or tangential force (acting along the longitudinal axis of forearm and through the joint). Note the magnitudes of these forces are represented by the lengths of the vectors. If reverse muscle action would occur (proximal bone moves rather than distal bone), the spurt and shunt roles of these two muscles would also reverse. Why?*

Voluntary movement has been observed by Travis and Hunter to be a continuation of a tremor without interruption of the tremor rhythm. The elementary unit of a slow, controlled movement is the tremor. If a short movement is attempted, its amplitude is determined by that of the tremor. Ability to make movements more and more minute is limited not by sensory methods of control, but by the fundamental tremor element. Stetson and McDill have determined that the magnification of the visual field does not improve the delicacy of minute movement.

Slow, controlled movements result from a slight increase in the algebraic sum of the number of muscle fibers contracting in the positive muscle as against the number of fibers contracting in the antagonist muscle group. The limb moves in the direction of the group exerting the stronger pull, and tension of the two groups of antagonistic muscles is continually readjusted.

Rapid Tension Movements. A movement in which tension is present in all opposing muscle groups through the motion may be considered a movement of translation superimposed on fixation, with one group of contracting muscles suddenly initiating the movement, followed by contraction of the antagonistic group to stop the movement. Control of these faster movements cannot be attained more often than 10 times in a second, since modifying the course of a movement is possible only at the tremor terminations and not at other points in the movement. If the tremor cycles average 10 per second, then no modification of the movement could occur in less than one-tenth of a second. This limitation is imposed on the maximal rate of tapping. If the rate of tremor is 10 per second, then the rate of tapping cannot exceed that value. Travis has shown that a majority of movements of the faster type synchronize with the tremor cycle.

Rapid Ballistic Movements. A ballistic movement, begun by a rapid initial contraction of the prime mover, proceeds relatively unhindered by antagonistic contractions and is followed by a relaxation of the protagonist while the movement is still in progress. During a movement such as throwing a baseball, the antagonist progressively decreases in activity during the throw, indicating cocontraction. In comparison with the activity of the prime movers, however, the tension in the antagonists is slight during the ballistic type of movement. Some believe that as one becomes more and more skilled, the amount of cocontraction decreases. Ideally, for a maximal effort, no cocontraction should be present. There is some question whether true ballistic movements occur in sport skills.

One of the greatest differences between skilled and unskilled movements centers around changing tension movements to ballistic movements. Attempts to perform ballistic movements with muscles that are already fixed are fatiguing. Tension in one group of muscles necessitates an increase in the intensity of contraction of other sets. The spread of intensity results in rigidity, which is wasteful and restrictive.

In a ballistic movement, such as a golf swing, the moving limb swings rapidly about a joint, and the movement is terminated by co-contraction of the opposing muscles and the loss of momentum. It is important that the antagonist contract as late as possible so that force production is not sacrificed. If a movement is arrested by a strong contraction of the antagonistic group of muscles and as a result moves in the opposite direction, the movement is said to be oscillatory. Movements of great amplitude are more economical than those of small amplitude because of the intensity and continuity of muscular activity required to stop and start each phase of oscillation. A fast, shallow kick in swimming requires more effort to gain the same propulsive force than a slower, deeper kick requires. Hubbard has stated that fast action of a limb involves muscular contraction that acts as an impulse (Ft, force applied over a period of time). A limb once set in action by an impulse will continue to move by virtue of its own momentum until acted on by an outside force. The muscle, having developed energy in the limb, then tends to relax.

REFERENCES

Adrian, M. J. (1981): Flexibility in the aging adult. In Smith, E. L., and Serfass, R. C. (Eds).: *Exercise and aging: The Scientific Basis*. Papers presented at the American College of Sports Medicine annual meeting, Las Vegas, NV, May 1980. Hillside, NJ: Enslow Publishers.

Barham, J. N. and Wooten, E. P. (1973): *Structural kinesiology*, New York: Macmillan Publishing Co., Inc.

Basmajian, J. V. (1973): Electromyographic analyses of basic movement patterns. In Wilmore, J., editor: *Exercise and sports sciences*, vol. 1, New York: Academic Press, Inc.

Basmajian, J. V. and Macconaill, M. A. (1977): *Muscles and movement: a basis for human kinesiology*, Huntington, NY: R. E. Krieger Publishing Co., Inc.

Basmajian, J. V. (1979): *Muscles alive: their functions revealed by electromyography*, ed. 4, Baltimore: The Williams & Wilkins Co.

Bosco, C. and Komi, P. V. (1982): Muscular elasticity in athletes. In *Exercise and Sport Biology*. Champaign, IL: Human Kinetics Publishers.

Brunnstrom, S. (1946): Comparative strengths of muscles with similar functions, *Phys. Ther.* 26:59.

Butler, D. L., Grood, E. S., Noyes, F. R. and Zernicke, R.F. (1979): Biomechanics of ligaments and tendons. In Hutton, R., editor: *Review of exercise and sports sciences*, vol. 6, Philadelphia: The Franklin Institute Press.

Dudel, J. (1978): Muscles. In Schmidt, R. F., editor: *Fundamentals of Neurophysiology*, 2nd ed., New York: Springer-Verlag.

Elftman, H. (1938): The force exterted on the ground in walking, *Arbeitsphysiologie* 10:485.

Elftman, H. (1939): The function of the arms in walking, *Hum. Biol.* 11:4.

Elftman, H. (1940): The work done by muscles in running, *Am. J. Physiol.* 129:672.

Evans, F. G. (1957): *Stress and strain in bones*, Springfield, IL: Charles C. Thomas, Publisher.

Evans, F. G. (1971): Biomechanical implications of anatomy, In Cooper, J. M., editor: *Selected topics in biomechanics*, Chicago: The Athletic Institute.

Evans, F. G. (1961): *Biomechanical studies of the musculoskeletal system*, Springfield, IL: Charles C. Thomas, Publisher.

Frankel, V. H. and Burstein, A. H. (1970): *Orthopaedic biomechanics*, Philadelphia: Lea & Febiger.

Frankel, V. H. and Nordin, M. B. (1980): *Basic biomechanics of the skeletal system*, Philadelphia: Lea and Febiger.

Frost, H. M. (1957): *The laws of bone structure*, Springfield, IL: Charles C. Thomas, Publisher.

Frost, H. M. (1967): *An introduction to biomechanics*, Springfield: IL, Charles C. Thomas, Publisher.

Fulton, J. F., editor (1955): *Textbook of physiology*, Philadelphia: W.B. Saunders Co.

Gowitzke, B. A. & Milner, M. (1976): *Understanding the scientific bases of human movement*, 2nd ed., Baltimore: Williams & Wilkins.

Hall, C. B. and others: *Normal human locomotion* (film series), La Grange, IL: Associated Sterling Film.

Hill, A. V. (1927): *Living machinery*, New York: Harcourt Brace Jovanovich, Inc.

Hill, A. V. (1927): *Muscular movement in man*, New York: McGraw-Hill Book Co.

Hill, A. V. (1951): *The mechanics of voluntary muscle, Lancet* 2:947.

Hill, A. V. (1965): *Trails and Trials in Physiology*. Baltimore: Williams and Wilkins Co.

Holland, G. J. (1968): The physiology of flexibility: a review of the literature, *Kinesiol. Rev.*, pp. 49–61.

Hubbard, A. W. (1960): Homokinetics: muscular function in human movement. In Johnson, W., editor: Science and medicine of exercise and sports, New York: Harper & Row, Publishers.

Huxley, H. E. (1958): The contraction of muscle, *Sci. Am.* 199:67, Nov.

Kapandji, I. A. (1970): *The physiology of the joints: Vol. 1 Upper Limb* (translation), New York: Churchill Livingstone.

Kapandji, I. A. (1970): *The physiology of the joints: Vol. 2 lower limb* (translation), New York: Churchill Livingstone.

Kapandji, I. A. (1974): *The physiology of the joints: Vol. 3 the trunk and the vertebral column* (translation), New York: Churchill Livingstone.

Kulig, K, Andrews, J. G. and Hay, J. G. (1984): Human strength curves, *Exercise and Sports Sciences Reviews* 12.

Leighton, J. R. (1957): Flexibility characteristics of three specialized skill groups of champion athletes, *Arch. Phys. Med. Rehabil.* 38:580.

Logan, G. A. and McKinney, W. C. (1977): *Anatomic kinesiology*, Dubuque: Wm. C. Brown Publishers.

Luttgens, K. and Wells, K. F. (1982): *Kinesiology: scientific basis of human motion*, 7th ed., Philadelphia: Saunders College Publishing.

Mautner, H. E. (1956): The relationship of function to the microscopic structure of striated muscle: a review, *Arch. Physiol. Med. Rehabil.* 37:286.

Mautner, H. E. (1956): The relationship of function to the microscopic structure of striated muscle: a review, *Arch. Physi. Med. Rehabil.* 37:286.

Morris, R. (1955): *Coordination of muscles in action: correlation of basic sciences with kinesiology*, New York: American Physical Therapy Association.

Rasch, P. J. and Burke, R. K. (1963): *Kinesiology and applied anatomy*, Philadelphia: Lea & Febiger.

Schotellius, B. A. and Schotellius, D. D. (1978): *Textbook of physiology*, ed. 18, St. Louis: The C.V. Mosby Co.

Stetson, R. H. and McDill, J. A. (1923): Mechanism of different types of movements, *Psychol. Monogr.* 32:18.

Travis, L. E. (1929): The realtion of voluntary movements to tremours, *J. Exp. Psychol.* 12:515.

Travis, L. E. and Hunter, T. A. (1927): Muscular rhythms and action currents, *Am. J. Physiol.* 81:355.

Viitasalo, J. T., Komi, P. V., and Bosco, C. (1984): Muscle structure: a determinant of explosive force production? In Kumanmoto, M., editor: *Neural and Mechanical Control of Movement*, Kyoto: Yamaguchi Shoten.

Weiner, N. (1953): *Cybernetics*, Garden City, NY: Doubleday & Co., Inc.

Wright, W. (1928): *Muscle function*, New York: Paul B. Hoeber, Inc.

Zernicke, R. F. (1986): Movement dynamics and connective tissue adaptations. In *Proceedings of the Symposium on Future Directions in Exercise/Sport Research*, Champaign, IL: Human Kinetics Publishers.

4

The Human Movement System

Early kinesiologists and biomechanists likened the movement apparatus of living bodies to a lever system. Bones were the levers that were rotated by means of muscles and external forces. Anatomically, each animal and human is born with muscle attachments at particular sites. During body growth and development, the muscles increase in strength, the bones become larger and longer, particularly in the case of the appendages, and the weights of the body segments change. Therefore the effectiveness of the lever system will also change. During extremely rapid growth periods, such as during puberty in humans, the lever system may seem unwieldy and unfamiliar to the person. The individual must learn again how to use the body. This was evident among the top Olympic-caliber female gymnasts, who were champions at age 14 and appeared less skilled 1 or 2 years later because of changes in distribution of segmental weights and because of longer levers.

This chapter is designed to explain lever systems and their functions; to show application of effective and efficient use of the muscle-bone lever systems; and to provide a method for analyzing those lever systems which are operating at a given point in time.

ELEMENTS OF A LEVER

A lever is a machine, a device, for transmitting energy; it is able to do work when energy is transmitted through it. In the human body, energy derived from muscular contraction is applied to the bones resulting in movement of the body segments. These segments may transmit energy to external objects more advantageously than is possible without a lever system.

The lever is commonly defined as a rigid bar that revolves about an axis or a fulcrum. In the body the location of the axis or the ful-

97

crum is readily identified as a line (axis) passing through, or a point (fulcrum) within, the joint in which the movement occurs. Since these joints have widths, and since the bones forming a joint have one or more contact points, such as condyles, the concept of an axis of rotation is more reasonable than that of a fulcrum.

Identification of the rigid bar may be more difficult if the word bar suggests a straight mass whose length is considerably greater than its width or thickness. The word rigid, too, may present difficulties if it suggests an undivided, continuous mass. One should realize that external levers can vary in shape and in structure. A hammer can be used as a lever in both driving in and pulling out a nail. Yet the hammer neither is a straight bar nor does it need be an undivided mass; the head need only be securely attached to the handle. Even the common crowbar, often cited as an example of an external lever, although usually one continuous mass, could be an effective device for transmitting energy if it consisted of two or more segments bound together firmly enough to withstand the forces to which it might be subjected.

The student of kinesiology (biomechanics) must realize that body levers may vary in shape from the traditional rigid bar. One or more bones may be bound together by muscles firmly enough for them to function as a single mass. For example, the bones of the upper and lower arms can be held together by muscles crossing the elbow joint; the bones of the entire arm, the shoulder girdle, the vertebrae, and the pelvis can be held together by muscles crossing all intervening joints. These variations from the common concept of external levers may suggest that lever identification in human movement is difficult. It will be simplified if the forces and the types of lever systems are classified according to the spatial relationships of the effort and resistance forces, and the axis. There are two basic types of lever systems: (1) the type in which the forces act at points on both sides of the axis, as in a teeterboard, and (2) the type in which the forces act only on one side of the axis, as in a door that rotates about its hinges. This latter type is usually subdivided into two types, depending on which of the opposing forces, effort or resistance, is closer to the axis.

These three types of lever systems are depicted in Fig. 4-1.

Note that the lever with the space arrangement E-A-R is referred to as a first-class lever system. The second-class lever system has the arrangement E-R-A, and the third-class system has the arrangement R-E-A, in which the lever is viewed from the distal end to the proximal end. The elements of the lever systems are enumerated as follows:

1. The axis, A, is depicted as a real or imaginary line passing through the joint and about which the rigid mass of the limb (lever) rotates. The axis will always be perpendicular to the plane of movement of the lever.

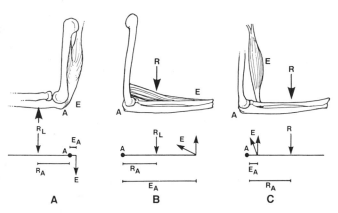

Fig. 4-1. *Types of lever systems. A, first class—axis lies between effort (E) and resistance (R); B, second class—resistance lies between axis and effort; C, third class—effort lies between axis and resistance. EA, effort arm; RA, resistance arm.*

2. The point of application of effort is the point at which the contracting muscle is attached to the moving bone.
3. The effort, E, is that force acting at its application site and is represented by a vector. The vector is the muscle—that which creates the movement volitionally.
4. The effort arm is the moment arm for the effort, that is, that distance from the axis to the site of muscle attachment. All the parts of the rigid mass of the lever between the axis and the point of application of effort compose the effort arm. However, the measurement of the effort arm is the perpendicular distance from the axis to the effort, not the curvature or other conformation distance along the bone.
5. The point of application of resistance is the point at which the external object, or the center of gravity of the mass of the lever, is applied.
6. The resistance, R, is that force acting at its application site which is represented as a vector having the opposite direction to that of the effort. In the case of the first-class lever system, the direction is the same, but the effect on the lever is opposite. For example, if the effort direction and site of application cause clockwise rotation, the resistance would cause counterclockwise rotation.
7. The resistance arm is the moment arm for the resistance, that is, that distance from the axis to the resistance vector. All the parts of the rigid mass of the lever lying between these two points compose the resistance arm. Again, the measurement of the resistance arm is the perpendicular distance from the axis to the resistance vector. Thus all three lines—axis, resistance vector, and resistance arm—are mutually perpendic-

ular. Note that in Fig. 4-1 all the axes are horizontal, the resistance and effort vectors are vertical, and the moment arms (resistance and effort) are horizontal, but at right angles to the axes. Movement occurs in the plane of the effort and resistance vectors.

In descriptions of body levers, the points E and R will not be precisely located. The attachment of a muscle will necessarily cover more than one point, or there will be two or more muscles involved in the lever system. An average position must be selected arbitrarily. Likewise, R may also cover more than one point, and usually there are at least two resistances; one is the weight of the segment, and the other is an external object. The axis, too, may cause some problems in analysis, since the axis may be a line of intersection of the body and an external object, such as the foot with the floor or the hands with the vaulting horse. Also, some bones may be moving along more than one axis simultaneously. Isolating each movement with the corresponding locations of E and R is very complex. This lack of precision should not hinder the understanding of the lever action in the body nor the utilization of the basic concepts concerning lever systems in the analysis of human and animal movements.

Function of Bony Levers

As previously stated, the bony lever, together with the forces acting on this lever, is known as a lever system. If bone and muscle were isolated from the body, the lever system would resemble that depicted in Fig. 4-2.

Muscle M attaches to bone V and H. The action of the muscle is one of shortening. The result of this muscle shortening may be movement (rotation) of bone V and bone H, of only bone V, of only bone H, or of neither bone. If bone H is the distal bone, it is the bone more likely to move, since its mass is apt to be less than that of the more proximal bone V. Furthermore, since the distal end of bone H is free to move, the resistance of the lever to movement is minimal. The more

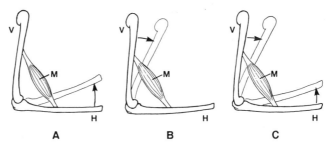

Fig. 4-2. *Effects of muscle (M) contraction on the lever system. A, produces movement of distal bone (H); B, produces movement of proximal bone (V),; C, produces movement of both bones (V and H). Under what circumstances does each occur?*

proximal attachment of bone V to another body segment adds additional mass to bone V; therefore bone V will probably remain stationary. Examples of these three movement possibilities are shown in Fig. 4-3.

When both bones move, the lever system actually becomes two lever systems, the muscle being the common force for each system. An analysis of the bone-muscle lever system is easiest if done on a planar level with two opposing forces. In reality, a complete analysis necessitates the investigation of moments of force in a world of three-dimensional forces. Referring again to Fig. 4-1, A, one can see that the muscle moment of force is equal in magnitude and opposite in direction to the moment of resistance created by the weight of the forearm, since no rotatory movement is occurring. As shown in Figure 4-4, the attachment of the triceps brachii can be estimated to be 15 mm from the elbow joint, whereas the center of gravity of the body segment is approximately 195 mm from the elbow joint. Therefore the muscle force must be 13 times that of the weight of the body segment (remember that the moments of force must be equal in magnitude to remain in a static state). The muscle force is calculated by means of the moment-of-force, or levers equation, which states that the product of the force acting perpendicular to a lever and its perpendicular distance (moment arm) from the axis of rotation equals the moment of force about the axis. Note that the line of the muscle vector, the distance from the muscle insertion to the joint, and the axis of rotation are mutually perpendicular to each other. Referring to the Cartesian coordinate system, y = muscle, x = moment arm, and z = axis. Note that the gravitational vector is also vertical, or in the y direction, its

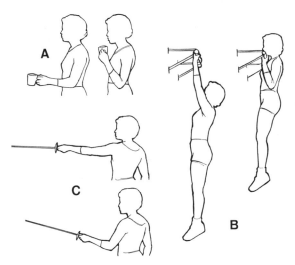

Fig. 4-3. *Examples of three movement possibilities as a result of contraction of biceps brachii. A, distal segment moves in lifting cup; B, proximal segment moves in chin-up because distal end is fixed; C, both proximal and distal segments move in fencing thrust.*

moment arm is x, and the moment of force, again, is about the z-axis but in the counterclockwise direction. What would happen to the amount of E required to hold the arm if a ball were placed in the hand? Hint: what effect does this have on RA? What if the object were moved closer to the axis at the elbow?

An example of the important concept of "mutual perpendicularity" is given in Fig. 4-5, which shows a comparison of the resistance moments produced in each of three options in holding a softball or baseball bat in the ready position for a pitched ball. In all options the wrists represent the axis of rotation, and the resistance arm is measured as the horizontal line (distance) from the extended line of the joint to the line of gravity of the bat. Note how the moment arm (RA) increases as the bat position changes from a nearly vertical position to a nearly horizontal position. The longer and heavier the bat (assuming that the center of gravity of the bat is in the same location, proportionally), the more muscle force will be required of the relatively small muscles acting at the wrist. Is it any wonder that the characteristic adjustment that batters make when their muscles are not strong enough for the task is to space the hands 15 to 25 cm apart? With this adjustment, the batter has introduced a first-class lever system into the ready position. The hand closest to the end exerts an opposite force to that of the weight of the bat, while the other hand, which lies between these two forces, acts as the balance point, or fulcrum. The mechanical advantage of the lever system is thus enhanced. The batter now uses the stronger muscles acting at the shoulder and elbow, as well as the weight of the upper arm, rather than relying on the muscles that cross the wrist.

Components of Muscle Force

Muscles rarely exert forces that are solely perpendicular (90 degrees) to the longitudinal axis of the bone; usually the muscles pull

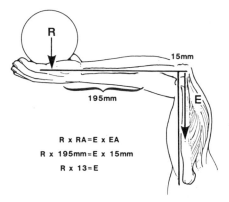

$$R \times RA = E \times EA$$
$$R \times 195mm = E \times 15mm$$
$$R \times 13 = E$$

Fig. 4-4. *Triceps muscle acting as a first class lever (R, resistance; RA, resistance arm, E, effort; EA, effort arm). The muscular effort required to hold the sphere is equal to 13 times that of the weight of the sphere. What implications does that have for activities involving the triceps muscle?*

THE BIOMECHANICS OF HUMAN MOVEMENT

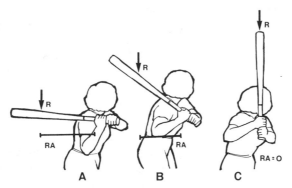

Fig. 4-5. *Three positions of bat during stance phase of batting. Resistance arms (RA) and resistance vectors (R) are depicted for ease of comparison of moments of force acting on wrists. The effort and effort arm must adjust to changes in RA. Measure the approximate effort arm and compare it to that of the resistance arms in each of the three positions.*

at angles of less than 90 degrees. Furthermore, the angle of pull changes as the angle at the joint changes. The force vector for the muscle, then, is diagonal to the longitudinal axis of the bone and can be resolved into its two components by using the graphic, or trigonometric, method described in Chapter 5.

Muscles, then, provide both a force that is capable of moving the bone and a force that acts on the joint. In most instances, the force acting on the joint acts to increase the integrity (stability) of that joint. This force is termed a stabilizing component, since it tends to draw the moving bone into the joint, that is, into a closely packed position. This force, which acts along the bone and has no moment of force, is also referred to as a reaction force, or tangential force. The movement component of force acts at right angles to both the axis and the bone and is termed a normal, or rotary force. When the bone to be moved is in a horizontal position, the movement component is a vertical force and the stabilizing component is a horizontal force.

There are instances in which the usual stabilizing force becomes a dislocating force; that is, it acts to pull the bone (lever) away from the second bone forming the joint. This occurs whenever the angle of pull of the muscle exceeds 90 degrees.

The stabilizing component of muscle force is important when the person or animal must exert great isometric forces or move at high speeds. These high speeds create great centrifugal forces, which act to pull the lever away from the joint. Dislocation would result if this stabilizing component and other assisting muscles did not exist.

Muscles possessing a larger stabilizing component than moving component are called shunt muscles. The angle of muscle pull is less than 45 degrees. Muscles having a larger moving component than stabilizing component are called spurt muscles, and their angles of pull are greater than 45 degrees. Although this classification is convenient, some muscles can act as shunt muscles with respect to their action on the distal bone and as spurt muscles with respect to the proximal bone. For example, in most activities of daily living, sports, and work, the brachioradialis functions as a shunt muscle. During the act of chinning, this muscle acts as a spurt muscle as it moves the proximal bone. Therefore, this classification is useful if one remembers to identify the moving bone and the point of attachment of the muscle on that bone (refer to Chapter 3). An important fact to remember is that the angle of the muscle attachment with respect to the bone is a changing angle; therefore, the amount of stabilizing and movement force also changes as the angle at the joint changes (Fig. 4-6).

A mathematic calculation of the forces acting in two static limb positions in which an object is held is given in Fig. 4-7. Note the use of trigonometry to measure the perpendicular moment arms of the resistance and the perpendicular component of the effort vector.

If the joint permits movement in a certain plane, the ability of the person to produce movement in that plane will depend on the following:

1. Number of muscles capable of moving the body part in that plane.
2. Force of each muscle and its angle of pull and cross section, and distance from the axis (joint).
3. Weight of body part(s) being moved and the distance of its center of gravity from the joint.

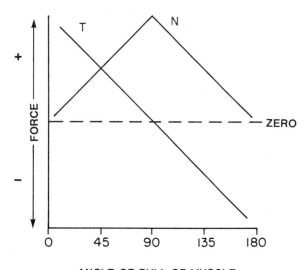

Fig. 4-6. *Relationship of stabilization and movement components of muscular force. (N, movement force which is normal or perpendicular to bone; T, stabilization force which is parallel to bone, either toward or away from joint.) Dislocating force exists at angles greater than 90 degrees, depicted below the zero line.*

THE BIOMECHANICS OF HUMAN MOVEMENT

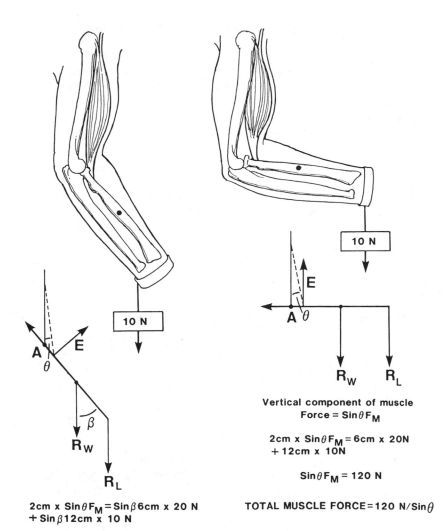

$$2\text{cm} \times \text{Sin}\,\theta\,F_M = \text{Sin}\,\beta\,6\text{cm} \times 20 \text{ N}$$
$$+ \text{Sin}\,\beta\,12\text{cm} \times 10 \text{ N}$$

Vertical component of muscle
Force $= \text{Sin}\,\theta\,F_M$

$$2\text{cm} \times \text{Sin}\,\theta\,F_M = 6\text{cm} \times 20\text{N}$$
$$+ 12\text{cm} \times 10\text{N}$$

$$\text{Sin}\,\theta\,F_M = 120 \text{ N}$$

TOTAL MUSCLE FORCE $= 120 \text{ N}/\text{Sin}\,\theta$

Fig. 4-7. *Free body diagrams for mathematical determination of amount of muscle force required to hold an object in two different positions.*

4. Weight of external objects attached to or held by the body part and their distances from the joint.
5. Number of objects resisting the movement.

Thus, it is the ratio of the moment of force produced by the muscles to the moment of force produced by the resistances that determines whether or not movement will occur when muscles contract. The formula is as follows:

R × RA divided by E × EA

- If the ratio is equal to 1, no movement occurs
- If the ratio is greater than 1, the resistance produces the movement.

THE HUMAN MOVEMENT SYSTEM

- If the ratio is equal to less than 1, the muscles produce the movement.

These calculations of muscle moments to produce movement presuppose that the body part is stationary and that the body part is accelerated from zero to an undefined acceleration. When a body part is moving, the movement itself is a force ($I\alpha$) because it maintains the object in its path and speed of rotation.

Muscle force required to stop the motion is equal to the force of the motion plus the resistance moments of force previously described. This relationship is logical because a moment of force greater than the resistance moment was required to cause a certain amount of movement, measured in units of acceleration. These types of calculations can be achieved by means of movie film analysis. Dillman was one of the first to estimate moments of force of muscles, which cause both acceleration and deceleration of a body part during running.

Single-Muscle Levers

The reader is encouraged to measure the moment arms and angles of muscle pull and to estimate the amount of muscle force required to initiate movement as presented in the following analyses of single-muscle lever systems. Any muscle force that produces a moment of force greater than the resistance moment will produce volitional movement.

Single-Muscle Levers in Sagittal Plane

Action of Biceps Brachii in Forearm Flexion. The action of the biceps brachii is illustrated in Fig. 4-8, in which the muscle is shown supporting a weight resting in the hand. The drawing might also be visualized as a "flash" representation of a phase of upward movement of the weight. If the movement starts with the upper arm and forearm at the side, and if the upper arm is held in that position as the forearm moves forward and upward, the forearm moves through the sagittal plane. The axis of movement will be a line that is perpendicular to the plane of movement and, in this situation, that passes through the elbow joint. This line will lie in the transverse and frontal planes, since a line may lie in two planes, and both of them are perpendicular to the plane of movement—the sagittal. The rigid bar includes the ulna and radius and the bones of the wrist and hand. The effort arm is that section of the radius and ulna that lies between A and the attachment of the muscle (approximately 3 cm in length). The resistance arm includes the bony mass extending from A to the center of the weight, including the total length of the radius and ulna, the wrist and metacarpals, and a portion of the proximal phalanges, approximately 20 cm in length. The lever is not a simple, continuous mass but consists of several bones bound together by muscles, tendons, and ligaments. The weight of the forearm and hand is not in-

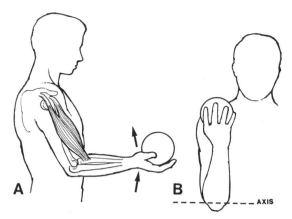

Fig. 4-8. *Action of biceps brachii in forearm flexion. A, sagittal plane; B, frontal plane with axis of rotation shown.*

cluded in the analysis. The arrangement is A-E-R, a third-class lever since the attachment of the biceps brachii lies between the axis and the resistance.

Since it is known that if the weight is to be supported, the length of A-E times the amount of muscular force must equal the length of A-R times the weight of the supported object, it can be seen that the amount of muscular force must be more than six times the weight of the object. For example,

$$E \times 3 \text{ cm} = R \times 20 \text{ cm}$$
$$E = R \times 6.67$$

For a resistance of 10 N, the muscular force must be 66.7 N. If the object were to be moved, the force must be even greater.

Note that in identifying the lever elements one needs to consider only the muscle attachment to the moving segment. It is the point at which energy is applied to the lever. The muscle must have another point of attachment, but that attachment is not part of the lever, although it is an essential part of the total machine. Under certain circumstances for the biceps brachii the upper arm is the moving lever as in executing a pullup. In most instances the forearm is the moving lever as in lifting an object.

Action of Greater Psoas Muscle in Thigh Flexion. The attachment of the greater psoas muscle to the femur is shown in Fig. 4-9. If this illustration is visualized as a phase in flexion at the hip, the femur is shown moving through the sagittal plane, and the fulcrum of the action is on an axis passing through the hip joint in the transverse and frontal planes. If the weight of the leg is 95 N, the muscle must oppose this force. However, the resistance arm is that section of the femur that extends from the axis to the center of gravity of the leg (approximately 36 cm), and the effort arm is only 6 cm. The effort arm is measured along the section of the femur that extends from the axis to the muscle attachment, since the leg is estimated to be horizontal. In Fig. 4-9, the angle of pull of muscle is estimated as 45 degrees. Since the sine of 45 degrees equals 0.707, the muscle force in the vertical direction is equal to:

$$E \times EA = R \times RA \text{ (for equilibrium)}$$
$$E \times EA = 95 \text{ N} \times RA$$
$$E(6 \text{ cm}) = 95 \text{ N} \times 36 \text{ cm}$$
$$E = \frac{95 \text{ N} \times 36 \text{ cm}}{6 \text{ cm}}$$
$$E = 95 \text{ N} \times 6$$
$$E = 576 \text{ N of vertical force}$$

To determine the total muscle force acting at a 45-degree angle, divide the vertical force by the sine of the angle. Thus the muscle force always will be greater than that required when the muscle acts at an angle normal to the bone (90 degrees). Thus:

Total muscle force = 576 N:0.7
Total muscle force = 823 N

In these calculations, the 823 N of muscle force required to support a leg weighing 95 N is equivalent to approximately 183 pounds of muscle force supporting a leg weighing less than 22 pounds. Thus the muscle must exert a force greater than 8 times that of weight of

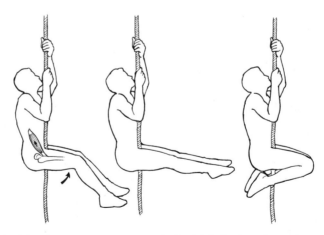

Fig. 4-9. *Action of greater psoas muscle in thigh flexion. Legs in partial flexion (RA = 36 cm). Calculate the muscle moment required with legs extended (RA = 46 cm) and legs in a tight tuck position (RA = 15 cm).*

THE BIOMECHANICS OF HUMAN MOVEMENT

the leg. One might estimate how much force would be required if the legs were held in a tuck position, with the center of gravity of the legs now being approximately 15 cm. If the legs were fully extended, as recommended for maximal difficulty, the resistance arm would be 46 cm. Is it any wonder that many persons cannot elevate their legs to the horizontal position and maintain this position? (This analysis is limited to only one muscle to simplify the mathematic processes.)

Action of Brachioradialis in Forearm Flexion. Flexion of the forearm resulting from contraction of the brachioradialis is illustrated in Fig. 4-10. The forearm moves through the sagittal plane, and the axis, passing through the elbow joint, lies in the frontal and transverse planes; the fulcrum is on that axis and lies within the joint. The lever includes the radius and the ulna; the effort arm includes that length of the bone which extends from the axis to the point of attachment of the muscle, a length of 15 cm. Since the center of gravity of the forearm-plus-hand lies closer to the axis than does the site of the muscle attachment, this is an example of a second-class lever system. This system could be one of great strength, except for the fact that the brachioradialis has such a small angle of pull that there is virtually no movement component to this shunt muscle.

Since the mechanical advantage of the brachioradialis is low, this muscle usually acts to stabilize a fast flexion or movement of a large load in which such stabilization is of prime importance. If a weight were suspended at the center of gravity of the segment, the arrangement would remain an E-R-A lever, that is, a second-class lever. If, however, the weight is moved to the hand, the arrangement could become an A-E-R lever, that is, a third-class lever. One would need to calculate the position of the center of gravity of the system (for example, arm plus hand plus weight) to determine the common resistance arm.

One can see readily how a performance may require great muscle effort or very little muscle effort merely by adjusting the placement of external weights on the body and by adjusting the position of the limb in space. For efficient movement the forearm and hand should be brought closer to the body, thus decreasing the moment arm for the resistances.

Action of Rectus Femoris in Leg Extension. A major joint action in kicking is leg extension. The action of the rectus femoris in kicking is illustrated in Fig. 4-11. The leg is shown moving through the sagittal plane; the fulcrum is in the knee joint on an axis that lies in the frontal and transverse planes. The rigid bar includes the tibia and fibula and those tarsal and metatarsal bones which are firmly attached to the leg bones from the ankle joint to the point of ball contact. The effort arm is that section of the bone which extends from the axis to the attachment to the tibia, a length of 12.7 cm (5 in), and the resistance arm includes those bones which extend from the axis to the center of gravity of the leg-plus-foot, a length of 35 cm.

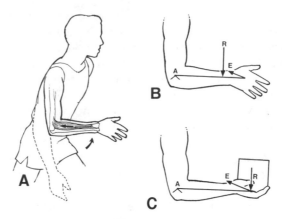

Fig. 4-10. *A, Action of brachioradialis in forearm flexion. B, brachioradialis in A is diagrammed as part of a second class lever system with the center of gravity of the forearm/hand as the resistance (R), the muscle as the effort (E), and the elbow as the axis of rotation (A). C, brachioradialis is part of a third class lever system when a heavy load is carried in the hand; RA now becomes longer than EA.*

Since the limb is not horizontal, components of the forces perpendicular to the moment arm are described as follows: (1) weight of leg times the sine of angle of leg with the vertical and (2) effort times the sine of angle of muscle with the forearm. At the point of contact with the ball, the weight of the ball will produce a resistance moment of force in addition to that created by the weight of the leg. The lever now includes the complete length of the body segment, since the ball acts at the distal end of the segment. In previous calculations in which no external forces existed, the resistance arm was measured only to the center of gravity of the body segment. One might say that the remainder of the lever did not exist. When objects are struck or projected, the entire lever, from an anatomic perspective, must be used in the calculations. (This concept will be discussed later in this chapter and other Chapters).

Single-Muscle Levers in Frontal Plane

Action of Latissimus Dorsi in Adduction of Humerus. The humerus shown in Fig. 4-12 is depicted as starting from 90 degrees of abduction and the forearm from 90 degrees of flexion, pointing directly forward. As the latissimus dorsi contracts, the humerus adducts and moves to the side of the trunk through a frontal plane. This shoulder action moves the forearm, although no action occurs at the elbow joint. The forearm moves through a frontal plane also, a concept that some students find difficult to visualize. Such students have found it helpful to perform the action and in doing so to note that as the distal end of the upper arm moves through a frontal plane, the proximal end of the forearm moves through a frontal plane parallel to that through which the upper arm moves. The distal end of the forearm and the hand move through frontal planes that are parallel to those through which the upper arm moves.

The fulcrum lies within the shoulder joint on an axis that is in the sagittal and transverse planes. The rigid bar of the lever includes the humerus, the radius, the ulna, the carpals, and the metacarpals. The actual resistance arm is the length of the upper arm, since the forearm and hand are the line of application of force passing through the elbow and are parallel to the axis at the shoulder. This moment arm, therefore, is a perpendicular line from the axis at the shoulder to the line of application of force. The effort arm is that portion of the humerus between the axis and the attachment of the muscle.

This analysis has dealt only with adduction of the arm. Since the latissimus dorsi also causes medial (inward) rotation, there will be a moment of force about an axis passing through the shoulder joint in the lateral-horizontal plane, and the humerus will move in the sagittal plane. A separate analysis of this movement or lack of movement, which is caused by the resistance of other muscles to this action of the latissimus dorsi, could be done.

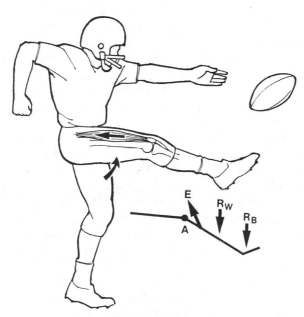

Fig. 4-11. *Action of rectus femoris muscle acting as part of a third class lever system in leg extension. The axis (A) is at the knee, the effort is at an ineffective angle of pull (E), the resistances consist of the weight of lower leg (R_w) and weight of ball (R_B). Note position of patella at lower leg near extension.*

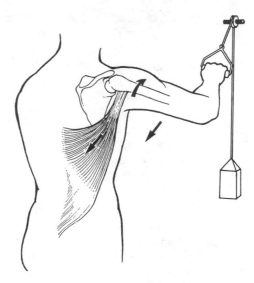

Fig. 4-12. *Action of latissimus dorsi in adduction of humerus. Note the large size of this muscle and its effective role in adduction, extension and medial rotation of the humerus.*

Muscle-Group Levers

Effort Arm for the Action of Muscle Groups. When more than one muscle contracts to move a segment, the point of application of effort is difficult to determine. In Fig. 4-13, three muscles are depicted, and the effort arm for the action of each is described. If the three muscles contract and pull on the femur at the same time, the amount of force that each exerts, as well as the point of attachment of each, must be known to determine the effort arm for the combined action. The amount of force exerted by each is not known, and to describe the effort arm and its length is therefore difficult or requires highly sophisticated techniques, such as magnetic resonance imaging. This is true for all situations in which the joint action is caused by the contraction of more than one muscle. The descriptions of single-muscle action have been presented only as a means of developing a concept of body levers. Until information regarding the pulling force of individual muscles is available, the biomechanist can only estimate the effort arm for muscle-group action. Modeling techniques have been used to estimate force production. Vectors are used to depict muscle angles of pull.

Action of Adductors in Lower-Limb Adduction. The action that occurs in moving a soccer ball to the left of the body is shown in Fig. 4-13. As the adductors contract, the lower limb moves through the frontal plane on an axis passing through the hip joint in the sagittal and transverse planes. The lever includes the femur, tibia, fibula, tarsals, metatarsals, and that portion of the phalanges which extends to make contact with the ball. The lever bones and length will be the same for the magnus, longus, and brevis muscles. However, the length of the effort arm will differ for the three. If each muscle is considered separately, each effort arm will include that portion of the femur which extends from the axis to the point of attachment of the muscle under consideration. The effort arm for the magnus is longest, and that for the brevis is shortest. In all three situations the resistance arm will include the bones and will be the length just mentioned in describing the total lever.

MUSCLE-BONE LEVER SYSTEMS OF THE HUMAN BODY

Several muscle-bone lever systems of the lower limbs are presented in Fig. 4-14. In certain cases, the vectors are drawn to illustrate the approximate lines of muscle force as well as the anatomic relationships of the muscles to the joint and bony lever. In other instances, the muscle-bone lever system has been separated into two illustrations because of the numbers of muscles acting at that particular joint. Since the muscles illustrated in Fig. 4-14 are expressed as a percentage of physiological cross-sectional area (PCSA) of one muscle, the vastus lateralis, one can easily compare the relative effectiveness of several muscles acting on the knee and hip. PCSA is an indicator of the strength of an individual muscle. Note that the vastus intermedius has only 55% of the PCSA of the vastus lateralis. The rectus femoris, a muscle assumed by many to be the major quadriceps force-producer, has only 42% of the vastus lateralis.

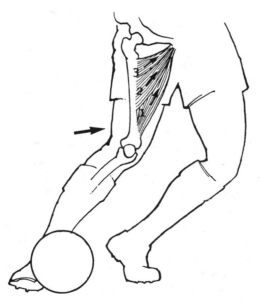

Fig. 4-13. *Action of adductors in lower-limb adduction. 1, adductor magnus; 2, adductor longus; 3, adductor brevis. The size of these muscles usually is greater than that of the abductor muscles acting at the hip joint.*

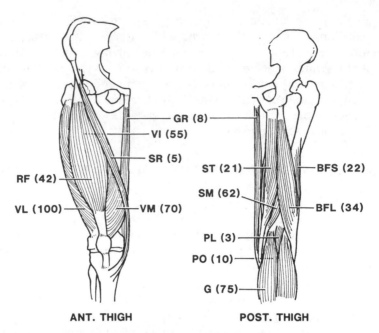

GR (8)
VI (55)
SR (5)
ST (21)
BFS (22)
RF (42)
SM (62)
VL (100)
VM (70)
BFL (34)
PL (3)
PO (10)
G (75)

ANT. THIGH   POST. THIGH

Fig. 4-14. *Muscles acting on shank, expressed as percentage of physiologic cross-sectional area (PCSA) of vastus lateralis (VL) the largest muscle. Several muscles are biarticular, crossing either hip or ankle, as well as knee. Relative effectiveness of each muscle may be estimated from PCSA values and attachment sites (direction of force and length of effort moment arms). VI, vastus intermedius; VM, vastus medialis; PO, popliteus; SR sartorius; RF, rectus femoris; GR, gracilis: SM, semimembranosus; ST, semitendinosus; PL, plantaris; BFS, biceps femoris, short head; BFL, biceps femoris, long head; G, gastrocnemius.) (Modified from Mastropaolo, J.:* Kinesiology for the public schools, *Paramount, Calif., 1975, Academy Printing and Publishing Co.)*

There is more information we can derive from the illustrations in Fig. 4-14. The muscle lines are drawn specifically to represent the muscles' angle of pull at the involved joints. Whereas the vastus intermedius and the vastus lateralis had larger cross-sectional areas, their angles of pull are very low. The rectus femoris pulls at a much higher angle thus producing a more effective force at the knee joint.

The angle of pull of some muscles is increased by anatomic pulleys. The patella acts to increase the angle of pull of the quadriceps muscles, thus increasing the effectiveness of the muscles' forces. Calcium deposits, which accumulate at the site of attachment of some muscles as a result of excessive use, can also increase the angle of pull. Further information concerning these muscle-bone lever systems is listed in Table 4-1. Since individuals may increase the cross-sectional area of selected muscle groups because of intense, habitual, and long-term exercise of a particular action, the data presented in Table 4-1 will not coincide with data obtained from these individuals. The table does, however, provide a basis for identifying the most effective—that is, the strongest or fastest—muscle-bone lever systems of a typically average, or normal, human body. The position of the moving body part in space and the plane of movement will determine which of these muscle-bone lever systems are potentially in a position to function. Knowledge of the anatomy of these systems will enable a person to select the most effective movement pattern. Additional anatomic data may be obtained from an anatomy textbook and applied to movement patterns.

Advantages of Third-Class Lever System

As illustrated in many of the figures in this chapter, the majority of muscles have their distal attachments near the joints. Therefore the body levers operate primarily as third-class lever systems. Since the muscle effort required in such a system is always greater than the resistance to be overcome, the body has a mechanical disadvantage when performing activities requiring the lifting of heavy loads. The mechanical advantage, MA, of a lever system can be easily calculated.

$$MA = EA/RA$$

Note that in third-class levers, EA is less than RA, so MA is less than 1.00, which is a poor mechanical advantage. Second-class levers, on the other hand, have longer effort arms than resistance arms, so MA is greater than 1.00 which results in a mechanical advantage. We make many adjustments in our everyday lives to increase our mechanical advantage. To gain more power in prying with a crowbar, we get a longer crowbar, which increases the length of EA, thus increasing the mechanical advantage. When carrying a heavy load, we hold it close to our bodies, which decreases the length of RA and increases the mechanical advantage. Can you think of other examples?

Table 4-1. *Physiologic cross-sectional areas (PCSA) of the largest muscles acting at the major body segments.*

Body Segment	Muscle	PCSA (cm$_2$)
Foot	Soleus	47.0
Shank (lower leg)	Vastus lateralis	41.8
Thigh	Gluteus maximus	58.8
Trunk (spinal column)	Levator scapulae	35.5
Hand	Flexor digitorum profundus	10.1
Fingers	Flexor digitorum profundus	10.1
Forearm	Triceps brachii, long head	14.1
Shoulder girdle	Levator scapulae	35.5
Trunk (respiration)	Diaphragm	35.8
Upper arm	Subcoapularic	10.8

Modified from Mastropaolo, J.: Kinesiology for the public schools, Paramount Calif., 1975, Academy Printing and Publishing Co.

THE HUMAN MOVEMENT SYSTEM　　　　　　　　**115**

Compensation for mechanical disadvantage is found in the arrangement of the muscle fibers into a featherlike structure. This increases the number of fibers in a given bulk, and since the strength of a muscle depends on the number of contracting fibers, the potential strength of the muscles is increased. With the increased strength, heavier and longer resistance arms can be moved.

There is an important advantage in possessing third-class levers; this advantage is speed. Given the same amount of shortening of a muscle and the same amount of time to produce this shortening, muscles that have the shortest effort arms will produce the greatest distance of travel of the distal end of the lever (Fig. 4-15).

Muscles with short effort arms usually will have an angle of pull that is mechanically more advantageous than that of muscles with long effort arms. Therefore, the design of the human body is one that enables the person to move the limbs rapidly, providing the resistance is not great.

In the sports world, teachers and coaches have capitalized on this human body design by adding to the length of the body lever some external levers of various lengths, but primarily of little or negligible weight. The effect of this additional external lever, such as a badminton racquet, is illustrated in Fig. 4-16. The outer end (the hand) of the shorter radius (38 cm), as it moves 90 degrees, will travel through 59.6 cm ([2 × 38 × 3.1416] divided by 4). (NOTE: The division by 4 is made in each case because the illustrated distance is one fourth of a circle.) If the movements were made in the same length of time, the linear velocity of the end of the longer arm will be twice that of the smaller, whereas the angular velocity is virtually the same. Naturally, the angular velocity will not be precisely the same for the two conditions; however, the decrease in angular velocity caused by the added weight of the badminton racquet is minute compared to the gain in linear velocity.

Adding additional segments and/or fully extending the joints increases the length of the resistance arm, resulting in greater linear velocities at the end of the levers. Individuals with longer limb segments therefore have an advantage in some activities. Baseball pitch-

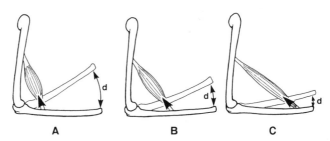

Fig. 4-15. *Given an equal amount of muscle shortening, the effect of length of effort arm on movement of distal end of moving segment can be estimated (d = movement arc of distal end). Relate these findings to spurt and shunt concepts and to speed and strength concepts.*

THE BIOMECHANICS OF HUMAN MOVEMENT

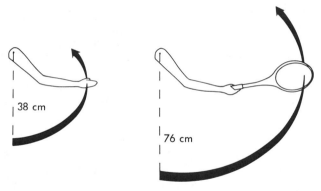

Fig. 4-16. *Effect of length of lever on angular displacement, and therefore on linear velocity of distal end of lever with and without an implement. Compare this figure to figure 1-5.*

ers are usually tall with long arms which aids in creating high-speed pitches. Tall, long-legged football kickers also have an advantage. There are times, however, we may wish to increase the angular velocity of the limb(s) at the expense of the linear velocity. Choking up on the baseball bat allows the batter to swing quicker against a fast pitcher. Can you think of other situations in which one shortens the resistance arm to gain angular velocity?

Two-Joint Muscles

Muscles that pass across two joints are called two-joint or bi-articular muscles. This arrangement provides another type of human muscular coordination in the use of body levers. The action of these muscles on the levers is similar to that of a pulley; the muscles act at each joint over which they pass. For example, the rectus femoris causes flexion at the hip and extension at the knee; the gastrocnemius helps flex the lower leg and plantar flexes the foot; the hamstrings cause flexion at the knee and extension at the hip. In addition, the flexors and extensors of the fingers might be called multijoint muscles, since they pass over the wrist and at least two joints of the fingers.

One outstanding characteristic of these muscles is that they are not long enough to permit a complete range of action simultaneously in the joints involved because of their location on two joints, either because the antagonist muscles prevent full range of action on these joints, or because antagonistic action occurs in the two joints (flexion in one and extension in the other). If the rectus femoris contracts, causing flexion at the hip, and at the same time the hamstrings contract to cause flexion at the knee, the pull of the rectus is increased at the hip because the muscle does not shorten as much as it would if extension took place at the knee. As an illustration, if there is a downward pull on a rope that passes over an overhead pulley, the tension will be transmitted in a reverse direction to the rope on the

THE HUMAN MOVEMENT SYSTEM

other side of the pulley. In the case of the flexors and extensors of the fingers, although the joints move in the same direction, the principle of pulley action is evident. Note the limited range of motion in the fingers as you try to make a fist while the wrist is already in full flexion. One of the main advantages of using the two-joint muscles is that they maintain tension without complete shortening. This advantage is not enjoyed by one-joint muscles, which lose tension as they shorten.

Two different patterns of action of two-joint muscles have been discussed by Fenn and by Steindler; these patterns are called concurrent and countercurrent. The simultaneous action of flexion (or extension) at the hip and knee is an example of a concurrent pattern. It has been described as follows: As the muscles contract, they do not lose length and therefore are able to maintain tension. In extension at the hip and knee, the rectus femoris muscle's loss of tension at the knee is balanced by an increase in tension at the hip. At the same time the hamstrings gain tension at the knee and lose it at the hip.

During certain phases in the kicking pattern the countercurrent two-joint muscle pattern is seen. If flexion occurs at the hip and simultaneous extension at the knee occurs, there will be loss of tension in the rectus femoris and gain of tension in the hamstrings. Thus, while one muscle shortens rapidly in an action, the antagonist lengthens to the same degree and maintains tension at both ends of the attachment. The result is an effective and coordinated movement.

This discussion does not minimize the importance of one-joint muscles. In a single-joint action they provide the needed force but expend more energy than do the two-joint muscles in the same action. On the other hand, when two joints are involved in the act, the two-joint muscles are more efficient. Elftman found that in running, although one-joint muscles could do the job, two-joint ones were more efficient; the expenditure of 2.61 hp (1945 watts) by the two-joint muscles could be compared with an expenditure of 3.97 hp (2962 watts) if single-joint ones were used.

ANALYSIS OF LEVER SYSTEMS

Speed of Body Segments

Little study has been done to indicate the speed with which body segments can be moved. Hill, the English physiologist, has said that in the human body the speed with which each segment moves is related to its length: the longer the segment, the slower its possible speed. This, says Hill, is a safety factor, and he compares these limits to the speeds with which glass rods can be oscillated. A short rod can safely be moved rapidly at a pace that would break a longer one. This relationship of speed to size is seen in the reported number of wingbeats per second of various birds. Hummingbird strokes are as fast as 200/sec; sparrow, 13; pigeon, 8; parrot, 5; stork, 2. The same relationship is shown in the rate of mastication (contractions per minute) of animals, reported by Amar: ox, 70; human being, 90 to 100; cat, 1962; guinea pig, 300; white mouse, 350.

Persons who have observed films of human action know that the wrist action is faster than the action of other joints acting during gross movements. The hand often is not visible without a blurring as it is moved particularly be flexion at the wrist. Less information exists concerning the rapid movements of the fingers during such rapid movements as are used in playing muscial instruments, particularly the flamenco guitar. The speed of various joints given in Table 4-2 represents some of the data reported in kinesiology literature. The fastest movement is that of an internationally ranked woman badminton player.

Linear velocities of distal ends—and therefore of any object projected or struck from the distal end—will be directly related to the length of the lever. One can expect high angular velocities from rotation about the wrist, but linear velocities of the fingers and of balls projected by means of this action will be low. Conversely, low angular velocities from rotation about the shoulder produce high linear velocities of the hand and of balls projected by means of this action. These relationships are shown in Table 4-3, which represents attempts by physical education students to project a ball as rapidly as possible either by using different levers or by modifying the effective radius of a hinged lever (consisting of several joints, as in the arm). The moment arms were measured, and the range of motion was predetermined. The ball was released in a horizontal direction, and the distance of projection and height of ball at the time of release were recorded. Since gravity acts to cause the ball to drop to the ground at a known acceleration, the time of flight of the ball could be calculated by using the following formula:

Table 4-2. *Angular speeds of body segments reported in biomechanics literature.*

Action	Rad/sec	Degrees/sec
Fexion at wrist	477	3000
Flexion at wrist with tennis racquet in hand	318	2000
Flexion at shoulder during standing long jump	255	1600
Extension at hip, knee, and ankle during standing long jump	236	1480
Transverse rotation at left hip in overhand throw (right hand)	115	720
Wrist flexion with forearm rotation during badminton smash	952	6000

THE HUMAN MOVEMENT SYSTEM 119

$$t = \frac{2(\text{height})}{\text{gravity}}$$

(This is a rearrangement of h = 1/2gt²)

Linear velocity of the ball was then equal to the horizontal distance of projection divided by the time of flight. One may assume that the linear velocity of the ball is equal to the linear velocity (tangential velocity) of the hand. Thus determination of the angular velocity of the hand, as well as of the other angular velocities of the other levers that were used, can be obtained by means of the following formula:

$$\omega = \frac{V_t}{r}$$

where r = moment arm, Vt = ball velocity, and ω = angular velocity.

Body Segment Positioning

A change in the length of the radius is well illustrated by a change in the position of the forearm when the hand is moved by medial rotation of the humerus, a joint action that occurs frequently in throwing and striking skills. To understand these changes better, go through the following movements. First, take a position in which the forearm is fixed in 90 degrees of flexion and the upper arm is abducted 90 degrees and laterally rotated, so that the forearm, pointing directly upward, is vertical. From this starting position, rotate the humerus medially so that the forearm is rotated forward and downward in the sagittal plane. The action of the humerus is more difficult to see, but it is also rotating in the same direction and the same plane as the forearm. The axis is a line passing through the shoulder joint and extending in the same direction as the humerus and roughly along its middle. The radius line must pass through the hand (the point of application of force) to the axis. Thus, the radius is perpendicular to the humerus. The length of the radius will be approximately equal to the length of the forearm (possibly 25 cm). Next, take a starting po-

Table 4-3. *Relationships of moment arm (MA), angular velocity (ω), and linear tangential velocity (Vt).*

Axis	MA (meters)	Distance of Projection (meters)	V$_\tau$(m/sec)	ω(rad/sec)
Hip	0.99	0.66	5.9	6
Shoulder (extended arm)	0.76	0.56	5.3	7
Shoulder (flexed arm)	0.36	0.36	5.0	14
Wrist	0.20	0.20	4.8	24

sition in which the upper arm is in the same position as in the first movement but the elbow is fully extended and the hand is facing upward. Now rotate the humerus medially so that the hand faces forward and then downward; try to eliminate any pronation of the forearm. The radius will now pass through the hand to the axis line, which must be extended through the forearm and hand as well as through the humerus. The length of the radius (represented by half the diameter of the hand) will be 2.5 to 5 cm (1 to 2 in). If the same angular velocity of medial rotation of the humerus were used in the two situations, the linear velocity of the hand would differ (refer to previous equation). The hand in the first movement would be moving 10 times faster than in the second movement since the radii are in a ratio of 10:1. Flexion at the elbow can vary from 0 to approximately 140 degrees. The linear velocity of the hand will be least in the instance of no flexion; velocity will increase as flexion occurs. Velocity will be greatest at 90 degrees, and beyond 90 degrees velocity will again decrease.

Because medial rotation of the humerus is an outstanding element in the human overarm pattern, because its angular velocity is one of the fastest of the joint actions, and because beginning biomechanics students often fail to recognize it, special efforts should be made to develop the ability to identify this action of the humerus in complex skills. To identify relative positions of upper arms and forearms as medial rotation occurs is also important. This rotation of the humerus on its long axis is usually accompanied by pronation of the forearm.

In studies in which the contribution of various body levers to the total force have been measured, the point chosen for observation has been the release in throws and the point of impact in strikes. All segments between that point and a moving joint are parts of the resistance arm. Thus in a throw the resistance arm for hip rotation would include the pelvis, the spine, the shoulder girdle on the right side (for the right-handed performer), the humerus, the bones of the lower arm, wrist, and hand, and the bones of the fingers up to the center of gravity of the projectile. In spinal rotation, the resistance arm would include the same segments except for the pelvis; the shoulder joint would include the segments moved by spinal action except for the spine and shoulder girdle. For all joints acting in the throw, the point of application of force is the center of gravity of the projectile; for all strikes, it is the point of impact.

The length of the moment arm for any lever and the speed with which it is moving will change during the force-developing phase — for example, in the forward swing in throwing and striking. However, the direct contribution is a result of the length and speed at the time of release. At that instant each acting joint can be considered a separate lever. For example, hip rotation will move the hand, as may spinal rotation and all other joints between the hand and the hip. The linear velocity of each can be determined, and if the measures are accurate, the sum of these linear velocities should equal the velocity of the object projected. This method of evaluating (measuring) of the contributions of each lever will be illustrated as specific skills are analyzed in later chapters.

Anatomic Differences

As is well known, individuals differ in length of skeletal parts. A child's bones are shorter than those of an adult; those of the average woman are shorter than those of the average man. Even individuals with equal total body heights may have varying arm and leg segment lengths. If all persons can move segments at the same angular speeds, those with longer limbs will have greater linear velocities. Some authors have suggested that the distance of the muscular attachment from the joint will differ in individuals. The greater this distance, the longer the effort arm, but the advantages of this length depend on the relationship between the lengths of the effort and resistance arms. If the forearm were 24 cm long and the attachment of the biceps 2 cm from the fulcrum, the ratio of resistance arm to effort arm would be 12:1. If in longer segments the effort arm, although increased in length, remained in the 12:1 ratio, no advantage would have been gained. However, an individual in whom the length of the effort arm is proportionately greater than the total length of the arm, and whose muscle strength ratio is also 12:1, will be able to lift heavier weights. Possibly this gain in ability to lift weights because of a proportionately longer effort arm will be accompanied by a decrease in angular velocity. If, when the effort arm is longer, the muscle shortens to the same degree and for the same length of time as when the effort arm is shorter, the distal end of the bone will be moved a shorter distance in the same time, with a resultant decrease in angular velocity. Little information on individual differences in proportionate lengths of effort arms is available, but the possibility of such differences suggests the need for investigations that might explain differences in strength and speed of joint actions.

Moment Arm Measurements for Levers Common to All Patterns

Moment arm lengths for the hip, spine, and wrist are illustrated in Fig. 4-17 with tracings of the body position at the time of release or impact in (A) an overarm throw such as a football pass, (B) an underarm throw, (C) a push such as the shot put, and (D) an overarm pattern such as a tennis serve. These tracings also illustrate changes in body levers because of different relative positions of segments.

On each tracing, a vertical line has been drawn through the left hip joint to represent the axis of rotation in that joint. In all four cases, that rotation will include in the resistance arm the pelvis, spine, right clavicle, humerus, radius and ulna, and the bones of the wrist, hand, and fingers; in the tennis serve the racket, as an extension of

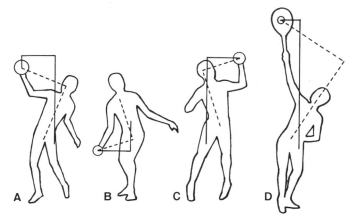

Fig. 4-17. *Length of movement arms in various patterns of joint action. A, football pass. B, underarm throw. C, shot put. D, tennis serve. Hip moment arm is shown by unbroken horizontal line from hip axis to center of ball. Spinal moment arm is indicated by broken horizontal or diagonal line from spinal axis to center of ball. Wrist moment arm (not shown) can be drawn from the horizontal line through the wrist to the center of ball. How does the performer increase linear speed of the hand and racquet by means of other body segments?*

the hand, is also included. The moment arm lengths will differ, depending to a minor degree on the length of the individual's segments but much more on the position of the segments at the time of release or impact. Horizontal lines perpendicular to the line of flight have been drawn from the axis to the center of the ball. The line of flight is assumed to be directly forward. Although the picture sizes differ to a small degree, for the illustration here all are assumed to be the same: 1 mm on the tracing is considered to be equivalent to 2.5 cm of actual measure.

MINI-LAB LEARNING EXPERIENCES

1. Measure the moment arms in Fig. 4-17 and discuss relative contributions of the trunk body segment.
2. Set various weights (books, arm weights) on a table and lift each as follows:
   a) Facing the table, grasp the object with: (1) arm at 90-degree flexion of forearm and (2) arm extended (180-degree at elbow).
   b) Facing away from the table repeat 1 and 2.
   c) Side to the table repeat 1 and 2.

Discuss difficulty with respect to muscle force within the same conditions and muscle force among the three conditions.

REFERENCES

Dillman, C. (1970): A kinetic analysis of the recovery leg during sprint running. In Cooper, J. M., editor: *Biomechanics symposium,* Bloomington: Indiana University.

Elftman, H. (1940): The work done by muscles in running, *Am. J. Physiol.* 129:672.

Fenn, W. O. (1930): Work against gravity and work due to velocity changes in running, *Am. J. Physiol.* 93:433.

Frankel, V. H. and Nordin, M. (1980): *Basic biomechanics of the skeletal system,* Philadelphia: Lea and Febiger.

Hill, A. V. (1927): *Living machinery,* New York: Harcourt Brace Jovanovich, Inc.

LeVeau, A. B. (1980): *Williams and Lissner biomechanics of human motion,* Philadelphia: W. B. Saunders Co.

Mastropaolo, J. (1975): *Kinesiology for the public schools,* Paramount, CA: Academy Printing & Publishing Co.

Steindler, A. (1955): *Kinesiology of the human body under normal and pathological conditions,* Springfield, IL: Charles C. Thomas, Publisher.

5
The Mechanics of Human Movement

Since we live on earth, and anything we encounter in space will be evaluated with respect to our environment on earth, it is vital that an understanding of the laws governing motion on earth is achieved by the human movement analyst and students of movement science. These laws are usually referred to as Newton's Three Laws of Motion. This type of mechanics, therefore, is referred to as Newtonian mechanics, also known as classical mechanics. Newtonian mechanics is the physical science that encompasses movement or motion of material bodies of ordinary size moving at speeds that are slow compared to the speed of light. Quantum mechanics, the physical science that evolved from Einstein's Theory of Relativity, may be more commonly applicable to human movement in future years, but such information will not be included in this book.

Readers with a strong background in physics, and therefore mechanics, will need to rethink mechanical principles in the light of living materials and motion. Since both the human body and its tissues are anisotropic, that is, their anatomical, physiological, and mechanical characteristics vary from one region of the tissue to another, living bodies cannot be treated exactly as one would treat non-living objects such as basketballs, airplanes, and machines. Likewise, readers with strong biology backgrounds, particularly anatomy, will need to view biology from a mechanical perspective.

The fundamental concepts of mechanics as applied to human motion will be explained. Applications will be limited since further examples are included in other chapters of the book.

All concepts included in this chapter are applicable to all movements of all persons under all circumstances on earth. The importance, however, of each concept will vary with respect to type of movement, characteristics of the persons performing the movement, the goal of the movement, and the environment in which the movement is performed. Free-fall and gravitational concepts are of primary concern during sky diving and gymnastics dismounts. Concepts of rotary motion are of greatest concern during swinging movements. Concepts of leverage are vital to strength activities, whereas, concepts of momentum and energy are more important during collisions. Some concepts are totally ignored by young, healthy, strong individuals. If, however, an arm is injured or paralyzed, concepts are utilized to develop successful adaptations. The concepts of lift and drag forces are negligible during normal walking speed conditions. They become important during sailing, swimming, ski jumping, and racing. As you read this chapter, match the concepts to activities according to primary importance.

HOW TO CONDUCT MINI-LABORATORY EXPERIMENTS AND ENGAGE IN LEARNING EXPERIENCES

Since the human being does not repeat a movement precisely identical to a previous movement, we often have difficulty "proving" that Newton's Laws of Motion apply to human beings. It's very easy to conduct experiments with balls of different sizes, densities and masses and to predict outcomes of collisions, of projecting the ball into space and of dropping the ball. If we ask two persons to "bump into each other," we cannot predict what will happen even if we know their masses and their approach velocities. Each is apt to change speed (increase or reduce it) prior to impact, change orientation of body parts, and change points of contact. Thus, repetitive actions will be dissimilar. Likewise, asking most persons to execute a somersault in tuck, pike, and layout positions, initiating each with identical angular momentum, is asking the impossible. Persons can reduce the dissimilarities with diligent practice, but few can achieve as great as 90% similarity.

This holds true for comparisons of the forehand drive in tennis using different racquet models and string tensions. It is more successful to test the racquet with a machine-propelled ball, then to test the racquet in the hand of a human being.

Thus, experimentation must include careful observation of all aspects of the testing situation in order to isolate factors influencing results.

If the person changes the initial conditions through inconsistent force productions, the test must be repeated, another subject selected, or limitations identified in the discussion of results.

MINI-LAB LEARNING EXPERIENCES

Scalar quantities are single quantities.
Vector quantities are double quantities.

Tensor quantities are triple quantities.
What are pulsar and quasar quantities?
Place the following in the correct category:

1) Direction
2) Direction + Magnitude + Time
3) Direction + Magnitude

List the units of measurement for the previous examples. (Refer to Appendix.)

THE FUNDAMENTAL CONCEPT

There is one fundamental concept that encompasses the understanding of mechanics of human motion. This concept is stated as follows:

Forces cause predictable and measurable responses (counter-forces, movements, reactions, deformations) of the human body and objects interacting with the human body. The nature of these responses are dependent upon the characteristics of these forces and of the human body, its parts, and the interacting objects. Furthermore, these responses can be predicted if the magnitude of the force, the point of application, and the direction of the force are known and measurable. In addition, the prediction is more precise if the masses of the bodies involved, their form, shape and density, and the center of mass of each body are known.

Within this context, then, Newton's Laws may be paraphrased as follows:

First law: If there are no forces, there is no movement.
The sum of all forces equals zero.

$(\Sigma F = 0)$

Second law: The magnitude of force is positively related to the acceleration produced in a body and inversely related to the mass of the body being accelerated.

$(F = ma)$

Third law: Each force produces an equal and opposite force

$(\bar{F} = -F)$

MINI-LAB LEARNING EXPERIENCES

Using a felt pen, write a number on each side of a block of wood and place the wood on a table or desk.

a) Strike one side of the block with a ruler or rod.

Observe the direction of movement and/or deformation in block or striking implement.

Repeat by striking each side of the block and observing the effect.

Record the results and discuss the concepts governing the responses.

b) Using a pool (or billiard) table, cue, and ball, repeat the experiments. Strike the ball through its center and also off-center.

c) Vary the force applied in striking the objects in parts a and b.

It is easy to state that a force was the cause of some movement or deformation; however, recognition of the nature of the force may be a difficult task. A starting point is to categorize forces into two types, internal forces and external forces. The common external forces that act on human beings and animals are the force of gravity (weight of body and other objects), the ground reaction force, friction, water buoyancy, drag, and lift forces. These latter two are present during motion through fluids, air and water being of most interest to human beings. The forces encountered during a collision, whether between two or more persons or a person and an object, might be termed the force of motion. Such forces are a result of momentum being changed during the collision and may be explained by Newton's Second Law.

Internal forces are no different in concept than external forces, but they tend to be less predictable and less simplistic. Muscles are the primary source of internal forces. Muscles do not always exert their forces directly to the receivers (bones and joints). Instead, tendons often are the transmitters of forces produced by the muscles. Usually these internal forces are categorized as compression (pushing together), tension (pulling apart), shear (sliding across the surfaces), torsion (twisting), and combinations of these (most commonly, bending, which consists of compression on the concavity of bend and tension on the convexity of bend). At the joints the forces are identified as reactions to the forces of gravity (weights of body segments forming the joint and any weights attached to these body segments), forces of motion (ma for linear motion and $I\alpha$ for rotary motion), and forces from muscles, tendons, and ligaments.

It is readily apparent that internal forces are not easily measured or understood. We usually isolate the forces acting on the various tissues or measure these forces on cadavers, animals, or human beings with prostheses. Thus our knowledge of internal forces is from limited data, compared to that of external forces.

MINI-LAB LEARNING EXPERIENCE—FORCE OF MOTION

You can experience the force of motion upon a joint if you swing your arm in a circle in the sagittal plane (as close to it as is possible when the arm approaches an overhead position). You will feel the numbness in the hand due to the movement of the blood toward the distal end of the fingers. You will also feel an ache in the shoulder due to the pulling of the arm away from the scapula. Look at your hand after repeating the swing at slow, moderate, and fast rotations.

Linear acceleration can be experienced at the instant of stoppage of an elevator. The body parts vibrate. Internal parts of the body appear to move independently within the shell of the body. A queasy feeling in the "pit of the stomach" may occur.

UNDERSTANDING THE VECTOR QUANTITY OF FORCE

Since forces must be defined with respect to two quantities (direction and magnitude), they are considered to be vector quantities, and as such, the simple arithmetic processes utilized with scalar quantities are not applicable. For example, the scalar quantity of distance (measured in one quantity—meters, feet, inches, degrees, etc.) can be added, subtracted, multiplied, and divided. The values for two or more forces, however, cannot be added unless all forces are acting in the same direction. Thus, weights can be added, since the forces are all vertical, whereas the forces of five persons on different parts of the circumference and pushing against a huge ball (cageball) cannot be added unless the directions are considered. Adding merely the magnitudes of the forces results in an erroneous answer.

There are two common methods of vectorally adding forces: the trigonometric method and the graphic method. These methods also are commonly used to investigate the effect of one or more forces upon a body. The fundamental concept of both methods is that of resolving the force vector into two components, each of which can then be compared to any other resolved force vector. Based upon a spatial frame of reference, vectors are resolved into vertical and horizontal force components, if the force acts in one plane. If the force acts in three dimensional space, "cutting through two or more planes," the vector is resolved into three components: one vertical and two horizontal, all of which are orthogonal to each other.

Based upon an anatomical reference frame, forces are resolved into normal and tangential components. The normal component acts at right angles (normal) to the body part, such as a head wind striking the body. The tangential component acts parallel to the body (shearing or tangential), such as the force of friction during sliding activities. Since most forces act at angles to the normal/tangential or vertical/horizontal, vector resolution techniques are required to identify optimum magnitudes and directions of forces. Most researchers and movement analysts assume two-dimensional force vectors and resolve the force vector into two components. In many cases, the assumption that the component in the third plane is negligible is a valid one. Three-dimensional vector resolution is best performed with the aid of computer algorithms. Two-dimensional resolution is depicted in Fig. 5-1.

The trigonometic method is based on the principle that right triangles of various sizes with identical angles will be proportional to each other. This means that the ratio of one side of the triangle to another side will always be identical among such triangles. Therefore, the equations for determining the components of a force acting at a known angle are as follows:

H = F cosine
V = F sine

Where H is the horizontal component (it also would be the tangential component in the anatomical reference frame) and V is the vertical (it also would be the normal force in the anatomical reference

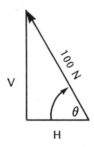

If magnitude (100 N) and direction (θ) are known, look in trigonometry table:

H = 100 N cosine θ

V = 100 N sine θ

Fig. 5-1. *Trigonometric resolution of vector components perpendicular to each other. Measure the angle and use the trigonometry table in the appendix to solve for the vertical and horizontal components.*

THE BIOMECHANICS OF HUMAN MOVEMENT

frame) component. Cosine and sine of the angle are found in Appendix B.

If a normal force component of 4000 N were recorded on a target as a karate blow was delivered at a 20 degree angle from the normal direction, the true force could be calculated by rearranging the equation:

$$V = F \sin \theta \text{ into } F = \frac{V}{\sin \theta}$$

Calculate the force of the normal force of the blow.

MINI-LAB LEARNING EXPERIENCES

Compare the normal and tangential forces in the following situations:

1. A force of 600 N is applied to a football at an angle of 45 degrees.
2. A force of 600 N is applied to a football at an angle of 88 degrees.
3. A force of 600 N is applied to a football at an angle of 20 degrees.

Assume that the football is set vertically and the angle is with respect to the longitudinal axis of the football.

The graphic method consists of diagramming the force vector on graph paper as depicted in Fig. 5-2. A scale is selected, such as one graph unit equaling 10 N. Horizontal and vertical lines are drawn and the 90 degree angle of intersection marked. At some point from the horizontal line, the angle of the direction of the vector is drawn using a protractor. Along this line, beginning at the intercept with the horizontal line the vector is drawn to scale. For example, in Fig. 5-2, 100 N equals 10 graph units. Measure the horizontal and vertical components (from the 90 degree angle to the intercepts of vector).

If two or more forces act on a body, the forces must be vectorally added to determine the resultant magnitude and direction of the summed force. This can be accomplished graphically by drawing the vectors as shown in Fig. 5-3. The tail of the vector is placed at the arrow of the other vector, and each is oriented in the prescribed direction. The resultant (summed) force is drawn from the arrow of the last force vector to the tail of the first force vector. It is measured with respect to magnitude and orientation.

An alternate method, of course, is to separate each force vector into its components. For example, all normal force vectors are added

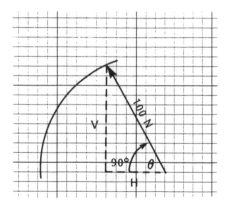

If trigonometry table is
not available:

1. Draw vector of 100 N
   magnitude at angle θ
   with the horizontal

2. Construct right triangle

3. Determine H and V by
   measurement

Fig. 5-2. *Graphic resolution and measurement of vector components perpendicular to each other. Compare your answers to those calculated for figure 5-2.*

together; all tangential force vectors are added separately. These two component vectors are drawn tail-to-tail, forming a 90-degree angle. The resultant force vector is then the hypotenuse of the right triangle drawn by connecting the arrows of each component vector.

A greater depth of understanding of the effects of forces upon the human body can be attained if forces can be measured and subdivided into pertinent components.

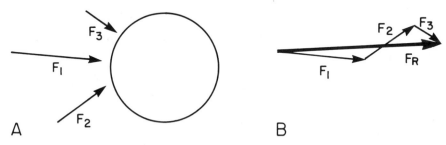

Fig. 5-3. *Graphic determination of resultant force (F) when several forces act on a body. A, three forces drawn according to direction and magnitude: F1 = horizontal force (zero degrees) of 150 units (these can be newtons or pounds); F2 = 40 degree directional positive force of 100 units; F3 = 35 degree directed negatively of 50 units. B, geometrically summating the three forces and drawing the resultant force (R) of 275 units at a 10 degree positive angle. Compare your answer using trigonometry to solve for the resultant force and for the horizontal and vertical components.*

FRICTION

Friction is the resistance that opposes every effort to slide or roll one body over another. Friction may be a hindrance or a help in sports and work performance. Some general facts about friction include the following:

1. Static, or starting, friction is greater than moving, or sliding, friction.
2. Although many factors are involved, generally friction depends on the velocity, load, condition, and nature of the two surfaces that are interacting with each other.
3. In most practical sports situations, friction tends not to depend much on the velocity of the sliding surfaces.
4. Friction depends on the nature and condition of the contacting surfaces because of the following:
   a. Friction is less when the surfaces are smooth and hard.
   b. With dry surfaces, friction is approximately the same regardless of the size of the area of contact.
   c. Friction is approximately proportional to the area of contact with well-lubricated surfaces.

Thus, a simple equation to use to calculate friction and the coefficient of friction is as follows:

$$R = B \times F_n$$

R = friction force, B = coefficient of friction, and F_n = normal force.

Another way to present this is as a ratio, as follows: the force pressing the surfaces together is represented by N (normal force) and R (force needed to overcome friction); therefore, $R/N = B$ where B is the coefficient of friction. The smaller B is, the less friction is created. On the other hand, the larger B is, the more the surfaces cling together, and the larger the force that will be required to cause slippage.

Sometimes it is advantageous to produce surfaces that have a high coefficient of friction; at other times it is advantageous to do just the opposite. Therefore, the concept of optimal friction is an important one. One must select the two materials that will interact according to the needs of the situation and goals of the performance. Each situation has an optimal amount of friction in which optimal performance can occur. Some coefficients of friction have been calculated for shoe-playing surfaces, (.4–.5), but much of what is known about friction and the world of human and animal movement has been obtained through trial and error. Examples of player and equipment adaptation with respect to the element of friction are as follows:

1. Ashes are put on automobile tires when driving on snow to increase friction so that sufficient traction against the snow can be secured.
2. In wet weather, a small amount of silica sand placed on the hands of a football passer may facilitate throwing the football more accurately because the coefficient of friction will be increased. However, wet, wrinkled socks inside a football player's shoes do the same thing and are likely to cause blisters.
3. Basketball players attempting to play on a floor that has been covered with wax for a dance may require the soles of their shoes to be irregular with indentations so that there is sufficient friction between the soles and the floor surface to enable the players to move adeptly.
4. Table tennis paddles that have a rough, irregular surface enable players to put more spin on the ball because of the increased friction.
5. Surfaces such as the new, nonsmooth cement rings used for shot putting and discus throwing prevent the performer from slipping too fast when moving across the ring. Cleats and spikes on athletic shoes have the same effect. Moreover, the placement of the cleats and spikes affects the amount of friction created.

When the problem of slippage is too great and the surfaces cannot be changed, the performer will have to keep the center of gravity more nearly over the base of support. The performer will have to take short steps, should avoid too much body lean, and may have to drop the center of gravity as low as possible by squatting. In this way, the athlete will be able to remain in a playing posture and to perform at reasonable efficiency.

Because of the condition of a surface (for example, slick and wet), it is possible to "spin the wheels" too fast, and the coefficient of friction will be insufficient for the object, such as a car or a person, to move forward successfully. The two surfaces must be in contact with each other long enough for traction to take place. Moving at a slower speed enables this to occur.

Since frictional force is produced by the interaction of two materials, the coefficient of friction refers to this interaction, not to one material or the other. If one surface can be tilted to produce an incline, the angle at which the second surface slips (slides) on this incline can be measured. The tangent of the angle can be determined by referring to Appendix B. This tangent value is equal to the coefficient of friction value. Frictional force is then determined by using the formula previously given, $R = B \times N$.

Frictional force may be determined directly by measuring, with a spring scale, the force required to cause one surface to slide on a second surface.

Friction Concepts

a) The greater the friction, the greater the muscle effort to oppose it.
b) The greater the friction, the greater the reduction of speed in human body or object.
c) Friction in one movement can be utilized in a successive countermovement.

The force, R, represents the friction force that is always present whenever materials or bodies—solids, liquids, or gases—move with respect to each other. Since friction is an ever-present force during locomotion, as well as during all movements of living things, an understanding of the factors that determine the magnitude of the frictional force and the coefficient of friction for two interacting surfaces is vital to an analysis and understanding of movement.

different surfaces, such as a rubber mat or carpet, on the ramp and repeat the experiment.

b) Glide down a snow-covered hill on skis in the cold morning (frozen snow) and in the mid-day sun (slushy snow).

c) Push a cart or piece of furniture across the room on a tiled floor, then repeat in a room with a carpeted floor. Try a low-pile, smooth-surfaced carpet and deep-pile, uneven-surfaced carpet.

d) Slide on a smooth surface (linoleum, tile, heavily-waxed wooden floor, or marble) with leather-soled shoes. Select three other shoes with different surfaces.

e) Devise an experiment to determine friction between implements held in the hand.

For each of the above experiments, state how you might estimate the magnitude or the relative difference in friction among the various conditions and surfaces. Attempt to calculate these using the previously presented equation.

RELATIONSHIP OF NEWTON'S THREE LAWS OF MOTION TO TRANSLATION

Whether or not motion occurs is directly related to the magnitude of force. Newton's first law, the law of inertia, states that a body at rest will remain at rest until some force of sufficient magnitude to overcome its inertia acts on the body. This law also applies to bodies moving at a constant velocity. An explanation of this law will be made initially with respect to translatory motion in the vertical direction. The inertia of a body is known as its mass. Mass is measured in kilograms (newton-second^2/meter or (Nsec^2/m) in the International System of Units (SI), also known as the metric system, and mass is measured in kilograms (newton-second^2/meter) or in slugs (lb-sec^2/ft) in the English system. A small letter m is used to denote the existence of mass in equations.

Vertical Motion

An upward movement can occur only if the force (F_y) acting on a mass is greater than the weight of the body (w). This can be proved by the application of Newton's second law, which states that the acceleration, and thereby the motion, of a body is directly related to its mass. In equation form, this principle is written as follows:

$$F_y = ma_y$$

where force (F) in the y direction equals the mass times the acceleration (ma) in the y direction.

In the case of more than one force, the symbol Σ is used with the above equation to indicate the "sum of all the forces." Stationary bodies standing on a floor have the acceleration of gravity acting downward on them. If a person stands on the ground, the ground exerts a force (measured in newtons ([N]) equal to the force of gravity (w) but opposite in direction. This is in accordance with Newton's third law, called the law of interaction, or the law of action-reaction. The former title is preferred because the latter implies a difference in time between the actions (forces), when in fact the reaction occurs simultaneously with the action. Given the situation, then, of a person's standing on the floor; since the two forces are acting in opposite y (vertical) directions, and since the forces are of equal magnitude, no movement will occur.

Linear Motion in Any Direction

It is evident that linear acceleration will not occur and will not produce translation of the body if the $F = 0$. Since movements occur in three planes, or in a three-dimensional world, the forces may be identified as F_x, F_y, and F_z, according to the Cartesian coordinate system mentioned in Chapter 4. All these forces must equal zero for translational equilibrium to exist. If F_z and F_y equal zero, but $F_x = 200$ N acting on the body, then a body weighing 490 N will be accelerated laterally in the direction of F_x at a rate of 4 m/sec^2. The process of determining this is as follows:

Step 1: Always draw a free body diagram (FBD), that is, depict the body in some simple shape and draw all external forces acting on it. Draw the vectors to scale—large forces are longer than small forces (Fig. 5-4).

Step 2: Determine in which of the directions—x, y, and z—the sum of the forces equals zero. NOTE: If diagonal forces exist, resolve these forces into F_x, F_y, F_z.

Step 3: Determine which sum is not equal to zero and solve the equation

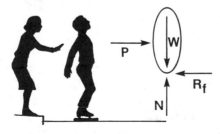

Fig. 5-4. *Depiction of life situation by means of free body diagram. Forces acting on body are represented by force vectors. This method provides convenient identification of probable effects on body (P, force of push; W, body weight. N, normal force; Rf, friction force.) The friction force equals 10 N and the pushing force equals 210 N.*

THE MECHANICS OF HUMAN MOVEMENT   **137**

$$F = ma.$$
$$F_y = 0 \quad F_z = 0 \quad F_x \neq 0$$
$$F_x = ma_x$$
$$F + R = ma_x$$
$$210\,\text{N} + (-10\,\text{N}) = 490\,\text{N}/9.8\,\text{m/sec}^2 \times a_x$$
$$200\,\text{N} = 50\,\text{N sec}^2/\text{m} \times a_x$$
$$4\,\text{m/sec}^2 = a_x$$

The acceleration is forward in the x direction.

This basic law of motion, expressed as $F = ma$, indicates that a body will experience linear acceleration when the F does not equal zero. For example, during the act of jumping, the reaction force is greater than body weight because muscle force is causing the body to accelerate upward. By calculating the acceleration, one can use the preceding equation to determine the unknown reaction force. The difference between the body weight and the reaction force is equivalent to the effective muscle force. The greater the muscle force, the greater the acceleration, and therefore the greater the vertical distance of the jump. Furthermore, if two persons of different masses utilize equal amounts of muscle force, the person of lesser mass will be able to create greater acceleration than the person of greater mass. This is known as the inverse relationship of body mass to acceleration. Note these examples and the basic equation. $F = ma$ summarizes only the external forces. Internal reactions, causing deformations of body tissues or resistance at joints and muscle forces, are not considered.

RELATIONSHIP OF LAWS OF MOTION TO ROTARY MOTION

When the Newtonian laws of motion are applied to rotary motion, moment of force is substituted for force, and moment of inertia is substituted for inertia in the equation: $F = ma$. With the acceleration no longer linear but angular, the equation becomes:

$$\Sigma M = I\alpha$$

where M = moment of force; I = moment of inertia; and alpha (α) = angular acceleration. Moment of force (M) is defined as the product of the force and its moment arm, that is, the shortest distance from the axis of rotation to the point of application of force. (Review chapter 4.) Moment of inertia (I) is defined as the rotary inertia or resistance to rotation. It is calculated by multiplying the mass by its radius (distance from the axis of rotation to the center of mass). The units are as follows:

M = newton meters
I = newton second^2/meters
α = radians/second^2

Note the radian is a dimensionless unit and will not be retained.

The determination of whether rotary motion will occur is directly linked to the question of whether the point of application of force is other than through the center of gravity of the body. In the preceding examples of translation, the assumption was made that (1) the forces were acting through the center of gravity of the body or (2) any moments that might have existed were being ignored. In Fig. 5-5, however, the forces act distances d_1 and d_2 from the turning point, which is both the center of gravity of the object and the axis of rotation of the object. The forces produce a turning effect, which is termed a moment or identified as torque. Since in Fig. 5-5 the sum of the forces

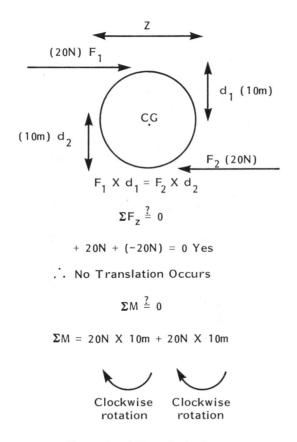

Fig. 5-5. *Use of free body diagram to determine whether or not translation, rotation, or both translation and rotation would occur for a given situation. In this situation, a clockwise rotation will occur but no translation will occur.*

is equal to zero, no translation occurs. If d_1 and d_2 did not exist—that is, if the force acted through the center of gravity of the object—it is evident that the sum of the moments would also be equal to zero, since the moment is calculated by multiplying the force by its perpendicular distance of application from the axis of rotation (center of gravity). Although the concept of moments of force is thoroughly discussed in Chapter 4, the fundamentals are presented in the following solution to Fig. 5-5.

If the moment of inertia of the object is determined to be 4 Nsec^2/m, then the angular acceleration of the object will be 10 rad/sec^2. This is determined by the following equation and solution:

$$\Sigma M = I\alpha$$
$$40 \text{ Nm} = 4 \text{ Nsec}^2/\text{m} \times \alpha$$
$$40 \text{ Nm}/4 \text{ Nm/sec}^2 = \alpha$$
$$10 \text{ rad/sec}^2 = \alpha$$

NOTE: Since the radian is a dimensionless unit, it is written after the value of alpha. One radian is equal to approximately 57 degrees, or 360 degrees divided by 2π. Thus 10 rad/sec^2 is equal to slightly more than 570 degrees/sec^2.

This example of two equal and opposite forces that act at equal distances from a point but produce the same direction of rotation is called a force couple.

The internal reaction forces are not considered in this free body diagram of external forces. For example, the interaction between the force and the surface of the object is not considered. The assumption is made that no force is lost (absorbed, converted into heat, etc.) in the act of pushing. The force represents the net force after any lost force is subtracted.

Internal forces must be considered whenever forces act upon the human body since different body parts will respond depending upon the site of application of the force.

For example, in football the tackler may apply the force at the head, chest, center of gravity of the body (hips), thighs, or ankles of the ball carrier (Fig. 5-6). If the force is at the crown of the head, the head is accelerated backward with rotary motion, producing a reaction force at the atlas (rotary point of head). Although there is little effect on the rest of the body, there is a high potential for neck or spinal cord or column injury. If the same force is applied at the chest, the ball carrier experiences rotation of the body above the lumbar region. Since the mass of these body parts is greater than the mass of the head, the acceleration is not as great as with the head. The reactive moment of force, however, occurs in the vulnerable lumbar region of the spine, which again produces a risk of injury to the body. In both cases, since the feet are in contact with the ground, there may be little or no movement of the lower body. Application of this same amount of force through the center of gravity of the body will produce

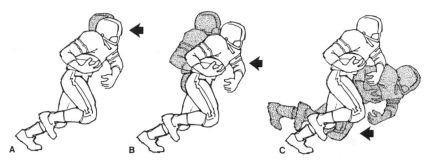

Fig. 5-6. *Identical forces acting on different parts of body produce different moments of force. Straight-line vector is point of application of force. Shaded body part is resultant rotation of body parts caused by moment of force. Note that either the joint caudal to force or the center of gravity of entire body acts as axis of rotation for moment of force.*

backward translation of the ball carrier, with no rotary accelerations of body parts. If the force is applied to the thighs or ankles, rotary acceleration again occurs. In this case, the feet are removed from contact with the ground, and the body rotates about its center of gravity.

Linear and Rotary Acceleration Principles

1. Linear acceleration of a body will not occur unless the sum of the forces acting on a body is greater than zero.
2. Rotary acceleration of a body will not occur unless the sum of the moments of force acting on the body is greater than zero.
3. As the force (or moment of force) acting on a body increases, the amount of linear acceleration or angular acceleration of that body will also increase.
4. If the same force (or moment of force) acts on two body masses, the larger mass will experience a lesser acceleration.
5. The net result of all forces and all moments of force must be added vectorially to determine whether or not acceleration is produced.

Changing the Moment of Inertia

A given force acting on a body to produce rotation can create varying magnitudes of angular acceleration merely by adjusting the body segments to create varying magnitudes of rotary inertia. Since the moment of inertia is dependent on the distance of the center of gravity of the mass from the axis of rotation, this distance can be shortened by changing the angles at the joints. For example, angular acceleration is greatest when the leg is swinging forward and the angle at the knee is as small as possible. Conversely, the angular acceleration is least when the leg is swinging forward with no flexion at the knee.

This concept is important because nothing comparable occurs with linear motion. The mass is usually a constant when linear acceleration is being produced. The moment of inertia, however, can be changed, thus allowing a body part of constant mass to be rotated at a faster rate of speed even though the same amount of force is applied at the same point on the body.

CENTRIPETAL AND CENTRIFUGAL FORCES

A unique force in all rotary movements is centripetal force. This force maintains the circular path of the body or body part. The force is directed radially, that is, toward the center of the rotation. The calculation of centripetal force is derived, once again, from the basic equation $F = ma$. Since centripetal force (C_p) represents a radial acceleration force, this acceleration can be derived from the following equation:

$$C_p = mr\omega^2$$

where m refers to mass, r refers to radius of the circle or arc of rotation, ω refers to the angular velocity.

Centripetal force can also be calculated from another equation, since there is a relationship between linear and angular motion. In this case the linear velocity at the distal end of the segment in motion is utilized in the following equation:

$$C_p - m\frac{Vt^2}{r}$$

where Vt refers to the velocity tangent to the arc of movement and at the distal end of the rotating segment.

This latter equation is probably best known since insufficient centripetal force will cause rotating objects to "fly off at a tangent to the arc at release." The force of this fly off is termed centrifugal force. It is the counterforce to centripetal force, and is computed by means of the same equations used for computing centripetal force.

Concern for controlling centrifugal forces is paramount in gymnastics activities. The gymnast uses special built-in finger flexion gloves to produce gripping force to combat centrifugal forces. Failure to do so may result in falling from apparatus, such as high bar or uneven parallel bars.

MINI-LAB LEARNING EXPERIENCES

Study the equation and determine who is at greater risk of flying off the high bar, all other factors being equal; a six foot-tall or four foot-tall gymnast? You might wish to use a hypothetical constant tangential velocity and also velocities proportional to the height differences (3:2 ratio).

THE BIOMECHANICS OF HUMAN MOVEMENT

High centrifugal force values result in numbness in distal segments during and after swinging movements. Pain at the proximal joint (axis of rotation) often results, since the muscles attempting to stabilize the joint and the ligaments are stretched.

Observe movement skills of recreational sports performers. You will note that the speed at which many of these performers execute their skills is less than optimum. Bowlers swing their arms and roll the ball at speeds ineffective to produce the required "pin action" for consistent strikes. Tennis serves and drives are executed with moderate speed arm swings. Softball players throw the ball without explosive force. Running is at slow to moderate speeds. Although many reasons may account for such low speeds, one major reason is unconscious, or conscious, fear of injuring the joints. Did you ever stop to think, much less estimate, what the centrifugal forces would be during sports movements? Table 5-1 includes estimates of centrifugal forces acting at the shoulder joint of a person with an arm 0.6 meters in length and a mass of 6 kg during softball pitching at five speeds.

What do these values mean? Let's compare these values to those reactive forces produced at the shoulder joint during a single arm hang from a high bar or holding a suitcase equivalent to one's body weight. Although these static situations are not producing centrifugal force, there is a comparable tensile force acting to pull the humerus from the scapula. This force is equal to the body weight. In the hanging position, this force is actually body weight minus the weight of the arm.

Don't these static activities feel uncomfortable to the shoulder? Naturally, the ability to tolerate such high forces during throwing is possible because the forces are of very short duration, often less than 50 ms.

FORCES IN AIR AND WATER ENVIRONMENTS

As a body applies a force to, or interacts with, air or water, the particles of air or water are disturbed and experience a change in speed and direction in direct proportion to their resistance to the body. This resistance, which is in keeping with the law of interaction, produces what is termed a drag force. The amount of resistance of the

Table 5-1. *Estimated centrifugal force during softball pitching (pitcher's arm is 0.6 M and has a mass of .6 kg).*

Speed of Ball		Centrifugal Force (N)
m/sec	ft/sec	
7	20	49
13	40	169
20	60	400
27	80	729
33	100	1089

THE MECHANICS OF HUMAN MOVEMENT 143

fluid is dependent on its energy, which is influenced by pressure, velocity, and position with respect to the body encountered by air or water. The basis for the understanding of the human body's interacting with the fluid, whether air or water, is Bernoulli's principle, which states that fluid pressure is decreased whenever speed of flow is increased.

Air and water flow past a symmetric object, such as a smooth ball, with a minimal disturbance in the flow pattern. This laminar flow, with little turbulence, is depicted in Fig. 5-7. Resistance may therefore be considered negligible, especially in an air medium; the fluid does little to alter the path of the object. Laminar flow will have different velocities, and the line of flow closest to the surface of the body will be the slowest. This difference in velocity will be dependent on the size of the shear stress, that is, the surface friction. For example, the skin of the dolphin offers an infinitesimal surface friction compared with human skin. (Swimmers often shave their hair to reduce friction.)

Contrast the laminar flow of Fig. 5-7 with the turbulent flow of Fig. 5-8. In Fig. 5-8A, the object is asymmetric, and the flow separates from the object and produces eddies early in its flow past the object. This turbulence creates greater resistance to the movement of the object through the fluid—air or water. In fact, the eddies can create suction forces, which produce a backward force. Drag resistance is also increased in this situation as compared with that of Fig. 5-7. Drag is the force normal to the surface of the object on which the force is exerted. Thus the forward parts of the object encounter a resistance to forward travel. This resistance is known as drag force because it opposes motion.

Drag force exists with all bodies, of all shapes and sizes, traveling through air, water, or other fluid. Rough, deformed, or less streamlined bodies will experience greater resistance than will those bodies said to be "aerodynamically designed."

The fluid flow across the object in Fig. 5-8B has minimum drag force since the surface area encountering the fluid is a narrow edge with a backward slope. Lift force, however, is created on this sloping top surface. Lift forces are common as an airplane wing encounters the air and an effectively pitched hand of a swimmer pushes against

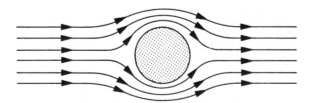

Fig. 5-7. *Streamlined or laminar flow of fluid (or air) as a result of interaction with smooth-surfaced sphere. The object is affected equally on all surfaces and has a normal flight pattern.*

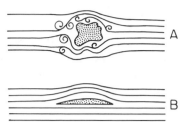

Fig. 5-8. *A, turbulent flow of fluid (or air) as a result of interaction with asymmetric, rough-surfaced, irregular object. Such turbulence inhibits the normal flight of object. B. Flow of fluid (or air) as a result of interaction with streamlined object. Such flow results in a lowered pressure due to higher velocity of fluid flow above the concave surface.*

the water. During such situations, the flow of the fluid over one surface is faster, creating a low-pressure area, than over the other surface, for which there is a high-pressure area. Thus the airplane or discus is lifted upward, and the swimmer may be moved forward or laterally depending on the position of the hand. This lift force always acts at right angles to the drag force, which is parallel to the direction of movement of the body or body part being analyzed. Both forces occur at all angles of tilt of this streamlined body except (1) at a 90 degree angle of inclination, in which only drag occurs, and (2) at a zero-degree angle, at which lift occurs. Thus, at the 45-degree angle of incline, the body will experience equal amounts of lift and drag. The special effects of drag and lift forces will be discussed further in Chapters 12, 13, and 16.

MINI-LAB LEARNING EXPERIENCES

Surface-area drag in air and in water are based upon identical concepts. Investigate these concepts by comparing the relative drag and its effect upon performance.

1. Experience the effects of changes in surface area exposed to fluid, either air or water, and measure these surface areas. Rank the relative drag (based upon perception of force) in the following conditions with the arm starting vertically at the side of the body:
   a) Flex and extend the forearm ten times with the hand slicing the air, with the arm rotated outwards so the thumb and index finger are acting as the frontal surface area.
   b) Repeat these experiments in the water.
   c) Alternately flex and extend the forearm with the palm of the hand acting as the surface area interacting with the air.
   d) Repeat experiment c in the water.
   e) Repeat a and d with a hand paddle strapped to the hand.

THE MECHANICS OF HUMAN MOVEMENT   **145**

2. Measure drag forces. Attach a spring scale to different-sized pieces of wood and pull horizontally through water. Measure the force on the scale for each condition and measure the surface area of the leading surface. Compare the surface areas and the drag forces. Place all values in tabular form for ease of comparison.

Repeat the test by pulling one piece of wood with different orientations. Repeat the test by attaching rough surfaces to the wood.

Although special names have been given to the forces in air and water, they can be divided into normal and tangential forces and related to the previously described explanation of forces. Drag force can be considered a reaction force as a result of action of the body on the water. For example, as a rower pushes against the water with the oar blade, the water pushes back on the oar blade. This drag force prevents slippage, or movement backward of the oar, and causes the boat to move forward. Another normal force present in water has been termed the buoyancy force of water. This force supports a body in the water, causing the body to float if its density is less than that of water. This concept is explained also in Chapter 16.

A further application of the principle of Bernoulli is noted in many ball-throwing, striking, and kicking activities. For example, in the case of a golf ball, backspin imparted to the ball by the golf club helps to create high- and low-pressure areas and thereby a drag-lift differential. This effect has also been called the Magnus effect, after a German engineer who is credited with first noting the curved path fol-

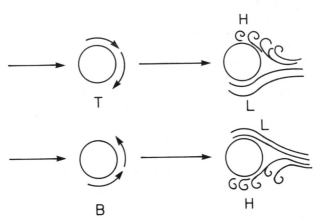

Fig. 5-9. *Flow patterns produced by spinning balls as viewed sagittally to path of travel. T = topspin and turbulent, high pressure flow pattern at top of ball causing topspinning balls to fall more rapidly than normal. B = backspin and turbulent, high pressure flow pattern at bottom of ball causing backspinning balls to rise more than normal. Rotations of right and left spinning balls can be visualized with the figure as an overhead view.*

THE BIOMECHANICS OF HUMAN MOVEMENT

lowed by a cannonball to which spin had been imparted before it became airborne. This rotation, seen in many projections of objects used in sports, usually is created by striking or otherwise exerting a force eccentric to the object. This creates rotation about an axis within the ball, and the ball veers right or left, up or down, or diagonally. This phenomenon is explained by the fact that as a body rotates, it tends to have the fluid next to it move with it, and the air or other fluid just beyond this so-called boundary layer is influenced. As the object travels through a medium such as air and meets the oncoming air, a high pressure is then developed on the side of the direction of the spin and a low pressure on the opposite side. The ultimate result is a curved, rather than a linear, path. (See Fig. 5-9.)

MINI-LAB LEARNING EXPERIENCES

Drop objects of different surface areas from various heights above a body of water at least 60cm deep (approximately 2 feet). Use such objects as rubber diving bricks, indoor (rubber coated) shot put and discus, and a rubber hammer. Objects of non-symmetrical shapes can be dropped with two or more orientations to the water.

1. Measure the time from release to striking the bottom of the water.
2. Observe the entry into the water and the movement of water during descent of the object through the water. Describe the flow pattern.
3. Explain and apply results.

MINI-LAB LEARNING EXPERIENCES

1. Sew or glue pieces of colored yarn to a strip of elastic binding or a strap. Fit the strap around the palm of the hand as shown in Fig. 5-10. Place the hand in front of a fan, in the following positions:
   a) fingers toward fan;
   b) palm toward fan;
   c) back of hand toward fan (dorsum of hand);
   d) 45-degree angle to fan.
   Observe the pieces of yarn and describe what happens to them. Explain the results with respect to basic principles of fluid mechanics. Apply the information obtained.
2. Perform the experiments in #1, modifying the placement of the yarn. Place the yarn on different parts of the body, such

THE MECHANICS OF HUMAN MOVEMENT   **147**

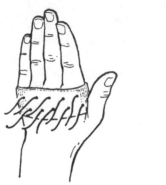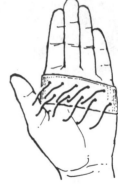

Fig. 5-10. *Pieces of yarn glued to hands to investigate flow patterns during swimming strokes.*

as the foot and the head. Once again, describe and explain the results, and apply them to some activity.

3. Perform the experiments of #1 and #2 in an aquatic environment. Move the body/body part through water and note the effects. Explain the results and apply them to the swimming situation.

DISPLACEMENTS WITH RESPECT TO TIME

When movement occurs, the most readily identifiable parameter is displacement: how far the body or body part was moved and in which direction, whether linear or rotary, the movement occurred. Pertinent measurements of angles and distances are shown in the following examples:

1. Length of stride during walking: Is the stride too short or too long for efficient movement?
2. Direction of foot angle with direction of locomotion: Can the foot exert the muscular forces effectively with the measured angle?
3. Height of jump: Is the jump average, below average, or above average according to achievement norms?
4. Direction of arm movement during throwing: Did the arm move toward the target?
5. Relationship of lean of trunk, position of legs, and other body parts: Are the distances and angles the same as those seen in highly skilled performances?

Displacement analysis, however, is not enough, since forces and, therefore, accelerations are ignored. For example, two balls may be thrown a distance of 9 m (30 ft), but one may take half the time to travel the distance than the other ball takes. Therefore, using the following examples, one can conclude that one ball projection is effective whereas the other ball projection is not:

1. The faster ball, if thrown to first base, will arrive to cause the batter/base runner to be "out."
2. The faster ball cannot be stopped by a soccer goalkeeper.
3. The faster ball cannot be intercepted by an opposing basketball player.
4. The pedestrian is able to cross the intersection prior to change in traffic light.

Displacement with respect to time is more important than displacement alone. Speed is the change in position (displacement) with respect to time if the displacement is not given a direction. If the direction is specified, the displacement with respect to time is called velocity. The equation for determining the magnitude of either is the same:

$$\text{Velocity} = \text{Change in position}/\text{Change in time}$$
$$= \text{Displacement}/\text{Time}$$

thus one may refer to the speed of a racehorse, a sprinter, or a sailboat as being a certain number of kilometers per hour or meters per second. The velocity would be in these same units, but in the horizontal direction, or at an angle of 20 degrees with the vertical, or in some other system denoting direction.

Angular velocities provide information concerning the ability to perform somersaults and move body parts fast enough for a given task. There is an interrelationship between linear and angular velocities. One example is:

$$V_t = r\omega$$

previously described in the section on centripetal force. Angular velocity can be resolved into two components. One component, parallel to the path in the arc at the instant of viewing, is the tangential velocity (V_t), since without the second component (radial velocity), the movement would continue on a tangent to the arc, in a straight line. The radial component is directed inward along the radius at each instant of time, to maintain the circular path of the limb.

Given the same angular velocity, the tangential velocity will increase as the radius increases. This definition of V_t is very important in throwing, kicking, and striking activities and will be discussed in Chapters 12 and 14. It is also important in the swinging activities of gymnastics.

Knowing the speed or velocity of the movement does not include information about the forces that created this speed or velocity. The

THE MECHANICS OF HUMAN MOVEMENT   **149**

rate of change in velocity, however, equals the acceleration, from which one can calculate force: F = ma. The equation for determining the acceleration of a body is as follows:

Acceleration = Change in velocity/Change in time = V/t

The relationships of displacement, velocity, and acceleration with respect to angular motion appear in Fig. 5-11.

The following are known relationships concerning displacement, velocity, and acceleration, whether angular or linear:

1. When the amount of displacement increases from one time period to the next, the velocity increases.

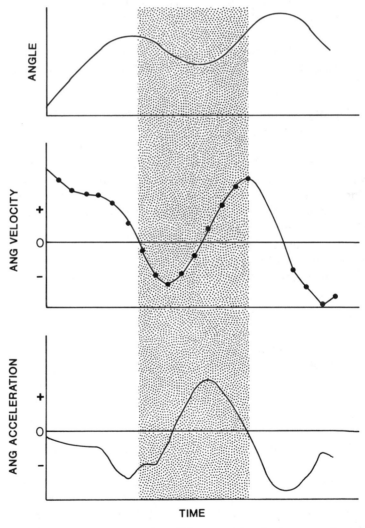

Fig. 5-11. *Computer plots of film data. When angular displacement is maximum or minimum value, angular velocity is zero. When angular displacement slope is greatest, angular velocity is maximum and angular acceleration is zero.*

THE BIOMECHANICS OF HUMAN MOVEMENT

2. When the displacement remains constant from one time period to the next, the velocity is constant and the acceleration is zero.
3. When there is a reversal of direction in displacement, the velocity will be zero at the instant of reversal.
4. At the instant of maximum velocity, the acceleration is zero.

These relationships are seen readily in an analysis of running. The displacement of the body from the first stride to the fifth increases as the time for each stride becomes less. Thus, the velocity increases, and since the velocity is not constant, positive acceleration occurs. At some point in time, the length of stride and the velocity become constant; the acceleration ceases and becomes equal to zero. Minute changes probably occur in all forms of locomotion at the instant of foot plant and push-off, but these are being disregarded. The runner maintains this constant velocity, with zero acceleration, until the end of the race, at which time acceleration (change in velocity) occurs.

Although the total body kinematics just described for a runner may be defined easily, the same statement cannot be made with regard to the kinematics of the body segments. Accelerations and decelerations of the limbs continue to occur even when the total body moves at a constant velocity. Since limb accelerations are angular in nature and are derived from angular velocities, there are two components of angular acceleration that define in linear terms: tangential and radial. Their directions are the same as those described for tangential and radial velocities.

Analysis of the kinematics of projectiles is easy if all forces are considered to be negligible except the force of gravity. The acceleration of any projectile then becomes the acceleration of gravity (9.8 m/sec^2 as an average value) in the vertical direction. A convenient equation for determining the kinematics of a projectile is $s = 1/2\ at^2$, where s = distance in the vertical direction, a = the acceleration of gravity, and t = time. Although the formula $s = vt + 1/2\ at^2$ can be applied more universally than $s = 1/2\ at^2$, there is always some point during the flight of the projectile, whether a ball, a human body, an animal, or another object, at which the vertical velocity will equal zero and the descending flight pattern will begin. Since the vertical velocity is equal to zero, the term vt in equation is also zero.

If the descent of the projected object is timed, the maximum vertical distance of projection may be calculated. For example, if a ball requires 1 second to fall to the ground from its highest elevation from the ground, this elevation is equal to 4.9 m.

When objects are projected horizontally, with zero vertical velocity, one can measure the height above the ground at the time of projection. Time is equal to the square root of 2 s/a, that is:

$$t = \sqrt{2\ s/a}$$

THE MECHANICS OF HUMAN MOVEMENT   **151**

Then the velocity of the projectile in the horizontal direction can be determined, since the horizontal distance traveled, divided by the air time, will equal the horizontal velocity. The horizontal distance is easy to measure. Concepts and examples of Projectile Motion appear in the appendix.

MINI-LAB LEARNING EXPERIENCES

1. Select a smooth-surfaced plank 3 m long and set it on an incline.
2. Place a smooth-surfaced ball at the top of the incline and release the ball without applying force.
   a. Using a stopwatch or an automatic timing device, record the number of seconds from release of ball until it rolls the 3 m.
   b. Repeat the test until reliability is satisfactory.
   c. Measure the angle of inclination of the plank.
   d. Measure or calculate the height of descent (H) of the ball. This can be determined trigonometrically by the following equation:

   $$H = \sin \theta \ (3 \text{ m})$$

   which is the same as that explained in appendix B: Opposite side = Sin θ (hypotenuse).
   e. Using all these data, show that gravity is a constant force producing a constant acceleration of 9.8 m/sec^2. Remember the following equation:

   $$s = 1/2 \ at^2$$

   or

   $$a = \frac{2s}{t^2}$$

   f. Repeat the test, using two different angles of inclination of the board. The same results should occur.

These displacements with respect to time provide insight into the kinetics of movement. As has been shown previously, an estimation of the forces acting on the body may be determined by measuring the acceleration of the body and multiplying this value by the mass of the body. If the force is known (measured by means of dynamographic devices), one can estimate the resulting acceleration of the body. Thus the outcome of the performance or the effectiveness of the muscle coordination may be assessed or predicted.

Additionally, the force platform can be used to measure force with respect to time, not merely force. It is now necessary to approach the analysis of movement in a holistic manner and view force as an action occurring in a known period of time and through a known distance of application. Thus force itself exists as a temporal and spatial entity and should be viewed as such to more completely understand movement.

IMPULSE-MOMENTUM

Although the external forces, such as gravity, that act on living bodies frequently possess constant magnitudes, rarely do any of the forces produced by the living body in motion have a constant magnitude. Each force acts for a period of time ranging from short to long in duration. Muscle forces required to maintain a static position may be of the same magnitude over a short period of time, but variation in muscle force during movement of a body segment almost always occurs. This variation is due to such factors as the angle at the joint, the speed of movement, the length of the muscle, and the position of the limb in space at each particular point in time. Furthermore, most human and animal movements require more than one contracting muscle or group of muscles. Therefore, several forces are created when different body parts move in a prescribed sequence and with a specific speed. This utilization of several body parts in time is called coordination, which also may be referred to as a summation of forces, development of momentum, or creation of kinetic energy.

SUMMATION OF FORCES

The principle of summation of forces is as follows: the force produced during movement of one body segment will be added to the force produced by the next body segment, and so on until the final action. The most effective timing of these forces has not been investigated thoroughly for all movements of humans and animals. Evidence, however, is conclusive that each force should occur at the time of maximal velocity of the preceding action during sequential summation. An investigation of velocity of motion is therefore necessary and can be approached through the following example:

A girl of elementary-school age creates muscle force for a short duration of time to accelerate her leg. The foot of her swinging leg contacts a soccer ball and applies force to the ball for a very short period of time. This causes the ball to accelerate, which creates velocity and displacement.

This physical phenomenon can be depicted as a cause-and-effect relation by using the equation $F = ma$ and modifying it to represent the force acting over a period of time (t):

$$\int Ft = \Delta mat$$

The product Ft is called impulse, or impulse of force, and its units are newton-seconds (Nsec). Since velocity equals at, the equation can be rewritten as follows:

$$\int Ft = \Delta mV$$

The product mV is termed linear momentum, and its units also are newton-seconds. This equation is known as the impulse-momentum equation. A given impulse will create a given momentum.

In actuality, the equation is more complex, since acceleration represents a change in velocity with respect to a change in time, not merely the relationship $a = V/t$. Readers acquainted with calculus will recognize the following rewriting of the equation as the integral Ft being equal to the change in momentum:

$$\int Ft = m_f V_f - m_i V_i$$

The subscript $_f$ refers to final momentum, and the subscript $_i$ refers to initial momentum. The integral (Ft) merely means the area under a force-time curve is a graphic representation of the amount of force occurring at each point in time over a selected period. Three such curves are depicted in Fig. 5-12. The areas of the rectangles of force-time can easily be determined by multiplying the length of time by the magnitude of force. In Fig. 5-12A, the force was a constant 100 N for 0.4 second, whereas in Fig. 5-12B, a greater force, but still constant, was applied for 0.2 second. The situation in Fig. 5-12C is the more common force-time curve seen with human and animal movements and is the more difficult area to measure. The areas of all three situations are identical in that the person applied an impulse of 20 Nsec to the ball. Despite the difference in maximal force production, since the impulses are identical, the velocity of the ball will be identical for all three situations.

Therefore, the product of force and time of application of the force will determine the amount of momentum that can be achieved. The human body makes a compromise between the development of maximal force and maximal time of application of force. If the person allows too much time, such as using a full-squat position before jumping, maximal force cannot be achieved because the muscles are in a disadvantageous angle for exerting force upward. The time of execution of the propulsive action of leg extension will be too long. In long jumping, the jumper must have enough time on the takeoff board to complete the leg extension. Too short a time will be ineffective. Likewise, too long a time will cause the person to decrease the hori-

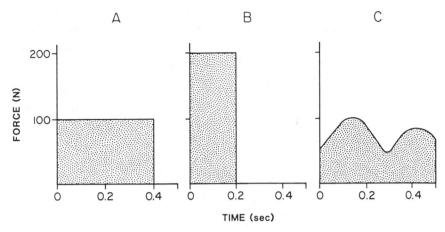

Fig. 5-12. *Theoretical identical impulses of 40 Nsec, but with different amounts of force and different durations of application of force. Most human and animal production of impulse resembles the variable magnitude of force application depicted in C. This is one reason human movement analysis is more difficult than analysis of motions of machines and other inanimate devices.*

zontal speed acquired during the run and therefore to decrease the force. Thus the ability to generate maximum impulse is dependent on anatomic considerations such as muscle strength, length and position of limbs, and position of limbs, as well as the ability to coordinate the movements (neurologic integration). Maximum impulse will be achieved by the best, or optimum, combination of force and time of application of force. Impulse creates velocity in a particular mass. Since a certain impulse will create a certain momentum, the greater the mass, the less will be the velocity. All the principles listed with respect to F = ma are applicable to the impulse-momentum equation.

The development of both the force platform and computerized cinematographic analysis have made it possible to analyze the impulse and momentum of performances and, from the point of view of safety, the impulse and momentum of impacts, or collisions.

CONSERVATION OF MOMENTUM

Linear Momentum

Impacts, or collisions, of two bodies result in a change in momentum for each of the two bodies. This phenomenon has been called a transfer of momentum but is better defined as a conservation of momentum, which is simply a rephrasing of Newton's third law, the law of interaction (action-reaction). The law of conservation of momentum states that when two or more objects collide with each other, the total momentum after impact is equal to the total momentum before impact. For example, when a bowling ball traveling at 7 m/sec and weighing 98 N strikes a stationary pin weighing 9.8 N (these higher-than-normal weights are given for ease of subsequent computations), the momentum of the ball and of the pin after impact will be equal to the momentum of the ball and the pin before impact. The pin, being the lighter of the two masses, will have the greater velocity after impact, but the ball will not experience much loss of velocity after impact, since its mass is 10 times that of the pin. As an illustration, if the pin acquired a final velocity twice that of the "before-impact velocity" of the ball, the changes in momentums and ball velocity would be as follows:

Before impact momentum = After impact momentum

$$m_{b1}V_{b1} = m_{b2}V_{b2} + m_pV_p$$

$$\frac{98N}{9.8m/sec^2} \times 7 \text{ m/sec} = \frac{98N}{9.8 \text{ m/sec}^2} \times V_{b2} + \frac{9.8N}{9.8 \text{ m/sec}^2} \times 14 \text{ m/sec}$$

$$70 \text{ Nsec} = 10 \text{ Nsec}^2/m \times V_{b2} + 14 \text{ Nsec}$$

$$56 \text{ Nsec} = 10 \text{ Nsec}^2/m \times V_{b2}$$

$$5.6 \text{ m/sec} = V_{ball \text{ after impact}}$$

The ball velocity decreased by 1.4 m/sec, whereas the pin velocity increased 14 m/sec. The momentum of the ball was 70 Nsec before impact and 56 Nsec after impact.

Since velocity is a vector, the assumption was made that the collision of the bowling ball and pin was a head-on collision and that all velocities were additive, that is, along the same line. If the impact had been at an angle, the momentums would have been resolved into two components (planar motion) or into three components (three-dimensional motion) to calculate the angles of deflection of both objects after impact. Because of the conservation-of-momentum principle, both objects will be deflected from their original line of motion because the impact will have a component parallel (shear force) to the object's original motion, as well as perpendicular (normal).

Success in the sports of billiards, racquetball, handball, and squash, as well as other games in which balls rebound from surfaces, is dependent upon the performer's ability to judge both the ball's angle of rebound and its speed of rebound. Although trial and error, as well as experience, may be prime factors in acquiring such judgment, the ability to solve the conservation-of-momentum equations and to explain the concept may provide the analyst with a means of shortening the trial-and-error method. The necessary skills will be thoroughly treated in Chapter 18. In addition, any spin force, friction force, and deformation of the two bodies during impact will introduce factors that will affect the measured velocities after impact. The bowling ball—bowling pin impact was as nearly a perfectly elastic situation as can be seen in any sport. An elastic situation is one in which no energy is dissipated in heat energy to deform the materials. The effect of not so perfectly elastic situations, such as when two human bodies collide or a tennis ball collides with a racquet, will be discussed in the work-energy section of this chapter.

Angular Momentum

Moments of force also act over a time period. The created momentum from the product moment of impulse (Mt) is termed angular momentum and is written as $I\omega$. The moment of inertia (I), or the resistance to rotation or turning, is measured as the mass of the object multiplied by the radius squared, of the rotating body. The ω refers to angular velocity. Since mass rarely changes within a movement, the importance of the radius in the determination of I is primary.

The same principles of linear momentum are applicable to angular momentum. The special case of conservation of angular momentum needs to be considered because this phenomenon often is seen in the angular motion of dancers, skaters, divers, gymnasts, jumpers, and other persons involved in airborne athletics, as well as in any person or animal using rotary movements. For example, a diver will tuck in the arm and legs, an action that concentrates the mass closer to the axis of rotation and thus decreases the moment of inertia of the body about this axis. Since angular momentum can be altered only by external couples or eccentric (off-center) forces, and since the tucking of body parts is due to internal forces, angular momentum is not affected and will not change. Thus angular velocity increases to maintain the constant angular momentum and to allow the diver to execute a turn in a shorter time. The dive can therefore be completed well above water level to provide for a nearly vertical and controlled entry into the water. In another example the ballet dancer and ice skater will start a slow-spinning motion with the arms held horizontally and then will bring the arms quickly to the chest area to increase the angular velocity of the spin. The reverse action with the arms will be used to slow the spin and initiate another movement.

Thus athletes, by changing the length of their body segments to redistribute their masses, are able to cause changes in their angular velocities (ω) because of the conservation-of-angular-momentum principle. The momentum remains the same, but the overall movement appears different to the viewer and to the performer because of the change in ω. These changes in ω produced by movement of body parts will vary with the body segment involved, as well as with different individuals. For example, the leg has a greater mass than the arm; consequently, movement of the leg will produce a greater change in ω. Long-limbed and heavy-boned individuals will be able to produce greater changes in ω than will individuals with short limbs or light-weight distal segments. If a person attempts to perform rotary movements with weights either held in the hands or strapped to different body parts, a more dramatic change in angular velocity will be noted with a redistribution of these weights than without weights, since there will be a greater change in the moment of inertia.

PRINCIPLES

1. Greater impulses of force applied to stationary objects produce greater changes in momentum and greater final velocities.
2. For the same impulse, the greater the mass of the stationary object the less will be its final velocity, since the momentum remains constant.
3. Given the same force, an increase in time of application of force will impart greater velocity to a body. In striking activities this may be possible and is referred to as "hitting through the ball."
4. Maximum impulse can be created by maximizing the force, by maximizing the time of application of force or by combining optimum force with optimum time. The latter strategy usually is preferred for movements involving locomotion or jumping.
5. Momentum is conserved in the collision of two or more objects; large masses will have low velocities compared to small masses after the collision.
6. Angular momentum is conserved within a body by an increase in the angular velocity as a result of a decrease in the moment of inertia, and vice versa.
7. Since a moving body possesses momentum, an impulse or force will be required to stop or reduce the speed of the body.
8. A body in motion would require no force to keep it moving in a vacuum. Since, however, friction or some other resistance always exists to some extent to reduce the velocity of a body in motion, equal and opposite impulses of force are required to counteract these resistances and thus maintain the momentum of the body. These impulses are minute compared to the impulse required to develop the existing momentum.
9. To capitalize on the momentum of one's body or body part, one must make each subsequent application of an impulse of force before the momentum has been reduced appreciably by resistances such as friction. Skilled swimmers apply this principle, as do other persons displaying what is termed rhythm, grace, and coordination.

MINI-LAB LEARNING EXPERIENCES

1. Using a twist board, piano stool, or revolving chair, turn a person on the device. Time the number of revolutions for the following positions:
   a. Arms held at sides while standing.
   b. Arms held at sides while standing; move arms to shoulder level while standing.
   c. Order of step b reversed.
   d. Weight placed in the hands and steps b and c repeated.

THE BIOMECHANICS OF HUMAN MOVEMENT

e. Twice the weight used in step d placed in hands, and steps b and c repeated.
f. Select other positions of your choice.
2. Estimate the changes in the moment of inertia (I) by calculating the angular velocity (ω). Remember that the angular velocity must be expressed in radians:

rad = revolutions per second $\times$ 2π

3. Draw conclusions concerning angular momentum and movement of body parts.

WORK-ENERGY

The work-energy approach is a viewing of the kinetics of motion from a different perspective than the impulse-momentum approach. The product of force and of the distance over which this force acts represents the work done by the force on an object. Thus the concern is with the distance rather than with the time of force application. When work is done, a change in energy results. Potential energy is the capacity to do work but no motion exists. Kinetic energy (KE) is the energy of motion. The work-energy equation is as follows:

$$\int Fd = 1/2\ mV_f^2 - 1/2\ mV_i^2$$

and the units are newton-meters (joules). The two velocities represent final (V_f) and initial (V_i) velocities.

The work-energy approach is useful in analyzing weight lifting and for analyzing and ranking movement tasks with respect to mechanical work and power. Collisions in which deformations are an important component of the interaction of two bodies, as in trampoline bouncing, also are useful for analyzing from a work-energy approach rather than from an impulse-momentum, or simple $F = ma$, approach.

The work-energy approach is as applicable to rotary motion as it is to linear motion, and one can explain the principle of conservation of energy in much the same way as the conservation-of-momentum principle. Conservation of mechanical energy does not always occur, however, since friction is a nonconservative force. Heat energy always results in situations in which friction exists.

Although applications will be discussed in Parts Two and Three, one of the most revealing applications of the work-energy concept involves the downward swing of an object, for example, a gymnast on the uneven parallel bars. Fig. 5-13 shows a taller person and a shorter person beginning a downward swing from a horizontal position. The taller person will take longer to reach the vertical position because gravity is a constant force accelerating the body downward. Since the

THE MECHANICS OF HUMAN MOVEMENT **159**

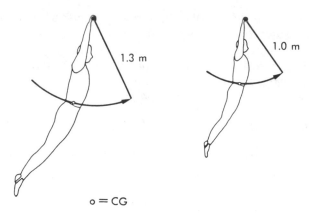

Fig. 5-13. *Different arcs of swing and vertical drops of center of gravity (CG) of two persons of different stature. If both body weights are equal, or if taller person has greater body weight than shorter person, taller person will do more work and develop greater kinetic energy than shorter person. Vertical drop (radius) multiplied by body weight equals work. Assuming the shorter person weighs 400 newtons, calculate the potential energy prior to the drop (P.E. = mgh). Calculate the velocity at the greatest kinetic energy (zero P.E.). Remember that the change in energy equals the work done.*

center of gravity of the body of the taller person must drop 1.3 m to reach the bottom of the swing, the shorter person will reach the bottom sooner. Work done by the taller person will be 1.3 m × body weight; that of the shorter person will be 1.0 m × body weight. Potential energy exists at the start of the movement; therefore, initial $1/2 \, mV^2$ = 0. Since the final kinetic energy is equal to the work done, if both persons were of equal mass, the taller person would experience greater downward velocity during the swing than would the shorter person, since greater work has been performed.

Each body segment creates its own kinetic energy independent of and interdependent with other body segments. Thus, work is done by each moving segment of the human body. Mechanical efficiency of the human body can be investigated by means of segmental-total body work and energy analysis.

MINI-LAB LEARNING EXPERIENCES

1. Place a ball on the floor, holding your hand in a position to push the ball forward.
2. Maintain contact with the ball for 10 cm, pushing with a constant force.
   a. Note the apparent speed of the ball.
   b. Record the distance the ball travels and the time of travel.
   c. Calculate the velocity of the ball.
3. Repeat step 2 but apply the force for a distance of 20 cm.
4. Weigh the ball.

a. Calculate its mass: N/9.8 m/sec^2 = weight/gravity
b. Calculate the kinetic energy for each situation: 1/2 mV^2
c. Calculate the force: F = KE/d (in meters)
5. Interpret the data: What was the effect of doubling the distance of force application? Did you hold the force constant?

POTENTIAL AND KINETIC ENERGY OF COLLISIONS

Characteristics of Elasticity

When two objects collide, the forces exerted on both objects tend to deform both objects. The property that enables a body to recover its original shape or volume is referred to as elasticity and is measured as the ratio of stress to strain, called Young's modulus of elasticity. Stress refers to the amount of force per unit area of collision, and strain is the amount of distortion (deformation) with respect to original size.

A scrutiny of the elastic properties of certain types of materials may be interesting and may have value in furthering one's understanding of the kinetics of collisions. Rubber, for example, is not perfectly elastic and therefore does not return to its original shape if distorted to the maximum. In fact, high-tempered steel and spring brass are much more elastic than is rubber. All gases act as perfectly elastic substances; for example, gas is used in pneumatic tires. Liquids are also perfectly elastic but difficult to compress. The inside of the best golf balls has a liquid core. When place-kicking, the toe of the shoe of the kicker often distorts the ball as much as one-third of its original shape. The baseball is temporarily flattened against the bat as much as one fourth. A golf ball may be distorted as much as one tenth or more and a tennis ball up to one half of its original shape.

Deformations are noted in shafts of long-handled implements such as rakes and hockey sticks but are not so noticeable in shafts of hammers, shovels, hoes, and short-handled implements. Some plastic used in the manufacture of sports and game equipment for children of elementary-school age may deform readily but may not easily regain their original shape. When used as striking implements, these plastics are ineffective because the striking implement deforms to a greater extent than does the object to be struck. Therefore, the ball does not acquire sufficient velocity for the child to experience success.

The characteristics of elasticity can be used to explain why a small boy can hit a tennis ball farther than a baseball, using a tennis racquet. The tennis ball can be compressed to the point at which it is considerably distorted. The strings of the racquet also are distorted (stretched). Potential energy is acquired. The ball and racquet remain together for a greater time (achieve greater impulse—Ft) and for a longer distance (achieve greater work—Fd); therefore, the mass of the ball will not deflect the racquet backward to any measurable extent.

The work done by the boy on the baseball, however, will not be sufficient to distort it and "carry" the ball. The greater mass of the ball also will resist the movement more than did the tennis ball. Golf instructors recommend that some women and small men not purchase golf balls with a liquid center because they will not be able to compress it to the same dgree that they can a ball, which has a rubber center.

Coefficient of Elasticity

The coefficient of elasticity is a number that has been derived to represent the characteristics of a collision between two objects. It does not measure the elastic properties of either material, but the interaction of the two materials. This coefficient of elasticity of two objects colliding with each other can be determined by the following experiment:

1. Drop a ball from a known height.
2. Measure the height of the rebound.
3. Calculate the coefficient of elasticity (e) by the following relationship:

$$e = \sqrt{\frac{\text{Height of rebound}}{\text{height dropped}}}$$

A second method is to measure the velocity (V) of the rebounding object before and after impact. The energy lost during the collision will be represented by the loss in velocity. The equation is as follows:

$$e = \frac{\text{V after impact}}{\text{V before impact}}$$

Racquetball, handball, and squash players increase the coefficient of elasticity (also called coefficient of restitution) between the ball and the rebounding surfaces by heating the ball. "Never play with a cold ball" is an adage to be followed, since the ball will not rebound as far, as fast, or as consistently as will a "hot ball." Different playing surfaces will also alter the rebound of balls. Plagenhoef has studied the characteristics of balls interacting with different surfaces in terms of both coefficient of friction and coefficient of elasticity and has found a variety of values with the same ball under different conditions, including different speeds of the ball as it enters the collision.

Handball players sometimes follow a procedure that has a bearing on this discussion. They soak a "stale" handball in hot water. The heat causes a rearrangement of molecules inside the handball, which will then bounce (for a while) as much as when it was new. Handball players also sometimes soak their hands in hot water to help prevent bruises. The fluid in the hands is brought to the surface and helps the skin to withstand blows.

The concept of stored energy because of easily deformed materials used for landing surfaces is an important one, especially in springboard diving, pole vaulting, and in trampolining. The material has the potential to do work on the performer by virtue of the distance through which the material has been deformed. As the material is regaining its original shape, the potential energy of the system is transformed into kinetic energy and the person rebounds from the surface. Divers change the fulcrum of the diving board and thus change the distance through which the board will deform. The result is more or less kinetic energy and a corresponding change in the height of the dive.

MINI-LAB LEARNING EXPERIENCES

1. Determine coefficients of elasticity for balls interacting with various surfaces. Use the following equation:

$$e = \sqrt{\frac{\text{Height of rebound}}{\text{Height of drop}}}$$

2. Test environmental factors such as the following:
   a. Heated ball
   b. Cold ball
   c. Underinflated ball
   d. Ball with attached padding

REFERENCES

Barham, J. N. (1978): *Mechanical Kinesiology,* St. Louis: C. V. Mosby Company.
Daish, C. B. (1979): *The physics of ball games,* London: English Universities Press.
Hochmuth, G. (1984): *Biomechanics of athletic movement,* Berlin: Sportverlag.
Hooper, B. G. (1973): *The mechanics of human movement,* New York: American Elsevier Publishing Co., Inc.
Merzkirch, W. (1979): Making fluid flows visible, *Am. Sci.* 67:330–336.
Rodgers, M. M. and Cavanagh, P. (1984): Glossary of biomechanical terms, concepts and units, *Physical Therapy* 64:1887–1901.
Schenck, J. M. and Cordova, F. D. (1980): *Introductory biomechanics,* 2nd ed. Philadelphia: F. A. Davis.
Townsend, M. S. (1984): *Mathematics in sport,* New York: Halsted Press: John Wiley and Sons.
Tricker, R. A. and Tricker, B. J. K. (1967): *The science of movement,* New York: American Elsevier Publishing Co., Inc.

6

The Human Communication System

Understanding of joint actions and the resulting lever actions is only the foundation for understanding and improving motor skill. The performer, the teacher, the coach, the therapist, and the industrial engineer must seek means by which the desired actions can become behavior. The action at joints depends on nerve impulses. Body segment movement, or fixation, is the result; nerve action is the means by which the result is achieved. This concept, still valid today, was expressed by Bard (1961): "The problem of behavior is essentially the problem of explaining how the central nervous system distributes messages to the muscles in such quantities and with such dispersion in time and space as to bring about the sequence of integrated motor events which comprise any normal body movement." Sage (1977) stated that:

> The observer of a smoothly coordinated motor performance usually does not realize that the performance represents a fantastically complex integration of many parts of the nervous system to produce the postures and movement patterns. In performing a basketball jump shot, a football forward pass or an intricate dance routine, the complete movement patterns consist of reflexes, simple movements, and complex movements with precise spatial and temporal organization, meaning that the appropriate muscles are selected and employed at just the right time.

Mountcastle (1974), in this same vein, stated the following:

> The motor systems of the brain exist to translate through sensation, and emotion into movement . . .

165

Movement is the end product of a number of control systems that interact extensively. Their complexity demands that we proceed logically by (1) defining the nature of movement in terms of muscles and joints, (2) presenting an outline of the motor systems so that the relation of the parts to the whole is apparent from the outset, and (3) explaining how "control" is achieved.

When the details of control of muscles by the nervous system are considered, the general structure of this system should be kept in mind. For convenience in discussion, the nervous system is divided into central and peripheral portions. This division does not imply a separation in function, but only in location.

CENTRAL NERVOUS SYSTEM

The central nervous system includes the brain and spinal cord. Both are well protected by the surrounding bones (the skull and the vertebrae).

Brain

The brain, protected by the skull, includes the parts of the nervous system that are the bases of voluntary muscular control, as well as many parts that control reflex behavior. The major portion of the brain consists of the cerebrum, the upper portion which is divided into a left and right hemisphere (Fig. 6-1). The surface of this portion is composed of gray matter that consists mainly of cell bodies rather than nerve fibers. The activity in these cells is the basis of consciousness and thought. Beneath this surface, the cerebral cortex, are nerve fibers and also other groupings of cell bodies, such as the thalamus and hypothalamus, and mixtures of white and gray matter, such as the reticular formation. Connecting these parts of the brain with the cord are the pons and medulla, parts of the brain stem.

At the rear of the brain and beneath the cerebrum is the cerebellum, which has an important function in movement. The cortex of this section, like that of the cerebrum, is composed of gray matter, whereas the interior is made up mainly of the white matter of nerve fibers. According to Schmidt (1978), the cerebellum is responsible for 1) programming rapid movements, 2) correcting the course of such movements, and 3) correlation of posture and movement. The basal ganglia, which are a group of nuclei located in the inner layers of the cerebrum, receive information from the reticular formation and motor areas of the cerebral cortex and transmit the information to the thalamus. It is responsible for initiation and execution of slow movements as well as facilitating and inhibiting a wide variety of movements. The motor cortex is not responsible for designing movement patterns, but is the last supraspinal station for conversion of the instruction to the motor program. It, therefore, serves as the coordinator or relay

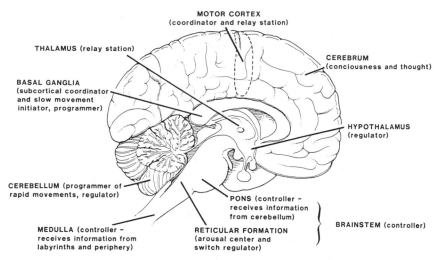

Fig. 6-1. *Human brain. The function of each area appears in parentheses. Note both the specialization and the integration of the different areas of the brain. We now know that the brain (and nervous system) has a high level plasticity enabling it to adapt activity in an area to losses in other areas.*

station for the information from other parts of the central nervous system.

The brain is often considered to be the computer or central processor of the human body. It also can be likened to the railroad station or air traffic control station where flow of traffic is regulated. Events are placed on hold, moved rapidly, interconnections are made, modifications in processing result, and all activity proceeds or is halted by the station's competence.

Thus it is only natural that sometimes the human body does not move as well as possible or does not move consistently from day-to-day. Fatigue, nutrition, lethargy, and other factors will influence the functioning of the brain. Conversely, the functions that occur frequently, such as walking, often appear to be performed without any effort by the brain. It is as if a memory program is activated automatically when walking occurs. According to Schmidt, spinal generators (complex neural circuits) may exist within the spinal cord and be responsible for simple automatic rhythmic actions such as gait.

The brain must interact with the peripheral muscles so that the bones can be moved. This is made possible by means of the spinal cord, which can be likened to the superhighways and airways of the world. The messages from the brain travel to the muscles, via the spinal cord, through the alpha motor neurons. The result is contraction or cessation of contraction (relaxation) of the muscle fibers.

Spinal Cord

Continuous with the medulla, extending through the spinal canal, and terminating at the upper border of the second lumbar vertebra is that portion of the central nervous system known as the spinal cord. Unlike the arrangement of the brain, the gray matter of the cord is in the interior section, in a configuration resembling the letter 'H' (Fig. 6-2). The ends of the 'H' are referred to as the anterior and posterior horns. Surrounding the gray matter are the white nerve fibers connecting various parts of the brain with the cord cells and connecting cells within the cord. The nerve fibers are grouped into tracts, the names of which often indicate the connected areas and also the direction in which nerve impulses are conducted, such as the spinocerebellar and the corticospinal tracts.

Neurons

Nerve fibers and cell bodies are not separate units, since each fiber arises from a cell body. Each cell body with its fibers is known as a neuron (see Fig. 6-3). Those fibers which conduct impulses away from the cell body are the efferent fibers, known as axons; those which conduct impulses toward the cell body are the afferent fibers, known as dendrites. Rarely does a neuron have more than one axon, and this one is usually longer than the dendrites; some axons are as long as 1 m. Often the neuron has several dendrites; near the cell these may be thicker than any axon, but they taper rapidly and branch repeatedly, forming a network of fibers at no great distance from the cell. Impulses do not pass from one neuron to another except at the point where the axon of one cell body is in close contact with the dendrites of another. This connection, known as the synapse, is found only within

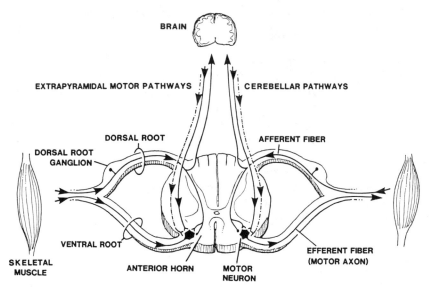

Fig. 6-2. *Cross section diagram of spinal cord with afferent and efferent fiber connections to the muscle. Single monosynaptic reflex loops involve entry and exit at the same level in the spinal cord, without utilizing the spinal cord vertical pathways. More complicated reflex and volitional loops require use of these vertical pathways.*

THE BIOMECHANICS OF HUMAN MOVEMENT

the central nervous system. These synapses occur at each level of entry into the spinal cord and throughout the brain.

PERIPHERAL NERVOUS SYSTEM

The peripheral nervous system includes the cranial and spinal nerves and the peripheral portions of the autonomic nervous system (Table 6-1). The latter controls the action of the viscera, glands, heart, blood vessels, and smooth muscles in other parts of the body and is not directly involved in the movement of skeletal parts. The 12 pairs of cranial nerves and 31 pairs of spinal nerves control the action of striated muscle and are thus directly involved in joint actions. The cranial nerves connect the muscles of the face and head and the central nervous system and also carry impulses to the central nervous system from the receptors of the special senses—the visual, auditory, olfactory, and gustatory senses—and from the more widely spread receptors of pressure, tension, pain, and temperature located in the face and head.

The spinal nerves are most directly involved in movements of the trunk and limbs. The 31 pairs are classified according to the area in which each enters the spinal column: 8 cervical, 12 thoracic, 5 lumbar, 5 sacral, and 1 coccygeal. (See Fig. 6-4.) Each group is numbered from the head downward. In general, the shoulders, arms, and hands are connected with the central nervous system by the fifth, sixth, seventh, and eighth cervical nerves and the first thoracic nerve; the trunk is connected by all the thoracic, lumbar, and sacral nerves; the hips, thighs, legs, and feet are connected by the second, third, fourth, and fifth lumbar nerves and first and second sacral nerve.

Each spinal nerve connects with the spinal cord by an anterior and a posterior root as previously depicted in Fig. 6-2. The posterior roots (afferent nerves) conduct impulses from the sensory receptors of

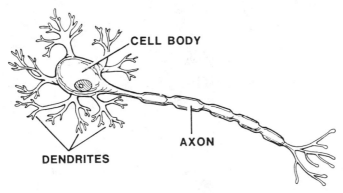

Fig. 6-3. *A typical neuron with its parts labeled. Think of this as a nerve tree analagous to the lung tree and arterial tree, with potential interaction with many other neurons via a synapse, also known as the traffic intersection of the nervous system. The richness of the dendrite tree may well be the key to recovery from neurological traumas.*

THE HUMAN COMMUNICATION SYSTEM **169**

Table 6-1. Cranial nerve identification.

Number	Name	Innervation Site
I	Olfactory	Nose
II	Optic	Eyes
III	Oculomotor	Eyes
IV	Trochlear	Face
V	Trigeminal	Face
VI	Abducent	Eye
VII	Facial	Face (tear ducts, tongue & ear)
VIII	Vestibulocochlear	Inner ear
IX	Glossopharyngeal	Tongue, Pharynx, Larynx
X	Vagus	Tongue & Neck
XI	Accessory	Neck
XII	Hypoglossal	Tongue

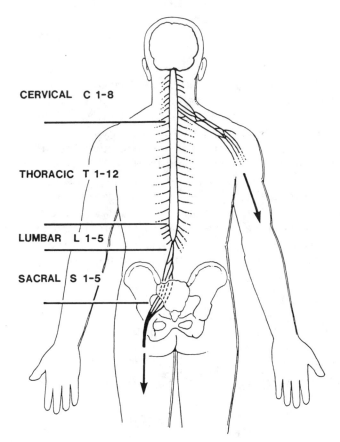

CERVICAL C 1-8

THORACIC T 1-12

LUMBAR L 1-5

SACRAL S 1-5

Fig. 6-4. The spinal nerves—C, cervical; T, thoracic; L, lumbar; and S, sacral. Note the body part being innervated with respect to each nerve. Dysfunction of a specific nerve causes dysfunction in movement coordination and control of the body part innervated by the nerve. Note also that lesions at the spinal cord destroy all spinal nerves arising from the spinal cord caudal to the lesion. Where could a lesion be and which nerves are damaged if a person were a paraplegic? State the same for quadraplegia.

those parts of the body with which the nerves are connected, and the anterior roots (efferent nerves) conduct impulses to the muscles from the central nervous system. Lesions and partial damage to the spinal cord result in loss of muscle function and/or control specific to the level of damage. For example, damage to the sacral nerve results in loss of function in the feet. (Refer to Fig. 6-3.)

MOTOR UNITS

Each efferent (motor) fiber in the spinal nerve arises from a cell body in the anterior horn and is connected with a muscle fiber in some part of the body. The majority of skeletal muscles have thousands of muscle fibers, but each is not supplied with a separate nerve fiber. Instead, the axon of the motor neuron divides into many collaterals just before and after entering the muscle; each collateral connects with a single muscle fiber, all of which contract simultaneously when an impulse is sent from the anterior horn cell. The entire neuron and the muscle fibers that it innervates represent an entity called a motor unit. By this arrangement part of the fibers in one muscle are able to contract while the remaining ones remain at their relaxed length. This arrangement for partial contraction of a single muscle is further facilitated by different degrees of strength in the stimulus needed to excite a neuron. A stimulus that is just strong enough to excite the most sensitive fiber is called a threshold stimulus, whereas one that is strong enough to excite all the fibers is called a maximal stimulus. Thus, logically a given muscle should be able to develop as many different degrees of strength (because of the contraction of fibers in a unit) as there are motor units represented in that muscle. If 100 motor units were present, 100 different degrees of tensions would be possible if progressive summation occurs. A variety of recruitment patterns, however, may be elicited. Therefore, seemingly infinite magnitudes of tension can be produced by a single muscle. The ability to repeatedly and precisely recruit optimal tension is a function of skill.

Since some muscle fibers are innervated by more than one motor unit, the strength of several motor units contracting simultaneously will not equal the sum of the strength of contraction of the individual units. The number of fibers innervated by a single axon varies with the precision of movement required by contraction of that particular muscle. It has been estimated that there is a ratio of 1775 fibers to 1 motor unit in the medial head of the gastrocnemius (which is responsible for large, gross movement). In the tibialis anterior the ratio is 609:1, and in the eye muscles the ratio is 5:1, since very precise movements are needed for effective vision.

Stimulation of Motor Units

If the muscle fibers in a motor unit are to contract, they must be stimulated by a nerve impulse from the cell body in the anterior horn cell. This cell, in turn, must be stimulated by impulses that come to it via its short dendrites. The dendrites, in turn, must receive impulses through the synapse that they make with many nerve fibers, both afferent (sensory) and efferent. These multiple connections make the motor mechanism of the central nervous system highly complex. The concept of this complexity is such that if the intention to move originates in the cerebral cortex, then at the time the nerve impulses from the cortex reach the anterior horn cell, the impulses from the cerebellum, from nerve cells in the brain below the cortex, and from the afferent fibers arising in other muscles and joints are also likely to be received.

The recruitment of motor unit firing for gradation of muscular force varies. Some believe that motor units are recruited by size. According to the Henneman (1980) size principle, the smaller units (small force, slow-twitch muscle units, innervated by small motoneurons) fire first and the larger motor units (larger, faster muscle units, innervated by larger motoneurons) fire last. Lower thresholds exist for the smaller motoneurons. Others say selective recruitment occurs; motor units are recruited according to the task, thereby being controlled by biofeedback. Rate coding is yet another theory. Motor units change their firing rate, increasing the firing rate for increased force demands. It appears that recruitment is important for low tension level skills and rate coding is more important for high tension level skills (e.g. weight lifting). According to Burke (1987), ballistic contractions are a result of synchronous activation of large portions of the motor unit pool.

RECEPTORS

Some comprehension of the complexity of the pathways by which a nerve impulse may reach a motor unit can be gained from consideration of the source of impulses. An impulse originates in the endings of nerve fibers that are specialized to be excited by certain changes in the environment. These endings, known as receptors, are each specialized to respond to certain changes only: those ending in the eye respond primarily to light; those in the ear, to sound; those in the mouth and nose, to chemical changes; and some near the body surface, to pressure. Impulses resulting from these changes may reach the cerebral cortex, and the excitations there have become known as sight, sound, taste, smell, and touch. The average person may be unfamiliar with the many other nerve impulses originating in other types of receptors, classified as (1) interoceptors, those located in the visceral organs; (2) exteroceptors, those responding to stimuli arising outside the body, such as sight, sound, smell, and external pressure; and (3) proprioceptors, those found in muscles, tendons, and joints, which respond to mechanical changes within the body. (The latter are of special interest in the study of movement.) A schematic of the role of receptors and central nervous system is presented in Fig. 6-5.

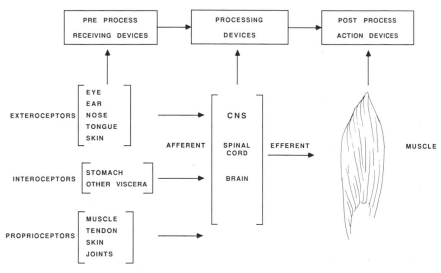

Fig. 6-5. *Schematic of the receiving, processing and action devices of the nervous system. Stimuli (signals) are received (picked-up) by various receptors, often by more than one simultaneously, and sent via the afferent network (A) to the central nervous system for sorting, planning, and programming. The designated response message is sent via the efferent network (E) to the muscle for action. Note that the muscle appears as the action device as well as the receiving device. Which substructures are specialized in the action part and which in the receptor? See figure 6-6 for answer.*

PROPRIOCEPTORS

Impulses originating in the proprioceptors may travel to the motor unit (via the spinal cord) and be responsible for joint actions that are not consciously directed. They can be the basis for reflex actions, for inherent patterns, for adjustments made during performance, and for learned skills. Proprioceptors are referred to as our "sixth sense" receptors. This "sixth sense" is termed kinesthesia. Several of these receptors have been identified and described, and they are discussed in the following paragraphs.

Muscle Spindles

As long ago as 1850, it was found that within muscles there are small groupings of fiber that differ in structure from surrounding fibers in the same muscle spindle. Some investigators thought that the muscle spindle might be the specialized receptor in which nerve impulses would be initiated by changes in the degree of contraction in the muscle. In 1894, Sherrington demonstrated that a nerve fiber from the spindle carries impulses to the spinal cord. We now know that the spindle is a two-way device, both receiving and transmitting impulses.

A representation (schematic drawing) of a muscle spindle is shown in Fig. 6-6. These receptors lie in between and parallel to the muscle fibers. Within a connective tissue sheath, or capsule, there are a number of muscle fibers know as intrafusal fibers. Other fibers in the muscle and not within the capsule are known as extrafusal fibers. Intrafusal fibers are much smaller and consequently produce much less force than the extrafusal fibers. Contraction of all the intrafusal fibers within a given muscle will not produce enough force for movement to occur. They do, however, have a very important function within the muscle spindle. This role is to adjust the bias or gain of the stretch receptor (further explanation is given later in this section). The center region of these fibers contains the nuclei (in a nuclear bag or nuclear chain fashion) and is noncontractile. According to Boyd (1960), in a cat's muscle spindle, the number of nucleii varies from 3 to 13, and in human beings, many more are found. Two types to nerve fibers are in the muscle spindle: 1) efferent, which carries nerve impulses from the spinal cord to the intrafusal muscle fibers; 2) afferent, which carries impulses from the muscle spindle to the central nervous system.

The afferent fibers are two types. They differ in diameter (the larger transmit impulses more rapidly than the smaller) and in type of ending on the intrafusal fiber. The primary (Ia), or annulospiral, ending of the larger type rarely branches as it approaches the intrafusal fiber; its ending winds around the fiber in the area of the nuclear sac much like a coil or spring. The secondary (II), or flower-spray, ending of the smaller afferent fiber also connects with the intrafusal fiber in the region of the nuclear sac, but it is farther from the middle than is the primary ending. There is only one primary ending on a fiber; there may be as many as five secondary endings, although only one is most commonly found. Whenever the nuclear bag area is stretched, nerve impulses are initiated in primary and sec-

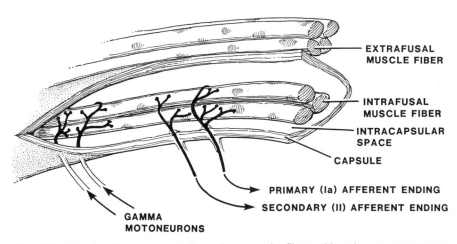

Fig. 6-6. *Schematic representation of a muscle fiber with relevant movement control parts. Note the efferent pathways for the muscle to receive the nerve impulse (message) from the central nervous system, and the afferent pathways for the muscle to send messages to the central nervous system.*

THE BIOMECHANICS OF HUMAN MOVEMENT

ondary endings and transmitted to the spinal cord. The muscle spindle then, is a type of stretch receptor.

Efferent nerve fibers to the spindle, known as gamma motoneurons, are small in diameter; they connect with the intrafusal fiber above the nuclear sac area, where the muscle fibers have contractile ability. Thus when the gamma efferent nerve impulses reach the intrafusal fibers, the latter contract, stretching the central nuclear sac area. Since the number of intrafusal fibers as compared to the number of extrafusal fibers in the muscle is small, this contraction appears to make little or no contribution to movement; its function is stimulation of the spindle afferent fibers, which now can be seen as sensory, or at least afferent, receptors. Firing of the gamma efferents, then, acts to set the bias on the stretch receptor, thereby adjusting its sensitivity, much like eliminating the "play" in a steering wheel. The muscle spindle can be activated by one of two ways: 1) stretching the nuclear bag region by muscle stretch, and 2) stretching the nuclear bag region by contraction of the gamma efferents.

When afferent impulses are initiated in the spindle and transmitted to the spinal cord, they have the possibility of reaching many parts of the body via the complex synaptic connections and nerve pathways in the cord. Some may be carried to the extrafusal fibers in the muscle, in the spindles of which the impulses originated; some may influence the contraction of other muscles acting on the same joint, bringing into action the assistant prime movers and synergistic muscles (Chapter 3); some may inhibit the action of antagonist muscles. Such afferent impulses may also activate anterior horn cells in many parts of the spinal cord and thus affect the movement and position of many segments; some may initiate activity in the nerve cells of the brain stem, subcortical brain areas, and cerebellum. Afferent impulses are the basis for the numerous possibilities for complex reflex acts and for the involuntary joint actions that are a part of voluntarily initiated motor acts. These possiblities support the statement that the mind orders an act and leaves the details of execution to lower levels of the nervous system. Without question the muscle spindle plays a major role in movement; by responding to contraction in the active muscles, it serves as a coordinator throughout the action.

Golgi Tendon Organs

Golgi tendon organ receptors (GTOs) are found in the tendons close to their muscular origin and in the connective tissue of the muscle. The end of an afferent nerve fiber is surrounded by layers of tendon fibers enclosed in a connective sheath. Within this encapsulated mass the nerve ending branches: when the tendon or connective tissue is stretched, the pressure on the nerve ending initiates impulses that will be conducted to the central nervous system. The GTOs are also stretch receptors; however, they respond to stretch in the tendon produced by excessive muscular contraction. Acting as a protector mech-

anism, the GTOs help to avoid tearing the muscle by a forceful con
traction. The result of their activation by a series of neural connections
via the spinal cord is relaxation of the muscle. For example, to relieve
a "charley horse," one attempts to stretch the muscle which is cramped.
Since the muscle is contracting during the cramp, the stretch then
occurs at the tendons. The result: relaxation of the cramped muscle.

Pacinian and Ruffini Receptors

Pacinian corpuscles are widely distributed in the fascia of muscles, especially beneath the tendinous insertion of muscles at the joints.
They are also found in the deeper layers of the skin. The nerve ending
is surrounded by concentric layers of fibrous tissue, within which the
nerve branches. Pressure will be exerted on the nerve endings due to
joint positions and when muscles contract or are stretched. Pacinian
corpuscles only respond for a very brief period of time; they therefore
are a source for information on rapid changes of position. Ruffini endings are located in the joint and also respond to pressure. This receptor, however, is slow in adapting and thus is a source for information
on continuous states of pressure. Combined information from the pacinian corpuscles and the ruffini endings is used to "feel and know"
the movement and position of the limbs of the body.

Skin Receptors

Skin receptors, which respond to touch and pressure, are also activated by changes in joints and muscles; they change the amount to
pressure on the skin and in the area of the movement. The nerve
fibers connected with these receptors reach the spinal cord by way of
the posterior branches of the spinal nerves. They branch as they enter
the cord, conducting impulses to anterior horn cells at the same level
or to higher or lower levels of the cord. These impulses may result in
reflex or subconscious movements. Some impulses may be conducted
to the cerebellum and may influence the coordination of movements
that are initiated by efferent impulses originating in this section of
the brain.

VOLITIONAL CONTRIBUTION TO MOTOR ACTION

Motor acts are often initiated by a decision (activity originating
in the cerebral cortex). That decision does not include conscious, detailed direction of the joint actions that will be needed. Studying motion pictures of our own performance, we often observe movements
that suprise us. The mind orders "whole," and the details occur without conscious direction. The neuromuscular system selects its own
methods of achieving the goal set. It is through practice with feedback
from many sources that learning occurs. According to Burke (1986),

The ability to perform at the limit of physical capacity is the essence of competitive sport. This must involve training not only the muscles, which are marvelously adaptable, but also the nervous system, which is no less so. Optimum usage of muscles may well require strategies of usage for which the usual sequence of recruitment is poorly adapted.

It is important that individuals practice new skills, or skills they wish to improve, at the same speed and under the same conditions as the performance is to take place. The recent works by Grimby (1986) and many others show that motor units are recruited differently and in different patterns based on the task. If our motor system is to "learn" the new skill, it must be practiced accurately.

A national women's golf champion was asked what she thought about as she prepared to take a shot. She answered, "I see the shot, then feel it, and then I do it." (Further questioning revealed that "seeing" meant visualizing the needed height and distance.) A basketball coach of national repute was asked how he developed skill in shooting from the free-throw line. His reply was identical to that of the golfer. He asked the players to visualize the high point of the shot and feel it before beginning the movement. A British scientist believes that it is more important to know what to do than how to do it and suggests that the less a performer knows about the details of the act, the more efficient that act is likely to be.

The lack of cortical control of specific joints and muscles is supported by the investigations of Gellhorn (1953), who reported that stimulation of certain points of the motor cortex results in definite patterns of movement. Among these are such combinations as (1) flexion at the elbow, extension of the wrist, and protraction of the arm; (2) extension at the elbow, flexion at the wrist, and retraction at the shoulder; and (3) flexion at the knee, dorsiflexion at the ankle, and extension at the elbow. Furthermore, Gellhorn found that the same parts of the body could be moved when different cortical points were stimulated: the movement of the lips in speaking and in mastication can be activated from different cortical points, as can flexion of the thumb and closure of the hand, which involve the flexors of the thumb. The concept that movements rather than muscles are represented in the cortex has received increasing emphasis in the last two decades.

The specific movements activated in the cortex are characteristic of the species; they are not unique for each individual. It seems miraculous that even though there are millions of nerve cells in the central nervous system and millions of muscle fibers in the human body, and even though muscles and nerves develop independently in the embryo and during infancy, the connections that develop between muscles and nerves are normally common to all individuals. An explanation for these common connections is given by Sperry (1959), who says that as nerves develop from the central system, each nerve has a predestined terminal contact point and is guided to this point by a chemical environment. Each nerve fiber as it grows develops numerous ramifications through which it makes contact with numerous cells, but chemical affinity determines which of these ramifications will develop into specialized synapses capable of transmitting a nerve impulse. Among the supporting experiments that Sperry presents is one in which he transposed the nerves connecting the skin of the left and right hind feet of rats. After the nerves regenerated, a mild shock to the sole of the right foot caused the animal to lift the left. During the experiments; some of the animals developed a sore on the stimulated foot, and they then hopped about on three feet but raised the uninjured foot. In another series of experiments, the optic nerve of the newt was cut, and the eyeball was rotated 180 degrees. After recovery, the animal responded to visual stimuli as if they were seen upside down. The severed nerves had evidently grown attachments to those sections of the eye to which they were normally connected. Observations such as those of Gellhorn and Sperry provide explanations of the common patterns of human action that are observed to occur without conscious control or awareness.

INVOLUNTARY DETAILS OF MOTOR BEHAVIOR

The involuntary details of common human motor behavior can be attributed to reflex action and inherent motor patterns. Observers of infant behavior, notably Gesell (1940) and McGraw (1943), have reported the age range within which certain reflex acts appear. Their observations may be interpreted as follows: as the infant matures, the reflex action comes under voluntary control and appears as part of a volitional act. The stepping actions that an infant 2 to 3 weeks old will make when held upright with the feet contacting a surface continue to operate reflexively in voluntary walking. The weaving of reflex patterns into voluntary movements may well explain the involuntary details of volitionally initiated movement patterns. Many reflexes continue to exist throughout life, such as the Babinski Reflex to stroking the sole of the foot.

Stretch Reflexes (Myotatic Reflex)

The knee jerk, patella-tendon reflex, is perhaps the most widely recognized human reflex. A sharp blow on the tendon at the knee results in a sudden stretch in the knee extensor muscles and initiates a nerve impulse in the afferent nerve fibers of the muscle spindles, which conducts the impulse to the spinal cord and then to the gray matter of the anterior horn cells where the afferent fibers synapse with dendrites of anterior horn cells. The impulse is then conducted via the axon of the motor cells to the muscle fibers of the knee extensors, and as these contract, the leg is rapidly extended. This type of response is also elicited when the pressure of the tendon is a steady pressure rather than a sharp blow.

The voluntary concept and the reflex can be visualized in an act such as holding a weight in the hand with the forearm flexed 90 degrees. The intent of the performer is to maintain this angle, with the mind ordering the act in its entirety. The stretch on the elbow flexion signals to the muscle the number of motor units needed. If the weight is increased or decreased, reflex information via the muscle spindle provides the needed adjustment in strength of contraction. The sensitivity of this response can be adjusted with the gamma efferents. When a person knows he/she is to receive a sudden change of weight, there will be little change in the elbow flexion due to the high sensitivity of the stretch receptors. However, if weight is added when the person least expects it, the response will be slower and the change in elbow angle will be much greater.

The stretch, or myotatic, reflex is widely distributed in the body and is especially well developed in antigravity muscles. In the description of the mechanical aspects of standing, the center of gravity of the body is known to be normally in front of the ankle joint. Gravitational force would pull the body forward, causing ankle flexion. The resulting stretch on the ankle extensors initiates the nerve impulses that control the amount of contraction needed to maintain the position that the performer intends. If the forward lean approaches the limits of easy balance, stretch increases and the stimulation to the ankle extensors increases, and the increase in muscle contraction pulls the body back. The intent to stand keeps the ankle joint within a range of flexion that is not consciously controlled. This is termed the gamma bias. With high-heeled shoes, the amount of stretch in the ankle flexors must be adjusted to accommodate the changed position.

This slack is taken up by the gamma efferents in the muscle spindles.

If the intent is to walk, run, or jump, the degree of ankle flexion is increased, as shown in Chapters 9, 15, 16, which illustrate joint actions. Ankle flexion is permitted to the extent necessary for the specific act. Then the ankle joint may be held stationary as the foot is raised and later extended at an angular rate that exactly parallels that of the metatarsophalangeal action. Basically these joint actions are the same in the unskilled and the skilled. Some mechanism common to both must be in control. This mechanism is the stretch reflex.

In throwing and striking patterns, it is likely that the rapid backswing, by means of the stretch reflex, produces contraction of muscles needed for the forward swing. Based upon observations of muscle action, it is known that the muscles responsible for the forward swing begin their contractions before the limit of the backswing is reached. These contractions not only stop the backswing but also increase the nerve impulses initiated by the stretch and thereby increase the speed of the forward movement. This sudden activation of the muscle spindle will result in a more forceful, yet sometimes jerky, contraction. For skills requiring more precision, a slow backswing and/or a pause at the end of the backswing will reduce or eliminate this phasic response. This can be seen in the execution of the golf putt where a slow, controlled backswing is used.

MINI-LAB LEARNING EXPERIENCES

Hold your arm horizontally abducted. Slowly swing the arm backward. Note what happens at the end of the swing. Repeat this action, progressively swinging faster and faster. Note the response. Explain the mechanism responsible for the response.

The myotatic reflex is the simplest of those observed in human beings, since often only two neurons are involved. Other, more complex reflex actions that involve action in more than one level of the spinal cord have been observed. These may result in movement of more than one joint and in some cases movement in the contralateral (opposite) limb. A painful stimulus applied to the foot or hand activating the pain receptors will result in withdrawal of that limb by flexion of more than one joint (the flexor, or withdrawal, reflex). This action will also initiate impulses that contract extensors in the opposite limb, which are needed to maintain balance (the crossed-extensor reflex). For example, a person stepping on a nail will flex that leg and extend the other leg to keep from falling.

Righting Reflexes (Labyrinthine Reflex)

The reflexes that act together to maintain equilibrium are known as the righting reflexes; they act in normal standing when the adjustments are barely noticeable and also when there is greater threat to balance. When balance is threatened, many body parts, especially the arms, may be seen moving vigorously and widely. These efforts to bring the body's center of gravity over the feet, needless to say, are not always successful. A righting reflex is the response of the head to a loss in its upright position as a result of body movements changing the orientation of the head. For example, the reflex occurs as a lifting of the head when novices attempt a forward dive into a swimming pool.

Tonic-Neck Reflex

An interesting concept can be drawn from observation reported by Hellebrandt and co-workers (1961). When a weight was lifted by wrist flexion and wrist extension, it was observed that under stress other segments of the body were moved and that head movements resembled those of the tonic neck reflex. This reflex is noted in children and usually is volitionally controlled in adulthood. The tonic neck reflex is a response of the limbs to a rotation of the head. The turning of the head to the side is accompanied by movements in the upper and lower limbs (Fig. 6-7). On the side toward which the head is turned there are adduction at the shoulder and extension at the elbow in the upper limb and flexion at the knee in the lower limb. On the opposite side there are abduction at the shoulder and flexion at the elbow in the upper limb and extension at the knee in the lower limb.

The resulting position is that seen in the fencing lunge (lower limbs) and thrust (upper limb). After observing the appearance of the head movements, Hellebrandt and co-workers found that voluntarily turning the head to the working side increased the work output and turning the head to the opposite side decreased the output. The head position evidently affected the number of nerve impulses sent to the wrist muscles. Thus, it is evident that the position of segments other than those acting in a given pattern can affect performance.

The neck and labyrinthine reflexes are among the most important reflex mechanisms in sport and gymnastic skills; for example, divers and tumblers use head movements to facilitate body spin, to flex or extend the limbs and trunk when these movements are desired in a stunt, and to attain correct position at the finish.

Reflexes may facilitate or inhibit volitional movements. For example, the tonic neck reflex inhibits the forward tuck somersault motion because cervical flexion causes the lower limbs to extend. This same reflex facilitates the backward tuck somersault because cervical extension causes the lower limbs to flex. When the head is turned to the side away from the striking arm in racquet sports, the tonic neck reflex causes arm flexion, which causes the person to "miss the ball." The old adage "Keep the eye on the ball," is well founded.

Gardner (1969) also states that understanding reflex mechanisms is valuable when successful performance requires voluntary inhibi-

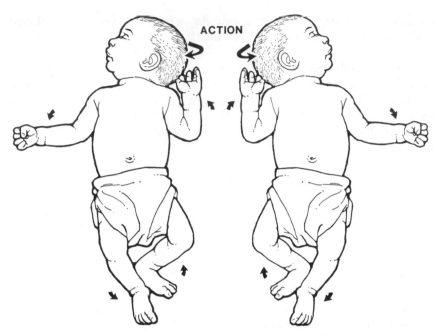

Fig. 6-7. *Tonic neck reflexes. The turning of the head is an action that elicits a response of the upper and lower extremities as shown by unlabeled arrows. Can you see why the turning of the head away from a working arm would increase the strength output of that arm? Although you can volitionally repress this reflex, can you think of ways you might want to allow it to happen to enhance a performance?*

tion of the associated joint actions, such as pivoting in the golf swing without swaying. She makes this point succinctly by saying, "One must inhibit 'what comes naturally.'"

Inherent Motor Patterns

Although reflex actions are inherent patterns, a division is made here to distinguish those which have a conscious purpose from those which are reactions to stimuli that arise in some part of the nervous system other than the cerebral cortex. Thus withdrawal from intense heat occurs without conscious intent; the withdrawal is often said to occur before one is aware of the pain. A reflex response does not vary, whereas a purposeful inherent pattern, characterized by basic similarities, is not stereotyped. If the human overarm throw is an inherent pattern, the details of performance may differ in individuals and in the same individual at various times, but basic similarities will be present. These responses are not learned: they appear without learning. One writer used the term action or behavior pattern and defined it as the traditional series of steps by which an objective is achieved. (This definition is closely related to this text's classification of human patterns according to purpose.) The writer also states that an action pattern is as typical of a particular species as is the structure of the animal, and that sometimes species are identified by their action patterns.

Inherent Motor Patterns in Human Beings

As human throwing, striking, and locomotion patterns are studied, common elements are evident. Of course, these elements could be learned, but they can be seen in the performance of young children who have had no instruction. We can state with confidence that even children who have an opportunity to observe skilled performers would not be aware of details of action. Selected tracings taken from a detailed study of the overarm throwing pattern of David, a 33-month-old boy appear in Fig. 6-8. He had no instruction in throwing; yet the elements of skillful performance are present. In A he is seen as forward movement begins. The weight is on the right foot; the left is lifted from the floor; the pelvis is rotated to the right over the supporting foot; the head faces in the direction of the throw. In B the left foot has been placed forward to facilitate rotation of the pelvis over that limb; the position of the throwing arm has changed little. In the 0.23 second between B and C, lateral rotation in the left hip has turned the torso in the direction of the throw, and rotation of the humerus has carried the elbow ahead of the ball. This is an interesting aspect of timing—forward rotation of one segment and simultaneous backward rotation of another. It is interesting to speculate what the actions would be if they were attempted by conscious direction. Two elements that would be seen in a more skillful performer are lacking: (1) no vertebral action is in evidence—the torso acts as a unit—and (2) the humerus has not held its position in the transverse plane but has been adducted. The position at release is shown in D, 0.03 second after the action shown in C. Rotation of the torso has continued, the humerus has rotated medially, the elbow has extended slightly, and

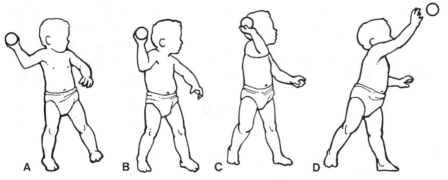

Fig. 6-8. *Tracings based on film of overarm pattern of boy 33 months of age who had no instruction. Joint actions and their sequences resemble those of highly skilled performers and are thought to be an inherent basic pattern of movement. Analyze the spatial characteristics of this throw with respect to axes of rotation, planes of segmental movement, and sequencing of segmental movements.*

THE HUMAN COMMUNICATION SYSTEM

the hand has undoubtedly flexed. The observer can only marvel at the coordinations that result from the intent to throw. Mature underarm and sidearm patterns were also demonstrated by this boy and other boys of preschool age. No observations were made of girls.

Locomotor patterns (walking, running, jumping, and leaping) are performed by young children. As everyone knows, the complicated coordination of walking and running develop without instruction. Detailed observation leads us to speculate that the young child's nervous system controls movements within the limits that ensure balance. As running movements first appear, at no time are both feet off the ground. The forward foot is on the ground before the rear foot leaves. With experience, the flight phase develops, and as skill is improved, the proportion of time of the flight phase during the running stride increases. As a two-footed takeoff for a jump is attempted, the nervous system of the young child refuses to allow the center of gravity to move forward unless one foot is moved ahead to receive the weight. This tendency can be seen at all ages perhaps because of lack of experience in attempting a two-footed takeoff. This pattern reappears with older persons (70- and 80-year-olds) who are asked to run and have not done so for many years. Projecting the body from one foot seems to be the natural, innate pattern.

Another tendency to preserve balance has been observed in the use of the arms in the standing long jump. Effective use consists of a forward swing in the sagittal plane on takeoff and a backward swing during flight, followed by a forward swing on landing. Researchers utilizing movie film have shown that elementary-school children and college women whose jumps are shorter than those of their peers do not swing the arms in the sagittal plane. Rather, the arms are held in horizontal abduction throughout the jump. (This resembles the action patterns of birds, whose wings are stretched to the side as they take off for flight and also during landing as the legs reach forward.) Unlearned joint action can also be observed in young children. A child under 3 years of age was observed as he jumped from a height equal to his own body height. The legs had been fully extended on takeoff; yet during flight the legs flexed to bring the feet forward for landing. This was not a learned movement; it was the first experience in that situation. What but inherent patterning could be the basis for the action?

Lorenz (1950) has stated that undoubtedly animals in general inherit behavioral traits. To suggest that human behavior follows a different pattern would be illogical. It differs only because of the greater human capacity to modify details of motor inheritance.

LEARNING MOTOR PATTERNS

If motor patterns are innate, one may logically question the need for learning. There are at least two apparent reasons for learning motor patterns. One is that even innate patterns improve with practice, and if patterns are not practiced during the time at which they appear naturally, they will never reach their full potential. Riesen (1950) reports that newly hatched chickens kept in darkness for 14 days after hatching failed to peck at spots on the ground when brought into the light. He concluded that prolonged lack of practice can interfere with the development of instinctive reflex behavior. He also reports that vision in chimpanzees will not be normal if the eyes are not exposed to light for an extended period after birth. Hess (1958) has shown that the instinctive following of a moving object, characteristic of the young of many animals and known as imprinting, is most strongly developed in mallard ducks if the experience occurs within 13 to 16 hours after hatching.

Since children at an early age, certainly before 6 years, have the basic patterns of throwing, striking, and locomotion, it is possible that if these patterns are not experienced at the time the nervous system is ready for them to be experienced, they will never reach their full potential. Ranson and Clark (1959) suggests this possibility when he says that the neurons of the nervous system of an adult human are arranged in a hereditary pattern but many of the details are shaped by the experiences of the individual.

The second reason for learning is that basic human patterns should and can be modified for specific situations. If the individual is aware of success or failure after performance, the pattern can often be modified without any conscious direction of joint action. This can be illustrated by experience with the previously mentioned 33-month-old boy. The boy had a running pattern, and an attempt was made to modify the run into a leap. A verbal description of how to do a leap was not attempted; instead a rolled mat was placed in the runway, and the boy was asked to clear it as he ran. In the first attempt, he took off from a running step and landed with both feet on the mat. No comments were made, and he attempted a second trial. This time he took off from the mat; he had moved the takeoff too far forward. The third trial was successful; he cleared the mat and landed on both feet (Fig. 6-9). He was then asked to continue running after clearing the mat. He then achieved a one-footed landing, which initially was not in balance, but which improved with successive trials. He had in mind a definite purpose as these adjustments were made; that intent was sufficient to modify joint action when he was aware of his failures. His mind had ordered a "whole" but had left the details of execution to those parts of the central nervous system below the level of consciousness.

In addition, this boy was led from a modification of the walking step into a standing long jump. When he was asked to execute a two-footed takeoff, one foot came forward to catch his weight. In an attempt to devise a situation that did not resemble so closely that of walking, he was placed on a platform 8 inches above the floor and asked to jump off the platform. He was able to jump without diffi-

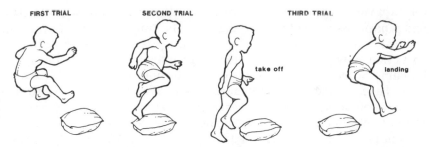

Fig. 6-9. *Motor adjustments made by boy 33 months of age as he attempted to clear obstacle. Although given no instruction he succeeded on the third trial, after first landing on the obstacle and next striking the obstacle during the takeoff phase. On all trials he utilized a pattern common to that of long jumpers taking off on one foot and landing on both feet.*

culty, although he had a tendency to lead with one foot. The height was increased to 15, to 20, and to 30 inches. The joint action of the lower limbs as he jumped from these heights took on the pattern of the standing long jump. Evidently the mind had developed the ability to order a given "whole." If the boy had been asked to jump toward an object held over his head, he could also have performed a standing jump for height. This conclusion is valid for other children, as well, since a purposeful intent brings into action the necessary joint movements. The learner can modify the innate patterns if the situation calls for the needed adjustments. The function of the teacher is to set up a situation that calls for the needed response.

Inexperienced jumpers can learn to develop the arm swing more rapidly if verbal suggestions are given. Young children of school age who fall backward on landing can swing their arms forward after verbal direction. After the suggestion to reach forward with the arms is given, this goal often results in a forward loss of balance on landing. Verbal suggestion adds a new goal—that of concentrating on a moving segment while one is executing a basic pattern. This is possible because the mind can be aware of movement.

The understanding of inherent motor patterns and reflex patterns is necessary to optimize the learning process. The biomechanist and the physical educator interested in studying, teaching, analyzing, and/or perfecting motor skills must know the effects and involvement of these patterns. Whether it be refining or modifying an inherent movement pattern, learning a novel task which may involve the inhibition of an innate reflex pattern, or the need to maximize a reflex pattern, knowledge of the basics of motor behavior is crucial.

PERCEPTION OF MOVEMENT AND POSITION

Usually a person can describe with substantial accuracy the position of various parts of his or her own body, even with closed eyes.

The skilled basketball player knows as soon as the ball is released whether the free-throw movements felt right and if the ball is likely to enter the basket. As stated previously, a skilled performer feels the action before executing it. This concept has been utilized in teaching through visualization and mental practice (also referred to as mental imagery). A number of motor-learning researchers have shown that a skill can be improved with mental practice, that is, by recalling the feel of the action and substituting successive recalls for physical practice. These recognitions of positions and feel are examples of memory of previous motor experience and of recalling activity in the cerbral cortex that accompanied motor acts and cerebral activity initiated by proprioceptors. Recently, commercial learning packages have been developed based upon this concept. These packages consist of repetitions of skilled performances that can be visually imaged and used as a supplement to physical practice of the skill.

Many kinds of memories are developed from cerebral activity— memories of sounds, sights, smells, touch sensations, and tastes. Each type of memory results from activity that was stimulated by a nerve impulse from a corresponding type of receptor. Memories of sound develop from impulses initiated in audioreceptors. Visual memories are recalled from those initiated in vision receptors. Yet, as far as is known, the nerve impulse initiated in one type of receptor does not differ from that initiated in any other type, as the impulse travels nerve pathways. The difference in recognition in the cerebral cortex results from the location in which the activity occurs. Cerebral activity initiated by visual receptors is in the lower rear of the cortex. Impulses from proprioceptors arrive in the cortex in a fairly large area that extends from the upper middle surface downward (Fig. 6-10).

The entire body is represented in Fig. 6-10, but the size of representation does not correspond to the size of body parts. The area that receives stimuli from the thumb is as large as that representing the trunk. The cortical representation parallels the density of sensory innervation from that part. When movement occurs, impulses are sent to that part of the cortex which represents the moving segments. The resulting cortical activity becomes associated with a specific movement, is recognized as accompanying the movement, and is the basis for memory of the act.

It is not known that impulses initiated in all types of proprioceptors reach the areas of the cortex shown in Fig. 6-10. When Sherrington demonstrated in 1894 that a nerve fiber from the muscle spindle conducted impulses to the spinal cord, it was thought that these impulses would reach the brain and be the basis for the cerebral activity that resulted in perception of movement and motor memory. Recent investigators agree that impulses from the spindle do go to the spinal cord but question whether they stimulate activity in the cortical area shown in Fig 6-10 It is thought that on reaching the spinal cord, these impulses may be directed to many muscles involved in the act, including the muscle in which they originated. In other words, these impulses coordinate the movement rather than develop memory or awareness.

Memory and awareness develop from impulses that originate in the proprioceptors found in tissue surrounding joints—ligaments, joint capsules, and adjacent connective tissue. As impulses from these receptors enter the spinal cord, they travel on neural fibers that extend up the posterior portion of the cord and terminate in the medulla, where they synapse with dendrites of cell bodies of neurons located in the medulla. The fibers of these neurons cross to the opposite side of the brain as they ascend, thus conducting impulses originating in the right side of the body to the left side of the brain and vice versa. These fibers terminate in the thalamus and synapse there with a third neuron, which conducts the impulses to the brain areas shown in Fig. 6-6. Feedback information regarding one's position of body parts and movement is known as kinesthesis. In addition to aiding us in the maintenance of balance, this feedback is the basis for how we learn motor skills. Without proprioceptive and other feedback information, accurate motor programming would not be possile.

REACTION TIME AND MOVEMENT TIME

Many sports rely on one's ability to respond as quickly as possible in a given situation. Examples are reacting to the gunshot at the beginning of a race or responding to the movement of an opponent or sport object as in guarding a basketball player or in stopping a soccer ball shot on goal. Much research has been conducted in the study of reaction time (RT), which is the time from the presentation of a stimulus to the beginning of the overt response, and movement time, which is the time to complete the action. A study of one without the other is not valuable from a practical point of view. For example, responding to an oncoming car requires reacting to visual stimuli and moving the body clear of the car.

Reaction time is comprised of several components: sense organ time (time needed for the sense organ to perceive the stimulus), nerve conduction time (time needed to conduct the impulses to and from the spinal cord), brain time (time needed for receiving, translating, and interpreting the message), and muscle development time (time needed for the muscle to develop the force needed to cause movement to occur). Brain time is the longest time interval and has the most variation depending on the situation.

Many factors affect one's reaction time. There is an optimum foreperiod (time interval between the presentation of a warning stimulus and the presentation of the stimulus) of between 1 and 4 seconds. If the stimulus arrives too quickly, the person is unprepared; if it arrives too late, readiness fades. Reaction time also varies with different sense modalities. Visual reaction time is slower than auditory and kinesthetic or proprioceptive reaction time (due to additional neural connections of the former). There are some problems in comparing

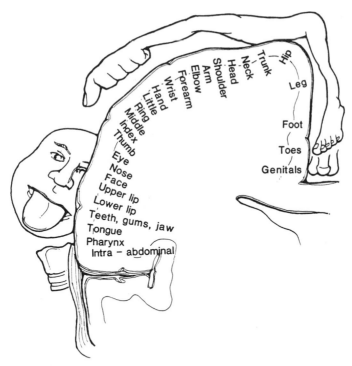

Fig. 6-10. *Topographic representation of somatic sensibility in postcentral human gyrus. Mapping of the brain continues to be done to better understand brain-body-mind interrelationships. (From Penfield, W., and Rasmussen, T,: The cerebral cortex in man; a clinical study of localization of function. New York: The Macmillan Co., 1950.)*

different modalities, however, due to different scales and different intensities of the signals. Reaction time increases with increased intensity of the stimulus to a certain extent. There are obviously many factors that affect one's ability to react. In order to obtain one's best reaction time, optimum conditions must exist.

In addition to factors that affect the reaction time within an individual, there are other factors that affect RT between groups. Researchers have shown that groups varying in gender and age have different reaction times. The reaction times for males tend to be faster than for females, although the difference is slight. Additionally, with increased age up to late teens and twenties, reaction time improves. The time to react to a stimulus during adulthood tends to increase with age. Since active people tend to react slightly faster, one would expect that the increase in RT with age can be counteracted the more active a person stays throughout life. Researchers have shown this to be true.

Points to Ponder

What are the typical reaction times required in various situations in daily life? Certainly sport situations are replete with quick reaction requirements. In daily life, however, there are frequent times when falling objects need to be caught to prevent breakage, movement must be stopped to prevent injury, or balance recovered in order to land on one's foot. Measure the time it takes for a served volleyball to arrive at the receiver. How much time do softball batters (slow-pitch and fast-pitch) and baseball batters have before they must initiate their swing? How much time does a soccer goalie or field hockey goalie have to respond to a penalty kick or flick on goal?

With respect to movement time, can one run faster backward than forward? Is the foot faster than the hand? Relate hand and foot speed to applying bicycling brakes. Should we block a blow with the right arm or the left arm? Is it faster to stop a stopwatch with the thumb or forefinger? Will practice improve any of these reaction times? Knowing reaction time and movement time abilities and capabilities is important to optimize learning and improvement of skill, as well as to generate safe movement situations.

MINI-LAB LEARNING EXPERIENCES

Using an ordinary ruler and the force of gravity, you can easily measure your own reaction time. Have a partner vertically suspend the end of the ruler between your thumb and forefinger. Have your fingers close to, but not touching, the ruler. Without warning, the partner is to drop the ruler so that it slides through your fingers. Pinch the ruler as quickly as possible as it passes. Record the distance (D) of the drop in centimeters to the nearest millimeter. Using the following formula, calculate your RT in seconds:

$$RT = \frac{2\,(D/100)}{9.8}$$

For a more accurate measure of RT, take the average of three trials. An average college student's simple visual RT is approximately .18 seconds. Compare your reaction times with the left and right hand. Holding the ruler against a wall one can also measure the foot's reaction time.

NEURAL ADAPTATION

Neural adaptation refers to possible changes occurring within the nervous system that allow production of strength and power to be enhanced. According to Sale (1986),

Strength and power performace is determined not only by the quantity and quality of the involved muscle mass, but also by the extent to which the muscle mass may be activated by voluntary effort . . . Strength and power training may cause changes within the nervous system that allow an individual to better coordinate the activation of muscle groups, thereby effecting a greater net force; even in the absence of adaptation within the muscles themselves.

Electromyography research consists of important information concerning tension-load and tension-velocity relationships, fatigue, strength development, learning, and responses to training. For example, there is a positive linear relationship between muscle tension and load, as well as between tension and velocity of performance (see Chapter 3). Thus, various motor units and muscle fibers may be in a state of tension depending on the speed and strength necessary to perform the movement.

Tension to produce a movement with the right arm will show irradiation to the contralateral arm. Contraction of one muscle to lift a very heavy object will require tension in many other muscles designed to stabilize body parts. Tension in a beginner will differ from that in a skilled performer.

Initial strength gains in strength training occur much too quickly for any adaptation within the muscle to occur. Increased voluntary strength in untrained limbs have also been found. The effects of strength training result in increases of voluntary strength largely specific to the types of contractions used in the training. As strength increases, as learning occurs, and as proficiency develops, the amount of tension and number of muscles producing tension will change; that is, they will be reduced. Since these changes are not accounted for solely by physiological changes in the muscles, the concept of neural adaptation has been proposed. The nervous system adapts the muscular contraction patterns until the most efficient one is found. Patterns of muscle tension in the prefatigued states indicate that there are a variety of ways in which persons utilize their muscles during activities requiring endurance. The relationship of each pattern to the actual endurance-time performance has not as yet been determined.

Since this area of research is relatively new, one can only speculate that the training of the nervous system may be the most important discriminator of the highly skilled performer of movement. According to Sale,

A question that is often raised in connection with neural adaptation to strength and power training is why humans are designed so that some motor units are so difficult or impossible to activate fully unless diligent training is performed or a crisis situation is faced. The answer usually given is that protection is provided by inhibitions that prevent the making of truly maximal contractions frequently and at a whim. . . .

If ways can be found to increase one's concentration and effort in training so that complete neural activation of the muscle is possible, coupled with mechanically accurate execution of the movement, the highly skilled performer will be able to achieve all that is capable of being achieved.

REFERENCES

Bard, P. (1961): *Medical Physiology*, ed. 11, St. Louis: C. V. Mosby Co.
Boyd, I. A., et al. (1964): *The role of the gamma system in movement and posture*, New York; Association of the Aid of Crippled Children.
Burke, R. E. (1986): The Control of Muscle Force: Motor Unit Recruitment and Firing Patterns, in Jones, N. L., et. al., *Human Muscle Power*, Champaign, IL: Human Kinetics.
Desmedt, J. E., editor (1973) *New Developments in Electromyography and clinical neurophysiology*, volumes 1, 2, 3, Basel, Switzerland: Karger.
Gardner, E. B. (1969): Proprioceptive reflexes and their participation in motor skills, *Quest*, 12:1.
Gellhorn, E. (1953): *Physiological foundations of neurology and psychiatry*, Minneapolis: University of Minnesota Press.
Gesell, A. (1940): *The embryology of behavior*, New York: Harper & Row, Publishers.
Gowitzke, B. A. and Milner, M. (1980) *Understanding the scientific bases of human movement*, ed. 2, Baltimore: The Williams & Wilkins Co.
Grimby, L. (1986): Single Motor Unit Discharge during Voluntary Contraction and Locomotion, in Jones, N. L., et al., *Human Muscle Power*, Champaign, IL: Human Kinetics.
Hellebrandt, F. A. (1958) The physiology of motor learning, *Cereb. Palsy Rev.* 10:9.
Hellebrandt, F. A., Rarick, G. L., Glassow, R. and Carns, M. L. (1961): Physiological analysis of basic motor skills, *Am. J. Phys. Med.* 40:14.
Hess, E. (1958): Imprinting in animals, *Sci. Am.* 198:81, March.
Kumamoto, M., editor (1984) *Neural and mechanical control of movement*, Kyoto: Yamaguchi Shoten Publishing House.
Lorenz, K. Z. (1950): The comparative method in studying innate behaviour patterns. In Danielle, J. F., and Brown, R., editors: *Symposia of the Society for Experimental Biology, No. 4: Physiological mechanisms in animal behaviour*, Cambridge, England: Cambridge University Press.
Lorenz, K. A. (1958): The evolution of behavior, *Sci. Am.* 199:67, December.
McGraw, M. (1943): *The neuromuscular maturation of the human infant*, New York: Columbia University Press.
Moore, J. C. (1969) *Neuroanatomy simplified*, Dubuque, IA: 1969, Kendall/Hunt Publishing Co.
Mountcastle, V. B., ed. (1974): *Medical Physiology*, v. 1, ed. 13, St. Louis,: C. V. Mosby Co.
O'Connell, A. L. and Gardner, B. (1972) *Understanding the scientific bases of human movement*, Baltimore: The Williams & Wilkins Co.
Ranson, S. and Clark, S. L. (1959) *Anatomy of the nervous system*, ed. 10, Philadelphia: W. B. Saunders Co.
Riesen, A. (1950) Arrested vision, *Sci. Am* 183:16, July.
Sage, G. H. (1977): *Introduction to Motor Behavior*, ed. 2, Reading, PA: Addison-Wesley, p. 123.
Sale, D. (1980) Chronic plasticity in reflex pathways: effects of training, and disuse, paper presented at the Symposium on Spinal Regulation of Muscle, American College of Sports Medicine, Las Vegas.
Sale, D. G. (1986): Natural Adaptation in Strength and Power Training, in Jones, N. L., et al., *Human Muscle Power*, Champaign, IL: Human Kinetics.
Schmidt, R. F. (1978): Motor Systems, in *Fundamentals of Neurophysiology*, ed. 2, New York: Springer-Verlag, p. 198.
Sherrington, C. (1933) *The brain and its mechanism*, Cambridge, England: Cambridge University Press.
Sherrington, C. (1953) *Man on his nature*, ed. 2, Garden City, NY: Doubleday & Co., Inc.
Sherrington, C. (1961) *The integrative action of the nervous system*, New Haven, CT: Yale University Press.
Sperry, R. W. (1939) Action current study in movement coordination, *J. Gen. Physiol.* 20:295.
Sperry, R. W. (1956) The eye and the brain, *Sci. Am.* 194:48, May.
Sperry, R. W. (1959) The growth of the nerve circuits, *Sci. Am.* 201:68, November.

Part II   Analysis of Human Movement

The How, What and Why

7

Tools for Assessment, Improvement and Prediction of Movement

As might be expected, the tools used in the study of biomechanics of human movement are strong determinants of the types of analyses that will be possible. The nature, type, and magnitude of data will be limited by the tools selected. Quantitative force data, for example, is impossible to obtain through visual perception. Limited qualitative inferences concerning force, however, may be possible. The eyes "record" only temporal and spatial changes, and the brain translates these into a perceived essence of movement.

Many tools are available, at varying costs. Some tools are more sophisticated than others and require greater training for operation. But even the least sophisticated tool requires training in its use if maximum analysis data are to be achieved. The common tools (including instrumentation systems) are listed as follows:

1. Human eye and other senses;
2. Anthropometry: measurements of human body;
3. Timing devices;
4. Artificial optical devices (photography): single image, cinematography, stroboscopy, videography;
5. Electrogoniometry: joint kinematics;

6. Electromyography: muscle action;
7. Dynamography: force production;
8. Accelerometry: acceleration.
9. Modeling and simulation: computer manipulation of the human body.

Each of these tools or systems will be defined, explained historically, and described in detail. The reader will then be able to select the best tool or tools for the specific biomechanics analysis project. Additional resources are listed at the end of the chapter. In addition, a series of five instrumentation videotapes are available from the publisher of this book. These tapes include information concerning electromyography and electrogoniometry, high-speed cinematography, digitizing, force platform, analysis, and force insoles with telemetry.

HUMAN EYE AND OTHER SENSES

Published works and principles based on the analysis of movement of living things have been known in Western civilization since the era of the ancient Greeks. The Greeks were among the first to practice so-called scientific thinking, as opposed to that based on emotional and spiritual ideas.

Hippocrates (460–377 B.C.) advocated the concept that people should base their observations on and draw conclusions from only what they perceived through their senses (particularly those of touch, sight, hearing, and smell) without recourse to the supernatural. One of Hippocrates' contemporaries, the Greek scholar Herodicus, was interested in gymnastics (exercise through active volition) as a means of curing disease. In fact, he prescribed it for fever patients and was criticized by Hippocrates for doing so.

Aristotle (384–322 B.C.) has been called the father of kinesiology. Aristotle made his many observations in almost every field of science. Students of kinesiology have been especially impressed with his treatise Parts of Animals, Movement of Animals, and Progression of Animals.

The scientific awakening known as the Renaissance was perhaps initiated and epitomized by the work of Leonardo da Vinci who is given credit for developing the modern science of anatomy. He studied human structure, especially noting the relation of the center of gravity to balance and motion during different movements. He made these observations while he was developing a treatise on painting. To be sure that his drawings of the body were authentic, da Vinci secured and dissected hundreds of cadavers. He was adept in many fields and blended the artistic with the scientific in a way never since duplicated. According to several historians, da Vinci was the greatest engineer, biologist, and artist of his time. Robinson stated that da Vinci was one of the first to break away from the acceptance of Galen, an early Roman physician, as the only authority. He was severely criticized by his contemporaries because he did not blindly follow noted authorities. Leonardo da Vinci said:

> I do not know how to quote from learned authorities, but it is a much greater and more estimable matter to rely on experience. They scorn me who am a discoverer; yet how much more do they deserve censure who have never found out anything, but only recite and blazen forth other people's work (Robinson).

Da Vinci's observations on human action in a specific movement show his insight. He said, "He who descends takes short steps because the weight rests upon the hinder foot. And he who mounts takes long steps because his weight remains on the forward foot" (Hart).

Even today, observation of motion of living beings, dissection of cadavers, reading of published works, and perusal of clinical records of injury are methods of investigating movement empirically. The data obtained are often limited and qualitative in nature and quite often are erroneous as well. Because of these errors, the discarded "facts" of one era are replaced by another set of "facts" in another era of history (O'Malley and Saunders).

The other senses (auditory, olfactory, tactile, and kinesthetic) have not been used as commonly as the eye to analyze human movement. The human ear can be used as commonly as the eye to analyze human movement. The human ear can be used in much the same way as the human eye in identifying the components of the movement. In this case, the perceiver can record the temporal aspects via the time intervals between sounds. In addition, the relative forces of the movement may be perceived via the changes in loudness. The seismograph is a tool that has been used extensively to record sound vibrations and rank earthquake severity. Several decades ago, prior to our high technology in biomechanics, a series of seismographs were placed at intervals along a running track, and the speed of runners was calculated based upon the vibration pattern recorded on a kymograph (rotating drum of paper upon which a pen inscribed the deflections). Recently, acoustics are being used in medicine to better understand the biomechanics of body substances and parts, such as flow of blood, exchanges of air during respiration, and the contractions of the heart. Use of these devices has not entered the non-medical world of human movement analysis.

Tactile and kinesthetic senses probably are best used in self-analysis. An understanding of the contact components of a movement and the specific "body feelings" of a particular movement, however, could be valuable when attempting to improve patterns of persons who are mentally retarded, victims of strokes, athletes, and other special populations. Folk dances can be analyzed from a tactile perspective. Table 7-1 is an example.

A combination of the senses could be used to analyze this folk

Table 7-1. *Folk dance step pattern and the corresponding body part receiving tactile stimulation. Qualitative assessment of movement pressures can be made using this scheme.*

Movement	Body Part Receiving Tactile Stimulation
touch right heel to floor	heel
touch right toe to floor	toe
step side with right foot	sole
step side with left foot	sole
step side with right foot	sole
step lift left heel	toe
slap hands to thigh 3 times	anterior thigh, palms
clap hands	palms

dance pattern. The movements would be analyzed via the eyes and the rhythm would be recorded via the ear.

Anthropometry

Not strictly a biomechanics tool, anthropometry is used to obtain basic information concerning the structure of the human body so that this information can be used to estimate forces acting upon the joints and other body tissues and the forces produced by the dynamics. Anthropometry is the measurement of the human body. The body and its segments are measured with respect to lengths, widths, diameters, circumferences (girths), and areas. Ratios and proportions based on two or more of these measurements are calculated, and shapes, sizes, and topography identified. One of the earliest studies in anthropometry related to human movement, gait in particular, was conducted by two German scientists, Braune and Fischer in the 19th Century. In 1889, these two outstanding German anatomists published a comprehensive paper on an experimental method thay they had developed to determine the center of gravity of the human body. Adolf Eugen Fick (1829–1901) drew on their work; he eventually became one of the outstanding authorities in the field of joint mechanics. Today's concepts on posture appear to have had their origin in the experiments of Braune and Fischer. Earlier methods of locating the center of gravity of the human body had proved to be ineffective, and Braune and Fischer introduced modifications of some procedures. First, they conceived of a way of freezing a dead body so that it remained unchanged while they made mathematic calculations. Second, they compared the frozen posture of a cadaver with the posture of a living person and found the two postures to be markedly similar. They located the center of gravity not only of the body as a whole but also of each component part. They were the first to estimate the percentage of the weights of body segments. After they located the center of gravity of the total body of the frozen cadavers, they cut two of them into body segments and located the center of gravity of each. Much of their work involved the use of photographic apparatus to obtain the evidence they needed for locating the midpoints of a joint and the axes of rotation.

Segmental body weights and centers of mass of each segment are indispensable for determining solutions to modeling and simulation of static postures. Other inertial characteristics of the human body and its parts are required for modeling dynamic movement. These characteristics are the moments of inertia and radii of gyration. Selected values and detailed descriptions of anthropometric techniques appear in the chapter on occupational biomechanics and in the resources at the end of this chapter, most notably the anthropometric data bases and review articles by Hay. Common anthropometric tools are depicted in Fig. 7-1.

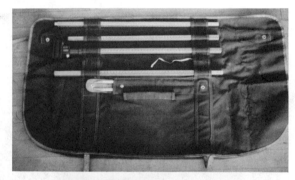

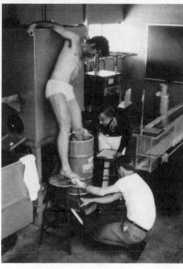

Fig. 7-1. *A. Anthropometric kit and its use in measuring body lengths, widths, and circumferences. Identification of anatomical landmarks is crucial if accurate measurements are to be obtained. B, Water immersion method for determining center of gravity and weight of body segment. In this procedure the scale is used to measure the weight of tank, water, and immersed body segment. How can the center of mass of the body segment be determined using this method?*

TOOLS FOR ASSESSMENT 199

TIMING DEVICES

A variety of timing devices (chronoscopes), including stop watches, counters, digital timers, switch mats, photo electric cells, real-time computer clocks, and laser tubes are being used to record speeds of the human being and its body parts. The outcome of movements (simple, complex, and sequential) is easily assessed. A chronoscope is started at a preselected instant in time, usually the initiation of the movement. At another instant in time, the chronoscope is stopped. Speed of movement is calculated by dividing the chronoscope time by the known displacement of the movement. An even simpler device is to use a radar gun for instant speed display. (See Fig. 7-2.)

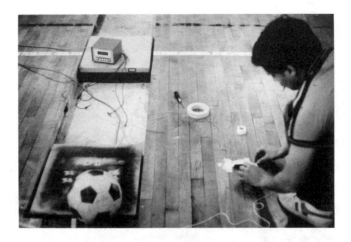

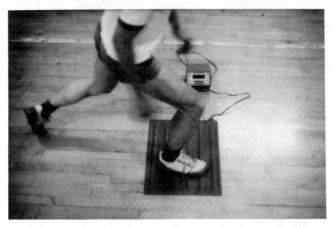

Fig. 7-2. *Timing devices are of many types including digital clocks interfaced with switch mats or photoelectric cells to open to start or stop the clock, as well as complex devices to record coordination or balance. (Compliments of Lafayette Instrument Company, Lafayette, Indiana).*

THE BIOMECHANICS OF HUMAN MOVEMENT

PHOTOGRAPHY AND CINEMATOGRAPHY

Since the flicker response of the human eye is 10–12 frames per second, the human eye cannot see the particulars of a fast motion. Furthermore, since the eye doesn't retain the total motion investigators turned to various devices to provide permanent images of movement.

A French physiologist, Etienne Jules Marey (1830–1904), was so interested in human movement that he developed photographic means for use in biologic research. In his works *Du Mouvement dans les Fonctions de la Vie and De Mouvement,* he explained and illustrated how this could be accomplished. Some of the translated works include the history of chronophotography and lectures on the phenomenon of flight in the animal world. Marey, as well as Robinson, was convinced that movement was the most important human function and affected all other activities.

Eadweard Muybridge (1830–1904), through his photographic skill, brought a new tool to kinesiological investigation. He was motivated by the work of Janssen, an astronomer who had been successful in taking sequential pictures of stars. Among the numerous Muybridge publications was an 11-volume work, Animal Locomotion (1887). A later publication called The Human Figure in Motion contains much of his original work. Using 24 fixed cameras and 2 portable batteries of 12 cameras each, Muybridge was able to take pictures of animals (Fig. 7-3) and people in action, and by using the zoopraxiscope he could mechanically move the pictures fast enough that actual movement was simulated. As an illustration of how an idea may be developed, Muybridge modified this device by mounting transparencies made from a series of his photographs on a circular glass plate. When the plate was rotated, individual transparencies could be projected by a projection lantern in the usual manner. A major refinement of the device was the addition of a second plate made of metal and mounted parallel to the glass plate on a concentric axis, but turning in the opposite direction. The metal plate was slit at appropriate intervals. When the two plates revolved, the metal plate served as a shutter. The persistence of vision between each slit gave the viewer the illusion of motion as each individual picture in the series was projected. As many as 200 transparencies could be mounted on a single plate, and the wheels, or plates, could be revolved endlessly, "a period limited only by the patience of the spectators."

The accomplishments of Marey and Muybridge paved the way for two German scientists, Christian Wilhelm Braune (1831–1892) and Otto Fischer (1861–1917), to study the human gait by means of photographic devices.

Photography has become sophisticated since those nineteenth-century experiments. Many investigations of human and animal movements are conducted by means of movie cameras (super 8mm, 35mm, or 16mm) capable of filming at rates up to 500 images per

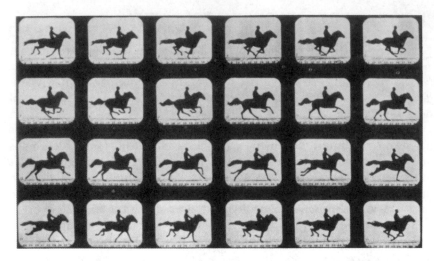

Fig. 7-3. *Motion of running horse. This is a classic psuedo-cinematographic product of Eadweard Muybridge in the late 1800's. The horse is Phryne L, whose length of stride was reported to be 6 m 2 cm (19 ft 9 in). (Courtesy Stanford Museum.)*

second, which is approximately 50 times the number of images the human eye can detect. Other cameras operating at 40,000-plus filming rates are utilized in collision and other impact studies of body deformation and destruction.

Single Image Photography

A single-image camera (126,35mm, portrait, etc.) may be used to analyze selected positions during a movement pattern. For example, the posture used to "address" the golf ball, to operate a typewriter, to get ready to swing an axe, or to prepare to lift a 900 N (202.5 lbs) barbell can be photographed and compared to other postures. A series of photographs of one movement pattern can be obtained with devices such as a graph sequence camera or an automatic rapid advance 35mm camera (Fig. 7-4).

Another common type of still photography, with the illusion of motion, is stroboscopy or intermittent light photography. Figure 7-5 depicts an example of the results of such a technique.

Stroboscopic photography uses multiple exposures on a single negative, which may be exposed to a brightly lighted or a dark background and to a subject. In the first case, the exposures are determined by the opening of the camera shutter at a set rate. An inexpensive technique for achieving a simulated shutter opening/closing sequence is to fabricate an external rotating shutter, as shown in Fig. 7-6.

In this case, the shutter remains open, and light illuminates the negative at intermittent intervals. For example, small electric light bulbs are attached to points on the body. These lights may be illu-

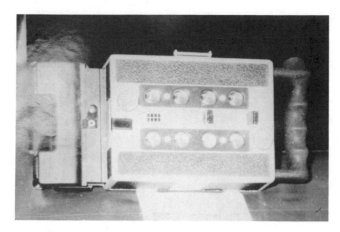

Fig. 7-4. *Graph sequence camera. This is an inexpensive way to obtain eight photographs at set time intervals. Newer 35mm cameras with rapid sequence advance can not achieve the short time interval of this multiple lens camera.*

minated continuously, resulting in a line of light on the photograph, or they may flash at a set rate, resulting in a series of dots on the photograph, (Fig. 7-7).

A stroboscopic light (true stroboscopy) may illuminate at set in-

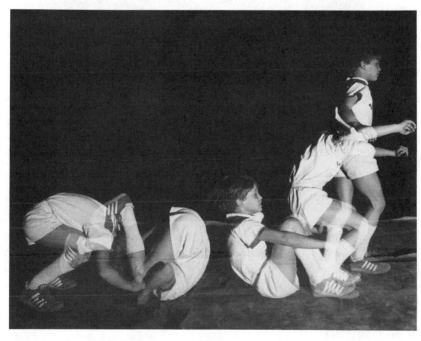

Fig. 7-5. *A stroboscopic photograph. Note the five distinct images taken at equal increments in time. Speed can be deduced by the position of the hair on the third image. Study the images and determine distances of travel and angles at joints that can be measured.*

TOOLS FOR ASSESSMENT

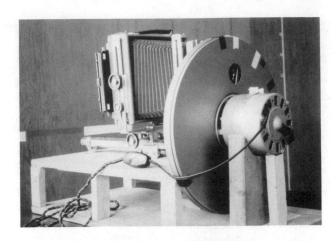

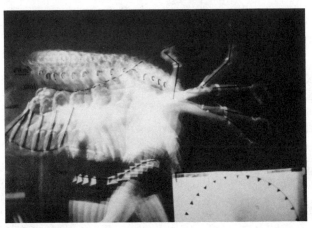

Fig. 7-6. *An inexpensive intermittent light photography system made from a portrait camera, a disk with one or more slits, an empty film reel cannister, and a motor to rotate the disk. The camera shutter is opened for the entire time of filming and light enters only when the slit of the disk rotates in front of the shutter. An example of a photo obtained from this system is included. Contrast this with figure 7-5.*

tervals the subject or reflective markers placed on the subject. This is by far the most expensive method since a large power supply is required to trigger the strobe light at successive short intervals of time. An interesting and comprehensive description of the history of high-speed stroboscopy by the "father of stroboscopy", Edgerton, can be found in the NATIONAL GEOGRAPHIC magazine, October 1987. The color photographs, alone, are worth the trip to the library.

Movie Cameras

Although "home movie cameras" exist, their use has been superceded by home video cameras. The home movie camera could be operated at 16–24 frames per second. The home video camera has the

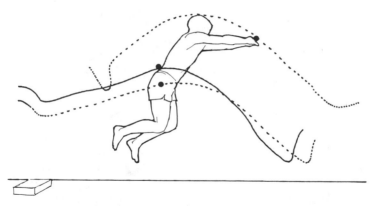

Fig. 7-7. *Light bulbs attached to joints of performer and filmed with stroboscopic techniques. The person carries a small battery pack to power the light bulbs.*

equivalent of 30 frames per second (Fig. 7-8). The movie film, however, can be projected on any wall, screen or plate of glass, or other clear matter. Therefore data can easily be traced from the projected image, at varying sizes, even lifesize. Despite the advantage of image-size capabilities, the filmed images from these low-speed cameras usually were blurred with most fast movements.

Moderate-speed cameras are relatively inexpensive and can be operated at 64–128 frames per second to eliminate the blurs of movements slower than, or equal to, brisk walking. Such operating speeds and shutters of 1/64th to 1/128ths of a second are adequate for analysis of many activities of daily living and work tasks.

High-speed cameras (Fig. 7-9), however, are common and required, though expensive, tools for sports biomechanics.

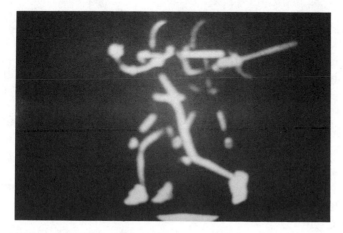

Fig. 7-8. *Photographic images taken from video monitor in playback pause mode. Note the two images representing the two fields of the image. (Image taken from Sybervision.)*

TOOLS FOR ASSESSMENT

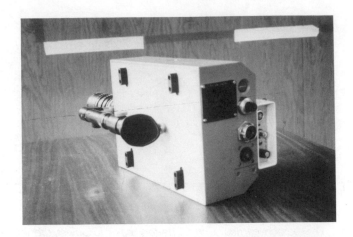

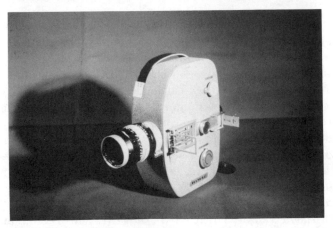

Fig. 7-9. *High speed cameras capable of operating at 500 images per second (LOCAM) and at higher rates (PHOTOSONICS). These cameras have built-in timing devices and can be phase-locked with other cameras for synchronized multiple image filming and synchronized with other data collection instrumentation systems.*

Many sports activities can be filmed at 80–150 frames per second if the shutter exposure time is short enough to reduce or eliminate the movement blur. If it is required to "capture" specific instances within the movement pattern, the camera will need to be operated at rates between 150–300 frames per second. Such applications, for example, include the filming of contact of a softball bat with a softball and the initial responses of the foot and leg to impact during the contact phases of a triple jump. Filming rates of 300–500 frames per second are required to precisely capture of collisions of 2 objects moving at high speeds, such as deformation of ball and tennis racquet strings during contact.

Filming rates are often expressed in units of Hz (cycles per second, derived from "electricity"). Thus 128 frames per second would be 128 Hz (128 cps).

3-D Cinematography

Since most naturally-performed human movements require a three-dimensional (3D) analysis, instrumentation systems have been deviced to capture, simultaneously, two or more views of the performance. This is possible via one camera and one or more mirrors or prisms, or via two or more cameras. The following set-ups have been most common:

1. One overhead mirror and one camera;
2. Stereophotogrammetry using 2 cameras in parallel (Fig. 7-10);
3. Three orthogonal cameras (Fig. 7-11).

Often the last set-up consists of the major plane-viewing camera being operated at a higher speed than the minor plane camera. For example, a sagittal view (side view) camera would be the major plane camera in the system of one frontal-view and one sagittal-view camera operating to film a long jump performance.

Cineradiography

Another form of photography used to film internal biomechanical research data is cineradiography. This technique consists of synchronizing a camera with a radiograph machine (x-rays) or fluoroscopic

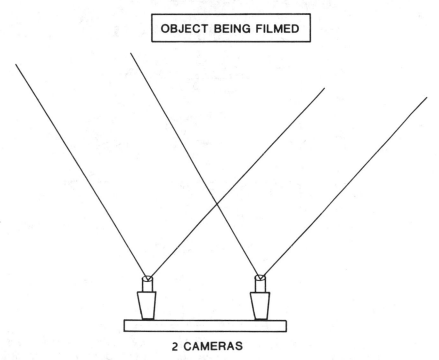

Fig. 7-10. *Stereophotogrammetry consists of two cameras placed parallel to each other. A typical set-up is depicted.*

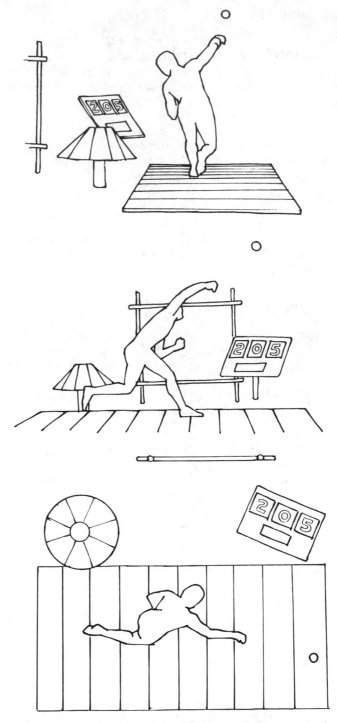

Fig. 7-11. *Rear, side, and overhead views taken to study overarm throw. Number 205 identifies subject and trial in series; note presence of cone-shaped timing device, as well as uprights and crossbars that establish vertical and horizontal lines to aid in measurement.*

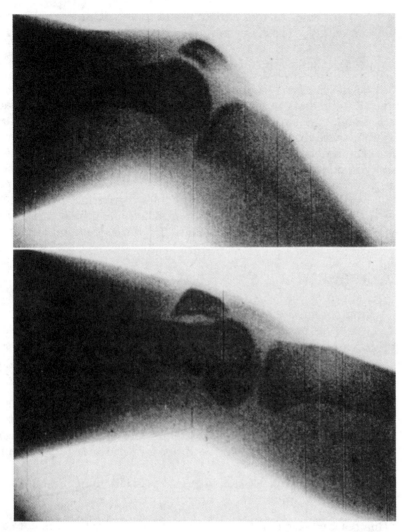

Fig. 7-12. *X-ray motion pictures of knee in kicking action. Note the displacement of the patella.*

machine. The bones are filmed in motion. Note the extreme position of the patella in Fig. 7-12.

Magnetic Resonance Imaging

The most recent tool to investigate the tissues and internal movements of the body is the magnetic resonance imaging (MRI). This is very expensive, but will become a major tool for computer modeling research. The exact position and status of a joint, for example, can be measured so that a "best-fit" prosthesis can be developed. Color is an important component of imaging and has been used extensively to identify positions and displacements of internal body organs and tissues. Excellent color images can be found in the SOMA articles cited and discussed later in this text.

Computerized Cinematography

Although analysis of single-image films or movie films may be conducted by means of physically tracing and measuring displacements of one image at a time and then calculating other motion variables from these displacements, since the late 1960's, researchers have utilized computerized film analysis systems. These systems have processing components for numerically and graphically printing displacement, velocites, acceleration, moments of force, centers of gravity, etc., as well as statistical data. A digitizing tablet is interfaced with a computer so that an almost infinite amount of data can be obtained in a short period of time, if the appropriate software is available.

VIDEOGRAPHY

Taking advantage of high technology is possible without a great deal of training or money, since videosystems are inexpensive and readily available to the practitioner, technician, and general consumer. The advantages of videography compared to cinematography are as follows:

1. The ability to synchronize two images on one screen, which is possible by means of a split-image, special-effects generator;
2. The direct and immediate transmission of the image to a computer, thus eliminating the human operator required in photographic analysis;
3. The direct playback capability, to provide immediate feedback to both the analyst and the performer.

One disadvantage is that the resolution of videotapes is not comparable to the highest quality of movie film, at least not presently at a reasonable cost.

Does high technology in videography exist? Oh, yes! As with cinematography, the changes in videography have been dramatic. Unknown prior to the 1950's, videography has nearly equalled or outdistanced cinematography in computerization, filming rates (20,000 Hz), and interfacing with other tools. Interfacing videography with a microcomputer is the least expensive high technology system for analyzing movement. The computer "grabs" an image and the human computer operator then digitizes the selected anatomical markers (Fig. 7-13).

A more expensive system consists of electronic digitizing, that is, non-human operated digitizing. The camera image "picks up" signals from devices of contrasting intensities that are electronically identified and located in space. The identifiable signals may be reflective

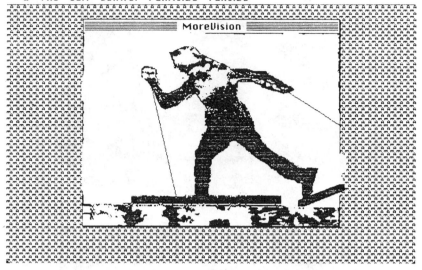

Fig. 7-13. *Video image grabbed by MacIntosh Microcomputer. The image can be reduced, portions enlarged, and it can be modified (for example, lines drawn connecting the joints of the body, background whitened) using the MacPaint or similar programs.*

tape illuminated by a bright light, light-emitting diodes, prisms of glass, tiny light bulbs or merely contrasting colors. The types and amount of data generated from these signals are limited by the electronic size of the computer and by the data analysis software. Examples of some of the high-tech video systems now available are depicted in Fig. 7-14. The human movement specialist can maximize the analysis of movements through knowledgeable selection of video components.

Camera

A color camera capable of indoor and outdoor use without extra lighting will be the most versatile. A shuttered camera, to eliminate the blur of regular videocamera images, is invaluable for sports movements, but not always necessary for most activities of daily living and work-skill analyses. Such shuttered cameras, however, usually require extra indoor lighting. Examples of images obtained via a regular videocamera and a shuttered camera (1/500th second exposure) are depicted in Fig. 7-15.

Microprocessors are standard equipment in many video cameras. Accessories also are available as add-ons. The advantages of these add-on devices are to title segments of the tape, to identify events, and to imprint a time-generated code on the tape. The images in Fig. 7-16 have time codes.

TOOLS FOR ASSESSMENT

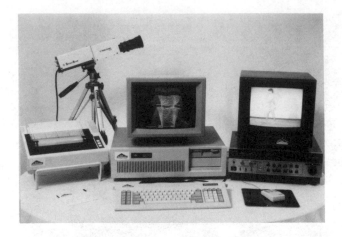

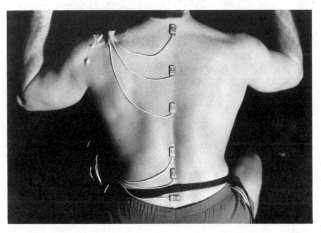

Fig. 7-14. *Examples of computerized video-type measurement systems. A, 2-D System, Courtesy of Peak Performance Technologies, Inc. B, light emitting diodes attached to subject for automatic 3-D position data input into a computer.*

Recorder

It is absolutely necessary to be able to still-image and image-by-image advance the videotape in the playback mode if time-effectiveness is sought. Any other recorder will involve too much trial-and-error and frustration to be efficient in selecting the appropriate images to analyze. There are 30 images per second on the commonly available recorder/playback units. Recently 60 fields per second (the ability to grab each of the two fields of each image separately) playback units have become available to the researcher. These are valuable for analyzing rapid movements, such as pitching a baseball, high jumping, and playing classical guitar.

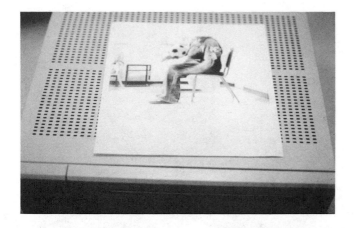

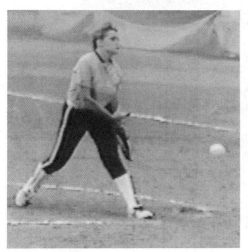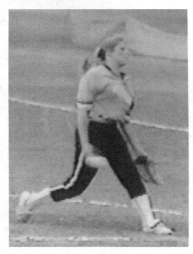

Fig. 7-15. *Reproductions of video images taken with regular video camera and high speed shutter video camera.*

ELECTROGONIOMETRY

Observation of joint action can be facilitated with the use of the electrogoniometer (also termed "elgon") which was devised by Karpovich in the late 1950's. The elgon is essentially a goniometer with a potentiometer substituted for the protractor. A goniometer is a device to measure (meter) angles (gonio), and consists of a potentiometer placed at the joint center, with two extensions attached to the body parts forming the joint. A potentiometer is a device similar to the volume control on a radio, that changes the resistance to the flow of electric current in a circuit. The degrees of movement in the joint to which the device has been attached can be read continuously and di-

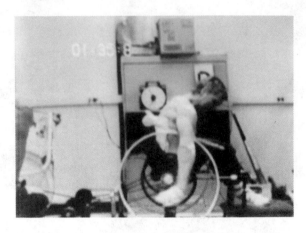

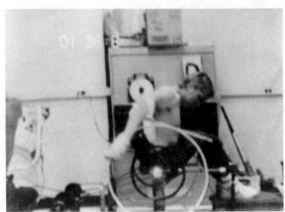

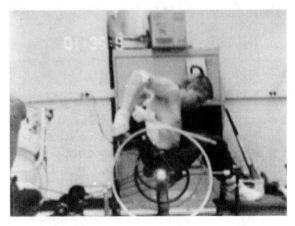

Fig. 7-16. *Video prints with time-generated code imprinted on sequenced images.*

THE BIOMECHANICS OF HUMAN MOVEMENT

rectly from an oscilloscope, recording paper or a computer, thus eliminating laborious measurement of each image of a photograph. The device has been used with other methods of recording movement; and has been especially useful combined with electromyography. A comprehensive description of the elgon and its application is presented by Adrian in the 1968 Kinesiology Review cited at the end of this chapter.

Three-dimensional electrogoniometers have been used in gait analysis in rehabilitation centers and laboratories and on the sports field. The advantages of electrogoniometry include the ability to record the action at the joint when it is not visible to the observer, such as during swimming and twisting movements. Another advantage is the instantaneous portrayal of angular displacement with respect to time. The electrogoniometry system can be linked to a computer to obtain angular velocities and accelerations. The use of a telemetry system (transmitting device and receiver with no wire connections, such as with radio and television systems) has been used to monitor joint angles of subjects from racehorses to swimmers to football players.

The goniogram, however, does not convey any spatial orientation of the limb, but solely the angle at the joint. There are other disadvantages, common to all devices attached to the body. The elgons must be fabricated of lightweight material, be non-interferring in nature, and fit the countours of the body. They must be attached to the average axis of rotation at the joint being studied and validated for proper placement for each joint. If many joints of the body are being investigated, the person will appear to be wearing an exoskeleton. An electrogoniometry system and the resulting goniogram (recording of angular displacement) are recorded in Fig. 7-17.

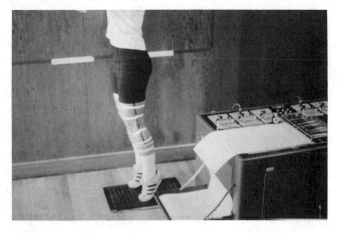

Fig. 7-17. *An electrogoniometry system, consisting of electrogoniometer (elgon), control panel, and recorder.*

ELECTROMYOGRAPHY

Muscle analysis based on anatomic position of muscles cannot be accepted as definitive of the action that occurs in the living, moving body. The fallacies of analyzing muscle action on the basis of anatomic position were demonstrated by Duchenne in the middle of the nineteenth century. On the basis of electrical stimulation of muscles, combined with observation of partially paralyzed subjects, he described the movements resulting from contraction of specific muscles as they functioned in living subjects. Unfortunately, his findings were not widely used in the United States, since they were published in French and were not readily available until translated in 1949 by Kaplan. By that time, investigators in the United States had begun to observe muscle action in living subjects by recording the electrical changes that could be observed by muscular contraction. The technique of recording, known as electromyography, has been greatly refined and, as complex motor acts are studied, will provide valuable information for the kinesiologist. The major current contributor to this development is J. V. Basmajian; his book *Muscles Alive* is a classic.

Electromyography (See Basmajian) is the process of recording electrical changes that occur in a muscle during or immediately before contraction. Necessary equipment for electromyography includes a device for picking up the electrical activity, a means for conducting the electrical impulses, and a device for translating them to visual form. The pickup devices are metal disks placed on the skin over the muscle or fine wires inserted into the muscle to be observed. Insulated wires conduct impulses from the pickup to the translating devices. Among the latter are ink writers, electromagnetic tape recorders, and oscilloscopes, from which photographs are made during the activity. The final form is a record, and electromyogram (EMG), similar to that shown in Fig. 7-18A.

Since the action potentials resulting from muscle contraction do not necessarily occur precisely when muscle contraction is produced, caution is needed in interpretation of the EMG. For exmple, the EMG signal always occurs before movement and is earlier in phasic than in tonic movements. Phasic movements will show fast-twitch muscle fibers to be active, whereas slow-twitch muscle fibers are active during tonic movements. Thus the magnitude of the EMG sign will be proportional to the velocity of the movement, since the magnitude of fast-twitch fiber action potentials is shown to be greater than that of slow-twitch fiber action potentials. In addition, the EMG magnitude also is directly related to the resistance to be overcome, or the amount of contraction utilized for static loading situations. Therefore, the amount of tension in the muscle is not exactly defined by the EMG.

Furthermore, to interpret an EMG, it is necessary to know which body segments have moved; in which joints actions have occurred, at what rates, and in what sequence; which muscles pass over these joints; and to which bones these muscles are attached. It is also necessary

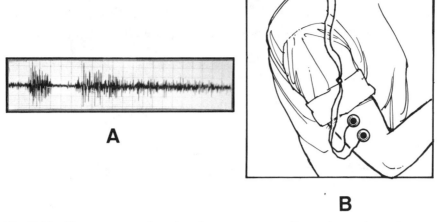

Fig. 7-18. *Electromyography. A, electromyogram; B, surface electrodes attached to performer.*

to know whether other forces were acting on body segments, especially gravitational force.

Note in Fig. 7-19 that the action of muscles differs during identical changes at the knee joint with a change in limb position with respect to gravity. Since EMGs do not provide kinematic information, other techniques of data collection are obtained at the same time. For example, photography (biplane is recommended) data will be used to show limb and muscle position in space and electrogoniometry (elgon at the joint being investigated) will be used to show angle at joint. Electromyography is a vital tool for muscle function analysis of postures and movement of all types and in all situations in life. This brief, simplified statement concerning electromyography does not convey one essential concept—that the competent, trustworthy investigator must have special technical skills. Such skills include the ability to select the best equipment for each study, to use the equipment, and to interpret the EMGs intelligently.

DYNAMOGRAPHY

Although dynamography has been used in industry and by engineers for many decades, there was virtually no use of this technique for analysis of human forces produced during sports situations prior to the 1960's. Dynamography is the technique of measuring the forces being produced during an activity. In the measurement of strength, primarily static strength, dynamography consisted of spring devices and cable tensiometers (Fig. 7-20).

Since the last decade, strain gauges have been placed on such devices as canoe and kayak paddles, athletic footwear insoles, ladders, bicycle pedals, and uneven parallel bars to determine the effectiveness of force production by performers using these devices. Strain

TOOLS FOR ASSESSMENT   **217**

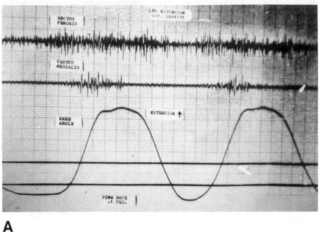

A

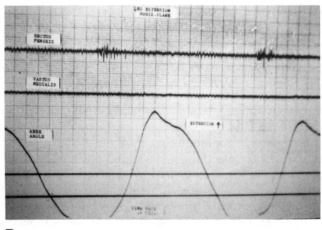

B

Fig. 7-19. *Electromyograms from identical muscles with body limb in two positions. A, Extension of lower leg is against gravity. B, Extension is in the horizontal plane. Note how gravity influences the role and tension produced in the muscle. The top tracing is electromyogram of rectus femoris muscle, the electromyogram beneath is of the vastus lateralis muscle, and the lower tracing is the angular displacement at the knee. Extension is represented as an upward trace.*

gauges are considered force transducers since they receive power from one system (power supply) and transfer their power (changes in force) to another system (a recorder). These devices are small, lightweight and can be fabricated for any purpose. A metal ring instrumented with four strain gages, for example, has been used to record the pulling forces of a performer being towed in water and to measure forces in a wire from which a metal ball was attached (Fig. 7-21A and B—hammer throw athletic event).

THE BIOMECHANICS OF HUMAN MOVEMENT

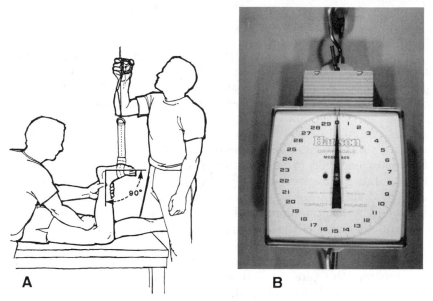

Fig. 7-20. *Mechanical devices to measure forces. A, The cable tensiometer is a versatile device used extensively for several decades by numerous researchers, including H. H. Clarke. B, The spring scale is not only useful for determining body weight, frictional force, but also as a strength recording device. with mechanical devices, especially.*

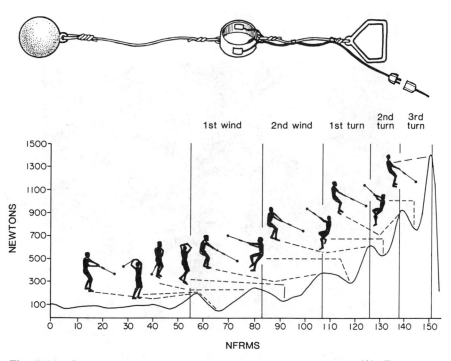

Fig. 7-21. *Strain gauge transducer used in the hammer throw (A). Force-time history of the tension on the cable (B). Notice the cyclic and incremental increase in force during the throwing sequence.*

TOOLS FOR ASSESSMENT

For the collection of large ground reaction forces, a more permanent, non-portable tool has been designed, the force platform. Force platforms have been built in many sizes, shapes, and designs, incorporating strain gauges or piezo-electric crystals to record force-time histories in three planes during such diverse activities as running, jumping, swimming, walking, and other locomotor patterns of human beings, as well as cats, dogs, horses, and other animals. Movements of athletes engaged in pole vaulting, shot-putting, sprinting starts, golfing, and gymnastics, among other sports, have also been measured by dynamographic techniques. Walking down stairs and down ramps and performing industrial tasks while standing on a force platform are other uses of the force platform. Some applications are shown in Fig. 7-22.

The force platform, although reported in 1938 as one of the tools for analyzing the gait of a cat walking on a treadmill, became the most exciting analysis tool of the sports world of the 1970's. It now is standard equipment in gait laboratories, mainly of a clinical nature, as well as sports biomechanics research laboratories. Improvements and modifications of the force platform concept have been made since its conception. Some of the more common innovations are described.

Foot plates

Force insoles (Fig. 7-23) have been fabricated and placed inside shoes in order to circumvent the problems of subjects not striking the

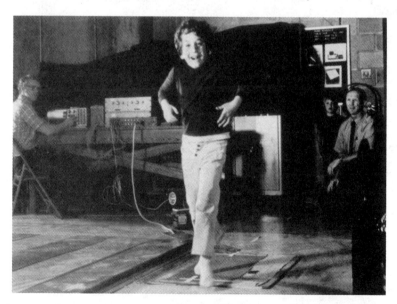

Fig. 7-22. *Force platform is in a well. Oscillograph light recorder and accessories shown on left are used in fast action. Handicapped children were used as subjects in this study. This is the common instrumentation for measuring external forces of the total body performance.*

THE BIOMECHANICS OF HUMAN MOVEMENT

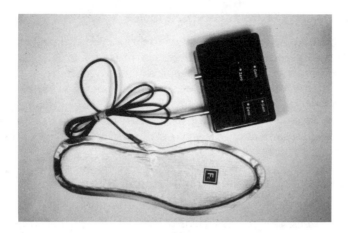

Fig. 7-23. *Force insoles to record vertical forces while worn in shoes. Constructed at Moss Rehabilitation Center. Further explained in Biomechanics Instrumentation. Video tape available from Benchmark Press.*

platform and not maintaining a natural locomotor pattern. Such portable devices, however, have not been perfected for 3-D recording. At this time, only vertical force measurements are practical. Similar efforts have been advanced in the animal world with instrumental horse shoes to investigate gaits of racehorses, as well as injured horses.

The use of anatomically-placed sensors on the feet was developed and termed clinical electrodynography. It is a diagnostic tool to identify function and dysfunction of the feet. The EDG force sensors are placed on the plantar surfaces of the feet at six locations (Fig. 7-24). The state-of-the art is such that the sensors must be validated with respect to reliability and must be carefully calibrated.

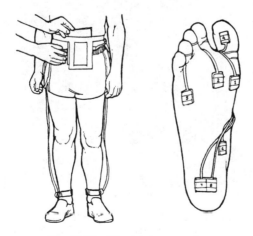

Fig. 7-24. *Electrodynography.*

Multiple Force Transducers in Plates

A series of thousands of transducers in one platform has been developed to record minute changes in pressure on the foot (Fig. 7-25). Needless to say, this highly sophisticated technology is expensive and requires complex software development and research know-how. The pictoral representation of data from such high technology, however, may become commonplace in the future and be used as a model for clinical assessments. This system, however, has the potential for the greatest amount of data.

Summary of Force Recording Instrumentation

The direct analysis of forces is not widespread but remains in the laboratory since it is not practical in natural settings of human movement. There is, however, a need to know the nature of forces occurring

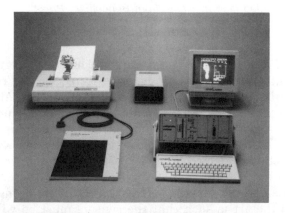

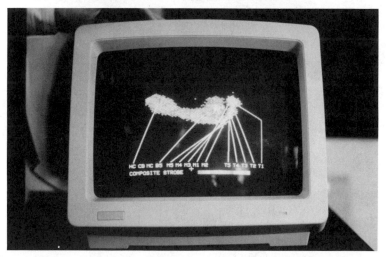

Fig. 7-25. *Other multisensor devices to record pressures throughout the surface area of weightbearing include the following: A, EMED-System (Courtesy of Novelgimbh, West Germany; B, Atlantis Scientific Corp. Indianapolis.*

during and actually producing a movement, especially with respect to implications for strength training and for general safety. In addition, the analysis of force-time histories (continuous force recordings with respect to time) is a means to differentiate between mechanical and anatomic factors of performance. For example, Fig. 7-26 consists of incorrect and correct application of force during a vertical jump. Incorrect application of force, however, produces greater velocity and a higher jump than that of a mechanically correct jump. Why? The reason is a simple one and relates to the proportion of muscle mass and body mass. The performer in Fig. 7-26B did not have a muscle strength-body mass ratio sufficiently high to produce an adequate impulse (product of force and time of application of that force). Consequently the velocity of projection was lower than that of the person weighing half as much, with almost the same amount of muscle strength. This is only one example of the many ways in which dynamography can be used to provide the necessary information to the human movement analyst to better understand a performance and thus be able to interpret the movement.

ACCELEROMETRY

The use of accelerometers, devices to measure acceleration, is an indirect measurement of force. Multiplying the mass that is acceler-

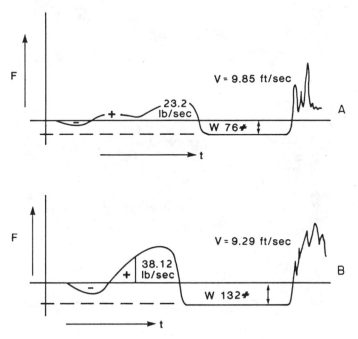

Fig. 7-26. Force platform recordings of two persons performing the vertical jump. A, unskilled, but lighter weight jumper produces greater effective impulse (as evidenced by greater velocity of projection) than skilled overweight jumper.

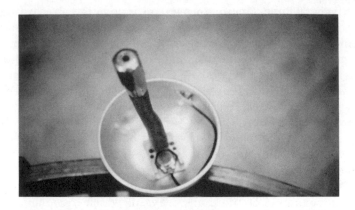

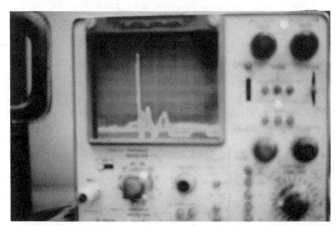

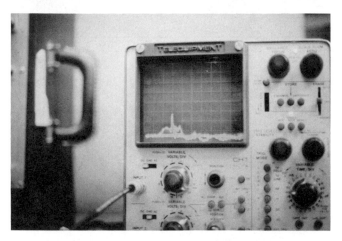

Fig. 7-27. *Accelerometer placed in guard of fencing foil to measure G forces. A, impact on sternum; B, impact on pectoralis major muscle.*

ated by the acceleration value will result in force produced or experienced by the mass. Accelerometers can be attached to the human body segments or to tools used, but placement and charting of the position of these accelerometers is crucial to the interpretation of data. Fig. 7-27 depicts an accelerometer placed in a foil guard and the impact recordings as a result of the foil striking flesh over muscles and flesh over bone. Note the higher impact force (G forces) with the bone impact site than with the muscle impact site.

Modeling and Simulation

Mathematic modeling of the anatomic characteristics of a living body can be combined with simulation techniques for the purpose of predicting performance achievements and developing new techniques of performance. Expertise in mathematics, anatomy, physics, and computers is required to bring these theoretical tools (modeling and simulation) to fruition.

Experimental data collected via the tools of cinematography, videography, anthropometry, dynamography, electrogoniometry, electromyography, and/or accelerometry are the foundation of the development of the model. The values for relevant parameters and their boundaries (possible ranges) are entered into a computer based upon the experimental data. Algorithms of motion (equations for calculations) are used in the simulation in which the movement can be varied with respect to speed, timing, ROM, etc. Software packages are commercially available to perform simulations and derive the biomechanically optimized model. In addition, CAD/CAM, CAEDS, or other computer-aided design programs are commercially available for stress analysis. An illustration of model images is shown in figure 7-28.

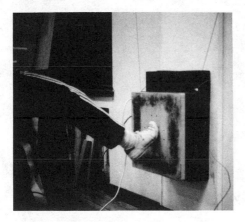

Fig. 7-28. *Models constructed using the computer aided engineering design programs. Karate kick against force platform. (Courtesy of Josef Loczi.) (Continued on next page.)*

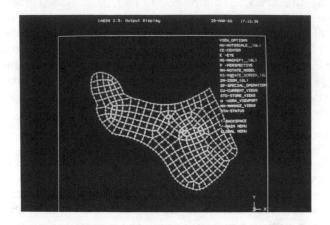

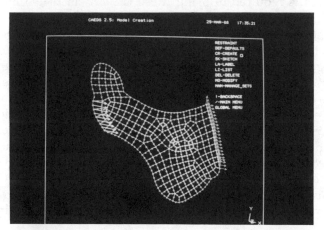

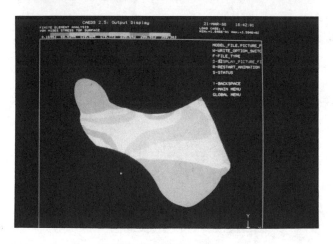

Fig. 7-28. *Continued*

THE BIOMECHANICS OF HUMAN MOVEMENT

SUMMARY

It is clear that the development of high technology has made it possible to gain a greater understanding of the biomechanics of human beings, both with respect to human movement and to the responses of human tissues to the forces acting upon these tissues. There are numerous other tools not readily available to those with knowledge or interest in biomechanics, including holography, thermography, CAT SCAN, and streak photography. All have had limited use, however, and may be of greater value in the future if cost and techniques become more favorable for general use.

Thermography results in a color display of hot and cold areas of the body to identify infection, blood volume, and stress.

It is important that the student and researcher of human movement select the tools necessary to solve their questions. There are many instances in which less sophisticated tools will be adequate for deriving the answers. Analysis is paralysis if instrumentation is an "overkill". If, however, more sophisticated equipment is required, there are several choices.

1. Purchase more sophisticated tools
2. Rent tools
3. Rent investigators with their tools
4. Become a part of someone else's data bank network and let them collect the data and you analyze
5. Change the question

REFERENCES

Adrian, M. (1973): Cinematographic, electromygraphic, and electrogoniometric techniques for analyzing human movements. In Wilmore, J. H., editor: *Exercise and sport sciences reviews*, vol. 1, New York: Academic Press, Inc.

Amar, J. (1972): *The human motor*, New York: Irvington Publishers, Inc.

Aristotle (1945): *Parts of animals, movements of animals, and progression of animals*, Cambridge, MA: Harvard University Press.

Atwater, A. E. (1973): Cinematographic analyses of human movement. In Wilmore, J. H., editor: *Exercise and sports sciences reviews*, vol. 1, New York: Academic Press, Inc., pp. 217–258.

Basmajian, J. V. (1973): Electromyographic analyses of basic movement patterns. In Wilmore, J. H., editor: *Exercise and sports sciences reviews*, vol. 1, New York: Academic Press, Inc.

Basmajian, J. V. (1979): *Muscles alive: their function revealed by electromyography*, ed. 4, Baltimore: The Williams, & Wilkins Co.

Carlsoo, S. (1972): *How man moves: Kinesiological studies and methods*, 1972, London: William Heinemann Ltd.

Chaffin, D. B. and Andersson, G. (1984): Bioinstrumentation for Occupational Biomechanics., In *Occupational Biomechanics:* New York: John Wiley and Sons.

Duchenne, G. B. (1949): *Physiology of motion*, Philadelphia: J. B. Lippincott Co.

Hirt, S., Fries, E. C., and Hellebrandt, F. A. (1944): Center of gravity of the human body, *Arch. Phys. Ther.* 25:280.

Journal of Physical Therapy, (1984) Vol 64, December (entire issue—Biomechanics Instrumentation).

Karpovich, P. V. (1930): Swimming speed analyzed, *Sci. Am.* 142:24, March.

Kluth, M. E. (1971): The effect of starting block height on the racing dive, unpublished thesis, Pullman, Washington State University.

Miller, D. I. (1971): Modelling in biomechanics: an overview, *Med. Sci. Sports* 11:115–122.

Muybridge, E. (1955). *The human figure in motion*, New York: Dover Publications, Inc.

Seireg, A. A. (1986): SOMA: *Engineering for the human body*, Baltimore: Williams and Wilkins.

Terauds, J., editor (1979): *Science in biomechanics cinematography*, Del Mar, Calif.: Academic Publishers.

8
Qualitative and Quantitative Assessment

Assessment of human movement may be conducted with the sophisticated tools described previously or with nothing more than the human eye and brain. Assessment, therefore, may be a rather superficial and grossly defined explanation of the movement pattern; or it may be a precise, analytically detailed numerical evaluation of each aspect of the movement. Although the eye and brain usually have been relied upon during teaching, coaching, clinical diagnostics, and other field situations, high technology is becoming a common part of these situations. Highly sophisticated tools of research are now at the disposal of practitioners, and can be utilized after a short learning period. As has been mentioned previously, there is an interrelationship between selection of tools and data acquisition. Traditionally, movie film has been the major medium by which investigators have analyzed, described, and quantified the temporal and spatial characteristics of human motion. In addition, movie film has been used to estimate the forces resulting from or producing the acceleration of the human body and its parts. Predictions of muscle force and reactive forces at the joints have also been based upon film analysis.

The desired types and amounts of data to be acquired, not the tool available, should dictate the selection of tools. There is a hierarchy of analyses based upon the broad categories of qualitative and quantitative analyses. This hierarchy is contingent upon the sophistication and amount of data that can be acquired, not which data are better (value judgment). These two categories actually should not be considered dichotomous. Analyses from the qualitative to the quantitative is actually a continuum in which the one merges into the other.

229

The nature of the analysis is a function of the goal of the analysis, and therefore of the problem to be solved.

QUALITATIVE ANALYSIS

This type of analysis can be subdivided into behavioral and relative analyses. The former has non-discreet data (information) such as: did the person move, sit, swing a hammer, lift a sack, throw a ball underhand, push a wheelchair, or remain immobile? Such investigation consists of categorizing performances into yes/no, successful/ unsuccessful, with difficulty/without difficulty, or similar descriptor cells.

When utilizing relative analysis, comparisons are made such as, comparisons of performances of two or more individuals, or comparisons of an individual performance and a standardized individual performance. For example, was the performance fast or slow, performed at an angle to the vertical, or requiring a movement greater than 90 degrees of flexion? Thus, relative qualitative analysis consists of non-precise quantification of movement performance.

QUANTITATIVE ANALYSIS

The most sophisticated type of analysis is quantitative. This necessitates the measurement of factors of the movement and ascribing numerical values to these factors. With respect to temporal factors, the analysis might include the duration (in seconds) of the preparation phase of the movement, or the time difference between one preparation phase of the movement and another phase, or the time difference between one body part beginning to move and another body part ceasing to move. With respect to spatial factors, the analysis might include the direction of the movement, the angle of the forearm with respect to the ground or the hand (in degrees), or the length of the step taken by a softball pitcher (in meters). The typical numerical quantities obtained via optical tools are displacement, velocity, and acceleration. Typical numerical quantity obtained through dynamographic techniques include force, impulse, work, energy, and power. Typical numerical accelerometer data are accelerations or "g" forces. Numerical values from EMG may be in electrical units (mV) or % of a criterion. Angular displacement data are obtained via electrogonimetry and angular velocity and acceleration derived mathematically or electronically. A comparison of qualitative and quantitative data with respect to the position of the feet during walking is depicted in Table 8-1. Precise changes, improvements or dysfunction can be assessed via quantitative data. Statistical comparisons with other re-

Table 8-1. *Types of analyses applied to an investigation of the feet during walking (support phase only.)*

TYPES OF ANALYSES
APPLIED TO AN INVESTIGATION
OF THE FEET DURING WALKING
(SUPPORT PHASE)

QUALITATIVE		QUANTITATIVE
BEHAVIORAL	RELATIVE	
FEET TOED-OUTWARD	RIGHT IS TOED-OUTWARD FARTHER THAN LEFT	10% TOED-OUTWARD

search data also are more readily possible with quantitative data than qualitative data.

NAKED-EYE OBSERVATIONAL PROCEDURES

Through years of trial and error the trained teacher or observer of movement learns to recognize many (but not all) skilled and unskilled movement habits. Some habits are sensed; some are recognized. However, only the most competent and keenest analyst is able to recognize what a performer does or should do to correct faulty movement. Such analysts also are able to encourage certain movement tendencies for optimum performance. It is almost impossible, without cinematographic or videographic records, to accurately view with the naked eye the distal ends of the limbs in a fast action. Both the starting position and the terminal position are seen, but the propulsive phase is almost always a blur. Yet, after an observer has had years of practice, some educated guesses are reasonably accurate and certainly are enhanced by biomechanic knowledge of starting and terminal positions, as well as performance outcome.

To be consistent and reliable both in observing performers who are learning motor skills and in evaluating movement for practical, diagnostic clinical, or research purposes (either in actual movement in a game or work situation or in action viewed from film), one must adopt a definite observational plan.

Plan of Visually Analyzing Walking

The viewing position is the first consideration when analyzing human movement visually and without instrumentation of any type. You must be able to see what it is you will hope to understand. Place yourself in an appropriate position to maximize your view. Usually, the best position is one that has the line of sight at right angles to the major movement plane. For example, walking would be viewed so that one side of the body is viewed. The changes in angles at the hip, knee, ankle, elbow, shoulder, and knee can be observed. The length of step and the changing levels of the body parts can be estimated, as well as the cadence of the walk. This observational position, however, is inadequate for observing medial and lateral deviations of the walker. A "head-on" view is necessary in order to note such movements as toeing-in of the feet, leg alignment at impact and at take-off, and lateral lean of the trunk. Thus, whenever possible, movement should be viewed from at least two perspectives.

Several trials should be viewed and mental images of each trial compared to determine consistency of performance. Consistent errors, as well as consistently correct movement patterns, can be identified only if multiple trials are viewed.

Observation is best conducted by a whole-part-whole method: the total body is viewed and then each of the major body parts are viewed. A videotape in which this method is described and applied to the analysis of locomotor patterns of physically handicapped persons is available from the publisher of this book. Spatial and temporal characteristics of each body part are estimated. The order of viewing may vary according to observer preference. For example, you might begin with the legs, then view the trunk, and then the arms during the "part" aspect of the observation. Another person may wish to observe from cephalic to caudal. Final observation of the total body would then be conducted to investigate the coordination or sequencing of movements of the various parts with respect to each other. A checklist to analyze walking appears as Table 8-2.

MINI-LAB LEARNING EXPERIENCES

Using Table 8-2, observe two persons and check the items that apply to each person's gait.

Since the eye can merely estimate the fast actions of the body, and can only capture images at approximately 10 per second, tools often are necessary for human movement analyses. If no tools are available, the start of the movement, the completion of the movement, and general pattern of the movement may be all that is possible to analyze with the human eye.

The preceding analysis is a qualitative description of the movement in spatial terms with limited temporal analysis. This checklist is best used as a clinical or developmental assessment technique.

The basic plan for analyzing walking was developed from a set of principles and a set of questions. These principles and representative questions are listed in the following sections. Both sets can be used as guidelines for developing checklists for analyses of other movement patterns.

Table 8-2. *Checklist to qualitatively assess walking*

Head vertically aligned
head inclined forward (flexion)
head inclined backward (extension)
head tilted to side (from front view)

Trunk vertically aligned
kyphosis
lordosis
trunk flexion
scoliosis (from front view)

Arm swing in opposition to legs
arm swing less than 45 degrees
arm swing greater than 45 degrees
rigid arm swing
kinematic chain-type arm swing
hands held in fists
equal Range of Motion (ROM) for both arms

Hip remains relatively at the same height (head may be viewed rather than
  the hip)
hip bobs up and down (head may be viewed rather than hip)

Shank vertical at initial contact
shank inclined backward at initial contact
push-off with shank vertical
push-off with shank inclined forward
equal ROM for both legs

Thigh remains below horizontal
thigh becomes horizontal
ROM at knee less than 45 degrees
ROM at knee greater than 45 degrees
foot held rigid
foot held in equinos
foot turned outward excessively
foot turned inward excessively
knocked-kneed
bow-legged

Initial contact with heel of foot
initial contact with flat foot
initial contact with ball of foot

Weight borne on medial part of foot
wieght borne on lateral part of foot
weight shifts borne effectively on foot

PRINCIPLES

1. It is difficult to identify fast action without first observing the origin of the movement. One must look at the large parts before observing the small parts of the body.
2. An observer can usually see only one part of the body in action at a time. One should then plan to observe the action of one part at a time—for example, the head or arms—before ana-

QUALITATIVE AND QUANTITATIVE ASSESSMENT   **233**

lyzing a motion. Several viewings of a performance are thus required.

3. The observer who is too close may be unable to see the action or may find it impossible to distinguish one part of the movement from another because of the speed of movement. Looking through (not at) the performer to include the entire background helps in gaining proper orientation. One might even look out of the corner of one's eyes part of the time to observe unusual actions.

4. The action should be viewed many times. The observer's analysis should not be made on the basis of only one or two observations because beginners and other unskilled performers rarely repeat one and only one error.

5. The powers of human concentration are such that an observer usually sees only what is expected to be seen. The observer must eliminate biases and learn to look for unusual clues to make an effective study of the movement.

6. One action is related to a previous action. Consequently, the total motion may be mentally traced from the termination back to its inception to discover how the action was performed.

7. It is valuable to observe the action from more than one vantage point—at a distance, close up, from above, from the rear, from the front, and even lying flat on the ground. Each position yields a different perspective.

8. The observer should have a visual-mental model of the skilled manner of performing the action and should attempt to compare the performance with this model. Garrett has suggested that a child model be used when analyzing movements of children. Likewise, a tall model, obese model, or paraplegic model should be visualized as appropriate to the performer.

9. Some actions are too fast for the naked eye to observe them accurately under any circumstances. Therefore, view the action in a slow-motion film or video. Then the movement may be identified by the naked eye.

REPRESENTATIVE QUESTIONS

1. Where is the center of the body while it is in action? A statement often used—"Look at the hub of the wheel before observing the rim"—is appropriate here. The center of the mass (center of gravity) of the individual(s) under study is the most slowly moving part (with the exception of the base of support) and the easiest to locate. It should be the orientation point for the observation of subsequent parts. The center should be located as accurately as possible.

2. What is the height of the center of gravity from the base of support? Is it low or high during the movement? Does it change

during the crucial part, such as at the moment of impact of the bat against the ball? Usually the center of gravity is high for quick, speedy action in a linear direction. It is low when great force is exerted or when stability is needed. The imaginary point of the center of mass should move in a parallel plane or steadily upward as the velocity increases.

3. If hip (pelvic) movement is essential, what are the extent and direction of movement during the action? In many sports, the failure to use the pelvis (hip region) properly is the difference between a skilled and an unskilled performance. When skilled performers are studied carefully, the hip region's leading of the rest of the body in action is very pronounced such as in the discus throw, the golf swing, lifting a bale of hay, swinging a sledge hammer, and other movements.

4. Where is the body weight at both the start and the finish of the action? Often the weight should be moved so that it is centered over the leading, or front foot as the action comes to a climax. Unskilled performers in golf, for example, often have their body weight centered over the rear foot as they contact the ball with the club head. In a throwing action designed for the purpose of gaining great ball velocity or distance, the body weight of the performer must be moving forward as the action is completed if the performance is to be effective.

5. What happens to the head during the action? The position of the head initially, as well as during and at the end of a movement, may be revealing. Usually the head should remain as stationary as possible during the action. A rapid change in its position may cause an undesirable change in the direction in which the body or its parts is moving. For example, the swing of the arms in batting may be altered upward if the head is raised, thereby affecting the resultant force on the ball. On the other hand, in twisting and tumbling actions, the head initiates the action and determines the direction the body will take. The position of the head may create a tonic-neck reflex response during industrial handling tasks, such as lifting or pulling a lever.

6. How do the shoulders move during the action? In most throwing and striking actions, the shoulders and head move almost as one unit. In most throwing and striking actions the shoulder is "turned" to promote effective performance. Yet in some movements, there is often a problem with a shoulder "dip." For example, the arc of the swing of a golfer may be altered during the course of the striking action, often causing an ineffective performance.

7. How wide is the base of support? In many movements, a narrow foot stance means that an unstable position has been assumed by the performer, and the total movement may be af-

fected adversely. However, a very quick step may be taken from a narrow base. A wide stance signifies stability, but an extremely wide base restricts quick movements.

8. In what direction do the feet move before, during, and after the action? The direction in which the feet move is usually the direction in which the action will take place.

9. How often will sway, dip, and unusual twists of the body occur during the action? A sway, dip, or twist of the body usually means that forces other than those moving in the desired direction are at work and most likely will diminish the total force. On the other hand, hip twist may cause the arm to attain a wide range of motion. One must differentiate between movements that position the body for the desired direction of force and movements that prevent the application of force in the desired direction.

10. What are the extent, direction, and pattern of the follow-through of the body, arm, hand, leg, or other body parts? The follow-through of the parts of the body after the main action has taken place is indicative of the direction in which the body moved and also may, in the case of the leg, for example, be indicative of just how much force was expended. For example, after a worker throws a bale of hay into a truck, what is the position of the center of balance?

11. In what direction (including path) do the arms and legs move during the action? Sometimes, in a striking motion, a performer moves one arm away from the desired direction and thus interferes with the effectiveness of the total action. Pulling the inside arm against the body in a golf stroke reduces the force that the arm is able to contribute to the swing.

12. What are the total range, the patterns, and the path of movement through which the body and appendages move during the action? Sometimes the range of movement is too wide to be effective. In others, the lack of enough range of motion hinders the performer. More force may be generated by a wide range of movement, but accuracy may be sacrificed, because the wider the range of motion, the more an error is accentuated.

13. How does the hand or implement act during the movement of impact in activities involving striking? Is the hand or implement, such as a hammer, axe, or golf club, moving so that the full portion of the hand or implement head contacts the object? If not, some force is probably lost.

14. What is the action of the wrist, hand, and fingers at the moment an object is contacted or released? Usually a trained eye can come close to detecting the uncocking of the wrist and the inward turn of the hand, which are components of skilled throwing or striking performance. The index and mid-

dle fingers supply the final force in throwing, especially when great speed is desired.

15. What is the angle at which the object leaves the hand or sports implement in a striking or throwing activity? Theoretically, the optimal angle for putting the shot or throwing a sphere a maximum distance is 45 degrees. Lesser or greater angles usually occur because of movement situations. Refer to Chapter 5.

16. Does the hand or implement cut across the object to be struck as the striking action takes place? Usually the follow-through of the body, and especially of the appendages and implement, indicates the manner in which the object was struck.

17. During a striking or throwing motion, are the eyes of the performer fixed on the object to be struck or on the target? A slight movement of the eyes toward the anticipated flight of the object, or the shifting of the eyes to some distracting influence as the action takes place, may move the head and consequently, the limb, due to the tonic-neck reflex or a lack of concentration. Such an action will change the arc of the swing of the arm or implement and thus may interfere with accuracy or force, moving the body away from the desired direction.

* * * * *

The above checklist questions are specific in nature. The following questions are concerned with general observations of the performer after details of the movement have been ascertained.

* * * * *

18. What is the total visual image of the performer as pictured by the observer? Is the action smooth, continuous, and rhythmic? Is there any unnecessary hesitation during the action? Usually smooth action means effective movement, but this is not always true. A performer may appear to be awkward in the action until a thorough study reveals that each phase complements the next. Thus the movement is effective because there is a continuously accelerating motion during the crucial portion of the action.

19. How effective is the total body movement? The analyst (observer) should be aware that the observed starting position is sometimes alternated as the action begins. This last-minute change affects performance and interferes with correct analysis if it is not taken into account. A starting stance is often changed just as the action begins to make the movement less effective or even more effective. In evaluating the movements of a performer, special attention should be given

to those actions performed at the time and in the position that are the most crucial to the total performance. For example, a baseball batter may have a peculiar, awkward stance at the plate, but just as the action of batting begins, the batter moves to a mechanically correct position in preparation for striking the ball. The awkward initial stance can be ignored.

ACOUSTICAL ANALYSIS OF RHYTHMIC PATTERN OF MOVEMENT

The rhythms of human beings in action are characterized by signs, motions, and sounds made by their bodies or parts thereof to express themselves in some manner. The word rhythm comes from the Latin word rhythmus and the Greek word rhein which means to flow. It also has a musical connotation because of the elements of accent, meter, time, and tempo. Thus the sounds and motions of a human being who is moving often have an orderly sequence of closely related elements called rhythm.

The organs and systems of the human body are capable of emitting signs that indicate to the skilled listener that certain conditions are present. As more sophisticated instruments are developed, a greater understanding of these rhythmic communications will become known. With an inexpensive microphone and tape recorder, the sound of the body may be recorded.

The examination of a sample of blood through the use of an electron microscope is information that the medical laboratory technician uses to detect the state of health or disease of a given individual. The beat of a person's heart, especially as seen in an ECG record acoustically "tells" the exercise physiologist valuable information about a person's heart and body functions, especially if subjected to a stress test.

The computer's role in the assessment, storing, categorizing and comparing of the rhythm of an action is almost unlimited. The records plotted by a computer can reveal so much more than the eye can see. We predict that the computers of the future will be able to "hear the rhythm of human movement" and diagnose it. The sounds made by the feet, hands, and implements used during physical activities can be recorded, analyzed, and then transcribed into musical symbols.

The easiest manner of analyzing the sound of the movement is to close the eyes (tune-out the visual stimulation) and listen. It is quite easy to differentiate between running, walking, galloping, hopping, and walking with a limp. Both loudness and tempo can be detected. Figure 8-1 includes the rhythm in musical notation for these forms of locomotion.

Verify these records by trying some activities yourself. The individual rhythms of shooting a basketball free throw are interesting

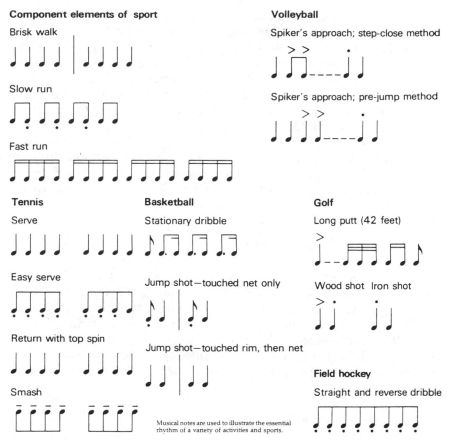

Fig. 8-1. *Rhythmic analysis of walk, run, and skills of selected sports. Ask a person with musical notation skills to help you beat the rhythms. Then try the movement skills to these rhythms. Does your natural rhythm fit these rhythms?*

to compare. Changes in acoustical patterns also are noticeable as a result of fatigue, stress, illness, and other factors.

Following is a summary of observations based on studying and analyzing the results of the rhythmic patterns of sports movements:

1. Every performer has a certain individual composite rhythm.
2. Each segment of each performer's body has a rhythm all its own.
3. The complete rhythm of movement is difficult to record.
4. In many activities, such as chopping wood, assembly line work, and typing, a person tries to "feel" the rhythm. In sports, such as boxing, the player tries to "feel" the opponent's rhythm. Couple dancing necessitates "matching own's rhythm to own's partner as well as to the music.
5. The tempo of a performer's rhythm is not necessarily smooth and even. It is often uneven but consistent in pattern.
6. Usually the tempo of movement is one of the biggest single

factors in distinguishing the skilled from the unskilled performer. Listen to, and identify these rhythms!

7. Most performers do not know what their rhythm is and only subconsciously recognize it. Lack of recognition may be the limiting factor in achieving consistency of performance.

8. There seems to be rhythmic pattern that is best for an individual to use. This pattern may be related to anthropometry, as well as, skill level.

9. As persons discover better and more effective ways to accomplish a task (perform a skill), they may develop different rhythmic patterns from the ones now used by top performers. (Additional information on this subject may be found in the article by Cooper and Andrews in Quest).

VIDEOGRAPHIC ANALYSIS

Since videography has now become commonplace and video equipment is purchased by one of every four families in the United States, the use of videography to provide both qualitative and quantitative analyses of human movement is not only practical but valuable. The video images should be obtained during several performances and from different angles, in order to obtain two or more orthogonal views if possible. Guidelines for analyses are given as follows.

Qualitative Videography

1. Observe the videotape and describe the movement with respect to space (planes of movement) and anatomy (joints used as axes of rotation and body parts being moved). Describe quality of movement—sustained, jerky, swinging type, limp, strong, fast, etc.

2. Estimate the time to perform selected phases of the movement pattern, estimate relative ranges of motion of body parts.

3. Focus upon different body parts and describe each one separately and then sequentially.

4. Compare the general pattern to a model (elite, average, self at another trial, etc.).

Quantitative Video Analysis

1. Trace the outline of the performer (drawing a contourgram) at selected instances during the performance as determined from the qualitative analysis. This can be done in several ways. The simplest and earliest form of analysis is image-tracing. A clear plastic sheet is affixed to the video monitor and the desired parameters are traced with a felt tip pen or crayon. The plastic sheet can be held or taped to the monitor (usually the plastic

self-clings to the screen) and the selected images traced in different colors, or with different line codes as depicted in Fig. 8-2. Each image can be traced on a separate sheet, always including a stationary object or reference point on each sheet and identifying the frame number (or time code).

The plastic sheets can be superimposed upon each other to study patterns. An alternative approach is to trace the stationary object once, and trace a series of images on the same sheet with reference to the position of the object. This is best if the movement is a locomotor one and the images will not overlap.

2. Draw point plots of the important landmarks, such as the displacement of hip, knee, and ankle during walking, ascending stairs, kicking, and dancing. (Fig. 8-3)
3. Draw line segments of the body parts, such as the upper arm and forearm during cross country skiing. (Fig. 8-4)
4. Determine the time period for each tracing by counting frames or using a digital time-generated code. This latter is standard equipment on some video cameras or as an accessory to the recorder.
5. Measure traced points and segments. Distances can be obtained between points. Angles can be measured with respect to the intersection of line segments or angles of inclination of line segments from the vertical or horizontal. These measurements can be taken by hand via rulers, protractors, and other drafting tools. A more sophisticated method is to use digitizing tablets interfaced with a microcomputer.
6. Calculate values. Calculate linear and angular speeds by dividing distances and angles displaced from image-to-image by time required to cause this displacement.
7. Calculate accelerations by dividing change in speed by the time required to cause this change.

The alternatives include the use of a camera to obtain a photograph or slide of the selected video image and trace from those media, or the use of a video printer to obtain an instantaneous print. Also, the images can be entered into a microcomputer. The most sophisticated video computerized systems have automatic input from the video camera to a computer.

Analysis of Video Prints

Using either the pause mode or play mode of the video recorder, press the print button to capture the image as a video print. The print can then be analyzed by ruler, protractor, planimeter or digitizer. An example of video print analysis obtained from videotaped performances of wheelchair athletes is depicted in Fig. 8-5. The beginning, release, and the ending of the throw of two different athletes can be compared with respect to range of motion and spatial orientations.

QUALITATIVE AND QUANTITATIVE ASSESSMENT   **241**

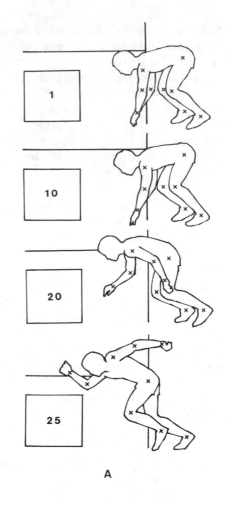

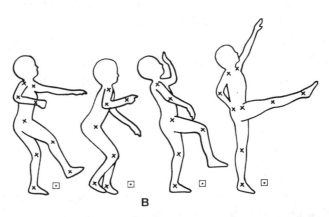

Fig. 8-2. *Two examples of contourgrams relative to inanimate object traced from video images. A, These have been traced on transparencies using a felt pen and then retraced with a pencil. B, This set was traced directly using the reflection of the video image on a semi-transparent digitizing pad (Hi-Pad model 1405).*

R = RELEASE
C = CONTACT

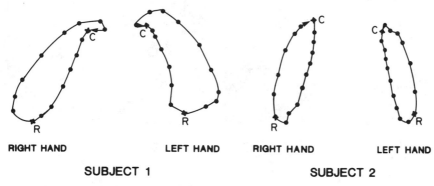

| RIGHT HAND | LEFT HAND | RIGHT HAND | LEFT HAND |

SUBJECT 1   **SUBJECT 2**

Fig. 8-3. *Example of point plots traced from video images. What information can you glean from these, not possible from figure 8-2?*

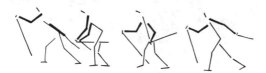

Fig. 8-4. *Example of line segment tracings of the upper extremities during cross country skiing. Is it easier to see the motion than point plots? What information can you measure?*

MINI-LAB LEARNING EXPERIENCES

Using Fig. 8-5, measure additional parameters: the angle of projection of the javelin. Identify the more skilled performance. Check chapter 17 for clues to the answer. The prints can be placed on a digitizing tablet and anatomical points digitized. In particular, analysis of the position of the center of gravity can be conducted.

Video-image Grabbing

Another method of transforming the videotape is to use a micro-computer. Garrett is a pioneer in this area, being the first to apply video "grabbing" to human movement analysis. Using sophisticated software and hardware, the selected image can be "grabbed," and then rotated, enlarged or reduced, enhanced, and otherwise modified and measured by the operator and printed. Both kinematic data and anatomical data, such as leg alignment and scoliosis can be collected for analysis. Footprints of boys and girls attending a youth sports camp

QUALITATIVE AND QUANTITATIVE ASSESSMENT   **243**

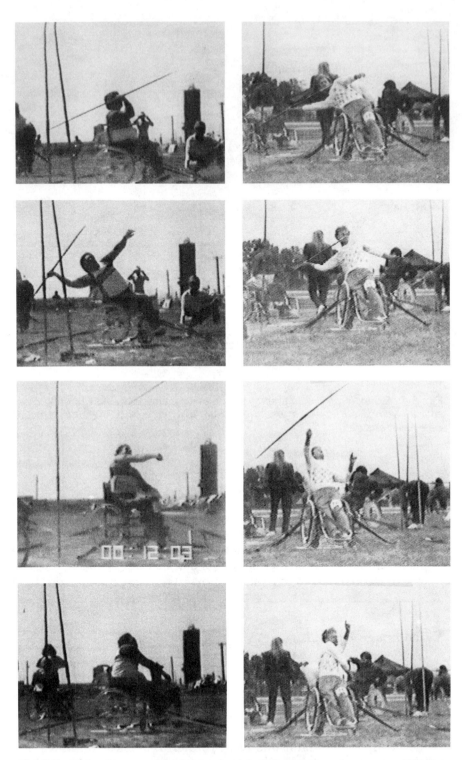

Fig. 8-5. *Video image print of two wheelchair throwing performances. Which is the more highly skilled? Why? Note the trajectory of the javelin.*

THE BIOMECHANICS OF HUMAN MOVEMENT

were reduced and enhanced via video-image grabbing technology. Selected reproductions are included in Fig. 8-6.

MINI-LAB LEARNING EXPERIENCES

Identify the types of feet and anomalies depicted in this figure.

Automatic "Video" Analysis

Figure 8-7 is another example of use of the microcomputer to analyze human movement. The angle at the hip, knee and ankle have been calculated and printed without operator measurement or digitizing. Such two-dimensional printouts are common. In addition, three-

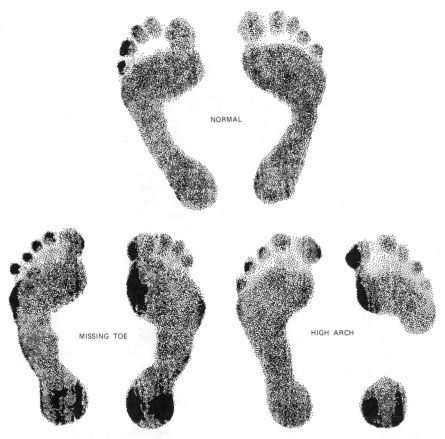

NORMAL

MISSING TOE

HIGH ARCH

Fig. 8-6. *Computerized footprints generated from video image grabbing, modifying, and printing processes with a MacIntosh system and Mitsubishi Video-printer. Note how easily one could measure surface area, unweighting area at the arch, and lengths and widths between selected points. More important these footprints can be included in a database for retrieval and comparisons. This is the poor analyst's imaging system!*

QUALITATIVE AND QUANTITATIVE ASSESSMENT   **245**

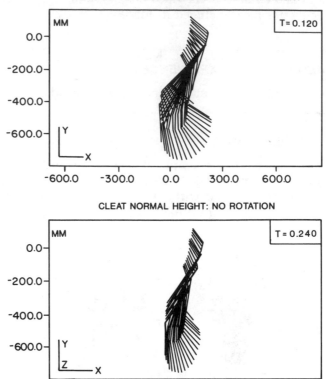

Fig. 8-7. *Computer generated line segments and angles from the Selspot system. Bicycling with cleats. The computer software has a subroutine to orthogonally rotate the output to any amount required. Some rotations are of greater value for the pattern than for the numerical values.*

dimensional kinematic printouts of all types can be obtained via more sophisticated software systems.

FILM ANALYSIS PROCEDURES

There are three basic methods available for obtaining quantitative data from film. (Refer to Fig. 8-8.) The oldest and most time-consuming procedure involves projecting the image onto a flat surface such as a wall. Segmental endpoints are then drawn onto graph paper attached to the surface. Care must be taken to ensure that the projection is at right angles to the drawing or wall surface; otherwise, there will be distortion of the image. One way to check this is to measure the dimensions of the four sprocket holders at the edge of the frame. If the projector is properly aligned, they should all be the same size. It is also necessary to mark stationary background references (two or more) on the paper to ensure that each frame is projected onto the same place on the drawing surface. Although this method does

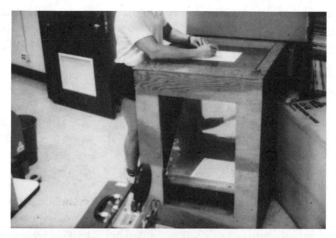

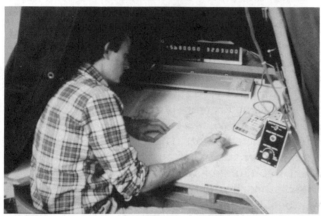

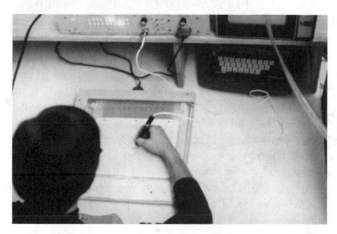

Fig. 8-8. *Film analysis systems. A, using s 16 mm L & W projector and mirror box to trace and measure 16 mm file images. B, using a Vanguard 16 mm projector head and Numonics acoustic digitizing tablet interfaced with Apple computer and University of Illinois mainframe computer to obtain spatial coordinates. C, Using a Hi-Pad digitizing tablet interfaced with an IBM computer to digitize film tracings or project the 16 mm film to tablet and digitize directly.*

QUALITATIVE AND QUANTITATIVE ASSESSMENT

have a number of disadvantages, it provides a large-sized image and therefore considerably reduces measurement error. Any stop-action, single-frame-advance movie projector may be used for this type of analysis.

The second and most widely used technique involves the use of a film Analyzer or fabricated mirror box used with a projector. The image is projected onto a ground-glass screen providing a magnification of 20 to 40 times the frame size. As with the first method, precautions must be taken to ensure that the frame orientation remains the same when the film is advanced (reference points). This method is acceptable as an excellent teaching aid and in the processing of small sets of data.

The third method, that of using a digitizing tablet, is the most commonly used today, especially for large data sets. The film is projected on a tablet, and a pen, cursor, or other device is used to mark the position of a joint or other points of interest on the tablet. A digitizer automatically displays the x- and y-coordinates of the point (Fig. 8-9). The investigator may copy the coordinates and calculate distances and angles, or the digitizer may be connected to a microprocessor or computer that stores the data points. Appropriate software performs calculations, such as, smoothing the data, and deriving velocities, accelerations and centers of mass. Although the computer may be used to determine all measured and calculated values, verification of these values (selected points, first trial, etc.) must be made. This not only saves embarrassment if absurd values are reported, but also assures an understanding of the parameters.

All these methods can be utilized with all types of films: 16mm, 35mm, 8mm, photographs, and slides. A combination point plot and contourgram is shown in Fig. 8-10 with the frames numbered and the calculations for ball velocity identified.

Angles

Any angles to be measured can be obtained through the use of a protractor if a film reader or projector is being used. If points are digitized, the software is used to calculate angular kinematics. The angles must be in the plane of the projection to be valid angles. When segments move out of the plane an angle should not be measured. It should be noted that by measuring angles at specific times it is possible to determine the angular velocity of the body, as well as its angular acceleration. This knowledge may lead to a better understanding of the relative contribution to movement made by each segment of the body.

Distance

It is important to realize that, in determining any distances determined from the film, they must be converted to life size, since the projection will be considerably smaller than true size. Consequently,

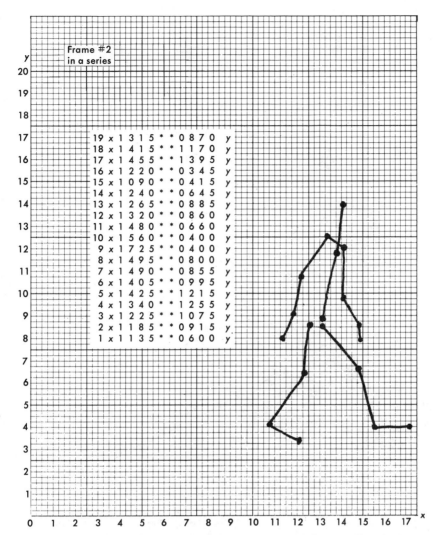

Fig. 8-9. *The x- and y-coordinate system used to analyze movement of soccer player. Graph paper can be used and measurement can be done without high technological instrumentation or any of the systems in figure 8-8 can be used.*

all measurements taken from the picture must be adjusted by using an object of known length in the picture. By comparing the actual size and the projected size, one can determine a multiplier that can be applied to distances measured on film.

Example 1. Assume that a 1-m measuring stick measures 10 cm (0.1 m) on the screen or tablet. It should be evident that 1 cm on the screen is equal to 10 cm in life. The actual computation of the multiplier is as follows:

> x cm on screen = Y cm in life
> 1 cm on screen = y cm in life/X

QUALITATIVE AND QUANTITATIVE ASSESSMENT **249**

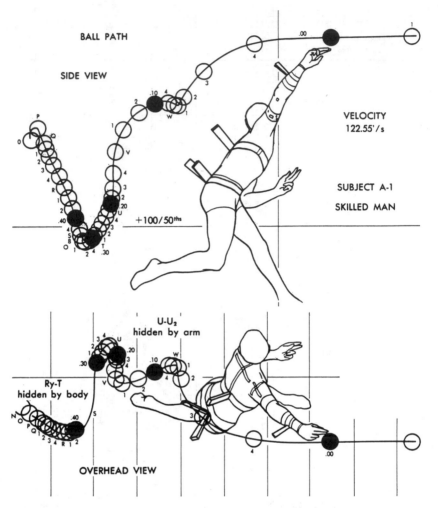

BALL PATH

SIDE VIEW

VELOCITY
122.55'/s

SUBJECT A-1

SKILLED MAN

+100/50ths

U-U₂
hidden by arm

Ry-T
hidden by body

OVERHEAD VIEW

Fig. 8-10. *Tracings from film to show path of ball. Circles represent equal time intervals. Note the fins to track rotations of body segments. Fins are also useful devices when only one camera can be used. (from Atwater, A. E.: Movement characteristics of the overarm throw, dissertation, University of Wisconsin, 1970)*

or

$$\text{Multiplier} = \text{life size/projected size} = 100 \text{ cm}/10 \text{ cm} = 10$$

Example 2. To compare English measurements, assume that a yardstick measures 3.6 inches on the screen. It should be evident that 1 inch on the screen is equal to 10 inches in life. The actual computation of the multiplier is as follows:

X inches on screen = Y inches in life
1 inch on screen = Y inches in life/X

or

Multiplier = Life size/Projected size

$$= 36 \text{ inches}/3.60 \text{ inches} = 10$$

Thus a measurement taken from the film in centimeters or inches must be multiplied by 10 to convert the distance to life-size units of centimeters or inches. (If life-size units in feet are desired, the multiplier is equal to 0.83 to convert screen measurements to feet.)

If a grid screen is provided in the film background, then displacement values can also be obtained by simply counting the number of grid lines crossed between frames. For example, assuming that you are using grid lines equal to 10 cm in life, and a body segment under study has moved through 16 grid lines, then the displacement would be equal to 10×16, or 160 cm (1.6 m). To use English measurements, assume that you are using grid lines equal to 4 inches in life, and a body segment under study has moved through 16 grid lines, then the displacement would be equal to 4×16, or 64 inches (5.3 feet). The use of a grid screen will help to reduce the possibility of perspective error.

Time

Since the camera is operating at a known speed, the time elapsed per frame can easily be determined. If it is moving at 128 frames/sec, the time per frame would be 1/128 second. If the camera speed is other than 128 frames/sec, then the time per frame is merely 1 divided by the number of frames per second.

Velocity

The velocity of an object or body part can be computed from the distance traveled and the time elapsed during the movement. Displacement can be secured by measuring the distance covered on the film and applying the multiplier or by counting the grid lines and multiplying by the actual width of the grid (in this case 10 cm or 4 inches). The time is obtained by counting the number of frames during that phase of the movement and multiplying by the computed time per frame. The following formula should then be used:

Example 1.

Distance = 16 grid lines $\times$ 10 cm = 160 cm/10 = 1.6
Time = 1/128 frames/sec $\times$ 14 frames = 0.109 second
Velocity = 1.6 m/0.109 second = 14.8 m/sec

Example 2.

Distance = 16 grid lines $\times$ 4 inches = 64 inches/12 = 5.3 feet
Time = 1/128 frames/sec $\times$ 14 frames = 0.109 second
Velocity = 5.3 feet/0.109 second = 48.62 ft/sec

Acceleration

Acceleration can be calculated by determining the rate of change in velocity as computed from the film. The data obtained, however, are not without error and in many cases are unreliable unless the original displacements have been smoothed mathematically before velocity and acceleration are calculated.

WHAT TO ANALYZE?

With respect to all these media, it is important to determine what should be analyzed. Determine not only the factors that will be measured, but also the types of comparisons that will be of value. Guidelines for doing so are as follows:

Table 8-3. *Rating scales for throwing and running mechanics. (Courtesy of Lois Klatt, Human Performance Laboratory, Concordia College, River Forest, Illinois).*

NAME _____ SPORT _____ DATE _____

THROWING MECHANICS

Mechanics	Rating	Comments
Preparation phase		
Rear hip rotation, extension		
Rear foot ground contact, power		
Front leg plant, counterforce maintenance		
Stride length, consistency		
Weight shift - rear to front		
Spinal rotation; flexion, lateral flexion		
Sequence of joint action		
Shoulder medial rotation; extension, adduction		
Path of ball, flat arc		
Complete follow-through in direction of throw		
Direction of forces, summation		
Balance position - release and follow-through		

Potential injuries
    Medial elbow valgu
    Medial elbow stress syndrome (compression of radial head)
    Elbow olecranon process, osteochondritis
    Shoulder - long head bicep, rotator cuff

Conditioning needs to include stretching and strengthening, an equal amount of strength, without stressing.

Rating Scale: **4** - very good, **3** - good, **2** - fair, **1** - poor, **/** - fine

Contributed by Lois A. Klatt, Human Performance Laboratory, Concordia College, River Forest, Illinois

1. Read the literature to determine what factors are important enough to analyze. Compare your reasons for analyzing the movement with those of the researchers.
2. Check with other experts to verify or modify what researchers deem to be important.
3. Use a checklist to rank or identify factors.
4. Measure the important factors.
5. Construct a template of the ideal and compare the performance with the ideal. A template is a pattern, model or form of the desired product. It is the criterion for comparison of the movement such as in Fig. 8-5 and Tables 8-1 and 8-2.

Table 8-3. *Continued*

NAME _____ SPORT _____ DATE _____

RUNNING MECHANICS

Mechanics	Rating	Comments

Frontal/Coronal Plane

Foot strike (heel, mid, toe)
  Knee and hip flexion

  Knee angle approx 170 degrees at contact

  C/g over base of support, breaking force

Mid-support phase - lowest c/g, knee approx 145° (diff approx 25°)

Take off (following - highest c/g - diff 4 inches)
  Extension of driving hip, knee, and foot

Rear - leg kick up

Stride length (longer inc speed - shorter dec speed; consistency)

Length ground contact relative to non-support phase (less - greater speed)

Pelvis posture

Trunk - straight line (back flat) through-out stride; body lean

Head erect, no strain anterior/posterior

Rhythmic leg movement (consistency)

Arm action; elbow 90°, relaxed; arms working in opposition - balance factor

Relaxed run; jaw easy; all body parts effortless

Sagittal Plane (support and non-support phases)

Foot plant relative to mid line - foot forces - pronation to supination, heel, outside border, head of metatarsals at time of push-off

Ankle pronation/supination (right/left)

Knee valgus/varus (right/left)

Hip inward/outward rotation, pelvis alignment

Direction of forces

Head and trunk/spine control, fixed position - arms and legs working independent of trunk

Rating Scale: **4** - very good, **3** - good, **2** - fair, **1** - insufficient

Contributed by Lois A. Klatt, Human Performance Laboratory, Concordia College, River Forest, Illinois

6. Construct a profile of the performance. Profiles are similar to templates, but usually consist of parameters of the movement or determinants of movement.

Checklists of the running and overarm throwing patterns appear in Table 8-3.

Note that measurements are not precise, but relative. Gross changes in movement patterns can be identified and developmental changes are easily recognized.

A template of skilled polevaulters was constructed by McGinnis. Selected factors are listed in Table 8-4. Individual polevaulters can be filmed and factors measured from their performances, and comparisons can then be made. Profiling is a striking way of drawing attention to inadequacies in performance. For example, in Fig. 8-11 the individual whose performance was profiled is below (less than the average) on two of the factors, average on three factors, and above average on one factor. Profiling consists of scaling the measurement scores to the average, norm, or ideal of a population. One can also use the individual's performance as the criterion profile. Thus, we would establish the baseline profile using Test 1 and compare subsequent profiles on later tests, such as test 2, 3, etc.) for longitudinal comparisons.

MINI-LAB LEARNING EXPERIENCES

Utilize photographs or tracings to analyze according to each item.

1. Example from field or clinical investigation—does this person toe out or toe in, does the body lean excessively or slightly, do the arms swing outward or forward, are the shoulders relatively level or definitely uneven? Is there asymmetry in the right and left limbs?
2. Example in the sport world—backhandspring with roundoff. Does the performer land with the body turned diagonally rather than in the direction of the movement, does the trunk lean laterally, does one person go lower than another, is the landing with a flexed trunk, does the person lose balance?
3. Example from ballet—are the arm movements asymmetrical, is the trunk out of alignment with flexion at the hip joint, does the person fail to elevate as high as desirable?
4. Example in work or daily living—driving an automobile. Is the driver hunched over the wheel, are the hands and tendons noticably depicting tension, is there a difference between the two persons depicted? (Playing a piano or using a microcomputer keyboard could be used as well.)

Each example can be taken from film or video or could consist of a series of photographs or contourgrams.

Table 8-4. *Means and standard deviations for 71 variables identified in a biomechanical analyses of 16 vaulters performing successful pole vaults above 5.5 meters. These may be helpful in profiling of polevaulters and predictions of performance potential or identification of performance problems. Some variables may be more important than others and variables are interdependent. This compilation, however, represents one of the more comprehensive biomechanical databases on a single skill. (Courtesy of Peter McGinnis, Northern Colorado State University, Greeley)*

APPROACH RUN

SECOND TO LAST STEP *(touchdown to touchdown)*

		M	S.D.
1.	Step length	2.20	0.14 m
2.	Velocity	9.43	0.34 m/s

LAST STEP *(touchdown to touchdown)*

3.	Step length	2.04	0.17 m
4.	Velocity	9.57	0.52 m/s
5.	Swing leg thigh angle at takeoff	64.3	6.3°
6.	Trunk angle at instant of last touchdown	88.4	3.7°
7.	Horizontal distance between center of gravity (CG) and toe at instant of last touchdown	59.0	8.0 cm

PLANT

(the instant when the pole strikes the back of the box)

8.	Pole angle	27.7	1.1°
9.	Trunk angle	87.5	4.2°
10.	Relative vertical extension of plant arm	89.0	11.2%
11.	Horizontal position of take off foot toe relative to top hand (- indicates behind hand grip)	41.0	14.0 cm
12.	Horizontal position of take off foot toe relative to box	3.94 m	12.0 cm
13.	Total time of support until plant	0.05	.02 sec

TAKE OFF (t = 0.00 sec)

(the instant when the take off foot leaves the ground)

		M	S.D.
14.	Horizontal velocity of CG	7.57	0.36 m/s
15.	Vertical velocity of CG	2.43	0.20 m/s
16.	Resultant velocity of CG	7.96	0.36 m/s
17.	Take off angle	17.8	1.5°
18.	Height of CG	1.28 m	5.0 cm
19.	Total mechanical energy of vaulter divided by vaulter mass	45.6	2.8 J/kg
20.	Relative amount of pole bend	4.2	1.5 %
21.	Pole angle	29.4	1.2°
22.	Trunk angle	79.0	6.1°
23.	Swing leg thigh angle	65.5	11.5°
24.	Relative vertical extension of plant arm	77.8	12.6 %
25.	Horizontal position of take off foot toe relative to top hand	16.0	9.0 cm
26.	Duration of pole support	0.07	.02 sec
27.	Duration of take off foot contact	0.12	.01 sec

SWING (t = 0.00 - 0.32 sec)

(from take off until the distance from the CG to the box is a minimum)

		M	S.D.
28.	Minimum distance between CG and box	2.62 m	10.0 cm
29.	Horizontal displacement of CG during swing	2.14 m	18.0 cm
30.	Vertical displacement of CG during swing	0.82 m	7.0 cm
31.	Duration of swing	0.37	.03 sec

Table 8-4. *Continued*

ROCKBACK (t = 0.32 - 0.79 sec)
(from end of swing until hips are above lower hand)

32.	Maximum relative amount of pole bend	30.6	2.4 %
33.	Minimum effective pole length	3.40 m	13.0 cm
34.	Angle of effective pole at instant of maximum pole bend	61.1	2.3°
35.	Time of maximum pole bend	0.48	.04 sec
36.	Minimum moment of inertia of vaulter divided by vaulter mass	810.0	150.0 g-cm^2/g
37.	Time of this minimum	0.60	.06 sec
38.	Horizontal displacement of CG during rockback	1.01 m	9.0 cm
39.	Vertical displacement of CG during rockback	1.46 m	24.0 cm
40.	Duration of rockback	0.43	.05 sec

EXTENSION, PULL AND TURN (t = 0.79 - 1.34 sec)
(from end of rockback until top hand release)

		M	S.D.
41.	Total backward rotation of body from plant	128.9	10.3°
42.	Time when backward rotation ends	0.78	.06 sec
43.	Maximum pole extension velocity	4.21	0.63 m/s
44.	Angle of effective pole at this instant	83.9	2.3°
45.	Time of maximum pole extension velocity	0.84	.06 sec
46.	Maximum vertical velocity of CG	5.04	0.38 m/s
47.	Angle of effective pole at this instant	85.9	2.0°
48.	Trunk angle at this instant	69.1	9.9°
49.	Distance between CG and pole at this instant (- indicates CG behind pole)	11.0	4.0 cm
50.	Time of maximum vertical velocity of CG	0.91	.06 sec
51.	Pole angle at instant of pole straightening	87.4	2.5°
52.	Trunk angle at instant of pole straightening	61.5	10.4°
53.	Time of pole straightening	1.09	.11 sec
54.	Time of lower hand release	1.09	.06 sec
55.	Horizontal displacement during extension, pull and turn	0.81 m	19.0 cm
56.	Vertical displacement during extension, pull and turn	2.02 m	25.0 cm
57.	Duration of extension, pull and turn	0.53	.10 sec

UPPER HAND RELEASE (t = 1.34 sec)
(the instant when the upper hand releases its grip from the pole)

		M	S.D.
58.	Pole angle	89.5	2.7°
59.	Trunk angle	46.5	8.2°
60.	Distance between CG and pole (- indicates CG behind pole)	46.0	14.0 cm
61.	Height of CG	5.49 m	17.0 cm
62.	Height of CG above top hand	0.87 m	15.0 cm
63.	Horizontal velocity of CG	1.49	0.51 m/s
64.	Vertical velocity of CG	1.78	0.81 m/s
65.	Work done from plant to release divided by vaulter mass	7.2	4.8 J/kg
66.	Excess kinetic energy divided by vaulter mass	2.65	1.94 J/kg
67.	Time of upper hand release	1.32	.10 sec

FLIGHT AND CLEARANCE

68.	Maximum height of CG	5.70	12.0 cm
69.	Horizontal position of CG at maximum height	-69.0	17.0 cm
70.	Difference between crossbar height and maximum CG height	10.0	9.0 cm
71.	Time of maximum CG height	1.51	.05 sec

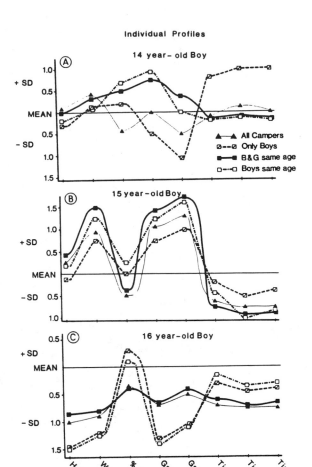

Individual Profiles

Fig. 8-11. *Profile of three young male cross country runners compared to their age group, and total group. The choice of a criterion, normative, or baseline profile will influence interpretation of performances of an individual. For which profile do these boys fare best? (Reprinted with permission from* Biomechanics in Sports III & IV, *edited by Terauds, Gowitzke, and Holt. Research Center for Sports. 1987. p. 310)*

BASIC DYNAMOGRAPHIC RECORD ANALYSES

Forces recorded with spring scales, cable tensiometers, or other displays of force, without respect to time, are expressed as maximum forces. If force-time patterns are recorded, such as depicted in Fig. 8-12, analyses may be a simple qualitative comparison of patterns (pattern recognition, usually an individual pattern compared to a criterion pattern). If quantitative analyses are made, these may be quite complete and include measurement of the total impulse (area under the curve), the maximum and minimum forces for each curvature, forces at specific instances in time, as determined by other experimental data,

QUALITATIVE AND QUANTITATIVE ASSESSMENT   **257**

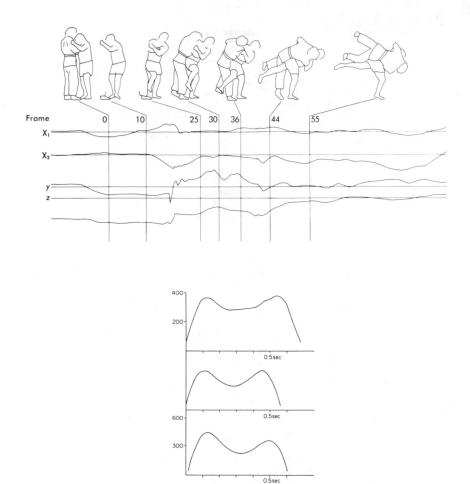

Fig. 8-12. *Contourgrams and three-dimensional force-time histories of judo throw, and walking at different speeds. Note how much easier it is to evaluate the kinetics of a cyclic and mostly planar movement than that of a three-dimensional movement, such as a judo throw.*

duration of total force production, duration of different parts of the force-time pattern, and time at which specific forces occur. In addition, the rise-time (slope of the curve) of force production can be measured.

ACCELEROMETRY

If the application of force is of short duration, such as during impacts as experienced in judo throw landings, jumping landings, and contact of a ball with a bat, an accelerometer may be the best transducer to use. The total peak forces expressed in G forces as well as the slope of the curve are common variables to analyze. Based upon these variables, a Severity Index was developed at Wayne State Uni-

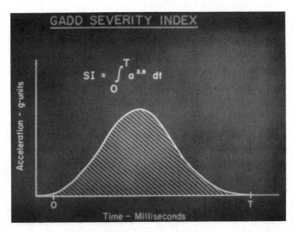

Fig. 8-13. *Measurement of impact deceleration via an accelerometer. The rise time, peak G force, the total impulse (area under the curve) and the severity index (area relative to possible trauma to body).*

versity as a criterion for potential head injury assessment. Recordings from an accelerometer appear in Fig. 8-13.

Electrogoniometric Analysis

Amplitude and duration of angular displacements are the most obvious measurements to obtain from the goniogram (recording from an elgon). In addition, the angles at key instances in time often are measured. Average velocities with respect to selected time intervals can be calculated and accelerations estimated. Patterns of changes of angles at the joint can be identified with respect to consistency and the norm. Measurement techniques are listed in Fig. 8-14.

MUSCLE ANALYSIS

Analysis of the active muscles during a movement can be conducted by means of electromyography, deductions from anatomical knowledge, and deductions from experimentally obtained kinematic data. Although none of these three methods is error free, analysis of the electromyogram is the most objective method. There is, however, the necessity of separating the artifact from the action potentials. Waterland and Shambes (1969) described this process quite well.

Analysis of the Electromyogram. The basic analysis is to determine whether or not the muscle is contracting and to estimate the magnitude of contraction. A comparison of two muscles, a flexor and an extensor muscle acting antagonistically to each other, can be made by observing the electromyograms in Fig. 8-15. Changes in the amplitude of the spikes of the electromyogram can be relatively assessed as being: none, slight, moderate, or marked.

Rather than compare raw signals of action potentials of the mus-

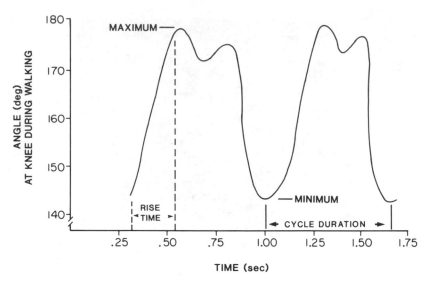

Fig. 8-14. *Goniogram and analytical process. The maximum and minimum angles are determined, the rise time is measured and angular velocity calculated, and the angles at key instants in time are measured.*

cle (EMG), most systems include an integrator so that the output will resemble the force-time curves described previously. There is a continuing summation of the action potentials when the signal is integrated as shown in Fig. 8-16. Another well-used analysis technique is to compare the EMG obtained during performance with the EMG representing maximum isometric contraction of that muscle. If performances require muscular contractions at low speeds, this type of analysis appears quite approprite. If fast speeds are produced during performance, the EMG values will be greater than 100% of the criterion (maximum isometric contraction). Data using this technique have been depicted in Fig. 8-17.

Muscle Figures

The ultimate evaluation of the electromyogram with respect to performance assessment is to create a muscle figure as shown in Figs. 8-18 and 8-19. The first figure was produced in the 1960's by Nemessuri, a well-known Hungarian biomechanist. The second figure is one of a series of analyses published by the National Strength Coaches Association. This particular set of muscle figures was produced based upon a combination of anatomical, cinematographic, and electromyographic interpretation.

COMPOSITE ANALYSIS

More and more, researchers are combining instrumentation to obtain a comprehensive analysis of a movement pattern. One of the more

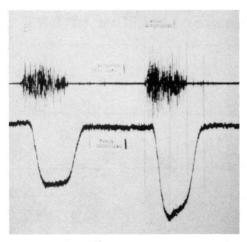

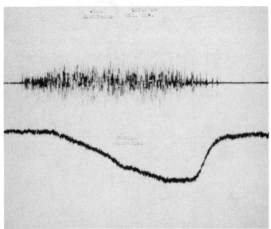

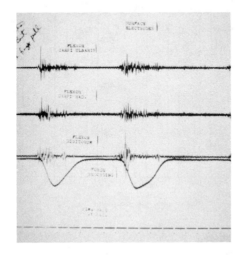

Fig. 8-15. *Is the muscle contracting or relaxing? How often is there marked con-traction, moderate, and slight contraction? This is the most qualitative method of analysis of electromyograms.*

QUALITATIVE AND QUANTITATIVE ASSESSMENT **261**

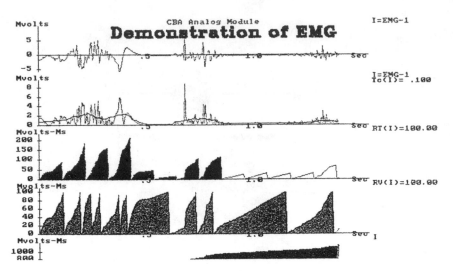

Fig. 8-16. *Integrated electromyograms (IEMG) are easier to interpret. Compare the area under the curve for two actions of the same muscle. Which activity required greater involvement of the muscle? How much greater? (Courtesy of Ariel Dynamics, Inc.)*

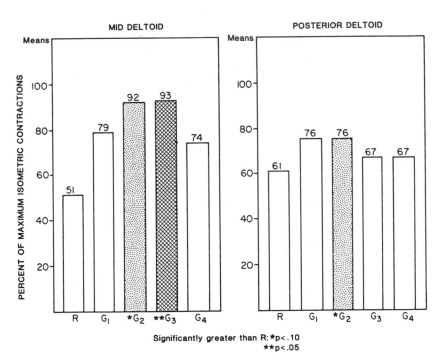

Significantly greater than R: *p<.10
**p<.05

Fig. 8-17. *Graphic portrayal of estimated muscle involvement during five styles of rope jumping. Muscle action potentials expressed in percent of maximum isometric contraction of middle and posterior heads of the deltoid muscle respectively are depicted. A gyro style rope with long handles and long rope was used.*

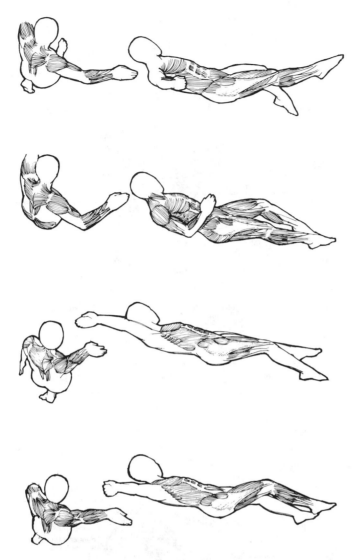

Fig. 8-18. *Identification of muscle involvement during different phases of swimming. Name the muscles. (Reprinted with permission from* Funktionelle Sportanatomie, *authored by Mihaly Nemessuri, Akademiai Kiado, Budapest, 1963)*

comprehensive approaches is to investigate movement from initiation to the brain until completion of the motor act. Study Fig. 8-20 and describe the process that occurs.

MOVEMENT ANALYSIS MODELS

Now that you have read the many ways to analyze movements of human beings, you might wish to have a model by which you choose

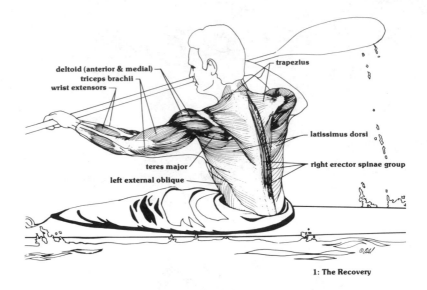

deltoid (anterior & medial)
triceps brachii
wrist extensors
trapezius
latissimus dorsi
right erector spinae group
teres major
left external oblique

1: The Recovery

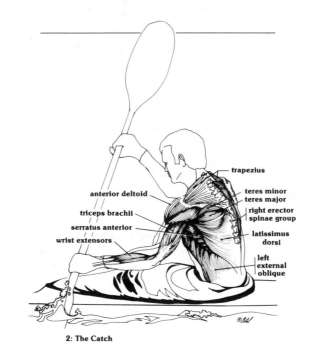

trapezius
anterior deltoid
teres minor
teres major
triceps brachii
right erector spinae group
serratus anterior
latissimus dorsi
wrist extensors
left external oblique

2: The Catch

Fig. 8-19. *Identification of muscle involvement during four phases of kayaking. (Reprinted with permission from* National Strength and Conditioning Journal, Vol 7, No. 5, 0ct.–Nov. 1986. Logan, S. and Holt, L. "The Flatwater Kayak Stroke," pp. 4–11.)

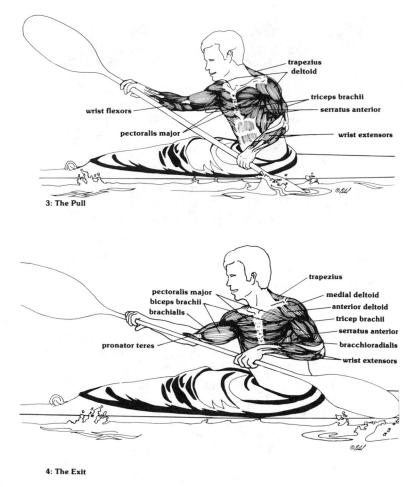

3: The Pull

4: The Exit

Fig. 8-19. *Continued*

what is important to analyze and the scientific plan by which you analyze. Three theoretical models will be presented: Possum, Factors-Results, Game Principles.

Possum

This model was proposed by Hudson and was developed based upon experimental evaluation of jumping skills. Possum is an acronym for Purpose/Observation System of Studying and Understanding Movement. The three guidelines she asks are:

1. What matters?
2. How is it measured?
3. How is it manipulated?

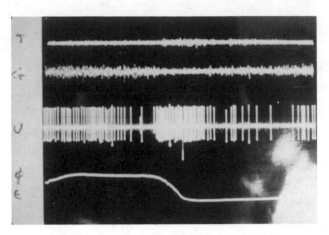

Fig. 8-20. *Multiple data recorded from EEG, electrogoniometry, dynamography, and electromyography. The sequence of onset of each event can be noted. A description of the sequence of neuromuscular phenomena can be written from this "picture worth a thousand words." Try it!*

The first step is to classify the movement with respect to purpose. Examples are generation of maximum force, maintenance of balance, and intentional loss of balance. Within a purpose category, there should be observable dimensions of movement that correspond with the correct execution of the task. That is to say, the observations that matter are those that can distinguish between levels of skill from the novice to the elite. If a variable is not useful in evaluating movement, then we consider it not to matter. Once an observation is deemed to matter, it must be measurable. Since most appliers of biomechanical information do not have access to high technology laboratories, it is considered beneficial for the observations to be measureable qualitatively with the naked eye. Once a measurement is made, the question becomes: Can this variable be manipulated? If the variable is crucial to performance but it cannot be changed, then we consider it not to matter.

Variables that matter (and can also be observed) for the vertical jump with a countermovement are listed below:

Specific Kinetic Observations

Force	*Torque*	*Use of Stored Elastic Energy*
• magnitude	• magnitude	• potential energy
• direction	• direction	• translational kinetic energy
• point of application	• axis of rotation	• rotational kinetic energy

Specific Kinematic Observations

Balance	*Range of* *Motion*	*Coordination*
• base of support	• starting position	• sequencing
• line of gravity	• ending position	• timing

Each variable is evaluated in relative terms based upon a continuum concept. Study the coordination continuum as follows:

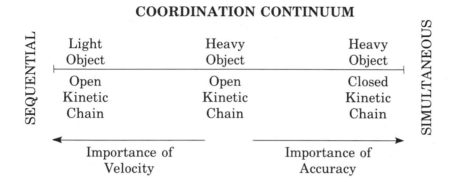

COORDINATION CONTINUUM

As velocity becomes more important, the kinetic chain becomes open and light weights are desirable.

A further example of observational coordination sequences are the three patterns of segmental coordination depicted in Fig. 8-21. With respect to vertical jumping, skilled jumpers use an observable simultaneous coordination pattern.

Two continuum POSSUM examples with respect to direction of force and magnitude of force are presented and analyzed with respect to vertical jumping. (See table 8-5.) The purposes are to remain stable over the base of support and to project the body vertically. By extending from the purpose continuum horizontally to connect with the observation continuum, the desired pattern of movement should be obtained. Therefore, if stability is desired, the line of gavity should be observed to fall within the base of support. And, if height of projection is desired, the initial path of the projectile should be vertical. With respect to magnitude of force, the purpose of maximum vertical jumping is to display maximum effort in a powerful manner with respect to the force-velocity trade-off. Moving horizontally from the power region on the purpose continuum, it can be seen that the beginning position of the range of motion should be in the middle, or from the results of skilled jumpers, slightly greater than 90 degrees. Also, a medium excursion should be taken to finish with complete extension. The pattern of coordination that connects with powerful efforts is simultaneous.

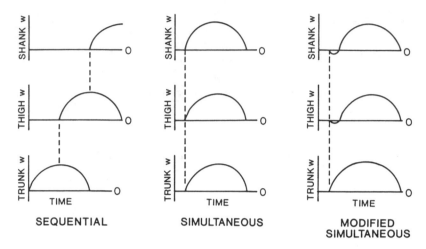

Fig. 8-21. *Three patterns of segmental coordination. Although other body parts might be represented when analyzing other movement patterns, only three are depicted here for a vertical jump in which arms are not used. Skilled jumpers utilize primarily the simultaneous pattern. Which coordination pattern is utilized by the segments of the upper extremity during throwing activities?*

Factors-Results

This is the name we are using to describe the qualitative model developed by Hay. In the recent book by Hay and Reid (1987) they describe the model as one in which the analyst identifies the result of the performance and then proceeds to list the factors which produce this result. Examples of results of common sports activities include the following: distance, time, height, points scored, weight lifted, and advantage attained. The result of throwing and some jumping activities is DISTANCE; whereas, running, swimming, and cycling activities has TIME as their result.

Hay then uses a hierarchial structure to depict the factors that determine the result. This hierarchical model is described for the standing long jump in Fig. 8-22. Note that the distance is determined by four sub-parts; the takeoff distance (how far the center of gravity is in front of feet), the flight distance (the distance during which the center of gravity does not fall below its elevation at takeoff), the landing distance (that distance reached by the feet beyond the flight distance), and the fall-back distance (distance to be subtracted). Except for the PHYSIQUE factor, the factors basically are motion factors (mechanics: velocity, speed, distance, force, mass, acceleration, resistance, such as water or air). This model is a deterministic model, in that each factor is determined by those linked to it from the next lower row of the hierarchy.

Table 8-5. *Examples of components of POSSUM Model developed by Jackie Hudson. Analysis of balance, projection, and maximum effort purposes are evaluated with respect to direction and magnitude of force. Observations are made and estimates of line of gravity, path, and range of motion are placed on the respective continuum. These estimates are then matched to each purpose continuum.*

Direction of Force

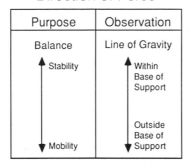

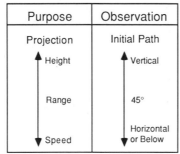

Magnitude of Force

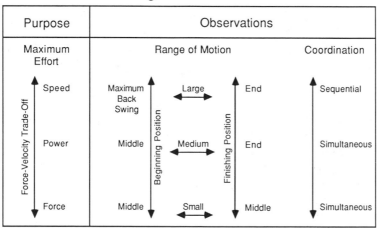

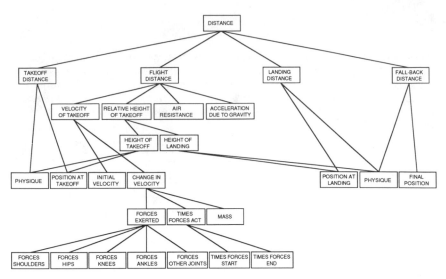

Fig. 8-22. *Factors-Results Model proposed by Hay for the standing long jump. Note the hierarchical structure. Each lower factor influences the linked factor above. Distance is the goal and four subcomponents of distance are influenced by 23 factors as diagrammed. (Reprinted by permission from James G. Hay and J. Gavin Reid,* Anatomy, Mechanics, and Human Motion. *N.J: Prentice Hall, 1988 p. 255)*

Game Principle Model

This model (See Fig. 8-23) is a holistic approach based on one by Higgins, and consisting of the following steps:

1) Describing the movement.
2) Setting the performance goal.
3) Identifying the anatomical, mechanical, and environmental considerations.
4) Setting forth the biomechanical principles for successful and skilled performance of the movement.
5) Assessing the performance with respect to these principles.

Step 1: Describing the Movement

This step consists of a qualitative and general description of the temporal and spatial characteristics of the movement as performed by the elite or expert performer. In addition, the forces involved in the movement are identified.

Example. Bowling could be described as a leisure-sport activity involving locomotion on land plus gross manipulation of a ball that will in turn be projected into space. The movements are primarily in the saggital plane. Rotations at the hip, knee, and ankle about the frontal-horizontal axes cause the body to translate forward four steps. The arm in which the ball is held swings in the sagittal plane, a half circle backward and a half circle forward. The total movement pattern

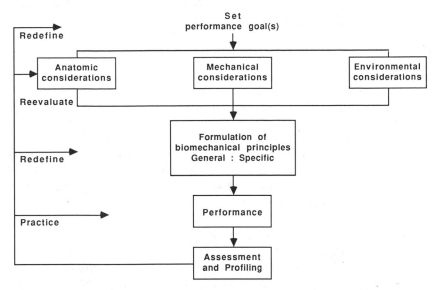

Fig. 8-23. *Game Principle Model developed by the authors. The goal of the movement is determined and the anatomical, mechanical, and environmental factors important to the movement success are listed. Basic biomechanical principles are formulated and movement is evaluated according to these principles. Profiles are constructed to aid in evaluation.*

takes approximately 2 seconds to perform. Movements appear to require little muscle force. The fastest movement is the arm swing, which appears to be pendular in nature, that is, influenced primarily by the force of gravity. The hand, fingers, and arm show a diagonally upward and lateral movement at the time of release of the ball. This movement is not precisely described by means of observational techniques. The locomotion shows an increase in speed until the final step, which is a sliding step. The person completes the action of bowling in a rather stable position behind a foul line. The ball rolls along the floor as a result of being released just after the low point of the swing during the sliding step.

Step 2: Setting the Performance Goal

Setting the performance goal is not always simple. There may be three different goals for three individuals performing the same movement. These goals temper the analysis of the anatomical, mechanical, and environmental considerations.

Example. A competitive breaststroke swimmer will not glide during the stroke cycle, whereas the swimmer desiring maximum stroke efficiency of energy output from each stroke will perform an optimum glide. The competitive swimmer wishes to accelerate from one stroke to the next. The recreational swimmer does not. In a like manner, the walking pattern of a cat changes when it stalks its prey. Race walking, walking on ice, and walking on snow shoes may have different goals, such as speed, balance and efficiency.

Step 3: Identifying the Anatomical, Mechanical, and Environmental
Considerations

A. *Anatomical Considerations*. The general size, shape and weight of the total body is investigated. In addition, strength and speed of the movement apparatus need to be estimated or measured to determine whether or not there are unique characteristics that must be considered. Unique characteristics should be noted and comparisons made with respect to age, sex, and other subgroups, such as members of a fencing team. Will extreme strength be required? Does the movement favor the short, lightweight person?

For example, a hemiplegic swimmer and a paraplegic swimmer will perform a swimming stroke differently from each other and especially from an able-bodied and neurologically sound person. Individual differences—whether high-level attributes or impairments—will influence what is biomechanically ideal for the given individual. In particular, the human individual might be an infant, a physically disabled person, a person over 80 years of age, a skilled ballet dancer, a professional tennis player, or some other person of unique or unusual characteristics or performance abilities.

B. *Mechanical Considerations*. Some of these considerations are unalterable unless movement takes place in outer space, such as on the moon, on Jupiter, or on an earth satellite station. Basically, the force of gravity rules or controls movements of animals and human beings, and even of planets.

Therefore, the first approach to the mechanical considerations is the magnitude, direction, duration, and point of application of force. If rotation is to occur, what is the moment of force required to produce and regulate the rotation? How many forces are present? Which forces will inhibit the movement, and how can their inhibitory roles be reduced?

The results of forces and moments of forces acting on a body will be the measureable and predictable velocities and accelerations of the body as it is moved in space. Analysis of these factors provides insight into the kinematics of the movement, but the final approach to the mechanical considerations is holistic. Here too the work-energy and impulse-momentum of the body are considered.

C. *Environmental Considerations*. What restrictions or restraints are placed upon the movement because of the implements, the climate, the terrain, and other persons? For example, in the work situation, the placement of facilities and equipment offers the greatest restraint to the movement pattern. In sports situations the impositions commonly consist of the rules of play. Movements would not be executed, and especially not terminated, in the manner they are if it were not for foul lines, height of nets, and intimidating actions of opponents.

Not to be omitted from environmental considerations is the internal environment of the performer. What is his or her motivation, state of mind, level of tension or level of relaxation? Although difficult to assess, the internal environment must be included in this set of considerations.

Step 4: Biomechanical Principles of Movement

A principle denotes a statement of fact about a phenomenon, a person, an object, or an event. Principles are formulated so that the complex movement of living bodies can be effectively reduced to simpler elements and thereby evaluated or described. Principles usually will state a relationship about two factors or will show a cause-and-effect relationship. For example, an understanding of equilibrium is derived from the following basic principle. A body will be in equilibrium if the center of mass remains above the base of support of the body.

Selection of the best combination of principles, or a compromise or an adaptation of general principles, is sometimes necessary because of the goal, individual impairment, or other unique anatomical, mechanical, or environmental consideration. For example, in golf one might sacrifice maximum distance for a gain in accuracy, especially with respect to distance, if two moderate-distance shots will equal one long drive and one short clip.

Example. In bowling the major principles would be as follows:

1. Moderate ball speed is required to achieve best pin action.
2. Ball speed can be achieved through summations of forces — approach, arm swing.
3. Muscular forces can be reduced if gravity is used as a facilitating force—use extended arm push-away to initiate downswing of arm, use trunk flexion to increase ROM and height of arm swing.
4. Accuracy is easiest if all movements are in the sagittal plane.
5. Greater kinetic energy is developed with a higher backswing.
6. Pin action (required especially for second ball) is best achieved through application of lateral spin on ball.

Step 5: Performance and Assessment

This step consists of isolating the components of the movement that cause success or failure and then relating those problems to the biomechanical principles. This process also involves the construction of profiles so that direct comparison can be made between the performance and a safe, effective, and efficient performance. Predictions of level of success and potential risk of injury are derived outcomes of profiling.

REFERENCES

Biomechanics Instrumentation Video Library, Indianapolis, IN, Benchmark Press.
Computer Software Movement Analysis Learning Modules, Indianapolis, IN, Benchmark Press.
Lanshammar, H.: *Gait analysis in theory and practice,* Sweden, 1985, Uppsala University.
Physical Therapy, December Issue, 4:12, 1984.

Part III   *Human Movement and Posture Biomechanics*

Concepts related to work, exercise, A.D.L.
artistic endeavors, disabilities, and the
developmental process

9

Developmental Biomechanics

Do two-year-olds, 20-year-olds and 90-year-olds walk, swing an axe, climb a ladder, and perform other movement patterns in the same way? Of course not. Movement patterns change during a person's life-span. Some of these changes will occur as a function of growth and development of the human body, and others are learned, via practice and education. Developmental biomechanics is the study of movement patterns and how they change due to interaction between human beings and their environment. During the early years, infancy and childhood sequential and orderly movement patterns emerge at predictable ages. Neurological development and physical development contribute to the nature of these movement pattern changes (and acquisitions). Thus, as with other living beings, motor development of human beings has a phylogenetic basis. The acquisition of skill in performing these movement patterns, however, appears to be founded upon learning theory, not hereditary theory.

The majority of research concerning motor development has been focused upon children. These studies have been descriptive in nature, with limited process-oriented experimentation. Since stage theory is the primary analytical model for the study of developmental movement patterns, it will be explained in the first section. Representative movement patterns of children and assessment of development stages will be described. Emphasis will be upon development of fundamental movement patterns and patterns of activities of daily living.

The second major section of this chapter will focus upon the aged population. Many questions have been posed, with few answers being agreed upon, concerning motor development of adults, especially persons over the age of seventy years. Descriptive data, however, exist and can be utilized to develop theories concerning changing movement patterns among the aged population.

Two other sections in this chapter have been included: diagnosis for effective teaching and motor control changes with age. Synthesizing the information in this chapter will enable you to be a pioneer in the acquisition of research-based knowledge in developmental biomechanics.

MOTOR DEVELOPMENT IS VIEWED AS A CONTINUOUS AND LIFELONG PROCESS

Motor development is one part of the study of human development. Charting of twins and children of psychologists occurred in the 1920's and 30's. Identification of the movement patterns and the age and order at which they appeared were reported. Qualitative descriptions of the movements composed the bulk of the research data. Wild (1938) was the first to propose the theory of stages of development of fundamental movement patterns. Her treatise on this topic was voluminous and was the foundation for most of the research during the next four decades. The University of Wisconsin faculty, and graduates of the university, have been the leaders in motor development with respect to children.

Stage-theory models can be classified into three types: stages, intratask component stages, and kinematic continuum stages. Although these have unique interpretations, the goals are identical. All theories include a hierarchial structure to depict progression toward maturation.

The most advanced stage theory, modified from Wild's stages, is that of Seefeldt and colleagues. Additional stages have been proposed to more nearly equalize intervals in the progression from one stage to the next. In addition, a biomechanical approach was used to describe each. Roberton and colleagues have proposed that the changes in throwing must be divided into substages, that is, each component of throwing will have a developmental sequence or series of stages. We propose that the action of the legs can be charted in stages independently of the action of the throwing arm. Using this classification, there would be a more finite number of stages defined than that suggested by Seefeldt.

Adrian, Toole, and Randall have proposed that movement patterns be considered as a continuum rather than as discrete stages. Here, too, the approach is a biomechanical one. The range of motion, planes of motion, and axes of motion are identified. If the goal is maximum speed or distance, then the level of maturation of the movement pattern is evaluated by the amount and complexity of space utilized. In addition the temporal aspects are evaluated, the sequencing of the body parts and the speed of these parts are reported. Again, maturation, the highest stage of development, refers to the fastest and the most effective timing of the body parts.

MOTOR DEVELOPMENT OF CHILDREN

Children's early motor development takes place in a sequential manner, from the reflex actions of the newborn to the more complex actions of the mature person. The first actions of the fetus as well as of the newborn child are reflexive and are primitive and postural in nature. Their purpose is survival; that is, they are done for securing food (sucking) or for protection (attempt at righting from a falling action).

There are various ways to classify voluntary movement. Gallahue and colleagues list such movements as follows:

1. Rudimentary movements follow reflexes and, in the opinion of some, build on them. The reflexes begin 5 months before birth and continue for about 2 years.
2. Fundamental movements begin at 1 to 2 years of age and continue until 7 years of age. They involve walking, running, throwing, and jumping, but are immature.
3. The complex sport skills begin at approximately age 7 to 10 years and are carried on into adulthood.

The reflexes are the first clues to later voluntary action. The stability patterns of creeping and crawling, followed by walking, and the manipulative patterns such as grasping, reaching, exploring, pulling, and twisting are the real basis for the later rudimentary and fundamental movements. The exact period for learning these skills varies considerably, but there is an age range at which these movements are best learned. Usually, they are learned in an unvarying sequential manner, regardless of the age range.

WALKING

The Walking Action

Steindler has stated that walking "is a series of catastrophies narrowly averted." First, there is a falling of the body forward; then the legs move under the body and prevent such an accident from occurring by establishing a new base of support with the feet.

Walking is a type of reflex action. The reflexes, such as righting and stepping, displayed by the infant are the very foundation on which walking is based. Reflexes are the first clues to later voluntary movement. The postural reflexes exhibited by the young child during the first months of life are evident during the standing and stepping actions induced by parents. They are the prelude to the walking action. The adult walking action is the very epitome of the horizontal of joint action and the synchronization of muscle action into a flowing movement. The action is beautiful to watch but extremely complex to analyze. It is a remarkable accomplishment, considering the design of the human body, which features a high center of gravity and a small base of support.

The first true walking steps begin between the ages of 10 and 16 months. The young child between the ages of 4 and 7 years usually is thought to walk with adult characteristics. Illness and consequent confinement for a long period of time may cause the walking act to be delayed or, in an adult, to have to be relearned.

Some of the phases of walking are altered in injured and permanently disabled persons. A continuous attempt is being made by biochemical researchers to develop artificial limbs that enable persons with pathologic conditions to walk as nearly normal as possible.

The bipedal position permits rapid initiation of the motion of walking. The center of gravity is easily displaced in the desired direction because (1) it resides high (at approximately the second sacral segment) over a small base of support and (2) the greater portion of the body weight is located in the trunk, head, and shoulders, rather than in the lower extremitites. This inherently unstable situation necessitates close cooperation of the neuromusculoskeletal system in the act of walking.

That the center of gravity is located above the main joint of support adds to the instability. The human body is classified as having three effective joints and two effective segments (the lower limbs) for speed and is not considered to have the most effective leg joints and segments in connection with balance. Thus, the human body is designed for rapid initial movement in walking and running but not for sustained speed.

There are two theories concerning the initiation of the step in walking. One involves the displacement of the center of gravity and then activation of both the step reflex and the righting reflex. The movement is termed "a falling/catching act," as previously noted. The other theory is that the movement of the center of gravity to its highest position—which is reached when the foot rises onto the toes—activates the gastrocnemius and hamstring muscles. They contract with the pulling of the heel off the ground, and along with the gravitational action on the center of gravity, activate the step. Each of these theories has its proponents.

Two phases of walking are in Fig. 9-1. The stance (support) phase, composed of heel strike, foot flat, heel off, flexion at the knee, and toe off is approximately 60% of the walking cycle, and the swing phase, composed of toe clearance and leg swing, is 40% of the walking cycle. Some of these percentages are changed in the stair ascent and descent, running, and jumping aspects of motion.

The stance phase encompasses the heel strike, midstance, and push off. The swing phase includes the beginning of the acceleration of the leg as the foot is lifted from the ground and the body weight is centered over the other foot. The swinging of the non-weight-bearing leg

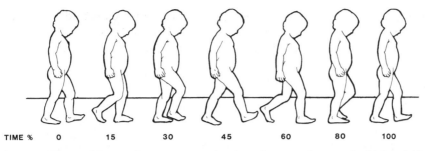

| TIME % | 0 | 15 | 30 | 45 | 60 | 80 | 100 |

Fig. 9-1. *The walking cycle: support and swing phase and percent of total stride at seven discrete positions.*

and its deceleration in preparation for the heel strike comprise the other portions of the swing phase.

Walking can be described as having two energy phases, a high- and a low-energy phase. The high-energy phase of walking occurs during the stance phase. This is explained by the fact that the descending leg is decelerated just before and at the time of the heel strike, thus preventing injury to the heel. In addition, the shock of the heel as it strikes is absorbed by the lower limb and the entire body, which requires energy. Since the shock absorption enables the body to be balanced during midstance, the energy cost is high. The leg abductors are very active during this time. Finally, the push off portion of the stance phase initiates the forward propulsion of the body and therefore is high in energy requirements.

The low-energy phase occurs during the acceleration portion (swing phase) of the walking cycle. The hip flexors and knee extensors help keep the heel from rising too high. Dorsiflexion of the toes at the midpoint of the swing in preparation for the heel strike prevents the toes from striking first. The hamstring muscles also expend energy to decelerate the leg during the latter stages of the swing. The question might be then raised: Why is this the low-energy phase? The reason lies in the pendulum action of the swinging leg, which takes considerably less energy than is expended at heel strike, absorption of shock, and push off. Gravity is working in favor of the pendulum swing by pulling the leg mass down toward the ground. The momentum gained at push off helps carry the leg through the swing phase.

It has been estimated that during a portion of the swing phase, the lower leg reaches a velocity of 32.18 kmph (20 mph). In running, this becomes 64.36 to 80.45 kmph (40 or 50 mph).

The most effective walking rate is approximately 70 steps/min for most individuals, but not for all. Amar has found that at just above 190 steps/min, it is more economical, in terms of energy, to run than to walk. This is true until a speed of just under 250 steps/min is reached.

The number of steps per unit of time varies with the speed of walking and the length of the lower limbs. Data collected by Morton and Fuller (1952) are presented in Table 9-1. Note the differences between the tall man's cadence and the shorter man's cadence.

MINI-LAB LEARNING EXPERIENCES

Test yourself at 100 steps per minute for a time of one minute. Determine speed of walking: measure distance traversed in that time and divide that distance by one minute. (Refer to Chapter 5 if necessary.) Convert your answer to mph or kmph and/or convert the speeds in Table 9-1 to feet/min or meters/min.

Can you calculate the average distance of each step? If you calculate distance per step for the two subjects (Table 9-1) and yourself, is there a relationship between body height and step length? Would another anthropometric measurement be a better indicator of predicted step length than body height? If you guessed leg length, you are correct.

Anthropometry influences the preferred or optimum step length and cadence (step rate or frequency of steps) an individual will choose. The step length multiplied by the step rate equals speed of walking. In studying the energy cost for 19 college women walking on a treadmill electrically driven at 3.2, 4.02, and 4.82 kmph (2, 2.5 and 3 mph), Baird found the optimum rate (ratio of the amount of work to the oxygen consumption) to be between 4.02 and 4.82 kmph (2.5 and 3.0 mph). Other researchers have hypothesized that human beings will naturally select an optimum cadence for efficient walking.

Table 9-1. *Relationship of cadence and height of person walking at various speeds. There is space for the reader to add personal data.*

	4.02 kmph* (2.5 mph)**	4.82 kmph (3.0 mph)	5.68 kmph (3.5 mph)	6.43 kmph (4.0 mph)
Cadence steps per minute male 1.76 m tall (5'8")	100	112	122	130
Cadence steps per minute male 1.98 m tall (6'0.5")	92	100	108	115
Cadence steps per minute **Reader**				

*.067 kilometers per minute or 67 meters per minute
**.042 miles per minute or 220 feet per minute

Kinetics of Walking

The action of the muscles in the foot-flat position is a cooperative one in which the quadriceps, femoris, hamstrings and gluteus medius, as well as the soleus, act during the supporting phase. The rise and fall of the body in a vertical direction is 5 cm (2 in.), and the percentage of body weight alternates between 80% as one foot leaves the ground, and 120% as the heel strike takes place at the time the foot descends. The path of the center of gravity is that of a sinusoidal, or smooth, curve; no sharp braking force is evident. There is side-to-side lateral and medial sway of about 5 cm (2 in.). The physically disabled person has greater rise and fall in a vertical direction (as much as 10 cm (4 in.) than the normal individual.

In addition, there is backward force as the heel strikes the ground during the end phase of deceleration of the leg. When the foot is flat, there is a forward force as the push off commences, as well as a torque as the foot twists about the hip joint. The axial rotation of the lower limb is such that it moves, in the swing phase, into internal rotation during the heel strike, and then at push off the external rotation takes place.

The muscles of the lower limb are busy firing in rapid order during the act of walking. Acting as stabilizers and shock absorbers, they contract over a short period of time and then relax. They cause extension, flexion, and internal and external rotation. They help decelerate and accelerate, and yet they fire in milliseconds and then remain quiet a great portion of the time. During the last portion of the swing and the first portion of the stance phase, 20% of the major muscle action occurs.

The body weight is centered on the heel, and then it moves forward toward the lateral edge of the foot and diagonally toward the undersurface of the big toe. The effect of moving the body weight in such a manner enables the walker to offset much of the recoil effect. The pressures on the various parts of a foot during the stance phase are depicted in Fig. 9-2. Although similarities can be found among individuals, each pressure pattern is unique to each person.

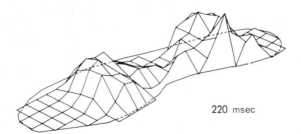

220 msec

Fig. 9-2. *Pressure pattern under foot of a person during support phase of walking. The largest pressures occur in the mid-heel region and across the metatarsals. Although other persons may produce similar pressure patterns, many persons will have dissimilar pressure patterns. (Courtesy Penn State University Biomechanics Laboratory).*

There should be an understanding of the contributions that each moving segment makes to the force that will move the body. For such an understanding, three concepts should be kept in mind.

Reversed Muscle Action

First, whenever the toes are not free to move (as in the case when they are in contact with the supporting surface and are supporting the body weight), each segment proximal to the toes is moved by reversed muscle action. Metatarsophalangeal joint action moves the foot, not the toes; ankle joint action moves the leg, not the foot; knee joint action moves the thigh, not the leg; hip joint action moves the trunk, not the thigh.

Gravity as a Facilitator

Second, gravitational force is a major contributor to segmental movements in locomotor patterns. When the body's center of gravity is not directly above the ankle joint, gravity tends to initiate movement at that joint. If the center of gravity is in front of the ankle joint, gravitational force tends to flex the foot. If muscles at the ankle contract and prevent such movement, gravity can raise the foot; if the action is moving the center of gravity forward, the heels will be raised; if the action moves the center of gravity backward, the fore part of the foot and the toes will be raised.

Pushing Action-Reaction

Third, locomotor patterns in walking are pushing patterns — pushing against the support surface. Some segments will move in a direction other than that of the desired line of force. Counteraction to the undesired movements must occur. In addition, as a segment moves, it carries with it all segments proximal to it. As the leg moves (when the foot is fixed) it also moves the thigh and trunk; as the foot moves, it moves the leg, the thigh, and the trunk. Therefore, the movement and position of a segment are determined not only by action of the joint at its distal end, but also by the movements of the segments distal to it. Before movements of a segment can be described or explained, both the movement of the immediately distal segment and the angle of the segment must be described (measured).

In summary, the main propelling force in the stepping-running-jumping pattern is derived from extension at the knee; to this is added the force of gravity, which rotates the entire body around the metatarsophalangeal joints. Extension at the ankle and hip keep the center of gravity in an advantageous position to move it in the desired direction.

DETERMINANTS OF WALKING

Saunders, Inman, and Eberhart (1953) have discussed the following six determinants of gait (walking) that continue to be cited:

1. Pelvic rotation. The pelvis rotates forward with the swing leg, and the center of gravity rotates forward on each hip as the step is taken. There is a total of 8 degrees of rotation, which reduces the drop of the center of gravity.
2. Pelvic tilt. The pelvis tilts downward during the stance phase of one leg, which tends to shorten the distance of the hip to ground and keeps the center of gravity from rising too much.
3. Flexion at the knee. It is to be remembered that as the heel strike occurs during midstance, the knee is at full extension. When the foot is flat, flexion begins at the knee (5 to 15 degrees); there then is extension at the knee and the flexion again at push off. The purpose of this flexing and extending is to prevent the center of gravity from rising unduly.
4. Foot and ankle motion. The foot and ankle help take up shock and smooth out the path of the center of gravity at heel strike. The foot is in dorsiflexion at heel strike, and as the heel off and toe off phases occur, the leg flexes, smoothing out the path of the center of gravity. The foot, ankle, and knee work together as a damper at heel strike.
5. Knee motion. There are two separate actions at the knee during walking. As the ankle rises during the heel off and toe off phase, there is flexion at the knee. The flexion at the knee serves as a shock absorber and reduces the degree to which the center of gravity rises.
6. Lateral movement of the pelvis. During walking, the lateral movement of the pelvis is 4.45 cm (1.75 in.) at each step. The femurs are adducted and the tibias are in slight valgus, enabling the body weight to be transferred downward to a nar-

row base without too much lateral motion (5 cm (2 in.)). (See Figs. 9-1 and 9-3.)

If walking starts from a stationary position, the first joint action to occur is flexion at the ankle. The reason is that there is a decreasing amount of tension exerted by the ankle extensors in the standing position when the center of gravity is in front of the ankle joint. When walking is initiated, the ankle extensors permit the center of gravity to move beyond the forward limit that is habitual in standing. The nervous system does not initiate a correction because one foot will be moved forward to receive the body weight. As the forward-moving foot is placed on the walking surface, the momentum of the moving body and the push from the rear foot carry the center of gravity over the new support. As each new foot contact is made, the momentum of the body is conserved by adjustments at the joints.

JOINT ACTIONS OF LOWER LIMBS

Joint actions of the lower limbs include those of the supporting limb and the swinging limb.

Joint Actions of Supporting Limb

Movement at the hip, knee, ankle, and metatarsophalangeal joints from the time the heel makes contact with the walking surface until the toes leave that surface is shown in Fig. 9-4. A graph such as this one presents detailed and exact information that if described verbally would require many times the space taken by the graph. Here one can see the direction of each change in angle at the joint (joint action), its degree in a given time, and the relationship between actions. Readers should develop the ability to interpret such graphs and to visualize the joint actions and the body positions shown at each time interval. In the illustration, notice that the heel makes contact at 0 second in

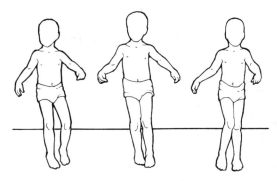

Fig. 9-3. *Walking as viewed from the frontal plane. (Note the changes in shoulder and hip with respect to the horizontal and the adduction/abduction movements of the legs.)*

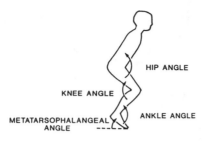

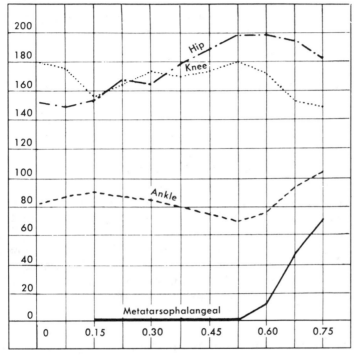

Fig. 9-4. *Joint actions during foot contact phase in walk of college woman. Time in seconds is shown at bottom—heel strike occurs at zero time, foot flat is at 0.15 sec., rear foot lift is at 0.50 sec, and toe lift is at 0.75 sec. Angles between body segments are shown in degree at left. Downward slope of lines indicates flexion, and upward slope indicates extension.*

time; then for the first 0.15 second, the ankle joint change is an increasing one, thus bringing the entire foot in contact with the walking surface. From this point, all joint actions will be reversed muscle actions: a decreasing angle at the ankle inclines the leg farther forward, an increasing angle at the knee moves the thigh, and a decreasing angle at the hip moves the trunk.

Because after 0.15 second the center of gravity is in front of the ankle joint, gravitational force will flex the lower leg; this action is controlled by the ankle extensors, which lengthen. Extension at the hip and knee will be the result of contraction of the entensors at these joints.

At 0.525 second, the leg has reached the desired degree of inclination (not consciously determined), and the ankle extensors contract with force enough to resist gravity, which now acts on the metatarsophalangeal joints and raises the foot from the surface. At point 0.60 second, the other (advancing) foot is making contact; then the center of gravity is moved over that foot by the forward momentum developed in the time from 0.15 to 0.60 second and by the final push with the toes and extension at the ankle of the rear foot. Note that the flexion is occuring at both the hip and knee in this final phase. Further explanation of the function of joint actions will be presented in the section on inclinations of the segments.

Joint Actions of Swinging Limb

After contact, the rear foot must be swung forward to establish the new contact. The swing, occupying 0.45 second, is accomplished by flexion at the hip. From full extension, the thigh flexes 34 degrees, bringing the thigh ahead of the trunk. Just before contact, the thigh extends slightly (3 degrees), to lower the limb for contact.

The angle at the knee, approximately 135 degrees as the foot left the ground, continues to decrease for a brief period—0.075 second. This action lifts the foot from the ground and also shortens the resistance arm for the hip action, thus reducing the energy needed for moving the limb forward.

The ankle joint, which was at an angle of 115 degrees as it left the ground, decreases (flexion of foot) immediately, lifting the forepart of the foot to clear the ground. Flexion continues until the last 0.075 second before contact. Then extension begins and continues until full foot contact is made.

Inclinations of Segments of Supporting Limb

In all locomotor and balance activities, a change in angle at any joint in the supporting limb changes the inclination of the segments above that joint. In standing, flexion at the ankle inclines the legs, thighs, and trunk toward the horizontal; extension at the ankle moves these segments away from the horizontal. In most forms of locomotion, simultaneous action is likely to occur in the joints of the supporting limb. This action may counteract the effects of distal joints or increase them. (See the discussion on locomotor patterns on land, in this chapter.)

The angle made by each segment with the horizontal in walking is shown in Fig. 9-5. The angles are those between a horizontal line drawn through the joint at the distal end of the segment and a line drawn through the segment. All angles are measured from the front except that for the foot, which is measured from the back. Foot measures shown begin at the time the foot is in full contact with the ground, and its inclination is therefore zero degree until the heel is raised. At 0.525 second, the heel leaves the contacting surface, and the angle of

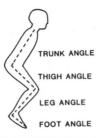

TRUNK ANGLE

THIGH ANGLE

LEG ANGLE

FOOT ANGLE

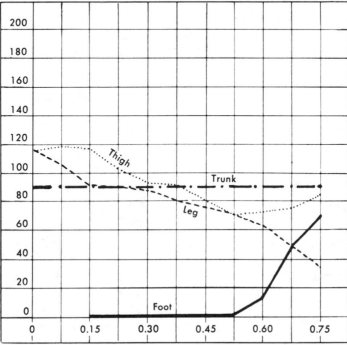

Fig. 9-5. *Angles of inclination of body segments (expressed in degrees at left) during foot contact phase in walk of college woman. Joint angles are depicted in figure 9-4. All angles are measured from front horizontal except those of foot. Note constant inclination of trunk, resulting from adjustment at hip joint to thigh inclination. Time in seconds is shown at bottom—heel strike occurs at zero time, foot flat occurs at 0.15 sec., rear foot lift occurs at 0.50 sec and toe lift occurs at 0.75 sec.*

inclination changes from zero degree to 72 degrees as the final push is made.

Leg inclination during full foot contact is changed by ankle action only. As flexion at the ankle occurs, it is paralleled by the change in leg inclination. However, when foot inclination begins to change at 0.525 second, foot inclination and ankle action affect leg inclination. As foot inclination begins, the change in angle at the ankle is at the same rate as the foot inclines; therefore, the inclination of the leg remains constant. If foot inclination is greater than the extension at the ankle, leg inclination will increase. These changes are shown in

Fig. 9-5. From 0.525 to 0.75 second, as a result of a 36-degree extension at the ankle and a 72-degree increase of foot inclination, the leg is inclined forward 36 degrees.

Inclination of the thigh is determined by the inclination of the leg and by knee action. Extension at the knee moves the thigh toward the front horizontal; forward inclination of the leg moves the thigh in the same direction. From 0.15 to 0.525 second, 26 degrees of extension occur at the knee and the leg inclines forward 20 degrees. The thigh during this time is moved 46 degrees toward the front horizontal. In the last phase of foot contact, the 50 degrees decreased angle at the knee moves the thigh away from the horizontal as the leg inclines 36 degrees. Thigh inclination during this period decreases 14 degrees.

Inclination of the trunk will be determined by thigh inclination and hip action. As the thigh inclines forward, the angle at the hip increases at the same rate, keeping the trunk at a constant angle. This is efficient mechanics, eliminating the effort that would be required if the trunk inclination changed.

MINI-LAB LEARNING EXPERIENCES

Using optical techniques described in Chapters 7 and 8, measure the joint angles and body segment angles of inclination in Figs. 9-1 and 9-3. Graph these angles and compare the stance phase angles with Figs. 9-4 and 9-5.

The joint actions just described provide the major forces in propelling the center of gravity in walking. At the same time, other joints contribute to the total movement. Among these contributions are rotation of the pelvis on the supporting femur due to medial rotation at the hip joint. These actions lengthen the stride. At the same time, the swinging limb is rotated laterally at the hip to keep the foot aligned in the desired line of direction. The torso is also rotated by spinal action to keep the shoulders facing the desired line of progression. As the speed of walking increases, the rotation of the spine is aided by shoulder action, with the right arm moving forward as the left foot advances.

Variations in Stride

Speed. The joint actions and segmental inclinations shown in Figs. 9-4 and 9-5 are those of a college woman walking at what she considered her average speed. As the speed of walking changes, the relative duration of the support and swing phases also change. In fast walking, the stance phase and swing phases are likely to be equal. In slow walking, gravitational force contributes less; the inclination of the leg decreases, and the length of the step is shortened. Whatever the speed, the same joints are acting, and each will be making the same type of contribution. However, variations occur in timing, range, and speed of joint actions.

GROUND REACTION FORCES DURING WALKING

The following information on walking was gathered by the use of a force platform capable of measuring vertical forces and horizontal (forward/backward and medial/lateral) forces:

1. Horizontal and vertical forces are exerted against the platform (ground) during walking; the ground exerts equal and opposite forces against the body.
2. A forward force is exerted on the ground as the heel strikes it. The reaction force is a backward force, braking the forward momentum of the body. This force is approximately 20% of the total body weight.
3. Beginning with heel strike to foot flat, the vertical vector increases in magnitude to 120% of the total body weight.
4. At mid-stance, the vertical force has decreased and is equal to 80% of the total body weight.
5. At mid-stance all horizontal forces are negligible.
6. After heel off, the vertical force rises again to 120% of the total body weight and decreases to zero as the foot is lifted from the platform.
7. From heel off to toe off, there is a backward push against the force platform, causing a forward reactive force (propulsive force) of approximately 20% of total body weight.
8. The foot pushes medially on the ground during heel strike and laterally on the ground during flexion at the knee.
9. Vectoral addition of vertical and horizontal forces can be seen in Fig. 9-6. The magnitude of the force is represented by its length and the angle of inclination from the vertical represents the rates of vertical and horizontal forces. Note the rather vertically oriented vectors throughout the stance phase.

MINI-LAB LEARNING EXPERIENCES

1. Ask persons to walk in response to a metronome, a drum beat, or recorded music (march, foxtrot, rock, jazz). Observe and tabulate limb and body movements for each condition. Use the checklist in Chapter 8 or construct your own.
2. Determine whether there are any differences in gaits of various persons wearing different types of shoes and clothing. Measure or estimate such variables as step length, range of motion at the ankle joint, and speed of walking.

DEVELOPMENTAL BIOMECHANICS   **291**

3. Record differences in gait patterns between injured and normal individuals.
4. Compare the walking patterns of young children and adults.

IMMATURE PATTERNS

Examples of the immature movements inherent in running, throwing, catching, kicking, and jumping are described in the next sections.

Running

During the early learning period for running, there is no observable flight phase, and the base of support is wide (the feet are spread; Fig. 9-7). The feet are rotated outwardly and laterally, and the stride is short. The center of gravity of the body is forward, and the action resembles tiptoeing rather than running. The arm swing is relatively rigid and is more lateral and horizontal rather than vertical. As maturity is gained, there is a definite flight phase with increased stride length and stride frequency. The support leg is more fully extended

COMPUTER AUTOMATED GAIT ANALYSIS – ORTHOGRAPHIC VECTOR PROFILE

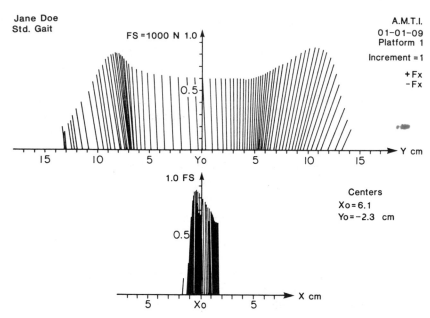

Fig. 9-6. *Vectoral force pattern of support phase of walking. The length of line represents magnitude of force and the orientation of the line represents angle with the ground.*

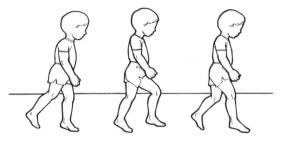

Fig. 9-7. *Child in running pattern. Note "tiptoe" style. There is no flight phase in this early stage of running.*

at takeoff, and the arms flex, extend, and move more vertically. (See also the discussion on mature running in Chapter 15.)

Throwing

In the early immature throwing action the movement at the elbow and part of the follow-through are similar to the mature action (Fig. 9-8). However, the center of motion is the elbow, with very little action elsewhere. The feet do not move, or at least there is no shifting of the feet into a step as the throw is executed. The axes at the shoulder, opposite hip, and spine are lacking. The throw is accomplished from a fixed, almost rigid position. (See the discussion on mature throwing in Chapter 17.)

Catching

In the early stages of catching, the head remains stationary regardless of the angle and height of the incoming object (ball). The hands remain fixed and slightly flexed and are not adjusted to the height path of the ball. At the point of contact with the ball, the hands have very little "give"; the momentum is not attenuated. Mature individuals who catch in this manner are said to have "board hands." There is very little if any flexion at the knees to help absorb the shock of the ball's velocity. (See the discussion on catching in Chapter 14.)

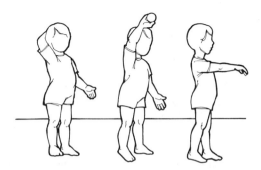

Fig. 9-8. *Immature throwing pattern. There is no step with leg opposite from throwing arm.*

Kicking

The young child initially makes very little movement of the upper body (arm and trunk) when kicking (Fig. 9-9). There is a very low amplitude of backswing, and often there is very little or no follow-through. The arms are kept to the side for balance. The kicking leg contacts the ball while it is deeply flexed. (See the discussion on mature kicking and striking patterns in Chapter 18.)

Jumping

The young child initially steps rather than jumps (Fig. 9-10). The pattern is a stride up or down as the situation dictates. Gradually the one- and two-foot takeoffs are learned. Frequently, in attempting to jump over a barrier, the young child merely jumps vertically rather than horizontally. The one-foot jump, after the step, is next in sequence, and then the two-foot takeoff is learned. A run and a step are combined in the leap. The ability to take off with one foot and land on two feet follows in the sequence. (See the discussion on mature jumping in Chapter 16.)

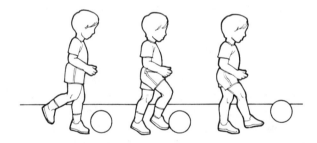

Fig. 9-9. *Immature kicking pattern. Note short backswing of leg.*

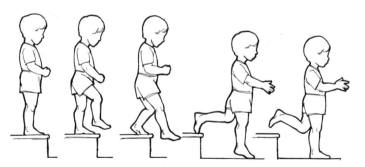

Fig. 9-10. *Child jumping down from step has an immature jumping pattern, since the action is actually a step down.*

ENVIRONMENTAL CONSTRAINTS FOR DEVELOPMENT OF MOVEMENT PATTERNS BY CHILDREN

Often the limiting factor in the development of movement patterns by children is the architectural design of the environment for adults. For example, ascending the descending stairs pose problems for three year olds. Compare the leg action of the child depicted in Fig. 9-11A with the leg action of the adult depicted in Fig. 9-11B. Why does the child have difficulty ascending the stairs? Measure the angles at the hip joint and at the knee joint.

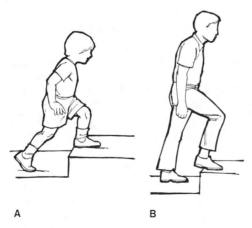

A   B

Fig. 9-11. *Ascending stairs: A, young child; B, adult. Compare the angles at the hip and at the knee during initial contact with lead leg. Compare angles at knee, ankle, and metatarsal joints of pushoff leg.*

DEVELOPMENTAL BIOMECHANICS   **295**

CLINICAL DIAGNOSIS SKILLS FOR EFFECTIVE TRAINING

One of the most important functions performed by the physical education practitioner is the observation and analysis of motor skills. In observing motor skills, the teacher, clinician, or coach conducts a systematic, visual inspection of the gross and fine aspects of the performance, and compares the observed movement patterns to a prescribed model or visual image. This process, entailing "decisions made by skill instructors regarding the nature of the learner's performance problems and the factors that give rise to them" (Hoffman, 1983, p. 36) has been termed "clinical diagnosis."

Clinical diagnosis is essential to effective teaching because it has six major functions in enhancing learning. These include:

1. Evaluation of motor skills by use of process measures;
2. Identification of developmental stages in the acquisition of fundamental motor skills;
3. Provision of accurate and precise feedback to the learner;
4. Development of teaching cues;
5. Selection of developmentally-appropriate learning activities and design of optimum learning environments; and
6. Application of clinical diagnosis to coaching contexts.

Each of these functions is described in the following sections.

1. Skills tests have traditionally been used to evaluate performance on the basis of product or end-result scores. Product measures refer to the description of outcome of the movement in terms of time, accuracy, or force; whereas process measures involve descriptions of the movement of the performer ("force-producing actions") (Safrit, 1981, p. 155). For example, skill in overhand throwing might be assessed by the number of balls thrown within a given time period; the distance that the ball was thrown; the accuracy of throws aimed at a target; or the velocity at which the ball traveled. These are four examples of product measures. All of these measurements, however, "fall short" in the sense that they provide no information about the form of the throwing pattern (i.e., the force-producing motions of the arms,

trunk, and legs). By means of process measures, the observer can determine the level of throwing proficiency displayed by describing the action of the humerus, forearm, and pelvis-spine, as well as the nature of the stepping pattern (ipsilateral or contralateral stepping, length of stride) and the presence or absence of a follow-through. Three stages of throwing proficiency which might be determined by process measurement are outlined in Table 9-2.

MINI-LAB LEARNING EXPERIENCES

Place the throwing performances (Fig. 9-12) in the appropriate development level using the scheme in Table 9-2.

One important factor that has limited the application of process measures in assessing motor skills has been the unavailability of instruments which could be easily applied. Instruments designed for evaluating fundamental motor skills were designed primarily for research purposes, and necessitated the use of sophisticated film analysis techniques. These instruments did not lend themselves to reliable observations in a live setting. Recently, Griffin (1984) and Cozzallio

Table 9-2. *Developmental levels of skill proficiency in overhand throwing.*

Body Segment	Level 1		Level 2		Level 3	
Arms	a.	Primarily a flinging motion from the elbow	a.	Humerus rotates to oblique position as ball is brought behind the head	a.	Arm swings backward in preparation
	b.	Elbow of throwing arm remains in front of the body			b.	Elbow of non-throwing arm is extended for balance in delivery
	c.	No forearm lag (elbow extends early)	b.	Arm swings forward high above the shoulder in delivery	c.	Thumb rotates medially downward in delivery
	d.	Fingers are spread at release	c.	Cocking of wrist occurs at completion of throw	d.	Fingers are close together at release
			d.	Forearm lags behind humerus in delivery	e.	Pronounced forearm lag
Trunk	a.	Body faces forward throughout	a.	Block rotation of trunk occurs (simultaneous rotation of hips and shoulders in preparation)	a.	Differentiated trunk rotation (hips-spine-shoulders) in delivery
	b.	Little or no rotation of shoulders and hips (remain facing target)	b.	Shoulders turn to face target in delivery	b.	Throwing shoulder drops slightly in preparation
			c.	Forward trunk flexion completes delivery	c.	Throwing shoulder faces target in follow-through
Legs	a.	No stepping	a.	Definite shift of body weight	a.	Weight is on rear foot in preparation
	b.	No weight transfer	b.	Ipsalateral stepping (same arm and leg move forward)	b.	Oppositional stepping (opposite arm and leg move forward)

Note: Children who are in transition between levels of skill proficiency may exhibit intersegmental variations (i.e., different levels of maturity are reflected in the action of the three body segments).

DEVELOPMENTAL BIOMECHANICS   **297**

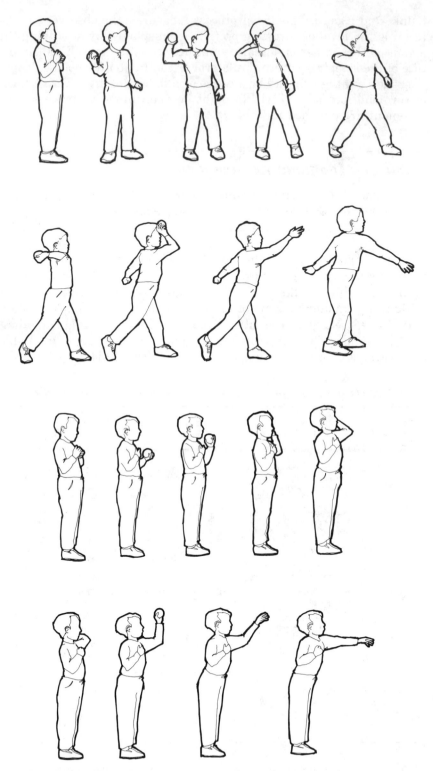

Fig. 9-12. *Sequential contourograms of throwing performances of two young boys.*

298   *THE BIOMECHANICS OF HUMAN MOVEMENT*

(1986) provided encouragement for the use of process measures in practical settings. In the first investigation, Griffin developed a process measure for throwing, striking, and kicking that was found to discriminate gender and grade-level differences, and correlated positively with product measures. In a similar study, Cozzallio developed a gross motor screening instrument for kindergarten that was found to be valid and reliable for use by classroom teachers. The instruments used in both of these investigations were checklists, which required the rater to match the observed motor patterns with established criteria. Similar checklists appear in Chapter 8.

2. The identification of developmental stages in the acquisition of fundamental motor skills is another teaching competency which requires proficiency in clinical diagnosis. A vast amount of literature consists of descriptions of the stages of development through which children pass in acquiring basic locomotor, manipulative, and axial movement patterns. Although most children do pass through similar stages in developing motor patterns, there is a great deal of variation in the rate at which they do so, and, thus, in the rate they mature. Therefore, process measures can provide a useful tool for allowing the teacher to identify children whose level of proficiency (immature to mature) deviates significantly from what is typically observed at a given age level. For example, a nine-year old child who demonstrated immature patterns in catching (e.g., avoidance behaviors, trapping the ball against the chest) would "signal the need" for remedial efforts. (See Fig. 9-13.)

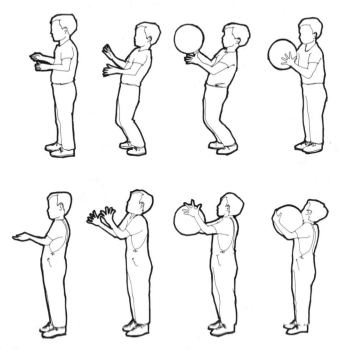

Fig. 9-13. *Sequential contourograms of catching performances of two young boys.*

DEVELOPMENTAL BIOMECHANICS

3. Provision of feedback, defined as "information generated about a response that is used to modify the next response" (Siedentop, 1983, p. 7), is another essential aspect of effective teaching which is enhanced by critical diagnosis. Sensory and proprioceptive feedback are intrinsically available to the learner and are obtained through visual, auditory, tactile, and kinesthetic cues. When this information is insufficient, however, the learner is dependent upon the teacher to provide augmented or supplementary feedback (Singer, 1980, p. 455).

Singer (1980, p. 282) has cautioned that the mere availability of feedback does not ensure improved performance by children. It appears that the "type, form, and receptivity to it" are factors which must be considered. A limited amount of research has been conducted in this area, but several researchers (Barclay and Newell, 1980; Newell, 1976; Newell and Kennedy, 1978) indicate that younger children benefit more from general feedback, while precise feedback facilitates the performance of older children. An extension of this finding is that teachers should provide feedback related to gross aspects of the movement pattern to young learners and those who display an immature movement pattern. In contrast, older and more skilled learners are able to cognitively process feedback that is more precise in nature.

4. In addition to providing a frame of reference for giving appropriate feedback, clinical diagnosis can guide the teacher in the identification of teaching cues. (Teaching cues are short phrases which direct the learner's attention to a specific aspect of performance, such as "racquet back, side to the net," as opposed to the product of the movement—"Did the ball pass over the net?"). Analysis of movement patterns from a biomechanical perspective results in the identification of scientifically correct-teaching cues. No cue is often more effective than a miscue. A correct cue, however, will be most effective.

5. Clinical diagnosis is an inherent process in the selection of developmentally-appropriate learning activities and the design of optimum learning environments. Rink (1985, p. 191) has emphasized that "a major problem in group instruction is that students function at different levels of ability in most tasks. . . ." Therefore, it is essential to determine the appropriateness of the content and the manner in which it is presented.

Consider, for example, the appropriateness of a game of kickball for a group of first graders. Prior to introducing the game, the teacher, through clinical diagnosis, observes that many of the children perform at an immature level in the fundamental skills of throwing, catching, and kicking. Demands of performing these skills in a dynamic game situation, with the added stress of competition, produces an environment in which the execution, much less the improvement, of these skills is unlikely. More appropriate tasks would be those in which the children perform the skills under static conditions or without the element of competition (e.g. throwing and catching with a stationary partner; kicking a stationary ball).

An innovative approach to helping children acquire motor patterns has been developed by Garrett. Cut-out figures or silhouettes drawn from photos or movies of children performing motor skills are used to help the children develop a clear visual image of the skill to be learned. By emulating the shape seen in the figure, children attempt to kinesthetically memorize the body position. Children might, for example, work in pairs and provide feedback to each other on the accuracy of their replication of the body position to be assumed in a sprinting start. Additional practice could be gained by asking the children to replicate the shape with eyes closed, or the teacher may provide formative feedback to the children in this manner.

6. Application of skill analysis to coaching contexts is the last major purpose for developing competence in clinical diagnosis. Effective coaching requires a thorough knowledge of the mechanics of correct performance of given skills and the development of a clear visual image by which to compare observed performance to a theoretical model. This visual image is the basis for error detection and precise and accurate feedback.

Clinical diagnosis is an essential element of effective teaching and plays a significant role in the enhancement of learning all motor skills. Hoffman (1983) has used the analogy of teaching and medicine to emphasize the importance of accurate diagnosis:

> As the physician's decisions regarding medical treatment are contingent upon his/her diagnosis of the patient's ailments, so are decisions regarding feedback, verbal prompts, or the nature of practice experiences contingent upon the instructor's diagnosis of the learner's performance deficiencies. Obviously, then, the teacher's ability to correctly ascertain the learners' problems . . . and allow that assessment to inform subsequent decision about the prescriptive part of teaching, would appear to be a major determinant of his/her effectiveness in helping learners attain the skill goal.

Biomechanical analysis can be the key to aid a teacher or other professional in effectively assisting a person in developing motor skills.

Four general guidelines are useful in the application of clinical diagnosis skills:

1. Become a student of mechanical analysis. Thoroughly analyze the mechanics of correct performance, and use this information to develop a clear visual image (theoretical model—biomechanically correct model) of the skill to be taught.
2. Develop comprehensive written plans to make sure that you give the learner an accurate presentation of the skill. Include precise performance objectives that describe in observable terms the level of performance that is desired, as well as skill analysis (brief summary of correct performance) and teaching cues that could be used.

3. Observe the skill performance carefully, with attention to those aspects of the mechanics that you have chosen to emphasize.
4. Provide precise and task-oriented feedback to the learner, based on comparison of the observed performance to the desired level of performance which you have identified in your objective.

WHO SAYS OLD PEOPLE CAN'T WALK?

At the age of 66, Hulda Crooks climbed Mt. Whitney. Hulda now has climbed that mountain 22 times, and, at the age of 91, climbed Mt. Fuji in Japan. Many cardiologists are now recommending that walking briskly at a constant speed of 3–4 mps has great health benefits. The breathing rate is increased noticeably. 1500 to 2000 calories can be burned in a week by walking two miles four times a week. There is a biomechanically correct way to walk in order to reap the greatest benefits and to reduce the possibility of adverse effects.

LOCOMOTOR PATTERNS AND AGING

The stereotypic gait of the older person in American society consists of slow, short, shuffling steps in which there is decreased range of motion at all joints and a "slumping" of the head, shoulders, and upper trunk. That this pattern is not typical for able-bodied older persons has been shown by Murray in her extensive investigations of walking patterns of both able-bodied and physically-impaired adults. Able-bodied males 60 to 65 years of age, for example, showed no differences in stance, stride width, swing, double-limb support, transverse, or sagittal rotations of the pelvis, hips, knees, and ankles, or movements of the trunk when compared to younger men. Shorter steps (3.1 cm), shorter stride lengths, and increased out-toeing (2.7 degrees) were the only significant differences noted. Since this was a cross-sectional study rather than a longitudinal study, one cannot be sure whether these differences were due to the age variable itself or to the sample within each age group.

Since individual differences in cadence, range, and speed of limb movements exist in every age group studied, the older person can be expected to be able to execute a walking pattern in the same manner as young and middle-aged persons. There are long striders and short striders, fast walkers and slow walkers, and persons with varying amounts of out-toeing and limb segment rotations among all age groups. Note the erect posture and "normal range and stride" of the 70-year-old woman depicted in Fig. 9-14.

If, however, Parkinson's disease or another pathological condition afflicts the older person, the gait pattern will be impaired. A "Parkinsonism gait" can be described as one with short, unstable, shuffling strides, with the body flexed at the hips and throughout the spinal column. Another type of gait pattern seen among the older pop-

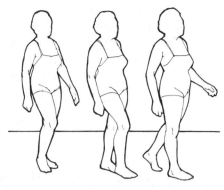

Fig. 9-14. *Normal walking pattern of able bodied 70-year-old woman. Note erect posture and normal opposition of arms and legs.*

ulation afflicted with labyrinthine dysfunction is that of a widened lateral stance and lateral sway or lurching of the body during changing of the base of support. Persons with total hip replacement, however, appear to be able to establish a normal walking pattern, as noted by research conducted by Murray.

Running

Although older persons are competing in Senior Olympic racing competition and in triathlons, the majority of older persons do not include running in their daily lives. An exception would be those who participate in sports and therefore engage in running required for such sports, as in tennis and softball. The speed of running is low for the average older person. The contourograms depicted in Fig. 9-15 represent the running force of women aged 60-80 years who engaged in swimming as a form of daily (or every other day) exercise. Is this a

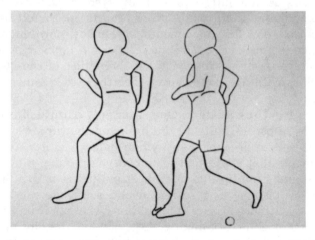

Fig. 9-15. *Sequential contourograms of running performance of older woman engaged in exercise swimming program.*

DEVELOPMENTAL BIOMECHANICS 303

jogging sequence or a maximum speed sequence? The women were asked to, and did, run as fast as they could. When comparing the kinematics of their run to the patterns of university track-team women who sprinted and paced, it was found that the older women ran at the speed the younger women paced. The kinematics were identical. If the older women's performances, however, were compared to the sprint performance, there was little similarity. What conclusions would you draw from these data, to answer the question: can older women run?

Jumping Patterns

Investigations of vertical jumping patterns of older women who had not executed the pattern since high school once again show no evidence of an age-related factor. The only difference noted between data from college-age women and from an older population was in the lack of speed of extension of the leg at the knee joint. The sequencing of limb movements and the force-time histories were similar for both populations. The lack of extension speed may be due to aging, disuse, ratio of slow-fast-twitch muscle fibers, or ratio of muscle cross-section to body weight. More research is needed to better understand the capabilities of older persons.

Age-Related Changes in the Motor Control Systems Which Subserve Performance and Skill Acquisition

Sense Organs. As we know from the changes in ourselves, or our older relatives and friends, the eyes and ears progressively change as we age. Close vision becomes more blurred, and we are not able to see as well at night or when the lighting is dim. Our depth vision becomes less precise also. Hearing may be impaired as well. Certain pitches may not be heard, or all frequencies may be affected. Other sense organs affected by aging include the vistibular apparatus and proprioceptors. As a result, balance is affected in standing and walking, climbing stairs, and turning. Our proprioceptors tell us how far we have moved, how fast movements were made, how much force we used to make the movement, and the positions of limbs in space. While we do not have specific evidence about the nature of change in these proprioceptors with age, we suspect that they, too, transmit signals to the brain.

Central Nervous System. One seemingly natural effect of aging is slowing of responses. Putting the brake on the car very rapidly, or catching oneself to prevent a fall when balance is low are common fast movements that are essential to everyday living. Slowing in response to a light stimulus and a sound stimulus are both affected with age. Other central nervous system declines include cognitive functions dealing with organizing information, whether it be new or old. A simple task such as organizing the events of the day may be difficult for some older adults. When memory must be used to attend to a specific input or stimulus, many older adults experience difficulties.

This specific deficit is called memory-driven attentional selectivity and is typical of the normal aging process. Other normal changes with aging include difficulties in putting new information into memory and retrieving or finding old information, especially if that old information is not so very old. These are deficits in encoding and retrieval and they affect most of us as we age. Storing information for a short period of time is also affected with age. Trying to remember the name of a person you met yesterday is an example of this short-term storage deficit. The older person's memory is also more susceptible to interference from other information stored in memory, as well as from noise or other stimuli in the environment. Many of these central nervous system deficiencies can affect learning and performing motor skills.

Muscular System. The natural aging process also affects the muscular system. There is a decline in muscle fibers, mass and muscular strength. Decreased flexibility also occurs and stability is affected by this change in the muscular system. There is also an increase in time of the antagonist muscle groups to relax prior to initiating a movement. All of these changes affect older persons in their ability to control movement.

Skeletal System. Whereas females are generally affected more than males by decline in bone mineral content and bone mass, an increased incidence of osteoporosis occurs for both sexes with the aging process.

Affects of Motor Control Systems' Decline on Biomechanics of Movement and Skill Acquisition

Sense Organs. The reduced and restricted utilization of vision greatly affects balance for the control of movement. This change in the visual system also limits one's ability to utilize feedback from the eyes for many daily living skills, as well as for learning new skills. Other less effective feedback systems must be used to maintain performance and assist in the learning of new skills. Accuracy of performance is greatly affected by visual impairment, whether the task be driving a car, lifting a pan of boiling water from the stove, or hitting a tennis ball over the net. Perceiving oncoming stimuli (balls in racquet sports or cars on the road) can be slowed and distorted. Stages of development for skill acquisition must change as a result of these changes in the visual system. The rate of skill acquisition for an open skill (environment changing) is slowed. That is, the capability of producing forces with the proper timing in response to an oncoming ball will be reduced and acquisition slowed due to this limited visual control. Although hearing is reduced with the aging process, the ears can become more important during the learning process for those who have more limited vision. A weakened vestibular apparatus can reduce the control of movement, which may limit displacement of the center of gravity. This reduction could, in turn, affect the capability to produce force.

Suggestions for the Practitioner. A restriction in vision need not prevent the older adult from learning new motor skills and performing old ones. Practitioners need to follow a few guidelines in order to assist clients in learning new motor tasks and maintaining optimum performance in spite of visual loss. Suggestions are: (1) Learn about each individual's visual impairment. Has it been corrected adequately? If not, deal with each person's problem individually. (2) Slow the stimulus (oncoming ball) in practice situations. Response to the ball will be delayed, so it is essential that its speed be reduced. (3) Provide auditory feedback to the learner who has visual impairment. For example, get your racquet back sooner to hit the ball earlier. (4) Provide other sources of auditory feedback, such as "Hit now!", or "You are lined up to the right for this shot—move your feet to the left by 2 inches." (5) Use bright stimuli such as orange balls or illuminescent paint or tape on the balls and boundaries of the court. With persons who have an impaired vistibular apparatus that affects balance, the practitioner could suggest brisk walking, or stationary bicycling or swimming for aerobic exercise instead of walking. Since ballistic skills may be impaired by this restricted balance control, encourage these persons to limit their range of motion so that the line of gravity stays well within the base of support. Of course, this may decrease force production but it may provide the performer with increased confidence that balance will not be lost.

Central Nervous System. Slowing of responses to stimuli will affect speed of movement in response to stimuli in open tasks (badminton, tennis, racquetball) necessitating competition with age peers who also have slowed responses. Accuracy becomes a more important component of the task than speed. Daily living skills may also be affected by slowed behavior. Performances of tasks such as turning the head to orient to someone who is speaking, catching a falling object, and braking a car may be slowed and impaired behavior may result. Cognitive function decline affects learning and maintenance of performance. For example, memory-driven attentional selectivity decline will affect one's ability to attend consistently to a portion of a new skill, such as, increasing the range of pelvic rotation in the golf swing. Encoding is also adversely affected with age, and this could potentially slow one's ability to learn new movement patterns for all newly learned motor tasks. Retrieval of previously-learned tasks may also be detrimentally affected since the proper motor program must be located and retrieved from memory each time we perform a task. If the performer has difficulty in retrieving the correct motor program, performance will be inconsistent and result in many errors. We cannot expect the consistent performance of youth nor can we expect a once-learned task (for example, an overarm throw) to exhibit its skillful youthful qualities. Portions of that task could be temporarily affected by lack of complete retrieval, interference from other similar tasks, or from a decaying trace.

Suggestions for the Practitioner. Changes in the central nervous system need not prevent the older adult from participating in physical activity. In fact, there is a growing body of research in support of the benefits of aerobic exercise to the central nervous system. Practitioners need to encourage the older adult to get involved in aerobic exercise and maintain a weekly workout program. Slowing of responding and memory changes may well be reduced by a consistent and vigorous aerobic program that includes maintaining the target heart rate for the recommended time. Slowing of movement is a natural response for many older adults who realize that their response speed has slowed. Encourage the older adult to play his/her favorite sport with age peers who also have slower responses.

The practitioner needs to be aware of the fact that declines in the memory system may affect the older adult's ability to remember events of the day or organize new information. These declines may also affect retention of motor skills. What was once a skillful movement for the young adult may show some inadequacies in old age because of changes in memory. Portions of the skillful motor program may not be retrieved at one certain time, one skillful aspect may decay more rapidly than others, and remembering to attend to one specific cue may be difficult. The practitioner should patiently remind the performer of aspects of the task that need attention. Search for a cue that the learner/performer can more easily remember. This may well be a different word cue for each individual. Teachers also should write cue cards for the performer so that the card could be used periodically as reminders. When the older adult learns a new skill, teachers need to use a great deal of content repetition and practice situations. This will tend to reinforce what was taught and prevent the older adult from forgetting essential cues. Utilization of many visual cues will also help the learner to remember better. Provide pictures of the task, show many demonstrations, and have the performer watch his/her own performance on videotape or in the mirror. The performer should look at body parts that move.

Muscular System. Decline in muscle fibers and muscle mass will limit force production capability, movement speed, and reaction to a fast stimulus. Strength will be affected. This would affect equipment standards and construction (for example, more flexible shafts for golf clubs might be required). Decrease in flexibility will limit the range of motion for most sports skills and many daily-living skills (reaching for the top shelf, bending for cleaning chores, stretching when gardening). Stability for riding a bus, climbing stairs, and carrying groceries may be affected by decline in muscle mass. Falls are more prevalent for older adults; women fall two times more often than men. Is it because of lower strength or poorly designed footwear for walking?

Skeletal System. Due to bone-mass loss, the center of gravity will be changed from younger years. This will place restrictions on motor control and may necessitate change in contemporary motor-skill technique. For example, stride length for brisk walking will have shortened for the person with bone loss in the spinal column and hip/femur area who must maintain a stooped posture.

Suggestions for the Practitioner. Changes in the muscular and skeletal systems will necessitate changes in motor behavior. Practitioners should not expect the older adult to produce the magnitude of forces in motor tasks that are achieved in youth. Limb speed (movement time) and total body speed can be enhanced, however. Since a strength training program can serve to promote increased muscle mass and strength, older persons should be encouraged to participate in a strength training program for their age group. Maintenance of range of motion for daily living skills must be promoted through daily stretching exercises. Changes in the muscular system also affect stability. The older adult should be encouraged to widen the base of support for many daily-living skills. For example, standing at the checkout line at the grocery, standing and talking, standing in the kitchen and then moving to perform tasks could be performed more effectively and safely from a wider base of support. A wider base of support should also be encouraged for motor skills and for other daily living skills in which the base of support is moving, such as in riding a bus. Encourage the use of handrails when they are provided. Wearing lower-heeled shoes should be advocated to promote better balance for the older person.

Biomechanical Requirements of Movement

In order to better understand the limitations of movement achievements by older persons, it is important to measure the characteristics of movement patterns. What are the temporal, spatial, and kinetic requirements of common movement patterns performed by older persons and movement patterns not normally a part of these persons' repertoire?

Speed requirements of walking can be related to the minimum required speed to cross a traffic intersection. Based upon research by Aniansson, 1.4 m/sec should be the criterion speed for walking. Average speed of "normal, functional walking" by a group of 419 70-year-olds was found to be less than the criterion speed. Aniansson calculated average speeds of 1.2 m/sec for males and 1.1 m/sec for females.

A small group of women age 58–80 were tested on their speed of walking normally and as fast as safely possible. Although this group also did not normally walk 1.4 m/sec or faster, their maximum walking speed was 1.9 m/sec, well above the criterion speed.

Klinger reported on the movement characteristics of twelve women aged 60 years and older who were actively involved in a regular exercise program. Videotapes were taken during performance of activities of daily living, exercises, and sports skills. In addition, electrogoniometers were placed at the elbow and knee to continuously record movements about those joints. A force platform was utilized for one of the performances, the vertical jump. The group could be qualitatively divided into a high- and low-ability grouping. The high-ability group members were characterized as moving faster, transferring body weight more easily, and showing a greater range of motion, more erect trunk posture, and better coordination, evidenced by greater continuity of sequencing of movements. A Rohler's Index (Wt./Ht.$^3 \times 10^7$) was used to determine if this anthropometric measurement correlated with the placement of persons into the two groups. The high-ability group had the lower Rohler's Indices, but one person in the low-ability group also showed a low R.I. The range for the high-ability group was 124–149 and for the low-ability group 124–173. The importance of strength and body mass was noted in the inability to some of the individuals to rise from sitting on a low block or the floor, although they were able to rise from a chair.

In an effort to relate the disuse phenomenon to aging changes, comparisons of angular velocities and displacements were made among the three types of activities. Movements at the knee during walking showed 40–60 degrees of flexion and peak angular velocities of 133 degrees/s–360 degrees/s. Although the sitting and rising activities required greater range of motion, the angular velocities at the knee were less than those measured during walking. Negligible ROM and ω were seen in the other activities of daily living. Vertical jumping, a sports skill, showed a minimum of 400 degrees/s and a maximum of 800 degrees/s angular velocity at the knee joint. In addition, the range of motion at the knee almost doubled when jumping. Force-time histories of these jumping patterns were similar to those found with college women. The major difference was in the inability to develop greater leg extension velocity, and thus greater impulses. For the category ADL, negligible angular displacements and velocities at the elbow were recorded during walking, sitting, rising from a chair, and simulation of putting on pants. Combing hair showed 42 degrees–95 degrees of motion and ω of 72 degrees/s–360 degrees/s at the elbow. Generally, movements of eating required 95 degrees of motion and speed of 200 degrees/s–400 degrees/s at the elbow. Floor mopping showed approximately 40 degrees of motion at 200 degrees/s at the elbow. Arm exercise patterns produce average angular velocities at the elbow of 500 degrees/s. Additionally, the velocity of forearm extension during some arm exercises was faster than some of the striking or throwing skills. For example, the elbow extensions in the backhand tennis were around 300 degrees/s. Typical velocities for throwing, however, were 800 degrees/s of extension at the elbow. The fastest extensions occurred during batting, the overhand badminton stroke, and overarm throwing. These velocities were greater than 800 degrees/s, although they varied greatly from individual to individual. The next fastest velocities occurred in the medicine ball throw and the tennis stroke, which were about 400 degrees/s. The velocities achieved by these older women in these sports skills were much less than the velocities reported for young skilled performers, but it should be noted that one-half of the subjects tested had no sports background, while others had not performed the skills for many years, some since high school. Additionally, even though the velocities were low, they were much higher than those achieved in the activities of daily living.

Based upon these results, exercises and sports skills, such as batting, throwing, jumping, and arm extensions, cause the limbs to move with greater velocity and through a larger range of motion than do the activities of daily living. To withstand strains and maintain life at a high quality, the older person must engage in activities requiring greater ROM's and velocities than necessary for ADL. Some of the implications of this study are: (1) Stress on bones is produced by muscle contractions. The stronger the contraction, the greater the stress; therefore, if stresses on the bone are less, disuse may be a major cause of early so-called aging changes in bone. (2) Lack of fast movement also reduces stress on the joints and may have implications for osteoarthritis. (3) Due to a lack of fast movements by the elderly, there are no phasic muscle contractions, and fast-twitch muscles are not used. (4) If the range of motion at the joint is less, a definite loss of flexibility may be experienced over time, which in turn leads to a further decreased range of motion.

ADL: THE FOUNDATION OF DEVELOPMENTAL BIOMECHANICS

The fundamental area of human movement analysis is ADL (activities of daily living). Herein lie the foundation for survival and the basis for many work and leisure activities, including sports and dance. A large number of an adult's waking hours are spent in ADL or activities of work. In fact, persons over 60 years of age spend almost all their time with ADL and engage in few, if any, other types of activities.

As one becomes older, the ADL becomes more difficult to perform, especially if these activities have been performed inefficiently—that is, in less than a biomechanically sound manner—in one's youth. The research in this area has been conducted mainly to identify problems of physically disabled persons, and dysfunctioning and unsafe conditions. In addition, ADL research is important to the construction of prostheses, braces, and other orthotic devices. Limited research exists concerning normal ADL analysis. The six major classifications of ADL are as follows:

1. Locomotion: walking, ascending and descending stairs, stepping into vehicles.

2. Changing levels: moving from chair to standing, moving from bed to standing, stooping, kneeling.
3. Lifting and carrying groceries, suitcases, and other objects.
4. Pushing and pulling: using a wheelbarrow, manual lawn mower, rolling pin, typewriter.
5. Working with long-handled implements: axe, hoe, broom.
6. Working with small implements: pencil, saw, hammer, knitting needles, eating utensils, hatchet.

In general, ADL consist primarily of movements performed at slow to moderate speeds, the majority of movements requiring little muscle effort. When the task could be strenuous, persons (especially older persons) will rest frequently or avoid performing the task.

Locomotion

Walking. A checklist is provided here to enumerate the basic considerations for the analysis and improvement of walking patterns of older persons in their homes and life spaces and of persons with physical disabilities.

1. Is the coefficient of friction optimum for prevention of slipping and for generation of force? If not, which surfaces can be changed?
2. Have the anatomic characteristics of the person changed since successful walking occurred and present walking dysfunction was noted? Assess the weight, specific muscle strength of "walking muscles," postural deviations, and neuromuscular functioning (such as balance) to determine which factors are probable causes of walking dysfunction. Determine a means for modifying the walking pattern or correcting the factor.
3. Do imposed environmental conditions, such as carrying packages, interfere with an otherwise skilled walking pattern? If so, use the principles of moments and the assistance of devices to alleviate the problem.

Ascending stairs. Ascending stairs poses a problem to many persons who have weak leg extensors. The leg is lifted by the contraction of quadriceps and other flexors at the hip, and the foot is placed on the next step, which is usually 23 cm higher than the preceding one. The body weight, then, must be lifted 23 cm. which has been selected as the optimum height for the average adult. The amount of leg lift and the optimum angles at the hip and knee joints will differ for individuals who have varying leg lengths. However, all persons show a greater range of motion at the knee, hip, and ankle during stair locomotion than during walking on level ground. Thus, muscle weakness will affect the stair-climbing pattern of obese and short persons to a greater extent than that of lightweight and tall persons.

Lifting the body requires that the center of gravity of the body be shifted from the rear foot to the new supporting foot and that the rear foot initiate plantar flexion. This plantar flexion will raise the center of gravity of an adult male with a size 7 foot approximately 8 cm. Thus, one-third of the total distance through which the body weight must be lifted may be achieved by this action. This action is not as effective for persons with smaller feet, notably children. The ideal sequential timing of extension at the hip and knee of the lead leg with respect to plantar flexion of the rear foot produces a series of acceleration forces caused by these muscle contractions. Thus, the summation of these forces facilitates the raising of the center of gravity of the body the necessary 23 cm to the next step. In this manner, a person can compensate for weak quadriceps muscles, which are the primary muscles used by many healthy young persons in stair locomotion.

Correct placement of the total foot on each stair tread is important for individuals who have balance problems. Unfortunately, some stairs do not have sufficiently wide treads to allow large persons, who often weigh more than average, to place the total foot on the tread. One must be careful not to place the foot so far forward that the toe catches on the lip of the step as the foot is lifted.

When placing the total foot on the tread, the muscles crossing the ankle joint can relax and the foot is in a neutral position. From this position, the foot dorsiflexes as the other leg enters the swing phase of ascent. From this dorsiflexed position the person can generate greater force because of the greater distance through which plantar flexion can be accelerated, compared to the person who uses the ball of the foot during the support phase of ascending stairs.

Another advantage of the neutral position of the foot is that it releases tension in the gastrocnemius and thereby facilitates extension at the knee. This facilitation occurs because the gastrocnemius crosses the knee, as well as the ankle. With the absence of tension in the gastrocnemius, the quadriceps can move the leg with less force than if co-contraction between agonists and antagonists existed.

There is, however, a critical speed of ascent at which most persons will prefer to use only the ball of the foot rather than the whole foot. Although this critical speed will vary with individuals, it represents the speed at which the person rapidly passes through each single-support phase; that is, there is no sensing of a static single-support position. The faster the speed of ascent, the more pronounced will be the absence of full foot contact. With speed, however, the likelihood of the person's ascending two steps at a time is great. A person may again use the full foot contact, since the height to which the leg must be lifted is lower with a full-foot landing than with any other type of landing. In addition, passive dorsiflexion of the foot can take place, thus shifting the center of gravity of the body forward and upward with little muscle effort.

Physical Disabilities and Ascending Stairs. Common modifications made by persons with physical disabilities when they are ascending stairs are of two types: (1) a handrail is used, and (2) the person marks time, that is, places both feet on each tread. The use of a handrail not only compensates for balance dysfunction but also provides a reactive surface for the hand. Arm extension thus produces another force for raising the body and compensating for weak quadriceps.

Persons who have had a stroke or other trauma that has resulted in the failure of one leg to function as well as the other should lead with the nontraumatized leg when ascending stairs. For these persons, total foot placement, strengthening of extensor muscle groups, and exact control of the center of gravity with respect to the base of support are important requirements for success in ascending stairs.

Descending Stairs. The problem imposed by the act of descending stairs are opposite those of ascending stairs. Whereas ascending stairs results in positive work (the product of body weight and height), descending stairs is negative work, since the muscles eccentrically contract to regulate the speed of descent caused by gravity. Once again, the line of gravity is shifted from one tread to the next via each foot, and greater stability is achieved with contact of the total foot than with the ball of the foot. The ball of the foot, however, usually makes the initial contact with the tread; thus, the body weight may gradually be lowered the final centimeters of the total distance of descent.

Persons may turn the foot for a diagonal placement if the foot is too long for the tread width. This pattern is noted frequently in persons running downstairs. However, in this case the ball of the foot may be the only part of the foot contacting the stairs. A person using a fast descent allows gravity to accelerate the descent of the body, thereby minimizing the amount of eccentric muscle contraction. The person has confidence that the end of the stairway will be reached before the acceleration causes lack of body control.

Physical Disabilities and Descending and Ascending Stairs. Persons with physical disabilities should lead with the disabled leg when descending stairs, since maximum stability is required on the upper tread during the lowering of the lead leg. The nondisabled leg can be lowered quickly as soon as the lead leg is supported. This action minimizes the amount of time during which the impaired leg is the sole support of body weight.

Certain principles are applicable for both descending and ascending stairs. The person maintains dynamic stability, utilizes forward and upward momentum to maintain momentum, and involves a sequencing of muscle contractions to create acceleration of the body in the desired path. Modifications are made in the pattern according to anatomic characteristics of the performer and environmental conditions. When the coefficient of friction is less than optimum, horizontal forces are reduced and vertical forces increased.

Changing Levels

Rising from a bed and chair and lowering oneself to these pieces of furniture involve the same general principles as described in locomotion on stairs. Weak quadriceps muscles usually are the limiting factor in the ability to rise from furniture. The lower the furniture, the more difficulty will be encountered by the person, since the person

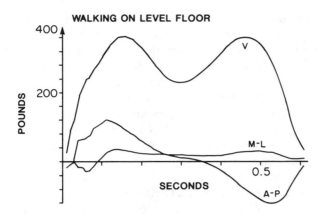

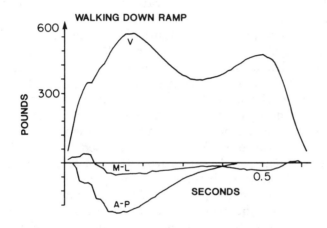

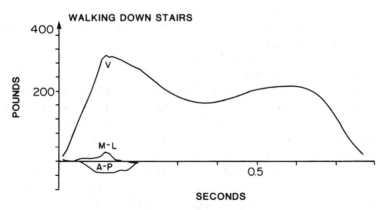

Fig. 9-16. *Force-time histories of supporting step during walking on the level, descending ramps, and descending stairs. Note the lack of anterior and posterior forces during the stair descent (A) since balance was considered crucial to this person. Note the differences in patterns generally among the three conditions. Can you postulate something concerning the kinematics of the gait from the force-time patterns?*

must perform more work (raise the center of gravity a greater distance) and will begin the movement at an unfavorable angle of muscle pull. In addition, the type of material and the construction of the furniture seat influence the method of rising. Mattresses and cushions do not provide a sufficiently rigid surface for the generation of reactive forces and therefore pose a greater problem than do rigid chairs.

The following general principles and movement analysis are useful for the improvement of the act of rising from furniture. The first action by the person desiring to rise from a chair is to move the center of gravity near the edge of the chair seat. Next, the person places one foot under the chair and one foot slightly in front of the chair legs. The person shifts the center of gravity over the new base of support, the feet, and stands by means of leg extension. If the muscles of the leg are not strong enough to raise the body weight at the initial angle of execution, the person may accelerate the trunk by alternating actions in the sagittal plane and may use the acceleration (which might be redefined as energy or momentum) of that body part to assist the muscles of the legs to create the necessary force to lift the weight of the body. In addition, the arms can be used to add a counterforce to the body weight by pushing against the chair or against the thighs. The latter action directly aids in extension at the knee joint.

Another example of the use of momentum of a body part to facilitate the performance of a movement pattern is found in the act of rising from a bed. Since the full length of the body may be distributed on the bed, the legs can be raised from the bed and then allowed to swing toward the floor with the help of gravity. This leg swing then raises the trunk to a sitting position. If the leg swing is facilitated by muscle contraction, the momentum of the leg swing may produce enough trunk motion to propel the person into a standing position with the help of a hand push against the bed. This technique utilizes both the strong muscles that cross the hip joint and the momentum of approximately one-third of the body mass to compensate for weak muscles crossing the knee.

Stooping, squatting, and sitting on the floor or ground are patterns common to scrubbing floors, placing items in drawers and cabinets, dusting furniture, picking up shoes and other items from the floor, and doing certain gardening tasks. With the advent of many laborsaving devices, some of these tasks have been eliminated from daily activity patterns, and others have even been eliminated altogether. There are instances, however, when stooping or sitting on the floor may be necessary and desirable. Most laborsaving tools do not find items that are dropped on the floor, do not clean the corners of the room, and are not worth the cost or effort for such tasks as putting one potted plant into the ground. These activities require greater ranges of motion at the hip and knee joints than walking and stair locomotion. Greater strength is needed to initiate the upward movement from the squat or sitting position on the floor than is required to rise from a chair or bed.

There are numerous ways to descend to and rise from the floor-sitting position. Persons over 70 years of age and young children select methods on an individual basis. Three patterns of young children are shown in Fig. 9-17. Older persons use all these patterns. The strength of the quadriceps with respect to body weight, the distribution of body weight, balancing capabilities, and previous experiences with success at the initial learning age are some reasons that may be cited for the particular method selected by a person. Several patterns are nevertheless possible because none requires maximum contraction of muscles. Therefore, persons can be inefficient until the task becomes one of maximum, or nearly maximum, effort because of a physical disability. Then efficiency is sought in the pattern. For example, efficiency is a necessary requirement in teaching a stroke patient to rise from the floor.

Since one side of the body usually is disabled after a stroke, the stroke patient should place the foot of the disabled leg close to the hips when attempting to rise from a seated position on the floor. The other leg is raised to a position supported by the knee and shank. The center of gravity is shifted to the foot, and the hands exert a push against the floor. If the leg is not strong enough to extend to the

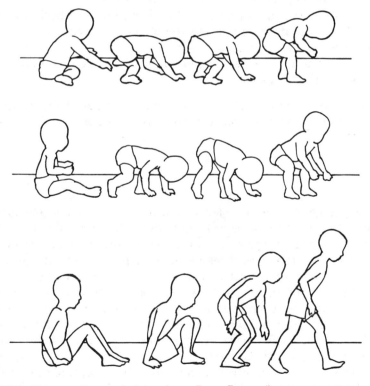

Fig. 9-17. Three patterns of rising from floor. Depending upon anthropometry, muscular strength, and balance, persons will prefer one pattern rather than another.

standing position, the person should grasp a piece of furniture to assist with extension of the leg, much the same as the handrail is used in stair locomotion.

A major concern of biomechanists is the incidence of injury to the knee as a result of squatting, kneeling, and stooping. As the squat position is achieved, the knee is placed in an open position, or what is sometimes termed a loosely packed position. This makes the knee vulnerable to dislocation and rupturing of ligaments or muscles crossing the joint. If these tissues are strong, it is unlikely that an injury will occur. There is, however, a danger of injury because of loss of balance or a deliberate twisting motion that would place excessive stress on the knee. The knee would then be injured because of the torsion, not the separation in the sagittal plane. Obese persons, persons who discover that they cannot rise from the squat position, and persons who attempt to perform movements requiring greater balance and strength capabilities than they possess are the most vulnerable to injury during squatting activities.

Persons desiring to perform the squat after not having attempted a squat for some length of time should test their ability to do so as follows:

1. If possible, perform the movement in water.
2. Assume the squat position while horizontal to check the range of motion and to eliminate the effect of gravity.
3. Assume a semisquat position.
4. With the assistance of a person, chair, or some other aid, assume the squat position.

At the first sign of pain, the movement should be discontinued until strengthening exercises can increase the stability of the knee joint.

LIFTING

The proper way to lift objects from the floor or other low position has been a topic in most kinesiology textbooks and industrial safety pamphlets because of the vulnerability of the human body to low back injury. Figure 9-18 shows three methods of picking up an object. The weight vector for the object and its moment arm from the principal axis of lifting motion can be drawn. Based on these facts, position A would have the least moment of resistance force and would have the least stress on the trunk, more specifically the lumbar region. Position B would primarily need lumbar extensor muscles to counteract the object being lifted. Depending on the weight of the object, however, either one or the other or both may be acceptable methods of lifting the object. Position C is never acceptable because it places stress on the posterior of the knee and stiffens the legs in a position of genu recurvatum (hyperextension at the knee).

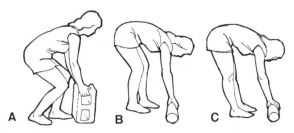

Fig. 9-18. *Three methods of lifting an object from the ground. A, least stress on spinal column. B, acceptable stress on spinal column. C, undesirable stress on knee and spinal column.*

If the weight of the object is light, either position A or B is acceptable, providing the person is not so heavy that the musculature cannot control the action of stooping and returning to a stand. The obese person is more apt to stoop rather than squat because the leg strength would probably be insufficient for rising from a squat. If the object is heavy, an obese person might not be able to achieve success with position A but could swing the object toward the legs, using position B in the manner of a weight lifter. The moment arm for the resistance is decreased, and then the object can be lifted with the back. There is danger in such a pattern because the swing may not remain in one plane and could therefore cause a twisting of the trunk and vertebral damage. Probably a combination of slight leg flexion and trunk flexion is the most effective and safest method of lifting heavy objects.

Chaffin has shown that there is a direct relationship between the amount of stress in the lumbar region on one hand and the horizontal distance of the object from the person's base of support and the vertical distance the object is moved on the other. (Refer to Chapter 12 for more information.) Therefore, the safest position is one in which the object is near the center of gravity of the body. This position minimizes the moment arm of the resistance.

Use of Implements

Long-Handled Implements. When human beings use long-handled implements such as rakes, hoes, brooms, axes, and shovels, the interfacing of the body size of the implement is an important consideration. For taller-than-average individuals, the commercially available long-handled implements may be too short for efficient use. The person must then assume a stooped posture that promotes excessive tension in the neck and upper back muscles, as well as possible tension in the lumbar region. Taller persons should thus adapt to the implement by performing the task with increased flexion at the knees and hips to maintain a more efficient trunk position. Shorter-than-average persons must adapt to the average-length implements by adjusting the placement of the hands.

DEVELOPMENTAL BIOMECHANICS   **319**

Long-handled implements require the user to establish the most efficient lever system possible, sacrificing movement distance for force improvement in many cases. For example, when using a long-handled shovel to lift a load of dirt, the person will separate the hands to produce a first-class lever system. The hand nearer the load will act as the fulcrum (axis of rotation), and the more distant hand will exert a force downward through a long distance (Fig. 9-19). Thus, the hand supporting the weight of the shovel and dirt is at or near the balance point of the system. The long moment arm of the handle of the shovel allows movement with a significant mechanical force advantage. Use of the large muscle groups—the leg muscles and the oblique muscles of the trunk—to lift and even to support the implement is also a means of utilizing the implement more efficiently.

In some instances, the person will push, slide, or pull the implement to move a resisting material, rather than lift it. These other actions, such as sweeping and raking, require less muscle effort and produce less work (and thereby less energy) than does lifting. The exception is the type of action in which there is an unusually high coefficient of friction for the materials involved, such as shoveling wet, heavy snow.

The act of chopping wood with an axe resembles many of the actions described in tennis serves and other overarm patterns used in sports. The use of the implement necessitates holding the handle near the axe head on the upswing to decrease the resistance moment arm and to increase control over the implement. The other hand is placed at the end of the handle. The body counterrotates, and the axe is lifted in a curved path above the head. The back hyperextends and the legs flex. On the forward swing of the axe, the body rotates, the trunk flexes, and the legs extend as one hand slides to meet the other hand at the end of the handle. This latter action increases the moment arm and thus the arc and velocity of the axe head as the axe swings forward and downward. Trunk flexion carries the force of the axe through

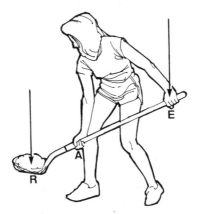

Fig. 9-19. *Lifting dirt with long-handled shovel. This is a first-class lever system. (R, resistance; A, axis; E, effort.)*

the wood as the muscle force and gravity combine to accelerate the weight of the axe head.

As with sports skills, the greatest acceleration occurs at the instant of contact, and the best performer accelerates the fastest or through the greatest distance. The taller and longer-limbed person has the potential for creating the greater force. However, since multiple levers are acting, the coordinated timing of these levers and the body's neuromuscular speed determine the effectiveness of the act. Thus, shorter persons might outperform taller persons even when using a less coordinated pattern. Note the path of the axe head for a tall person and for a short person chopping wood, as depicted in Fig. 9-20.

MINI-LAB LEARNING EXPERIENCES

1. One of the basic gardening activities is hoeing, an activity involving a long-handled implement. Describe the pattern of hoeing.
2. Given the following conditions, explain how the basic pattern just described could be modified.
   a. Condition A: hoe blade decreased in size by 50%.
   b. Condition B: ground made of hard clay.
   c. Condition C: handle reduced by 0.66 m.
3. List the key concepts and principles that necessitated the modifications you indicated in #2.

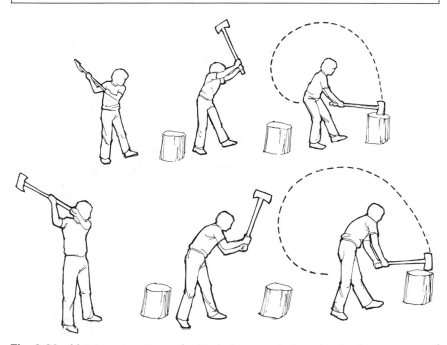

Fig. 9-20. *Movement pattern of axe during wood chopping by two persons of different stature. Note arcs of swing.*

Small Implements. Most ADL skills involve the use of small implements. One of the best approaches to the study of these movements has been developed by the time-motion analysts (human engineers). These persons have analyzed movements required in industrial tasks and have set guidelines and made modifications in the human-machine task or in the environment to improve the efficiency of the human-machine operation. (See Chapter 12.) Because of the financial need to obtain maximum production for minimum cost, including minimum cost in human years of productivity, the analysis of industrial tasks has a solid scientific basis. Scientific analyses of ADL involving small implements are needed if these same benefits of human productivity are to accrue in daily life. Older persons, the weak, or physically disabled especially need efficiency in their daily tasks. The young and strong need to learn efficiency to help others or help themselves, especially in later life.

The three basic components to be considered, once again, are time, space, and force. The direction, range, speed, and rate of sequencing of each direction of a movement task are studied to determine whether or not the values of each allow the person to perform the task with a minimum of force and a minimum of nonessential movements. In addition, the required posture for the task is evaluated by the same criteria. The last step in the analysis is to identify variations and inefficiency caused by anatomic differences.

For tasks in the home that will be repeated or performed for several minutes' duration, the following guidelines may be considered as biomechanical principles for efficiency:

1. Keep the distance of travel of the arms and hands in an area that allows the trunk to remain stable and without excess tension. The shoulders should be in a relaxed position, not elevated, retracted, or protracted. The arc of a horizontal plane depicting this travel would be approximately 120 degrees, with midposition being at the midline of the body and a radius of the length of the person's arm. The vertical space to be used is approximately the distance from shoulder to elbow. This vertical distance provides the optimum working position for the trunk and causes minimum lifting of the upper arms, thus facilitating a low energy output.

2. Whenever possible, use curved movements rather than linear movements requiring changes in direction. An increase or a decrease in the curvature of motion requires less force than stopping movement in one line and initiating movement in another line. The inertia of a moving body increases the efficiency in the former action but decreases efficiency in the latter action.

3. Horizontal movements have an advantage over vertical movements. The work against gravity is virtually zero in movements in the horizontal plane. One need only counteract the

mass of the limbs, since there are no vertical accelerations. Most movements that are slow to moderate in speed and that require little force are performed more efficiently with horizontal movements than with vertical ones.

4. When gravity can be used to facilitate the movement, vertical movements have an advantage over horizontal ones. The upward lifting of the arms is performed close to the body to decrease the moments of force. On the downward movements, the arms are moved away from the body and allowed to accelerate without muscle effort. Thus, gravity-assisted movements are very efficient. An example of such a movement is the act of hammering a nail into wood.

5. Allow the large (strong) muscles to perform the work task. Pulling motions are usually done best in the anteroposterior plane, and pushing motions are done in the horizontal plane (lateral movements). Women, especially, tend to have weak forearm extensors and thus are ineffective in pushing with the arms solely in the anteroposterior plane.

6. Perform essential movements only.

7. Establishing a rhythm tends to eliminate nonessential movements and to utilize the momentum of one phase of the movement to initiate the next phase. (See Chapter 8 for details concerning the use of rhythm in movements.)

Fatigue becomes a factor to consider with many ADL, hobby, and work tasks. The rate at which a task can be done decreases with time unless the optimum pace is set for the individual. This pace may have to be determined by trial and error, but the number of trials necessary to find the optimum place may be decreased by following these steps:

1. Ask the person to select a pace and rhythm.
2. Observe the person's performance, noting signs of excessive tension, such as shoulder bracing and head movements.
3. If tension is noted, ask the person to decrease the pace. If tension is not noted, ask the person to increase the pace.
4. Observe the performance again.
5. Make further corrections in pace if necessary.

Posture

Standing Posture for ADL. It has been suggested that the commonly used standing position for work tasks is a potentially harmful one, and it is one that has been reinforced in many school and work situations. This deleterious position is one in which the feet are together, the lower limbs are stiffened, and the upper body is in a flexed position. This posture produces sustained tension that may lead to loss of normal elasticity of the tissue, reduced circulatory efficiency, progressive reduction in the range of movement, and chronic general fatigue.

While working in a standing position, the tendency is to hyper-extend the legs and to create excessive tension in the chest and cervical regions. Persons should be taught to actively relax the muscles in the chest and neck and to flex the legs while performing work and ADL tasks. The feet should be separated into a forward and backward position for balance and reduced tension.

To avoid pooling of blood in the legs, excessive pressure on the blood vessels (which may cause partial occlusion of flow), and increased muscular tension, a person should move about frequently, at least every 10 minutes. A 10-minute rest during each hour of a repetitive task is recommended for more productive and safer performance.

Sitting Postures. Just as persons may assume, out of habit, a standing posture for long periods of time that is not efficient and may in fact cause postural deviations, persons may also assume undesirable sitting postures (Fig. 9-21). In some instances, the sitting posture is assumed incorrectly because of preference; in other instances, the furniture requires a particular posture. For many years, the design of seats in commercial airplanes produced a forward tilt of the head and discomfort in certain passengers due to upper trunk position and sitting height. Fortunately, these seats have been redesigned by some of the airline companies to eliminate the problem.

The soft-cushioned chair produces a different type of problem:

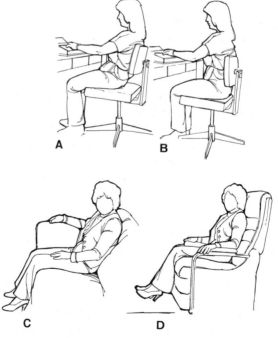

Fig. 9-21. *Effects of chair design on sitting posture. A, lordosis; B, erect trunk; C, no support for head; D, feet do not reach floor.*

pressure on thighs and lumbar curve. The straight-back chair provides the best support for buttocks, thighs, and back. The height of a chair also affects the comfort of the sitter. The feet should reach the floor, with a leeway of no more than a few centimeters. If the feet-to-floor distance is not optimum, persons may assume a slouch position (Fig. 9-21D) that is inefficient and places the body trunk in a potentially dangerous position. The abdominal muscles and the erector spinae muscles or both may contract to form a rigid bridge of the lower trunk in the lumbar region. Increased lumbar curvature (lordosis) may result from prolonged sitting in this manner.

What, then, is the best furniture design for persons with back problems? The furniture must provide support for the lower back, forcing the lumbar curve to flatten. Any number of designs can be used to achieve this goal, but the straight-backed, rigid chair designed centuries ago still remains one of the best designs, along with the newer reclining chair.

MINI-LAB LEARNING EXPERIENCES

1. Compare the two styles of typewriting shown in Fig. 9-22. Apply the principles of efficiency, and determine which style is more efficient.
2. Attach a pedometer or estimate the amount of walking or running performed by the following:
   a. Airline cabin crew members on one flight.
   b. Players in a basketball game.
   c. Yourself on a typical weekday.
3. Discuss the adjustments in equipment and technique that would be made by a carpenter having a choice of four hammers with two different head weights and two different shaft lengths. The carpenter would hammer nails for two hours each under the following conditions:
   a. Into a floor;
   b. Into a ceiling;
   c. Into a wall.

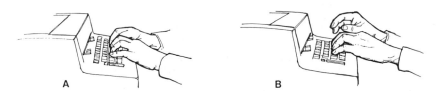

A   B

Fig. 9-22. *Two styles of typewriting. A, Hands and forearms are relatively stable, with muscles in continual state of contraction. B, Hands lift intermittently, providing periods of muscle relaxation, but also causing muscle effort to raise hands.*

REFERENCES

Andriacchi, T. P., Ogle, J. A. and Galante, O. (1977) Walking Speed as a Basis for Normal and Abnormal Gait Measurements, *Journal of Biomechanics*, 10:261.

Andriacchi, T. P. An Optoelectric System for Human Motion Analysis, *Bulletin of Prosthetics Research*, BPR 10-35, 18(1):291.

Aniansson, A. (1980) Muscle function in old age with special reference to muscle morphology, effect of training and capacity in activities in daily living, thesis, University of Goteborg, Sweden.

Armstrong, C. W. and Nash, M. (1983) Performance error identification as a function of visual and verbal training, *Abstracts of Research Papers* nv:48.

Baird, J. E. (1959) Energy costs of women during walking, thesis, University of Southern California.

Barclay, C. R. and Newell, K. M. (1980) Children's processing of information in motor skill acquisition, *Journal of Experimental Child Psychology* 30:89–108.

Bates, B. T., S. L. James and L. R. Osternig, (1978) The Use of Orthotic Devices to Modify Foot Mechanics, *Journal of Biomechanics* (under running), 11:210.

Beveridge, S. K. and Gangstead, S. K. (1984) A comparative analysis of the effects of instruction on the analytical proficiency of physical education teachers and undergraduates, *Abstracts of Research Papers* nv:78.

Biscan, D. V. and Hoffman, S. J. (1976) Movement analysis as a generic ability of physical education teachers and students, *Research Quarterly* 47:161–163.

Cavagna, G. A. and Margaria, R. (1966) Mechanics of Walking, *Journal of Appl. Physiol.* 21:271–278.

Cozzallio, E. R. (1986) The development of an assessment instrument for screening selected gross motor skills of kindergarten children, *Dissertation Abstracts International* 47:118A (University Microfilm No. DA8604166).

Espenschade, A. S. and Eckert, H. M. (1967) *Motor development*, Columbus, OH: Merril.

Gallahue, D. L. (In Press) *Understanding motor development: Infants, Children, and Adolescents.* Indianapolis: Benchmark Press, Inc.

Gallahue, D. L., Werner, P. H. and Luedke, G. C. (1975) *A conceptual approach to moving and learning*, New York: John Wiley and Sons, Inc.

Gangstead, S. K. and Moyer, S. (1985) A comparative analysis of the effects of skill specific training on the analytical proficiency of physical education majors, *Abstracts of Research Papers* nv:20.

Godfrey, B., Godfrey, K. and Newell, K. M. (1969) *Movement patterns and motor education*, New York: Appleton-Century-Crafts.

Griffin, M. R. (1984) The utilization of product and process measures to compare the throwing, striking, and kicking proficiency of third and fifth grade students, *Dissertation Abstracts International* 45:279A (University Microfilms No. DA8427302).

Halverson, L. E., Roberton, M. A. and Harper, C. J. (1973) Current research in motor development in children, *Journal of Research and Development in Education*, 6:56–70.

Hannah, R. E. (1980) Interpretation of Clinical Gait, Analysis Data, Human Locomotion I, Proceedings of Canadian Society for Biomechanics.

Hoffman, S. J. (1983) Clinical diagnosis as a pedagogical skill. In Templin, T. J. and Olson, J. K., editors: *Teaching in physical education*, Champaign, IL: Human Kinetics.

Imwold, C. (1984) Developing feedback behavior through a teach-reteach cycle, *Physical Educator*, 41(2):72–76.

Kelly, S. N. (1986) A description of information physical education teachers use to formulate feedback messages, *Dissertation Abstracts International* 46:2617A (University Microfilms No. DA8525480).

Klinger, A., Masataka, T., Adrian, M. and Smith, E. (1980) Unpublished report presented at AAHPERD Research Symposium.

Kniffin, K. M. (1986) The effects of individualized videotape instruction on the ability of undergraduate physical education majors to analyze select sport skills, *Dissertation Abstracts International* 47:119A (University Microfilms No. DA8526199).

MacGraw, R. and Foort, J. (1979) Tri-joint electrogionometric assessment of patients receiving knee implants, NHW Project 610-1128-Y, final report, Vancouver, B.C., Division of Orthopaedics, University of British Columbia.

Morrison, C. and Reeve, J. (1986) Effect of instructional units on the analysis of related and unrelated skills, *Perceptual and Motor Skills* 62:593–566.

Morton, D. J. and Fuller, D. D. (1952) *Human locomotion and body form*, Baltimore: The Williams & Wilkins Co.

Murray, M. P. (1967) Gait as a Total Pattern of Movement, *American Journal of Phys. Med.* 46:290.

Murray, M. P., Drought, A. B. and Korg, R. C. (1964) Walking patterns of normal men, *J. Bone Joint Surg.* 46A:335.

Newell, K. M. (1976) Knowledge of results and motor learning. In Keogh, J. and Hutton, R. S., editors: *Exercise and sport science reviews*, vol. 4, Santa Barbara, CA: Journal Publishing Affiliates.

Newell, K. M. and Kennedy, J. A. (1978) Knowledge of results and children's motor learning, *Developmental Psychology* 14:531–536.

Petrakis, E. (1986) Visual observation patterns of tennis teachers, *Research Quarterly for Exercise and Sport* 57(3):254–259.

Rarick, G. L. (1982) Descriptive Research and Process-oriented explanations of the motor development of children. In *The Development of Movement Control and Coordination,* Kelso, J. S. and Clark, J. E., eds.: New York: John Wiley and Sons, Ltd., pp. 275–291.

Roberton, M. A. (1976) Developmental kinesiology, *Journal of Health, Physical Education, and Recreation* 43:65–66.

Roberton, M. A. (1978) Longitudinal evidence for developmental stages in the forceful overarm throw, *Journal of Human Movement Studies* 4:167–175.

Roberton, M. A. and Halverson, L. E. (1984) *Developing children—Their changing movement a guide for teachers,* Philadelphia: Lea and Febiger.

Safrit, M. J. (1981) *Evaluation in physical education* (2nd ed.), Englewood Cliffs, NJ: Prentice-Hall.

Sanders, M. T. (1986) Effects of augmented feedback on the acquisition of a motor skill in two environmental conditions, *Dissertation Abstracts International* 46:3286A (University Microfilms No. DA8600049).

Saunders, J. B., Inman, V. T. and Eberhart, H. D. (1953) Major determinants in normal and pathological gait, *J. Bone Joint Surg.* 35A:543–558.

Seefeldt, V. and Haubenstricker, J. (1982) Patterns, Phases, or Stages: An analytical model for the study of developmental movement. In *The development of movement control and coordination,* Keslo, J. A. S. and Clark, J. E., eds.: New York: John Wiley and Sons Ltd.

Siedentop, D. (1983) *Developing teaching skills in physical education* (2nd ed.), Palo Alto, CA: Mayfield.

Singer, R. N. (1980) *Motor learning and human performance: An application to motor skills and movement behaviors,* New York: Macmillan.

Smidt, G. L. (1971) Hip Motion and Related Factors in Walking, *Phys. Ther.* 51:9.

Smoll, F. (1982) Developmental kinesiology: Toward a subdiscipline focusing on motor development. In *The Development of Movement Control and Coordination,* Kelso, J. A. S. and Clark, J. E., eds.: New York: John Wiley and Sons Ltd.

Steindler, A. (1955) *Kinesiology of the human body under normal and pathological conditions,* Springfield, IL: Charles C. Thomas, Publisher.

Vaughn, K. (1982) Biomechanics of Human Gait, An Annotated Bibliography, Printed and Published, University of Cape Town, South Africa, March.

Weismeyer, H. (1984) Picture analysis for classroom instruction or testing, *Journal of Physical Education, Recreation, and Dance* 55:72–3.

Wickstrum, R. (1977) *Fundamental motor patterns,* Philadelphia: Lea and Febiger.

Wild, M. R. (1938) The behavior pattern of throwing and some observations concerning its course of development in children, *Research Quarterly* 9:20–24.

Wild, M. R.: Unpublished Dissertation, University of Wisconsin, 1938.

10
Biomechanics of Exercises

Biomechanical assessment of exercise will reduce risk of injury and will maximize benefits of exercise. Exercises should be based upon biomechanical as well as physiological principles. For example, if the goal of an exercise is to strengthen the pectoralis major muscle, one cannot assume that the posture selected will, in fact, cause the pectoralis major to contract as the primary muscle. The exerciser must scientifically position the body parts in the planes of desired muscle function. Furthermore, the selected posture used to perform the exercise must not cause excessive stress to the spine. This possibility exists when performing the bench press (Fig. 10-1) in which two body postures are depicted, one in which the lumbar curvature is increased dangerously.

An important, although not often considered contribution of biomechanical assessments of exercise postures and movement patterns is reduction of the risk of injury during exercise.

Biomechanical assessments of exercise maximizes the benefits of the exercise. For example, if range of motion at a joint is to be increased, the movement must be performed in the plane of desired increase throughout the entire possible range of motion and with the adjacent body parts positioned to facilitate stretch. One cannot assume that this will be automatic. One of the most common examples of changes in plane of movement is noted during the exercise to increase range of horizontal extension at the shoulder. The arms begin the movement at shoulder level and usually drop during the backward stretch, rather than remaining at shoulder height. The "correct" and "incorrect" executions of this exercise are depicted in Fig. 10-2.

The goals of the exercises should be clearly defined, and the exercise pattern executed to ensure that the goals are met and that no deleterious side effects result, in order to insure maximum benefits with minimum risks of injury. The basic guidelines for biomechanical

329

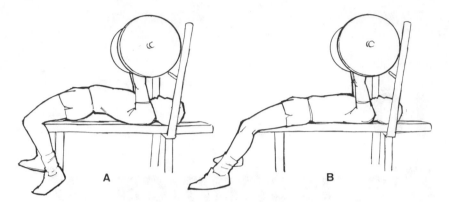

Fig. 10-1. *Two persons performing the bench press., Note the excessive lumbar curvature in A. This posture is less safe than that of B.*

design and evaluation of exercises will be identified with respect to four broad categories of exercises:

1. Exercises to improve strength and power of muscles, ligaments and bones;
2. Exercises to improve anaerobic/aerobic capacity;
3. Exercises to increase range of motion at the joints;

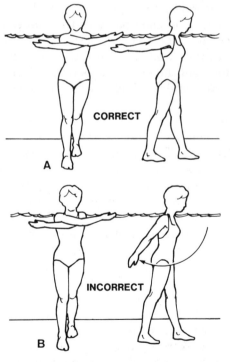

Fig. 10-2. *Horizontal extension exercise performed correct (A) and incorrect (B). B includes movement in a plane other than the horizontal and does not maximize muscular strength development.*

4. Exercises to increase neuromuscular functioning, such as agility, balance, and coordination.

GUIDELINES FOR BIOMECHANICAL DESIGN AND EVALUATION OF EXERCISES

A synthesis of basic physiology and biomechanics knowledge should be available prior to analysis of exercises. In addition, it has become evident that the inclusion of cultural, sociological and psychological perspectives is valuable in selecting the type of exercise for a particular population or individual. Usually there are several exercises that elicit similar benefits. Selection of the most appealing one will facilitate participation. Furthermore, since persons today want scientifically designed programs, motivation to exercise is greater if the exercises are biomechanically designed than if they have not had such scientific design. The basic guidelines for biomechanical design and evaluation of an exercise are as follows:

1. *State the goal precisely.* Is the goal to: (a) increase strength in a particular muscle, (b) increase range of motion at a particular joint and in a particular plane, (c) increase decision-making skills with respect to type of movement and timing of movement, or (d) to enhance kinestheses and balance? Be specific in stating the goal of the exercise.
2. *Identify the exercises that could fulfill the goal.* There are numerous sources in which exercises can be found. Select the most appropriate with respect to the population which will perform the exercises. Factors such as age, experience, strength, and convenience need to be considered. If no existing documented or published exercises appear to be appropriate, use biomechanical knowledge to define an exercise that would be beneficial.
3. *Determine the minimum characteristics of the person for success.* Based upon the literature or empirical research, identify the average strength requirement, ROM requirements, and other characteristics a person must possess to perform the exercise. Identify stress to joints and any other potential dangers to the person.
4. *Determine the body position required to initiate the exercise.* Define the body alignment and the posture necessary to fixate the body parts required to stabilize and facilitate specific movements.
5. *Describe exactly the movement to be executed.* Form a mental image of the sequence of movements.
6. *Identify probable execution problems.* Identify likely problems in executing the required movement. At which instances during the exercise is the person likely to arch the back, lean with

the trunk, or rotate a leg or arm in such a way that the benefits are reduced and/or potential for injury is increased?

7. *Evaluate the performance.* Ask the person to perform the exercise and evaluate the performance with respect to safety and technique. Modify performance if necessary.

8. *Determine duration, intensity, and frequency of exercise performance.* Ability to perform and to improve performance is based upon the triad of exercise prescription: DIF (duration, intensity and frequency). These three components will be explained in the following section, since they should be utilized in all exercise prescription. An acronym to remember is that "DIF makes all the difference" between maximizing benefits from exercise or exercising for nothing.

MUSCLE STRENGTH

Improvement of Strength

Since improvement of strength in bones and ligaments cannot be measured directly in living beings, this section will consist only of descriptions of the biomechanics of improvement of strength of muscles. The assumption must be made that the ligaments of the joints crossed by the contracting muscles, and the bones to which these muscles are attached, will be strenghtened concurrently with the strengthening of the muscles.

Exercises to improve strength may have as their goal an increase in strength for a particular sport competition, activity of daily living, or job-related skill; the rehabilitation of an injured limb; or the modification of upright posture. The following information should be used as guidelines for prescription of strength exercises:

1) The muscle or other body part to be strengthened should be identified so that the type of exercise that will produce maximum benefits can be selected.

2) The movement plane and the angle of the limb should be specifically defined and adhered to throughout the exercise, since changes in position may negate the original purpose and cause different muscles to function.

3) Finally, the resistance and the resistance moment of force should be quantified to determine relative difficulty of the exercise and probable degree of improvement.

Knowledge of moment arms and muscle angles of pull and the ability to estimate their magnitudes will allow the exercise directors and participants to determine the relative difficulty of each selected exercise. They will also be able to determine the safe initial load and to progressively increase the load according to the gains in strength. In this way, the optimum regimen for improvement of strength may be formulated.

The importance of these guidelines is illustrated by observing the two positions of a person performing a leg press on a machine such as the Universal Gym. Note the undesirable position in Fig. 10-3A and B, which necessitates a lighter load for success, as compared to the position in Fig. 10-3C and D, in which it is possible to move a heavier load. The person in A and B have an unstisfactory mechanical advantage for the hip extensors and an undesirable force vector against the foot plates.

The vectors along the shank in Fig. 10-3A and B are more vertical than horizontal, whereas the vectors in C and D are more horizontal than vertical. Therefore, the application of force in C and D is more perpendicular to the leg press lever (and the foot plate), thus producing more force in the desired direction of movement of the lever. Conversely, the force of the leg extension in A and B is wasted, for the most part, being ineffective in producing movement. The foot muscles are activated in A and B to compensate for inadequate leg angle. Unfortunately, these small muscles are inadequate in producing the equivalent force produced by the leg muscles.

Type of Strength Exercises

Strength exercises may be subdivided into isotonic (same tension), isometric (same length), and isokinetic (same velocity) exercises.

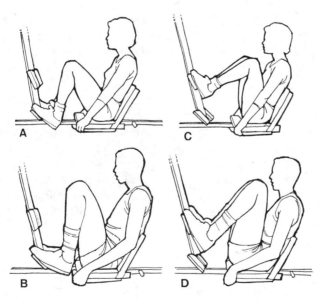

Fig. 10-3. *Two persons performing leg press on weight machine. Differences in body segment angles, muscle angles of push, and direction of application of force are different for each foot plate position and each individual. Drawing a vector through the shank in C and D best estimates the direction of force application. Note the use of the balls of the feet to change the angle of force through the shank axis.*

BIOMECHANICS OF EXERCISES 333

Isotonic Exercises. Isotonic exercises, though misnamed since muscular tension is not a constant magnitude throughout the exercise, are the most common. The exercised body part moves through an angular displacement, as when weights are used and in everyday tasks. Quite often, however, when weights are being lifted, the starting position is a weak position. Thus, the capability of the muscle at all positions other than the starting position is not even approached during this exercise. Furthermore, the person exercising in this manner is likely to accelerate the weight rapidly after the initial inertia is overcome, causing momentum to be the primary force throughout the remainder of the movement. Since muscle action is necessary merely to begin movement, strength is not developed in other segments of the range of motion to the same degree as at the start of the movement. To ensure maximum benefits from isotonic exercises, the performer should move at a nearly constant velocity rather than allow momentum to vary and facilitate the movement.

The use of free weights, such as barbells in weightlifting competition, is a classic example of the use of acceleration to enable the lifter to succeed. If the timing is exactly correct—that is, if the barbell has begun to accelerate upward—the lifter can change from a position in which the shoulders are above the bar to one in which the shoulders are below the bar. Full arm extension can then be used to lift the weight above the head. In other lifts, the bar may be swung toward the thighs to reduce the moment arm and to utilize the inward swing to overcome the inertia of the stationary bar.

When weights are lifted from a semisquat or full-squat position, there is a danger of injuring the joints (ankle, knee, hip, lumbar spine) because of the increased moments of force (torques) acting at these joints. One might suppose that the moments of force would increase proportionately with the increase in weight lifted. This linear relationship does not always exist with human beings. As the weight changes, the person changes the kinematics of the lift. Furthermore, all persons do not change their kinematics in the same fashion. Hay found that one lifter, in changing from a weight 60% of maximum to one 80% of maximum, increased the moment of force at the knee twofold, whereas another individual showed a decrease in the moment of force at the knee. Thus, the most important factor for safety and for improvement is the manner in which the weight is lifted.

MINI-LAB LEARNING EXPERIENCE

Utilizing the information in Chapter 5, identify the moments of force for each of the squat performers in Fig. 10-4. Which joint has greatest moment? Anthropometric data influences the performers since they shift body segment positions to maintain equilibrium.

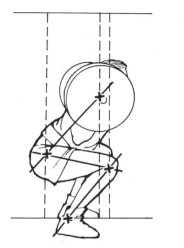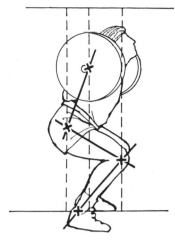

Fig. 10-4. *Squat performances by persons of different anthropometry. The weight line and moment arm from various joints are drawn so that the relative moment at these joints could be estimated.*

Increasing the resistance may produce different benefits or may pose different dangers than are found with the lighter resistance. For example, arm extensions with free weights or attached weights may not increase the strength of the triceps brachii because persons may rotate the arms outward and thus utilize the strong shoulder girdle muscles (rhomboids) to change the angle at the shoulder. This change in angle may cause the arm to accelerate so that the weaker triceps brachii can be assisted in producing extension at the elbow. Other compensations may include rotation of the body along its longitudinal axis and the use of the momentum of the body and the stronger arm to begin the arm extension. The weaker arm is therefore bypassed or allowed to extend only after upward acceleration has occurred. Body lean and other kinematic actions can be observed when compensation is made. EMG studies are useful also to determine which muscles are active in performing a certain exercise. When lifting free weights, the number of muscles required to stabilize the body are greater than when the body is fixed in a weight lifting machine.

Isotonic exercises described have been of the concentric contraction type. Plyometric exercises take advantage of eccentric contractions of muscles to facilitate performance. The portion of this contraction activated by muscle elasticity and by stretch reflex is not known, but both have been implicated (Kilani, 1988). Plyometric depth jumping is the most popular form of eccentric exercise. The person jumps from an elevation, lands and immediately jumps again. The act of landing and preparing to jump again involves eccentric contractions and muscular strength gains. Limitations on elevations and use of weights must be made to avoid injury to the joints. Trauma to the body can be estimated by performing these depth jumps onto a force platform.

BIOMECHANICS OF EXERCISES   **335**

Isometric Exercise. Although isometric exercises produce no actual work, they may be useful in strengthening muscle groups. In particular, persons who have broken or sprained a body part will find that isometric exercises are the only possible exercises to prevent atrophy of certain muscles enclosed in a cast. This type of exercise is convenient to perform and appeals to persons who do not wish to exert themselves unduly or perspire while exercising. Since occlusion of the blood supply to the muscle occurs, and since persons reflexively tend to hold their breath during isometric exercises, the duration of each muscle contraction should be short, preferably less than six seconds. Counting is a useful means of achieving normal breathing during isometric exercises.

Isometric contractions can be combined with yoga exercises and tension control programs, which will be described in later sections of this chapter. Isometric exercises have the following limitations: (1) Muscle strength improves primarily at the angle at which isometrics are performed, and (2) only slow-twitch muscle fibers are activated. Thus, it is unlikely that a muscle will be strengthened throughout the range of motion solely by the use of isometric exercises. Neither will all the muscle fibers be activated by isometrics; that is, fast-twitch fibers will not contract.

Isokinetic Exercises. The concepts of zero acceleration and graphic output of the force applied during exercise was incorporated into strength-conditioning programs in the 1960's. This system of exercising was termed isokinetics. Since the limb is not allowed to accelerate, muscle force must be used throughout the exercise. The addition of graphic displays of the force-time curve or force-angle curve insures that the performer attempts to apply muscle force throughout the exercise rather than "cheat through the move."

Isokinetic machines can be set to move at various specified rates for improvement of strength or power. Both the resistance and the speed can be varied, thereby providing a variety of work outputs. Since the same work output may be produced by using either a high resistance (force) with low velocity or a low resistance with high velocity, the product of force × distance × repetitions may be identical for a given time period.

Measurement of Strength Gains

Strength improvement can be measured by the resistance overcome (load lifted) or by the work done. During isometric exercise one can pull against a dynamometer and record the total force produced. No work can be calculated, since the load is not moved. According to the definition of work, the work was equal to zero (Force × Distance = Zero). The degree of muscle tension involved for the particular isometric contraction can be measured and compared to other persons' scores or to one's own progress chart.

During isotonic and isokinetic exercise, positive work accomplished is equal to the distance the weight is lifted, multiplied by the weight. In most reported calculations, no credit is given for lifting the body part itself, although this does require muscle force. Likewise, no credit is given for lowering the weight, since this work is negative and is caused by eccentric contraction of the same muscle used in the production of positive work. The total work performed is equal to the work done for one lift, multiplied by the number of repetitions of the lift.

In a strength exercise program, the total work output should increase gradually. For example, swimmers swim more laps, joggers run more kilometers, and persons walk longer distances to increase their work output.

Work. The intensity of the work performed in an exercise is determined by the amount of muscle effort required to move the external weight through a distance and at a specific speed. A viable method of estimating the intensity of an exercise is the calculation of work performed during the movement. In the leg press, the work performed is equal to the product of the distance the weight is raised and the magnitude of the weights. Work performance with respect to a given exercise usually differs among individuals. For example, the tall, long-legged person might raise a weight of 200 lbs. (454 N) a distance of one foot (0.28 M); whereas a short, short-legged person might only raise the weight half that distance. Thus, the work done would be only half as great. Total work is equal to the amount of work for each lift multiplied by the number of lifts (repetitions). In the case of the tall and short person, 10 repetitions would be equal to 454 N × 0.28 M × 10 for the tall person, and only 454 N × 0.14 M × 10 for the short person. Work is in units of Newton-meters. Equating the number of repetitions for all persons in an exercise class does not equalize the work done, but overtaxes some individuals and undertaxes others.

Not only may the distance the body is moved differ, but the resistance will differ. A heavier person will perform more work than a lighter person, despite the fact that each executes the same exercise. This difference may be only of slight importance if both individuals have appropriate muscle mass. If one individual has predominantly fat (adipose tissue) and another person has predominantly muscle, the inequality with respect to intensity of exercise is magnified. Thus, without a biomechanical assessment, optimum levels of duration and intensity cannot be achieved. The danger of excessive overload in strength training is probable. This is especially true in arm strength exercises, such as pullups and pushups. Pullups and pushups have always been easier for short-armed ectomorphic/mesomorphic individuals to perform. For example, male and female gymnasts are always at the top of arm strength performance scales. Refer to Table 10-1 for comparison of force required and work done by short, medium, and tall individuals (with corresponding arms lengths), both muscular and obese.

Exercise Equalizing Equation. In order to equalize work done, an exercise equalizing equation is proposed. This equation is based

Table 10-1. *Work performed by persons with different anthropometric characteristics. One chin-up and the maximum number of chin-ups.*

Subject	Arm Length (cm)	Body Weight (Newtons)	One Chin Up (Newton-Meters*)	Repetitions Performed	Total Work Done (NM)
Muscular	55	600	330	10	3300
Persons	48	500	240	15	3600
	39	445	174	20	3480
Obese	55	600	330	2	660
Persons	48	500	240	3	720
	39	445	174	4	696

*A newton-meter (NM) is equivalent to a joule.

upon the available muscle mass, the body weight, and the anthropometric lengths of the body. Unfortunately, muscle mass can only be estimated in the exercise situation. This is a limitation of the equation: however, it has greater validity than existing age and sex-related norms. The Exercise Equalizing Equation is as follows:

Work performed = [Number of repetitions × (weight lifted + body segment weight lifted)]

Adjusted lean body weight = equalizing factor % lean body weight

Adjusted work = Work performed × Adjusted lean body weight

The equalizing factor is .80 (average % lean body weight). Thus, persons with average lean body mass will have no adjustment in work performed. Persons with greater lean body mass (more muscular) will "receive credit for less work than actually performed", and persons with less lean body mass (obese) will "receive credit for more work than actually performed." Application of the exercise equalizing equation to these three cases is as follows:

fat = 20%, Adj. Work = 1.0 × Work
fat = 30%, Adj. Work = 1.1 × Work
fat = 10%, Adj. Work = 0.9 × Work

MINI-LAB LEARNING EXPERIENCE

1. Using the data from Table 10-1, estimate the work when performing the following:
   A. Pullups from leaning position in which two-thirds of the body weight rests on the feet.
   B. Pushups from a knee support position in which one-half of the body weight rests on the knees.

2. Assume that the lean body weight is 85% for the muscular persons and 70% for the obese persons. Using the exercise equalizing equation, calculate the adjusted work for exercises in #1.

This basic concept of individualized work also has implications when considering the amount of time (duration) spent engaging in a specific exercise. If 10 repetitions are required of all persons in an exercise class, some persons will take longer to perform these 10 repetitions than will others. This usually results in the muscles of slower moving and taller persons contracting for a longer period of time. If time is not increased, the taller person compensates (especially if the exercise is performed within time-constraints) with faster actions. These faster actions are performed at the expense of greater accelerations, consequently greater muscle force.

Improvement of Muscle Power

Strength alone is not sufficient; the improvement of power also is desirable. Power is the rate of doing work:

$$\text{Power} = \frac{\text{Work}}{\text{Time}}$$

As exercises are performed at gradually increasing speeds, the amount of resistance that can be overcome decreases. This is evident if one remembers that power also is equal to force multiplied by velocity. Power exercises are designed to improve the velocity at which loads of varying weights can be moved. Fast-twitch muscle fibers are activated during high-velocity movements, and all muscle fibers become involved as fatigue causes the velocity of the movement to decrease. Isokinetic devices have made it possible to assess power quantitatively and to exercise in a more scientific manner than was possible previously. However, these devices have limitations in speed; their maximum speeds do not approach those used in sports. Since so many of the sports movements require power, it is important to construct exercises to improve performances of individuals. Mastropaolo suggests that the person exercise at the level of power overload, that is, the load which is greater than the load for which maximum power was achieved.

Exercises for Anterior Muscles. Since the human being walks on two feet in an upright position, the anterior muscles of the trunk tend to be underdeveloped and weak. The abdominal muscles in particular are usually inadequate for protection of the lumbar curve of the spine during both heavy lifting and carrying a fetus. To understand the role of the abdominal muscles, ask a person to lie in the supine position. When a person is lying supine, the lumbar curve increases, and persons usually can place their hands under the curvature and encounter no resistance. This increased curvature causes an increase in compression at the posterior edges of the disks of the vertebrae. The rectus abdominis muscle can contract to tilt the pelvis and thereby decrease the curve and reduce the stress to the spine. If the abdominal muscle is not strong enough to reduce this stress, there is potential danger of damaging the disks.

One of the most common abdominal strengthening exercises is the sit-up, with its many variations. As the sit-up is initiated, the iliopsoas muscle contracts, tilting the pelvis into an increased lumbar curve and preventing trunk flexion. This lack of trunk flexion prevents the shortening of the moment arm of the part of the body being lifted from the floor. Only the anterior ligaments and muscles can oppose this resistance moment. Thus, the rectus abdominis contracts to decrease the lumbar curve, thereby facilitating trunk flexion during the sit-up and reducing the stress to the lumbar vertebrae.

Based on the equation of moments of force, a selection of graduated exercises may be done. Figure 10-5 illustrates the differences in resistance moments during various sit-ups. The resistance is equal to the weight of the upper body, that is, from the hip joint to the top of the head, including the arms. The moment arm measured by the distance from the hip joint to the center of gravity of the upper body according to the distribution of the body parts. When an external weight is added to the upper body, the total resistance is the sum of this external weight and the weight of the legs on the resultant resistance moments of force that are illustrated in Fig. 10-5.

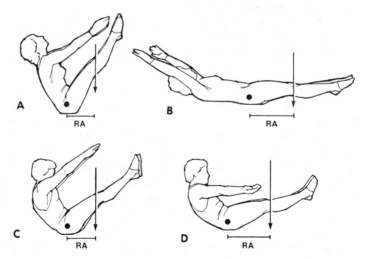

Fig. 10-5. *Differences in moment arms during V type sit-ups. (Arrows represent gravitational force acting on legs (weight of legs); RA, moment arm of resistance (hip to weight vector)). The moment of force acting counterclockwise on legs opposing the muscle effort can be calculated using RA = 45 cm (in D) and weight of legs = 325 N. Note that the moment arm in C is approximately three-fourths of that in D. Calculate the moment in C. If the woman weighs 590 N (130 lbs) and her legs are 40% of body weight, what would be the muscle moments for her?*

One must understand the anatomy of the body to know precisely what roles the muscles are likely to perform. In the example of the sit-up, the rectus abdominis does not create flexion at the hip joint or cause the sit-up action. It stabilizes the pelvis in the desired position to prevent injury to the spine, and it facilitates the flexed trunk position. The action of the iliopsoas and other flexors at the hip can be more nearly equalized with that of the rectus abdominis by performing sit-ups, and quite often this gain in strength is several times greater than the strength gain in the abdominal muscles. If the back is not flexed during sit-ups, little gain in abdominal strength results. Thus, rather than the complete sit-up, persons with weak abdominal muscles might well do head and shoulder raises, static "V" sitting positions, or sit-downs.

Instrumentation for Development of Muscle Strength and Power

Computerized variable-resistance exercisers have been described as a means of facilitating maximal muscular involvement and of optimizing exercise productivity. A computer or microprocessor is connected to an exercise machine and a person is tested on the machine for the purpose of diagnosing strength at various angles of various body parts. Baseline data are stored in the computer, and initial loads are selected by the computer. The computer can assign resistance values for various angles and degrees of strength. Force curves can be displayed and compared with other curves, and a new exercise program can be selected by the computer. Work output and power output can be recorded and displayed. (See Fig. 10-6.)

Programmable treadmills and strength devices are being used for rehabilitation programs, athletic conditioning programs, and physical fitness assessment in general. Physiological and biomechanical data

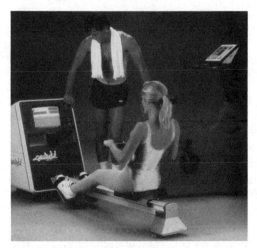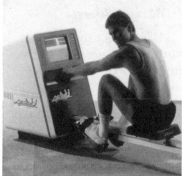

Fig. 10-6. *Computer interfaced programmable exercise machines.*

are recorded and used to profile the performances and to determine the exercise protocol. The growth potential of commercial equipment using computers or microprocessors or both to record, program, and modify programs of exercise is now the state-of-the art in exercise. Those should be exploited fully for the benefit of all exercisers.

RANGE OF MOTION

Range of motion (ROM) exercises are designed to increase the mobility of all joints of the body in all the planes possible for each joint. For maintenance of ROM, one may exercise faster and less often than if specific movements are to be enhanced. As with strength exercises, care must be taken to prevent an increase in performance in one plane or direction at the expense of performance in another plane or direction. For example, exercises to increase plantar flexion of the foot without concomitant exercise to increase dorsiflexion are likely to cause a foreshortening of the Achilles tendon or triceps surae muscle or both, and thus severely limit the amount of dorsiflexion possible. Such a condition causes pain in walking barefoot or uphill.

Most ROM exercises are designed to improve posture and symmetry of body. These exercises lengthen certain muscles, thereby increasing ROM at a joint, and attempt to equalize the respective roles of agonist and antagonist muscles. Since the shortened muscle is usually stronger than the lengthened muscle, strength exercises should compliment ROM exercises.

ROM exercises may be performed alone, with the aid of others who produce a force (passive exercise for the exerciser), or with the use of walls, towels, or other devices. In each condition, the movement may be conducted at various speeds and with or without the influence of gravity. Yoga exercises and other slow exercises are safe and combine an isometric strength advantage with the ROM benefits. With practice and continual exercising, persons beyond the age of 40 years can achieve ROM values not possible for them in the previous twenty years.

ROM and Speed

There is a potential danger when ROM exercises are performed with high velocities or accelerations. In these situations, either the muscle force or the force of gravity causes a momentum that may override the myotatic reflex, which normally protects the body from injury. In other instances, the myotatic reflex is elicited, causing a contraction in muscles that should have been lengthened. Thus, the purpose of the muscle lengthening exercise is defeated.

Muscle strain or complete separation can result when one attempts to increase the length of the muscle beyond its strain limit. Older persons, who have a decrease in the elastic component of the soft tissues, and persons who have fibrous tissue or calcium deposits are particularly susceptible to injury if ROM exercises are performed rapidly. Exercises performed while the body is under water are especially safe for these persons. Moderate speeds of movement and the use of gravity, under control, sometimes provides a means of attaining ROM goals not possible in slow movements.

ROM Benefits

The importance of biomechanically well-designed ROM exercises with respect to biomechanics cannot be underestimated. As with strength, the inability to perform normal ROM exercises at a specific joint may indicate severe restrictions on normal functioning and may prevent performance of some common ADL, work, or sports movements. For example, ROM limitations have prevented many persons from putting on and taking off shoes and stockings. Lowman has described numerous postural deviations and shown how each has a deleterious effect on athletic performance. Cardiorespiratory function and endurance, as well as movement efficiency of limbs, have been hampered. There is evidence that athletic performance may produce postural deviations that must be corrected through appropriate ROM and strength exercises.

MOST ADL and job-related patterns of movement tend to promote kyphosis (contracted pectoralis major muscles) and elevated shoulders. These characteristics also are noted in weightlifters and persons involved in other sports. Through an assessment of ROM restrictions, individualized ROM exercises can be constructed to correct unique anatomic characteristics.

PROGRAMMING FOR ROM

If based upon biomechanical principles, any range of motion exercise program would include exercises for every joint in the body, in each of the planes the joint allows an appreciable movement to occur. Range of motion required for sport, work, playing a musical instrument, performing basic activities of daily living, and other movement patterns must be assessed with respect to requirements prior to selection of exercises. Inadequate range of motion for the task should be identified, and priorities given to exercises which develop adequate ROM for the task. If the movements are sports movements in which high accelerations will be achieved, the exercises should be used to produce greater ranges of motion than the individual is capable of producing without assistance. This implies that another person or safety-controlled device would be used to place a gradual and slightly increasing force on the body part than that which is possible by the exerciser alone. If this is not practiced, the ROM exercise may never achieve the same ROM that occurs in the sport (since dynamic ROM is greater than static ROM), and damage to the soft tissues could result. The action of another muscle or force will tear a muscle; a muscle cannot tear itself. Lengthening of a muscle beyond its capabilities is caused by the forceful contraction of an antagonist muscle or by the force of gravity, or by another person.

NEUROMUSCULAR FUNCTIONING

Neuromuscular facilitation, or perceptual-motor exercises, involves the development or maintenance of balance, speed, agility, coordination, and other eye-hand or eye-foot exercises. During the early years of life, these exercises are necessary to assist the child in learning to move effectively. Late in life, disuse, pathologic conditions, or the aging process may create a need for persons to relearn these basics. Research with rats has shown that exercise increases the size of neurons and facilitates neuronal pathways of the central nervous system, including enhancement of the brain. Therefore, one might speculate that continued practice of coordinated movements might improve or at least maintain neuromuscular functioning during the later years of life.

Eye-hand coordination skills, reaction-time skills, movement time in all planes of movement possible, eye-foot coordination skills, and bilateral, contralateral, ispsilateral, and other combinations of upper- and lower-extremity patterns can be selected and made part of a daily exercise program. Additional benefits of strength and ROM will also occur with many of these perceptual-motor exercises.

One other type of neuromuscular facilitation exercise is that of tension control. Basmajian states that skilled persons know how to effectively reduce the tension levels in muscles that are not necessary to a movement. The unskilled person cannot do so, and excessive tension from undesirable muscle action interferes with the success of the movement. Woods has shown that the Jacobson method of tension control is effective in learning to regulate tension levels. Again, the biomechanical principles center on the perception of a moment of force, a quantity of work, or a postural deviation. The ability to recognize and regulate tension in one muscle is the basis for achieving efficiency in movement patterns.

The ability to replicate precisely a previous movement and to determine when and how fast to perform this movement can be evaluated using analysis tools described previously. Integration of this knowledge, together with biomechanical and motor control theory, can serve to determine whether or not an exercise incorporates the desired speed, coordination, balance, and agility characteristics.

AEROBIC EXERCISE

Why is biomechanical analysis a part of aerobic exercise? Although aerobic exercises are devised to enhance the functioning of the heart, lungs, and, in general, the respiratory and circulatory systems, the joints of the body cannot be ignored. Aerobic exercise often involves moderate to vigorous movements of a repetitive nature. Usually the same body parts move many times in the same manner. The same joints, muscles, tendons, and ligaments are stressed repetitively. Repeated stress, occurring frequently, at short intervals and with high magnitudes, has been termed the overuse syndrome. The body tissues can fatigue in the same way that a person feels fatigued. Such fatigue of tissues may result in tears, fractures, and other injuries. Such overuse has been noted in aerobic exercise, such as aerobics (exercise to music), jogging, rope jumping, swimming, running, and bicycling.

MINI-LAB LEARNING EXPERIENCE

Biomechanical analysis of these exercises is critical to reduce trauma to the body. Think about the movements in these types of aerobic exercises, and list the areas of the body most likely to experience trauma. The answers are after the next section.

Although the major two reasons for injury, excess repetitions and incorrect technique, are the same for all these forms of aerobic exercise, there is an important difference between aerobic dance (aerobics) and the other exercises. Aerobics often is a group activity. The other forms of exercise may be more individualized. Thus, aerobics has been chosen as an example of the application of biomechanics to aerobic exercising. Modification of the aerobics routine should be made based upon the anatomical characteristics of the class and the following biomechanical principles (used by permission of authors of *The Complete Encyclopedia of Aerobics: A Guide for the Aerobics Teacher*, Klinger, Adrian, Tyner-Wilson):

1. The greater the body weight, the greater the potential for injury.
2. Airborne activities produce greater forces to the body than do non-airborne activities.
3. Fast twisting movements of arms and upper trunk produce reaction forces in the lower back.
4. Stress is proportional to the surface area of the body receiving the force and to its magnitude.
5. The least amount of stress is placed upon the joint if the bones are aligned in a straight line.
6. The knee joint supports the least stress if it is aligned above the foot during all body support phases.
7. Alignment of the trunk above the pelvis provides the greatest potential for a balanced position.
8. The farther the limbs move away from the trunk, the greater the potential loss of equilibrium.

9. The longer the limb which is swinging, the greater the reactive force at the joints.
10. The faster the limbs move away from the trunk, the greater the potential loss of equilibrium.
11. The faster the swinging movements, the greater the reactive force at the joints.
12. The greater the body segment weight, the greater the muscular strength required to perform an activity.
13. The longer the body segment, the greater the muscular strength required to perform an activity.
14. The taller the person, the more time needed to perform the activity.
15. Safety can be increased or decreased by modifying the intensity of an exercise.

Answers for Mini-Lab Learning Experience:
Common Trauma Areas of the Body During Aerobic Exercise

Exercise	Body Sites
Jogging	feet, knees, back, shins, hips
Running	feet, knees, back, shins, hips
Rope Jumping	feet, knees, back, shins, hip, wrist, shoulders
Swimming	depending on the stroke, but usually the shoulders, back, and sometimes the knees
Bicycling	knees, buttocks, back, hips
Aerobic dance	feet, knees, back, shoulders, shins, hips

Rope Jumping

There are many styles and weights of jumping ropes. EMG has been used to rate the involvement of upper body muscles using these ropes (Chapter 8). Rope jumping can improve the strength of the upper body, as well as develop the cardiovascular system. The use of heavy ropes and heavy elastic ropes, however, could result in injury to the shoulders or wrists of low-strength individuals. Proper mechanics of turning and gradual increase in intensity of the rope jumping exercise will safeguard the individual from injury.

WEIGHT TRAINING

Weight training can be of two types: free weights and weight machines. The use of free weights is a more versatile way of strength development than weight machines. The body is less restrained, and a variety of types, sizes, and magnitudes of weights can be used. Muscles are required to stabilize proximal joints and to balance the body. The person must learn to adjust to asymmetrical strength variations. Thus, exercising with free weights is often advocated as the "natural exercise." Weight machines, however, have the advantage of reducing the risk of injury due to inability to balance or control weights. In addition, body parts can be supported and muscle groups isolated for strength development.

The general principles of exercising hold true with weight lifting. The position and amount of lordotic curvature must be evaluated. The use of a weight belt to fix the lumbar spine is a safety measure to provide reactive forces against a stable body segment. Increasing the abdominal pressure through respiration, exhaling on the forceful lift, has an estimated 10% benefit. Modeling of the body during lifting tasks in industry is pertinent to the analysis of weight lifting as an exercise or a sport. Refer to Chapter 12, Occupational Biomechanics.

ANATOMICAL CONSIDERATIONS

The selection of exercises should be based on scientific principles. As Flint has said, "Just because an exercise is commonly found in exercise programs does not assure its quality or qualify it for future use." There are kinetic hazards that may cause injury if they are not recognized. For example, when exercises are conducted in large groups on command or on count, taller persons tend to compensate. They do not execute the exercises completely and therefore receive little benefit, or these taller persons generate momentum during certain phases of the exercise that may cause injury. Figure 10-12 shows a typical dangerous position when squat thrusts are executed on a count of 4. The stress on the lumbar curve may be excessive and could cause serious damage. This is not to say that group and cadence exercises are never to be used, but the biomechanics of each exercise should be analyzed fully to guard against problems. Cadence can then be prescribed. Individualized exercises provide a means of regulating the duration, intensity, and frequency of the exercise program. These three components make the difference in whether or not the program maintains, improves, overloads, or has little beneficial effect. The force, time, work, and power can be calculated for each exercise, and progression can be determined on an individual basis. For example, two persons, one weighing 801 N (180 lb) and the other weighing 1080 N (240 lb), each of whom is more obese than muscular, would be doing different amounts of work when performing stair climbing, pushups, chin-ups, jumping jacks, and so on.

MINI-LAB LEARNING EXPERIENCES

1. Identify muscle groups which need strengthening in order to successfully perform in your favorite sport, in your work, or your daily life. Determine a strength progression series of exercises based upon biomechanics of work.
2. Select an activity in which balance is very important and determine an exercise progression to improve balance. Hint:

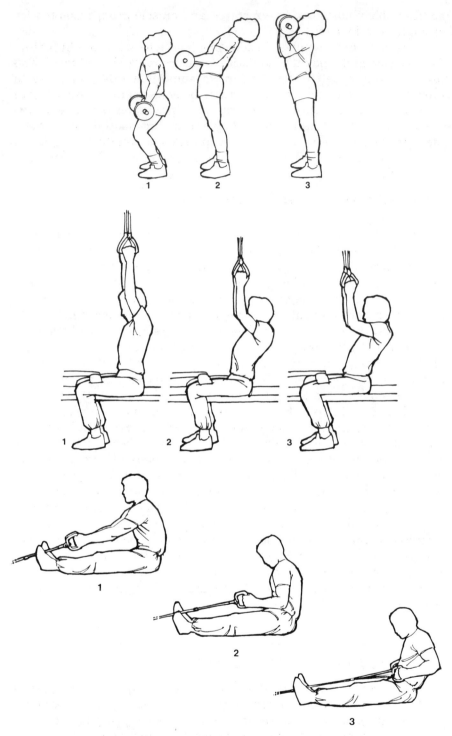

Fig. 10-7. *Postures used by the novice during exercising. Determine the postures in which the lordotic curvature is excessive and the body alignment is not vertical. These are unsafe postures.*

THE BIOMECHANICS OF HUMAN MOVEMENT

(a) Start from the largest foot base to the smallest foot base.
(b) Start from a static position to a dynamic position.
3. Is there any advantage in performing a sit-down compared to a sit-up? Hint: (a) Think about eccentric, concentric, isometric contractions. Construct moment arms.
4. Compare the requirements for anatomical alignment for the two types of pushups depicted in Fig. 10-13.
5. Develop a rationale for individualized exercise programs as opposed to programs in which all persons perform the same number of repetitions of the same exercise with the norm for each level of achievement based solely on age and sex.

EXERCISE EQUIPMENT EVALUATION

Each year, new products in the exercise area are developed and sold to the public, as well as to fitness centers, health spas, and other agencies. Biomechanical analysis of such products and performance techniques by persons using these products should be a prerequisite to the distribution of such products to the public. If this is not the case, the professional in charge of these products should evaluate them

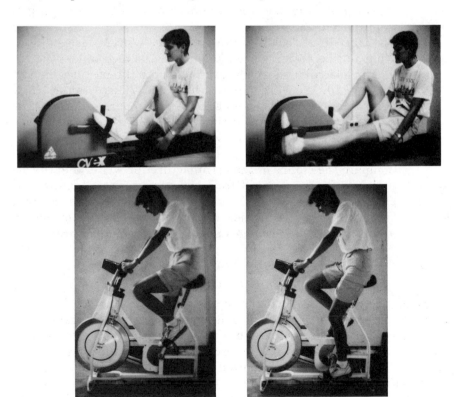

Fig. 10-8. *Exerciser on recumbent bicycle (A) and upright bicycle (B) ergometer.*

BIOMECHANICS OF EXERCISES 349

prior to purchasing or immediately after acquiring them. Although standards for testing fitness equipment are almost nonexistent, efforts are being made by the ASTM committees to develop standards. (Contact this national standards writing body at 1916 Race Street, Philadelphia, PA 19103.)

Practical guidelines for biomechanical evaluation of fitness equipment are listed, in question form, as follows:

1. Can persons of varying sizes use the equipment in a comparable manner? For example, if a bicycle ergometer is being evaluated, can a tall exerciser and a short exerciser adjust the bicycle to enable both persons to move their legs through comparable ranges of motion? See Chapter 12 for more information on this topic.
2. Can potential exercisers of varying fitness levels use the equipment? For example, if leg strength is low, is the initial resistance loading on the device too high? Conversely, is the highest resistance loading too low for a potential exerciser with strong legs?
3. Is the equipment stable, and otherwise safe to use? The equipment should resist pulling, pushing, and deliberate attempts to tip it. For example, will a recumbent bicycle tip if the exerciser grabs the machine to maintain equilibrium when getting up from the seat?
4. Do safety limits exist, or are guidelines written for safe use?
5. What unsafe postures are likely to be assumed unless the exerciser has guidelines? For example, note the postures in Fig. 10-7. Identify the position in which the spine and posterior trunk muscles are at risk. This can be done by comparing the amounts of lumbar curvature and estimating the line of gravity of the human body external load system.
6. What specific benefits can be derived from the equipment? Compare the claims of the manufacturer or writer and the actual benefits as deduced from the performance. Identify the planes of motion, axes of rotation, probable muscles involved (strength), range of motion (flexibility), sequences of motion (coordination), and changes in line of gravity (balance).

Biomechanical Evaluation of Bicycle Ergometers

The upright bicycle ergometer is similar to a regular bicycle except that resistances (effort) can be regulated. Ergometers, however, include different styles: upright and recumbent and arm cranking.

In Fig. 10-8A, a photograph of a person pedaling a recumbent bicycle, note the absence of the force of gravity to aid in extending the leg. The trunk is also supported and reactions can be used to aid in pushing. The ROM is similar to that of persons using an upright bicycle. Compare the leg alignment and ROM of persons pedaling in their 2 positions as shown in Fig. 10-8B.

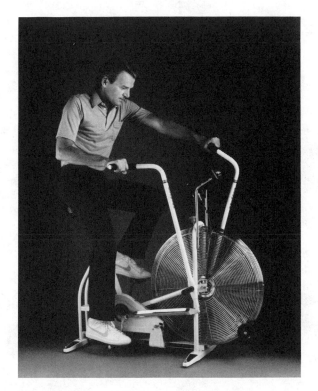

Fig. 10-9. *Schwinn aerodyne ergometer (courtesy of company.)*

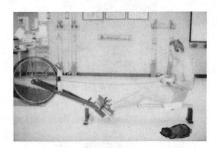

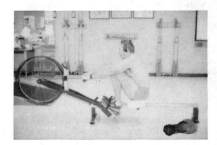
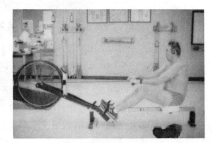

Fig. 10-10. *Exercising on a rowing machine.*

BIOMECHANICS OF EXERCISES 351

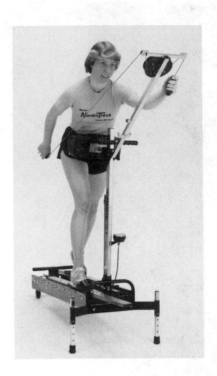
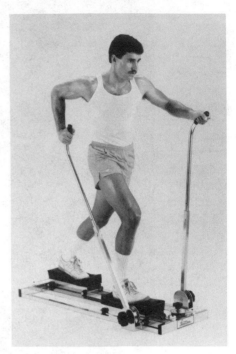
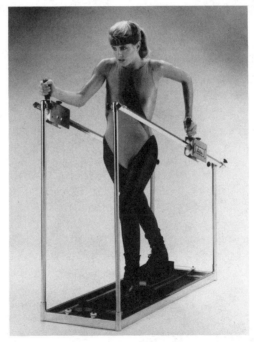

Fig. 10-11. *Exercising on cross-country ski ergometers. (Courtesy of Fitness Master Inc. and Nordik Track.)*

THE BIOMECHANICS OF HUMAN MOVEMENT

Another type of bicycle ergometer is depicted in Fig. 10-9. The arms flex and extend in a coordinated pattern with the alternating flexion and extension of the legs. Thus, cardiorespiratory fitness, leg and arm strength, and coordination are benefits from this machine.

MINI-LAB LEARNING EXPERIENCES

Biomechanical Assessment of Cycling

a. Quantitatively evaluate the probable ROM of the arms and legs using the ergometer in Fig. 10-9.
b. Compare these ROMs with those of Fig. 10-8.
c. Compare these ROMs with walking.

Biomechanical Assessment of a Rowing Machine

Analyze the sequence of rowing exercise photographs (Fig. 10-10). What is the ROM? What muscles appear to be active? How can you tell? Is there a potential risk of injury? What biomechanical principle could be followed to reduce this potential?

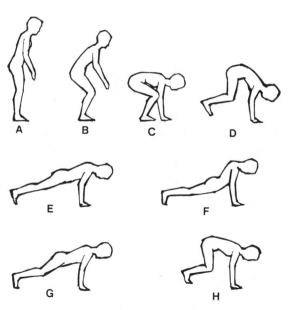

Fig. 10-12. *Note position of trunk when squat thrusts are done as fast as possible. The development of momentum creates a force that is greater than the muscular force to stabilize the pelvis and spinal column. Watch someone perform squat thrusts at three different cadences and note what happens.*

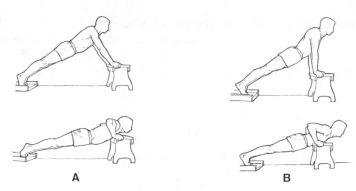

Fig. 10-13. *The initial up position and the down position of a male performing pushups on a bench with the arms perpendicular to the surface of the bench (A) and with the arms perpendicular to the line of the body (B). Note the inability to stabilize the pelvis and lumbar spine in one condition. Note the different ranges of motion required at the shoulder, elbow, and wrist in the two conditions.*

Biomechanical Assessment of a Cross-Country Skiing Exerciser

Evaluate the cross-country trainer depicted in Fig. 10-11. Compare the kinematics of the cross-country trainer with the arm-leg bicycle ergometer. What is the advantage of the standing posture?

SUMMARY

Exercise often is task and goal specific. If the goal is general fitness, guidelines exist and programs are fairly easy to construct. If, however, the goal is specific to a sport, a position in a sport, a particular occupation, a particular disability, or a specific movement, the construction of exercise programs is not easy. Too often the biomechanical assessments have not been conducted on the optimizing of the exercise. The skill, tasks, or movement to be improved is unknown. Therefore, foundation data are missing. If the actual movement kinematics of the time and space and the actual kinetics of muscle force are not known, a valid and optimum exercise program cannot be constructed. The greatest barrier to scientific exercise programs is the lack of such knowledge. Physical educators, with their background in biomechanics, can research the movements and help to develop scientific sports exercise programs. Likewise, all human movement specialists, be they physical educators, kinesiologists, biomechanists, coaches, physical therapists, or industrial engineers, can collect and share the required information for movement analysis. Only then can we construct safe, effective, and efficient exercise programs.

REFERENCES

Ariel, G. R. (1978): Computerized Dynamic Resistive Exercise. In Landry, F. and Orban, W. A. R. (Eds.). *Biomechanics of Sports and Kinanthropometry*, Miami: Miami Symposia Specialists.

Basmajian, J. V. (1979): *Muscles Alive: Their Functions Revealed by Electromyography* (4th ed.), Baltimore: The Williams and Wilkins Co.

Flint, M. M. (1965): Selecting Exercises, *JOHPER* 35:19.

Garhammer, J. (in press): Biomechanics of Weight Lifting and Training. In *Biomechanics of Sports*, C. L. Vaugham (Ed.), Boca Raton, FL: C.R.C. Press, Inc.

Kilani, H. (1988): Stretch-shortening Cycle in Human Muscle Contraction: The Role of the Stretch Reflex in Force Production in Various Vertical Jumps. Unpublished doctoral dissertation, University of Illinois at Urbana-Champaign.

Lowman, C. L. (1958): Faculty Posture in Relation to Performance, *JOHPER* 29:14.

Mastropaolo, J. A. (1979): Personal communication.

Wells, K. F. and Luttgens, K. (1976): *Kinesiology* (6th Ed.). Philadelphia: W. B. Saunders Co.

Woods, M. (1980): Tension Control, Unpublished report, Seattle, Tension Control Clinic.

Terauds, J. (Ed.) (1979): *Science in Weightlifting,* Del Mar, California: Academic Publishers.

11
Rehabilitative Biomechanics

What is rehabilitative biomechanics? Rehabilitative biomechanics is that part of biomechanics applied to the study of movement patterns of injured and disabled persons. Why is it important? How does it integrate with the occupational therapists, corrective therapists, physical therapists, and other health services and medical personnel? These persons identify dysfunctions among the population and design and structure programs to alleviate or compensate for these dysfunctions. The rehabilitative biomechanist can aid the therapist in analyzing movement patterns, predicting forces acting upon the joints, designing assistive devices, optimizing performance, and reassessing performance—after rehabilitative training. A team approach is required, although some biomechanists may also have therapeutic training, and can work more independently than those without training in both therapy and biomechanics. Some therapists have a basic background in biomechanics, but this background consists primarily of anatomical biomechanics.

The goals of rehabilitative biomechanics are as follows:

1. Define the biomechanical characteristics of the patient. Normal anatomy cannot be assumed. The anomalies must be identified. Muscle weakness must be assessed.
2. Evaluate movement patterns and postures of the patient and compare these to normal patterns.
3. Determine whether or not normalcy of function is a realistic goal. If not, determine the compensatory pattern to be used.
4. Evaluate the training program developed by the therapist.
5. Evaluate the use of assistive devices.
6. Assist with the design of assistive devices.
7. Evaluate the workspace environment.

The information in the first chapters of this book is the basis for fulfillment of these seven goals. Specific applications of this knowledge base, however, are described in this chapter. Common concerns with respect to training programs (exercises) will be discussed first, since exercise is the foundation for rehabilitation.

PURPOSES OF THERAPEUTIC EXERCISES

Although there have been many goals for therapeutic exercises, eight relate to biomechanics. These have been paraphrased as follows:

1. To reduce, prevent, or eliminate contractures due to muscle imbalances.
2. To increase strength in order to power devices and perform work.
3. To improve ROM.
4. To improve coordination.
5. To develop awareness of normal movement patterns.
6. To improve voluntary, automatic movement responses.
7. To optimally develop strength and endurance requirements so that deformities do not occur.
8. To improve power of muscles.

Specific biomechanical guidelines have been developed in order to attain these goals without risk to the patient.

Guidelines for Rehabilitative Exercises

1. Move the body part slowly in order to reduce acceleration to a negligible value.
2. Allow the muscles to contract throughout the range of motion. This is achieved by maintaining low velocities and therefore, controlling momentum.
3. Maintain alignment of body parts, since any change in alignment will change angles of pull and lengths of muscles, tendons, and ligaments.
4. Maintain balance of antagonist muscle groups. For example, if the exercise is to strengthen the biceps brachii, exercises should also be conducted to strengthen the triceps brachii.
5. Utilize one or more sets of exercises to improve and maintain the integrity of all structures and tissues related to the area of injury. This often includes the joints proximal and distal to the injury site.
6. Develop alternative exercises to reduce boredom and provide versatility for home and travel environments.
7. Maintain or develop aerobic capacity.

An example of an exercise protocol based upon the previously mentioned principles is described in the next section.

Rehabilitative Exercises for the Medial Collateral Ligament of the Knee

It is important that the muscles that flex and extend the shank at the knee be strengthened. Concomittantly, the ligaments must be protected. This is usually achieved by dorsiflexing the foot and locking the knee during certain aspects of the performance of the exercises. Why?

MINI-LAB LEARNING EXPERIENCES

Draw a simplified free-body-diagram of the knee in a position of near extension. Include the force vectors for the triceps surae muscle group and the medial collateral ligament.

Next, diagram the knee with the triceps surae muscles contracting to dorsiflex the ankle. What happens to the vector of the medial collateral ligament?

This also can be visually depicted by using two pieces of wood connected by two rubber bands representing the medial collateral ligament and the gastrocnemius muscle. The rubber bands should be attached in a relatively taut state of tension. The gastrocnemius band will then be stretched (greater tautness) to represent the contraction producing dorsiflexion of the foot.

Since the leg swings from the hip, the muscles crossing the hip joint should be strengthened, as well as the muscles and ligaments crossing the knee joint, when planning an exercise program to rehabilitate the knee. A series of exercises are analyzed in the following section to aid you in biomechanical analysis of the anatomy involved.

The first set is a series in which the load (resistance) is only the person's body part. The number of repetitions will be selected based upon the severity of the injury and the physical attributes of the injured person. For example, a long-legged individual, an obese-legged individual and a severely injured individual might perform three repetitions, whereas five would be the usual starting number for average persons.

Sit and Extend. Action: sitting on a table or chair with the knee at a right angle, the lower leg is slowly extended to the horizontal. The foot is in dorsiflexion throughout, and, at the end of the extension, the knee locks.

Analysis. All the quadriceps contract, and the strong rectus femoris initiates the action.

Long Sit Leg Extension. Action: The person sits on a table or

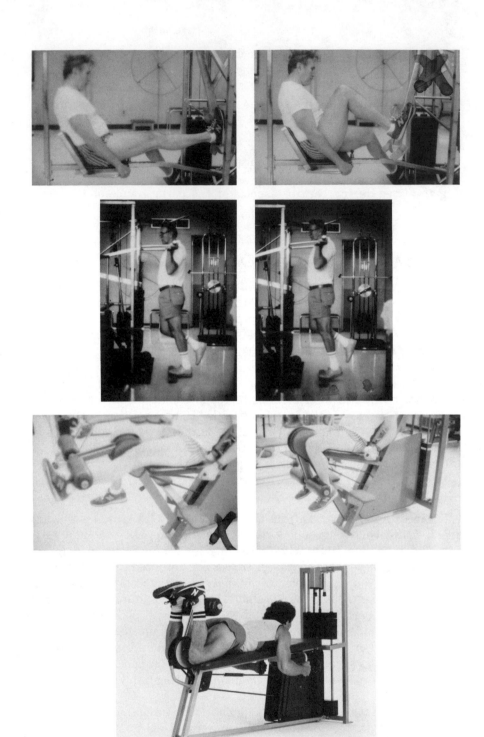

Fig. 11-1. *Different exercises and exercise devices to strengthen the knee and stabilize it. A, Single-leg presses on a weight machine. B, Toe raises on a single leg. C, Nautilus leg extensions. D, Hamstring exercise on universal gym bench. E, Orthotron. F, Fitron bicycle*

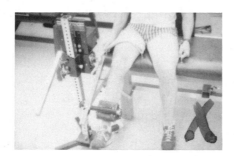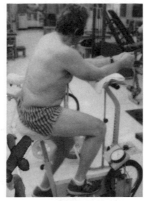

Fig. 11-1. *Continued*

floor with leg to be exercised extended and resting on surface. The knee is locked and the foot dorsiflexed as the leg is lifted (flexion at the hip) from the table. The other leg is flexed and the foot placed on the table near the knee of the extended leg.

Analysis. The rectus femorus muscles is virtually eliminated from functioning. The medial collateral ligament is protected as the vasti muscle groups are strengthened.

Prone Lying. Action: In the prone-lying position with the foot dorsiflexed, the leg is raised (extension at hip).

Analysis. To maintain muscle balance, the hamstrings and gluteus maximus muscles are being strengthened.

Prone Lying with Flexed Leg. Action: The leg is flexed 90 degrees, and the foot is dorsiflexed. Extension at the hip (lifting thigh from table) is executed.

Analysis. The hamstrings are virtually ineffective and the muscles crossing the hip are strengthened.

Side Lying Leg Lift. Action: Person lies on one side, flexes the lower leg, and lifts the injured leg in an abduction movement. The foot is dorsiflexed.

Analysis. Abductor muscles crossing the hip are being strengthened.

Side Lying, Upper Leg Flexed. Action: Person lies on one side, flexes the upper leg and lifts the injured leg in an adduction movement. The foot is dorsiflexed.

Analysis. The adductor magnus, brevis, and longus muscles crossing the hip are being strengthened.

Stand and Lift. Action: In a standing position, the person flexes the lower leg to the horizontal, maintaining a vertical position of the thigh. The foot is dorsiflexed.

Analysis. The hamstring muscles are isolated as the prime movers. This set of seven exercises are repeated with a two-pound weight at the ankle. This weight creates a second level of intensity, without overstressing the knee.

The next set of exercises incorporate strength machines or body weight in order to increase the load intensity (Fig. 11-1).

1. Single-Leg Presses on a Weight Machine. Extend and flex slowly.
2. Toe Raises on a Single Leg.
3. Nautilus Leg Extensions. Isokinetic concept—loads the muscles consistently throughout the range of motion and isolates the thigh muscles.
4. Hamstring Exercise on Universal Gym Bench. Maintain balance between muscle groups.
5. Orthotron.
6. Fitron Bicycle.
7. Other machines.

Analyze these devices and exercises with respect to specific value of each.

COMPENSATORY GAITS

Gait and Muscle Weakness

Variations from normal walking patterns are responses to pain, muscle weakness or paralysis, spasticity or contractures of muscles, sensory disturbances, and disease. In addition, habitual and peculiar walking patterns may result in structural changes in the anatomy. Thus, permanent walking abnormalities can result. All variations in walking may be classified as changes in timing, misalignment of body parts, and difficulty in executing the movement (slowed motion or co-ordination problems).

Research in rehabilitation of gait, mostly walking for the average population and running for the sports population, is one of the most widely conducted areas of investigation in the field of biomechanics. Gait laboratories consist of the most highly technological instrumentation that exists. Clinical analysis, however, remains a common fundamental approach to identification of gait problems and effects of rehabilitation upon gait.

Table 11-1. *Effect of Muscle Weakness and Contracture Upon Gait*

Muscle Weakness	Gait Change
Hamstrings	Hyperextension of leg occurs
Internal rotators	Leg externally rotated outward
Anterior tibialis	Drop foot (foot in calcaneovarus position and toes drag); may walk on toes to compensate

Muscle Contracture	Gait Change
Gastrocnemius	Equinus foot
Adductors	Scissoring of legs; feet will cross
Iliopsoas	Lordosis and trunk lean

A listing of weaknesses in selected muscles and resulting gait changes and limitations of motion is included in Table 11-1.

Validity of prediction of gait anomalies, as well as prediction of muscular weakness or contracture, is being investigated by means of biomechanical modeling of the anatomy and planes and axes of movement. A simplified example of modeling is described as follows:

The angle of pull of a muscle is always a vector in the plane of the muscle. Muscles lying in the same plane but on the opposite surface of bones will become slack as the contracting muscle shortens. Thus, if the posterior tibialis muscle is in constant contracture it will pronate the foot, collapse the longitudinal arch, and produce forefoot varus. The anterior tibialis becomes slack.

Refer to the Appendix of anatomical charts and set up other muscle weaknesses and contractures. Predict gait anomalies. Refer also to Steindler's book, listed at the end of this chapter.

Physical dysfunction may be such that a normal walking pattern is not efficient or safe. In such conditions, a variation may be taught, or self-discovered. Such a gait has been referred to as the "intermittent double-step gait"; it is used extensively as a temporary gait pattern, as well as a permanent pattern among the elderly, those with ununited fractures of the hip, hemiplegics, those afflicted with Parkinson's disease, those with knee disorders, and spasticity patients. The underlying problem is one of instability caused by loss of balance during the swing-through and/or support phase of the involved leg.

Thus, the person utilizing the intermittent double-step gait will pause after two steps have been taken. Since momentum must be controlled, shorter steps than normal are taken and the trunk is kept erect. Long distances will usually require a cane. Pretend that you have one painful knee and describe how you might use the intermittent double step gait with a cane. Next, compare the following description with your description.

Stage 1: The cane is used for supporting the body prior to taking the first step. The involved leg is behind the other leg, and the cane is at an angle of 45 degrees from the sagittal and coronal planes of the body. The involved leg is predominantly passive and takes a short step, bearing a minimum of body weight. The body continues to lean on the cane as the sound leg quickly takes a step. The cane then is moved forward as the person stands momentarily.

Stage 2: The person takes a cane movement directly forward rather than somewhat laterally. The two quick steps are taken without as much lateral trunk lean.

Stage 3: The person moves the cane and involved leg simultaneously. The double step is taken and the pauses are shortened.

Thus, many changes in gait can result from one part of the body failing to function effectively. Researchers have investigated the nature of compensation and its effects upon gait. One such investigation by one of the authors consisted of artificially inducing dysfunction (Tayler et al., 1967). A long leg brace was placed on the leg of a normal, able-bodied male. This brace could be adjusted to produce four constraints at two joints: (1) a rigid ankle, (2) a rigid knee, (3) a rigid ankle and rigid knee, and (4) a reduced range of motion at the knee. Electrogoniometers were placed at the knee and at the ankle of the unbraced leg to record the angular kinematics at these joints as the man walked with the previously stated constraints. Changes in the kinematics of the nonbraced leg occurred to compensate for dysfunction in other leg and are depicted in Fig. 11-2.

Ambulation Aids and Ground Reaction Forces

The type of ambulation aid to select for use is determined primarily by the amount of weight to be borne by the aid. Common ambulation aids listed in a heirarchy of weight-bearing potential, are the single cane, aluminum forearm crutch, two forearm crutches, two axillary crutches, and the walker. Canes are mainly used by those who require aid in balance since no more than 20–25% of body weight should be borne by the cane. Forearm crutches can support 40–50% of body weight. The axillary crutches and walker are used in early rehabilitation and in permanent disabilities in which 80% or more support of body weight is required. Crutches are useful, however, only if the arms can hold the crutches and keep pressure from the radial nerve, preventing crutch paralysis. Walkers are important if balance is also a problem.

How is the effective and safe weight-bearing pattern executed? How can the pattern be measured? Discuss these questions, and then refer to the hints in the minilab experiment after the following section.

Walking Pattern Using Assistive Aids

Cane. Step with involved leg only when cane and sound foot are on the ground. Use cane on contralateral side of body with respect to

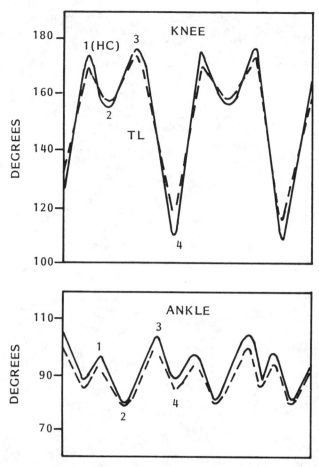

Fig. 11-2. *Compensations made by the non-braced leg to restrictions due to bracing. (From Taylor, et al., Effect of Restriction of Joint Movements in One Leg Upon the Action of Similar Joints of the Other Leg, J.A.P.M.R, Jan–Feb, 1967.)*

involved leg, in order to relieve compressive forces on hip of involved leg. (See Fig. 11-3.)

Four-Legged Cane. This has the same use as the single cane, but is used when greater stability is required, and the person walks slowly. Fast walking will cause persons to execute a rear-front two-point contact pattern with cane, thus nullifying the stability potential.

Forearm Crutch. This has the same use as the cane, except used when hand cannot grasp, and wrist is weak.

Two Crutches. This is a three-point gait with the involved leg and both crutches moving as one unit and the sound leg moving independently. (See Fig. 11-4.)

REHABILITATIVE BIOMECHANICS

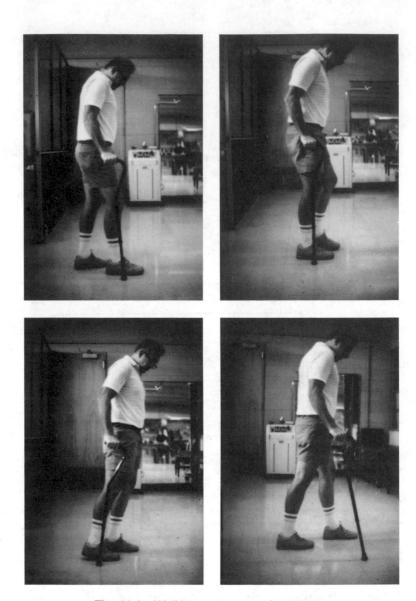

Fig. 11-3. *Walking sequence using a cane.*

MINI-LAB LEARNING EXPERIENCES

Use a force platform or a standard body-weight scale to record vertical ground reaction forces during walking with and without ambulation aids. Compare the following conditions:

1. Normal walking.
2. Contact the scale or platform with the cane during walking. Place hypothetical disabled foot on scale. Place sound foot on scale.

THE BIOMECHANICS OF HUMAN MOVEMENT

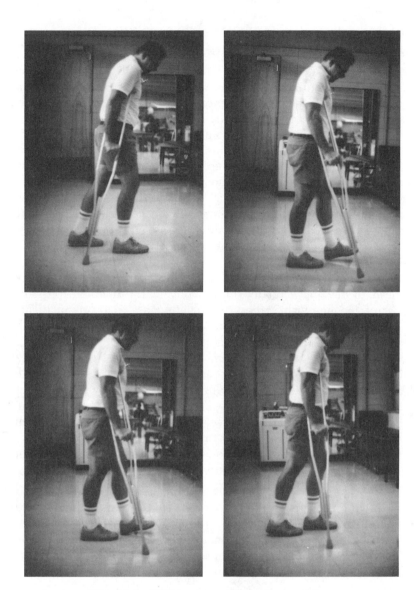

Fig. 11-4. *Walking sequence using crutches.*

3. Use a swing-through gait with two crutches, and contact the scale with the sound foot and then with one crutch.

Record the weight of the person, and check whether or not the reactive force on the cane was acceptable. Do the same for the crutches.

If a person had very little stability and great weakness in the legs, what gait pattern would be substituted for the three point gait? Explain the sequence of supports and what forces would occur.

TASK ANALYSIS OF THE PHYSICALLY DISABLED

The tasks to be analyzed are classified as activities of daily living (ADL), work activities, and leisure activities. ADL consists of loco-motor, self-care, management of devices, communication, and home-management activities. The self-care activities include such tasks as dressing, toiletry, and combing hair. Leisure activities comprise a vast continuum of activities ranging from sedentary activities to organized athletics. In the past, and predominantly today, performances of all these tasks by the physically disabled have only been qualitatively assessed. The most common method is a five-level ranking: (1) able to perform, (2) able to perform in certain situations (such as afternoon or under optimum friction conditions), (3) can perform with difficulty, (4) can perform with an assistive device, and (5) cannot perform. Unfortunately, limited analysis of the movement patterns has been conducted. Little information exists concerning the ranges of motion, strength, and technique requirements for successful performance. There is a need to develop a model for the physically disabled, possibly a number of models with respect to various classifications of disabilities. Only then will the disabled have an equal chance with the able-bodied to optimize their performance.

A number of principles are of value in the process of task analysis of disabled populations. One of the most important is that the disabled will compensate for loss of function in one body part. This imposes difficulty in recognizing the underlying problem. For example, the lack of strong quadriceps muscles when rising from a chair may not be recognized because of the "transfer of momentum" technique utilized to rise from the chair. The principles of transfer of momentum may be utilized in the following manner:

> The person rocks forward and backward, moving the trunk in the anteroposterior plane. Acceleration is developed, and at the appropriate time, the line of gravity is shifted forward and upward over the feet, and extension of the legs becomes possible. The technique employed by most able-bodied persons is not possible by many disabled persons.

A second, equally important, principle is that one anomaly creates a second anomaly. For example, unequal leg lengths may produce scoliosis.

Therefore, the goal is to reduce energy expenditure and to execute a safe movement. It is more important for the disabled to utilize leverage optimally, to apply the force effectively, and to use the large muscles to produce force in the desired direction and magnitude than it is for the able-bodied person.

Sample Analysis of an Activity: Pinch Process in Molding Clay for Pottery

The analysis has been subdivided into three sections: movement, muscles, and forces. (See Fig. 11-5.)

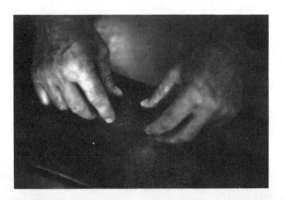

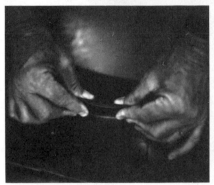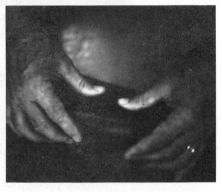

Fig. 11-5. *Pinch process in molding clay for pottery. The movements, muscles involved and forces acting during the molding of clay determine the rehabilitative benefits.*

1. The movement is localized to flexion and extension of the MP and IP joints of digits one and two, opposition and abduction of the CMC joint of the thumb, and flexion and extension of the MP and IT joints of the thumb. Movements at the wrist are mainly static or holding positions for the clay. Minor adjustments in radial and ulnar deviation, flexion, and extension occur as the hand moves around the pot. The back and neck are stable, as are the trunk and legs. Only slight movement occurs at the shoulder and elbow.

The ROM is minimal-to-moderate with respect to potential range. MP joints are in 60–90 degrees of flexion, and IP joints are in nearly full extension with minimal changes. The wrist angles change from neutral to as much as 90 degrees of ulnar deviation.

2. The major muscles contracting concentrically are the opponens pollicis, flexors pollicis longus and brevis, lumbricales, and flexors digitorum profundis and superficialis. Palmar interossei are in isometric contraction. The extensor digitorum communis, extensor indicis proprius, extensors pollicis longus and brevis, and abductor pollicis are primarily acting eccen-

trically during the pinch and concentrically during the release.

3. Muscle strength requirements are low to fair plus, this latter value occurring in the opponens pollicis. Since the number of repetitions and the cadence can be adjusted, the endurance requirements also are low. Gradation in strength to perform the task is not too practical. Stiffer clay can be used.

Wheelchair Propulsion and Hand Patterns

The mobility of a wheelchair user is directly related to the physical characteristics of the person, the characteristics of the wheelchair, the interaction between these two, and the interaction of person, wheelchair, and environment or use. In Fig. 11-6, these aspects are depicted, and the various factors that should be investigated and quantified are outlined.

This model is a valuable tool used by the biomechanist to determine whether or not the wheelchair fits the user, whether or not a person can perform better in one wheelchair than another, and to identify precisely the temporal, spatial, and force parameters of the movements of propulsion.

MINI-LAB LEARNING EXPERIENCES

Compare the speeds, movement patterns, and rolling friction of wheelchair propulsion of two different types of wheelchairs and two different-sized individuals. Use the ideas from Chapters 5 and 8.

Wheelchair athletes use racing wheelchairs, designed with low seats and more forward wheels than ordinary wheelchairs. The ordinary wheelchair is heavy and has been designed for stability. The arm action including the arc of propulsion of a person using a racing wheelchair is depicted in Fig. 11-7. Note the extreme shoulder angle at the instant of initiation of pushing action.

Head, shoulder, elbow, and hand patterns during a 30-second anerobic wheelchair ergometer test of a skilled, but non-elite racer are depicted in Fig. 11-8.

Can you identify which is which—10 sec., 20 sec., and 30 sec. points?

What are the distinguishing features of each?

Prosthetics and Gait of Amputees

Have you seen persons with artificial legs run, ski, play volleyball, and bowl? More and more researchers in rehabilitative engineering have begun to develop prostheses that can function with flu-

WHEELCHAIR EVALUATION

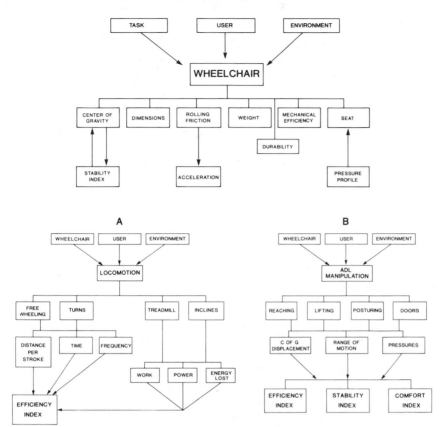

TASK EVALUATION
A. LOCOMOTION   B. MANIPULATION

USER EVALUATION

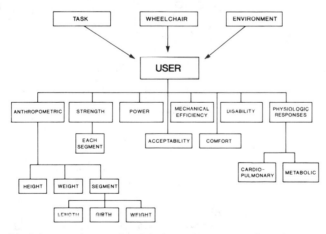

Fig. 11-6. *Model to evaluate wheelchair, task, user, and environment interrelationships to optimize mobility of wheelchair user.*

371

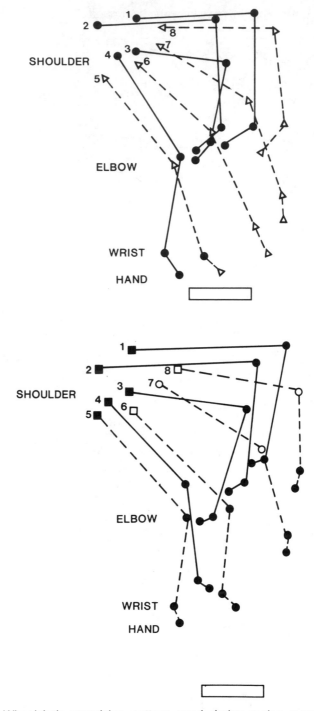

Fig. 11-7. *Wheelchair propulsion pattern used during racing events in track competition. Extreme ranges of motion at the shoulder during initial push against the handrim is cause for concern. Analysis of the angles is valuable to construct training programs to prevent injury. One these performances is skilled, the other is not. Can you determine which is which?*

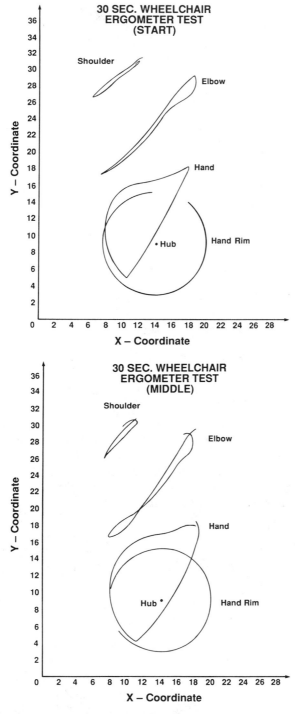

Fig. 11-8. *Changes in the kinematics of wheelchair propulsion during a 30 sec anaerobic test to exhaustion. S, shoulder; E, elbow; H, hand; N, neck. Sequence is as follows: 10 second point, 20 second point, and 30 second point. Were you able to guess?*

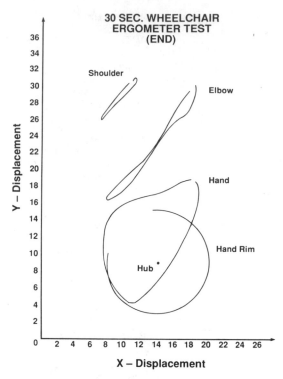

30 SEC. WHEELCHAIR ERGOMETER TEST (END)

Shoulder

Elbow

Hand

Hand Rim

Hub

Y – Displacement

X – Displacement

Fig. 11-8. *Continued*

idity and resiliency and through extreme ranges of motion and orientations. The Flex-Foot is an example of a below-knee prosthesis that stores and releases energy in a manner similar to a coil or spring. The heel-toe action of the natural footstep can be duplicated, and the flex of the material cushions the impact, stores the energy (through this deformation in flexion), and then springs back (releasing energy and acting as a propulsive force into the next step). The design is a simple one.

Based upon the listed mechanical properties, what value would this prosthesis have for walking, swimming, or jumping? What limitations do you forsee?

Design of Prostheses

There are two basic categories of lower limb prostheses: below the knee (BK) and above the knee (AK). Upper limb prostheses would be classified as below-elbow and above-elbow prostheses. Based upon the biomechanics of motion, the loss of function due to active links in the kinematic chain of motion is directly proportional to the number of links lost. Thus AK amputees have lost two links (foot and shank) in their kinematic chain, and BK amputees have lost only one link. A prosthesis is designed to duplicate normal functioning. This goal,

THE BIOMECHANICS OF HUMAN MOVEMENT

however, is dependent upon the patient's level of general functioning ability, the level of amputation, and practicality. Thus, the BK may be a single-axis foot attached by single plane hinges to the thigh, or the BK could be designed to allow inversion, eversion, and torque absorption. It is obvious that this latter design would not be appropriate for persons with amputations at near-patella level and with weak musculature at the knee level.

The more elaborate and more functional (simulating the functions of the living leg) the prosthesis, the greater will be the likelihood of maintenance problems and increased weight of the prosthesis. If the weight of the prosthesis is not identical to the living leg, imbalance will result. If the weight does not match the musculature to move the prosthesis, compensatory actions result. Because of the mismatches, many amputees walk with a lateral trunk lean. Some individuals over 60 years of age have required as long as two years to physically and mentally function effectively with an above knee prosthesis.

In order to walk with low-energy expenditure and with a flowing, non-interrupted cyclic pattern, the following artificial knee units have been designed:

1. Variable friction—Resistance is greater at the beginning and end of the swing phase and reduced during the mid-swing phase.
2. Hydraulic—This is adjustable to different speeds and swing and stance requirements and can function during bicycle riding.
3. Hydracadence—This is a special type of hydraulic unit with programmed swing phase, adjustable cadence control, and automatic dorsiflexion of foot at flexion of 20 degrees at the knee.
4. Computerized—prototype stage development.
   a. Dayton, Ohio—Muscular contraction of the sound limb is used to innervate the sequencing of musculature in the sound leg.
   b. Massachusetts Institute of Technology—Motion, resistance, and velocity data of one step of the sound leg are fed into the computer and stored. At the appropriate time, these identical motions are activated in the prosthesis (echo system).

Evaluation of Prostheses

The following seven criteria can be used in the evaluation of the prostheses:

1. Fit: Stump fit and proper sizing are essential to comfort and function.
2. Alignment: The prosthesis should be an extension of the upper leg.
3. Length: The length must agree with the contralateral limb.

4. Weight: Optimum weight for amputee to handle depends upon musculature.
5. Stability: The prosthesis position must be constant and dependable.
6. Tolerable Pressure: Too much pressure will cause sores, trauma, and complications.
7. Durability: Breakage during use should not occur.

The process of fitting of any prosthesis continues to be a problem and a serious one, for amputees. In many cases, if the prosthesis is fitted to the exact length of the other leg, it may be functionally too long or too short for the person utilizing an abnormal gait pattern. For example, if there is instability in the stepping pattern and the trunk compensates for this problem, the sound hip may be carried lower than the other hip during the support phase of walking. The prosthesis, then, is functionally too short. Lengthening the prosthesis may solve the problem for a short time, but as the person becomes stronger and the gait pattern improves, the prothesis then is too long. Thus, there is the necessity for assessment of the gait pattern on a frequent basis. Biomechanics analysis and documentation of the gait pattern becomes valuable to the rehabilitation staff.

ORTHOTICS

Prescription of orthotic devices to be worn in shoes has become a common practice ever since the running boom occurred in the 1970s. Injuries were estimated to be related to poorly designed shoes, weak musculature controlling the feet, and bony malalignments. Thus podiatrists, sports medicine personnel, and advertisers advocated orthotics of all types. Researchers have shown that orthotics can change the orientation of the foot and, therefore, the kinematics of the foot and leg during running. The primary use of orthotics is to prevent over-pronation of the foot, which creates stress at the medial ankle joint and to the medial collateral ligaments at the knee.

Not all people need orthotics, and not all orthotics are beneficial. McPoil showed that, during walking, an orthotic to correct forefoot valgus may have no greater value than a well-designed, well-fitted shoe. See Fig. 11-9 for force platform recordings.

MINI-LAB LEARNING EXPERIENCES

1. Walk and concentrate on the pressures experienced on the feet. Do you strike on the heel hard or soft? Do you feel more pressure on the second metatarsal or the first metatarsal? Record your perceptions.
2. Videotape your feet during walking. Analyze the movement patterns and estimate the muscles acting to cause the movements.

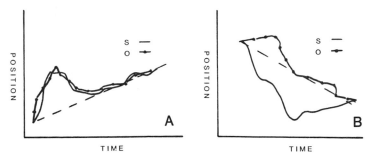

Fig. 11-9. *Force-time pattern during support phase of walking barefoot, with shoes and with orthotics inside the shoes. Orthotics have little value for this person with forefoot varus problem. (From T. McPoil dissertation, Univ. Il. at Urbana-Champaign, 1987)*

---

3. Repeat the preceding process with the following conditions. Place wedges of foam or plastic at the following sites of a shoe (either inside or taped to the sole):
   a. Under the big toe
   b. Along the lateral border of foot
   c. Under the medial heel.

Evaluate the results.

SURGERY

Removal of living tissue may alter the functioning of the human body. This is most noticeable with respect to knee surgery. Removal of half a meniscus at the knee joint ultimately results in degeneration of that joint. An unequal loading occurs since partial removal results in unequal levels within the ring of the meniscii. This is similar to the experience you had with the orthotics learning experience. Misalignment of the tibia with the femur will be directly related to the site and amount of meniscii removed. In addition, based upon animal research, degeneration (osteoarthritis) also is directly proportional to amount of meniscii removed. The use of artificial substances to replace the meniscii should reduce risk of osteoarthritis.

MINI-LAB LEARNING EXPERIENCES

Qualitatively analyze the three methods of transferring depicted in Fig. 11-10, A, B, C.

Describe the planes of motion, the axis of rotation, and the major muscles required in the transfer.

Draw force vectors and free-body diagrams for the propulsive phase in each.

REHABILITATIVE BIOMECHANICS 377

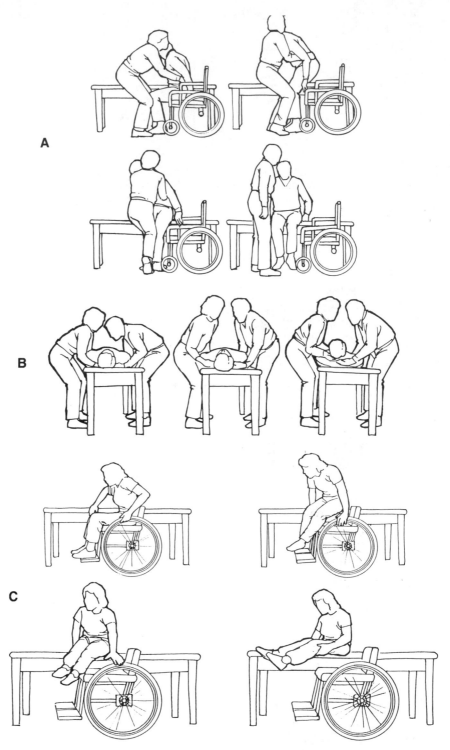

Fig. 11-10. *Three methods of transfers. Note the muscles and angle of push required for each of the types of transfers.*

378

Rank the amount of force required by the patient in each figure.

Identify high stress areas to the joints.

Indicate how you might quantitatively measure the forces at the propulsive phase.

EFFECT OF UNEQUAL LEG LENGTHS

Schuit investigated the effect of leg length discrepancies on ground reaction forces and lower-extremity joint angles during the stance phase of walking. Ground reaction force vectors and kinematic data were collected for 18 subjects wearing recreational footwear. Subsequently, appropriately-sized heel lifts were fitted into the shoes of the short leg for each subject and were worn for three weeks. After the test period, kinetic and kinematic data were again recorded. A significant increase was found for maximum vertical force for both legs after the lift was added. A significant increase in maximum medial force was found for the short leg, in both no-lift and lift conditions. Such medial

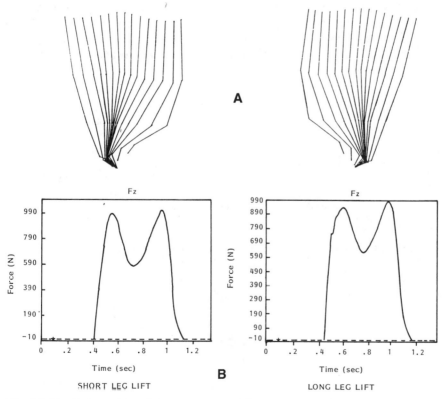

Fig. 11-11. *Data collected from persons with unequal leg lengths. A, angle of leg at heel strike; B, force-time curve. (Courtesy of Dale Schuit, dissertation, University of Il, at Urbana-Champaign, 1987)*

REHABILITATIVE BIOMECHANICS   **379**

and lateral differences are an indication of compensatory mechanisms acting to stabilize the body during ambulation. The increase in vertical force was no more than 10% and would also be reflective of the unequal leg-length adjustments.

MINI-LAB LEARNING EXPERIENCES

Measure the angles at the leg joints during the gait of persons with leg length discrepancies. (See Fig. 11-11.) Measure the maximum forces and compare the force curves.

MEDICAL HIGH TECHNOLOGY

Arthroscopy has been a major technique for preventing excess trauma to the joint during surgery. Use of this technique also is the primary cause of early mobility after surgery.

Other scientific discoveries have been instrumental in aiding the arthritic patient to regain mobility in the joints. Joint-replacement surgery is being conducted for the elbow, knee, hip, and interphalangeal joints. In previous decades, ankyloses were performed, that is, the joint was fused. Joint replacements (prostheses) have alleviated the ankyloses procedures. Rehabilitative biomechanics has become a high technology science.

REFERENCES

Jebsen, R. H. (1967). Use and Abuse of Ambulation Aids. *JAMA*, 199:1, pp. 63–68.
McKenzie, D., Clement, D., Taunton, J. (1985). Running Shoes, Orthotics, and Injuries, *Sports Medicine* 2:334–347.
McPoil, T. G. (1987). The effect of foot supports on ground reaction force patterns, unpublished dissertation, University of Illinois at Urbana-Champaign.
Palmer, M. L. and Toms, J. E. (1986). *Manual for Functional Training*. Philadelphia, PA: F. A. Davis Company.
Pedretti, L. W. (1981). *Occupational Therapy*. St. Louis, MO: C. V. Mosby Company.
Perry, J. (1967). The Mechanics of Walking, Part of the Proceedings of an Instructional Course—Principles of Lower-Extremity Bracing. *JAPT* Vol. 47:778–815. (also entire issue).
Peszcznski, M. (1958). The Intermittent Double Step Gait, *Archives of Physical Medicine and Rehabilitation*, 39.
Schuit, D. (1988). The effect of heel lifts on ground reaction force patterns and lower extremity joint angles in subjects with structural leg length discrepancies, unpublished dissertation, University of Illinois at Urbana-Champaign.
Steindler, W. (1957). *Normal and Pathological Gait*. Springfield: Charles C. Thomas.
Taylor, B., Adrian, M., and Karpovich, P. (1967). Effect of Restriction of Joint Movements in One Leg upon the Action of Similar Joints of the Other Leg, *J.A.P.M.R.* Jan.–Feb.

12

Occupational Biomechanics

Occupational biomechanics is not only a subdivision of biomechanics, but also one component of the broad area of human ergonomics: the study of the interaction of the worker and the industrial environment. Whereas human ergonomics encompasses the physiological, biomechanical, psychological, and environmental aspects of work, occupational biomechanics is limited to the anatomical (including anthropometrical), mechanical, and environmental aspects of the work task as each are related to the other. Work productivity and work safety are the two most important goals of the occupational biomechanist and the ergonomist. The emphasis is upon enhancing performance without compromising safety.

Chaffin and Andersson have identified six methodological areas of occupational biomechanics. (See Fig. 12-1.)

The functional anatomy and anthropometrical methodologies form the foundation for the other four: task analysis, mechanical-work capacity evaluation, modeling, and instrumentation. This foundation consists of defining the size, shape, and form of the human body performing the task, and the kinematic capabilities of the human body. For example, the range of motion at each joint with respect to space and time, and the optimum positioning of the muscle-bone-joint lever system to produce optimum or maximum force to safely, efficiently, and effectively perform the task will be determined.

Analysis of the task itself involves classification and time-prediction methodology. The elements of each task are identified with descriptors, such as reach, position, and grasp. The number and types of elements that comprise a task are tabulated and the predicted time to complete the task can be calculated. Tasks are classified to enable comparisons of commonalities and to develop heirarchial matrices. Such development consists of classifying tasks with respect to difficulty, body part utilized, and type of task. Prerequisite task training can be

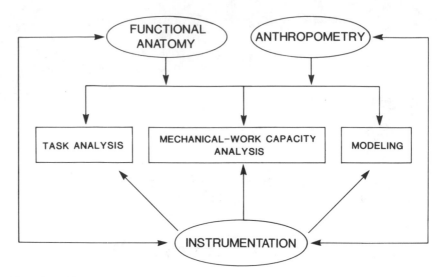

Fig. 12-1. *Relationships of methodological areas of occupational biomechanics. (Modified from Chaffin and Andersson,* Occupational Biomechanics. *New York: Wiley-Interscience, 1984, p. 1.)*

determined prior to the assignment of a worker to a task. This classification and prediction can be valuable knowledge for job placement counseling and determining salary scales.

The mechanical-work capacity evaluation methodology consists of determining performance levels based upon worker characteristics, such as strength, stature, and hand size. Although most of this evaluation has been conducted with physiological instrumentation, the amount of work or power produced prior to discontinuance, due to fatigue or exceeding a time limit, is another viable way of evaluating these parameters. Work and power requirements are evaluated with respect to muscular strength of the worker. Through biomechanical research, standards, with respect to frequency, load and performance technique, can be formulated based upon predicted stress to body tissues.

In order to conduct research in occupational biomechanics, instrumentation is required. Motion pictures were the basis for most time-motion studies of industrial tasks from the 1920's through the 1950's. Instrumentation now usually includes videography, electrogoniometry, accelerometry, dynamography, and electromyography.

Biomechanical modeling has been the most recent investigative methodology. As noted previously, modeling is a safe process for estimating forces acting on the performer and thus evaluating the potential productivity and risk of injury. Modeling of the worker, the environment, and the task as separate systems and then as one combined system is very productive.

What then are the most common concerns in occupational modeling investigations? The concerns, naturally, are the tasks in which there is the greatest injury rate, or greatest severity of injury. The lower back is the area of greatest concern and causes an economic drain in the work industry. Lifting and handling tasks, as well as sitting tasks, are the focus of many other biomechanical modeling investigations. Tool use (including tool design), because of the carpal tunnel syndrome, is also a major area of concern. Segmental and whole-body vibration jobs are also important areas of study.

ANTHROPOMETRY

As a result of extensive compilation of anthropometric data, standards have been formulated and are used as industry criteria for such items as heights and widths of chairs and work tables. Although ranges, rather than a precise numerical value, are frequently listed in these standards, the standards often will not incorporate persons at the extremes of the data distribution. For example, if you were 4 feet 6 inches or 7 feet tall, the standard chair would be biomechanically incorrect for your use. Persons at the 50th percentile with respect to anthropometric values will be able to function optimally in most work spaces.

Another use of anthropometric data in industry has been the setting of minimum physical standards for acceptance into specific jobs. Maximum or minimum stature, age, and physical fitness requirements have been introduced into such occupations as mililtary services, airline attendant, police officer, firefighter, truck driver, and restaurant server. By means of human performance analysis of the requirements of the task, we can determine whether or not the standards are justified. If the standards are not justified, persons may be considered discriminated against. This issue is a very important one in today's society.

Discrepancies exist between the standards and individuals for many reasons, some of which are ethnic background, nutrition, physical activity habits (remember bones grow in relation to the forces placed upon them through physical activity and other factors), and genetics. More importantly, the population from which the standards were derived affects the applicability of the standards. For example, the mean stature of the British population and the Swedish population differs by 4 cm, whereas the difference is 10 cm between Swedish and Japanese populations. Similarly, mean differences between statures of male and females is approximately 10 cm. Link-length differences between male and females are between 3 and 7 cm depending upon the link and the percentile of the population being compared.

Anthropometric tables have been constructed in which mean values and percentile values are listed. (See appendix.) These tables consist of link-lengths, such as, stature, widths, and lengths of body segments. Often, these link-lengths are reported as proportions of stature. Refer to Fig. 12-2.

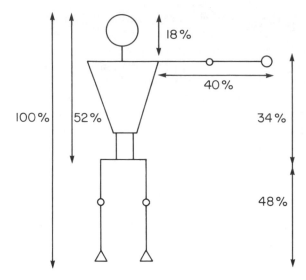

Fig. 12-2. *Proportionality of body segments with respect to total body stature.*

Other anthropometric measurements and their importance to an understanding of work performance are link-weight, link center of mass, radius of gyration and moment of inertia.

1. Link weights—proportional to muscle effort.
2. Link center of mass—proportional to muscle effort. Center of mass of the limbs is approximately 40% from proximal end, since their geometric shape is comparable to a frustrum (truncated cone). Center of mass of the head is in the center, since its geometric shape is a sphere. Center of mass of the trunk plus head is 20% from the caudal end, since organs are in abdomen and lungs are in thorax.
3. Radius of gyration—Radii of gyration are similar for the motion axes X and Y, but negligible (except for the head) in the Z motion axis. This latter motion is rotation about the longitudinal axis of the segment.
4. Moment of inertia—proportional to muscle effort to start and stop of a movement.

WORK SPACE (WORK STATION)

Biomechanical analyses must include the analysis of the workspace, since the workspace often determines the manner in which the task will be performed. There are three types of workspaces to consider: sitting, standing (including twisting), and locomotor spaces. Since the advent of the Information Society, sitting is by far the most prevalent work position. High technology and computer-related businesses have resulted in less reliance upon physical strength to perform occupational tasks. Ultra-efficient transportation devices bring objects to the worker's table, bench, or chair. In other cases, the jobs require video-display terminals and information manipulation. Few dentists now stand and twist their bodies as they work. A swivel adjustable chair is used to reduce the possibility of injuries due to twisting. Average, mean, or normative anthropometric data are used to determine the amount of space that can easily be utilized by the worker and to determine the dimensions of the inanimate objects incorporated into the workspace.

Examples of pertinent measurements and the biomechanically designed sitting workspace appear as Fig. 12-3.

MINI-LAB LEARNING EXPERIENCES

Use the following checklist to evaluate the acceptability of one or more chairs interfaced with three or more persons of dissimilar anthropometric characteristics.

Check list—check the items that apply to the person passively sitting in the chair.

feet flat on the floor
no portion of feet touch floor
toes or balls of feet touch floor
more pressure is felt on distal portion of thigh than on buttocks
thighs are horizontal
thighs are inclined upward from hips to knees
thighs are inclined downward
shanks are vertical
shanks are inclined

The optimum height of a chair is one in which the sitter can place the feet flat on the floor. There should be no pressure at the distal parts of the thighs, and the thighs should be inclined slightly upward. Rate the anthropometric characteristics of greatest importance to chair design. Check Fig. 12-4 to evaluate your ratings.

Let's look at the sitting posture from the perspective of long term sitting without undue stress to the spine. Did you know that the measured pressures on the lumbar vertical discs during sitting are higher

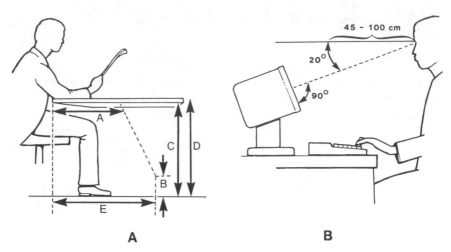

Fig. 12-3. *(A) Workstation and relationships of working desk surface and height to worker. A, minimum of 450 mm for working desk, and 300 mm for dataterminal table. B, 150 mm. C, minimum of 630 mm. D, 670–780 mm. E, minimum of 600 mm. (B) workstation and line of vision. (Modification from Ericsson Information Systems, from 1983, Ergonomic Principles in Office Automation p. 68. and 67.)*

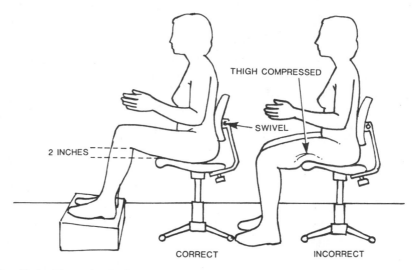

Fig. 12-4. *Biomechanically correct and incorrect sitting position and furniture. The highest point of the seat should be at least 2 inches below the popliteal crease of the worker. If necessary, this must be accomplished by a footrest. The backrest should swivel about the horizontal axis to align with the lumbar curve. (Modified from Tichauer.,* The biomechanical basis of ergonomics: anatomy applied to the design of work situations, *N.Y. 1978. p. 7.)*

than during standing at rest? The difference between these sitting and standing can be as much as 35% of the lowest measured sitting pressure. Changes in posture and changes in the chair configuration will result in changes in disc pressure. In fact, a 200% reduction in disc pressure can occur merely as a result of modifying each of three chair parameters: the inclination of the backrest, type of arm support, and the amount of lumbar support.

Naturally, human movement analysis cannot be performed on workers by invasively placing a force transducer in the spinal cord to measure disc pressure. This technique, however, has been performed in research settings and values appear in Table 12-1.

What is the basic biomechanical design concept related to chairs with back supports? The basic concept is that reactive forces are operating to transfer some of the weight of the body parts to these chair supports. Consequently, less weight is transmitted to the spine.

Note that the inclined backrest (110-120 degrees backward) is a favorable position. This position is similar to that used in the "hog motorcycles" and recumbent bicycles. Unfortunately, many work tasks cannot be performed in this position. Or can they? Could you design a workspace to capitalize upon this more efficient sitting position?

Pressure on the lumbar discs is determined by the angle at the hip, the lengths of hip muscles at that angle, the tilt of the pelvis, and the weight of the upper body. The 135-degree angle at the hip has been determined to be the normal position of balanced muscle relaxation. Thus, at an angle of 135 degrees, the natural curvature of the lumbar spine is maintained. An angle greater than this angle will increase the lumbar spine curvature and angles less than 135 degrees will reduce this curvature. (See Fig. 12-5.)

Table 12-1. *Disc pressure (expressed as percent of relaxed lean back position) when person sits in chairs with different configurations and performs different tasks. (Compiled and modified from Chaffin and Andersson, Occupational Biomechanics, 1984.)*

Backrest Angle (degrees)	Disc Pressure (%)
90	171
100	129
110	99
120	89

Trunk position	Disc Pressure (%)
Relaxed lean back (with back support)	100
Vertical	105
Relaxed (slouch)	123
Posterior slouch	125
Anterior lean (straight)	139
Anterior lean (slouch)	157

Task	Disc Pressure (%)
writing (arms on table)	124
depression of pedal	124
typewriting	146
lifting weight (arms horizontal)	170

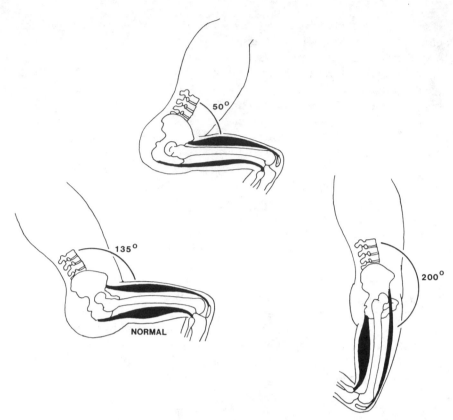

Fig. 12-5. *Relationship of muscle length and angle at the hip during sitting. A series of tracings from roentgenograms of the lumbosacral spine, pelvis, and femur of one individual were taken as the person lay in a lateral recumbent position. The hamstrings and quadraceps muscles are depicted to show the effect of the limited length of these muscles: rotation of pelvis and change in lumbar curve. Note the balance muscle position is 135 degrees. Greater than this angle results in increased lumbar curvatre. (Adapted from Chaffin and Andersson, 1984)*

ASSESSMENT OF MUSCLE ACTIVITY

Muscle activity levels may be an indirect measurement of stress at different levels of the spine or other joints of the body. Electromyographic investigations can also be conducted to ascertain the positions requiring the least amount of muscle tension during performance of the work task. For example, Hamilton recorded tension in selected neck muscles in response to positioning of the work document being read and entered into a computer. (See figure 12-6.)

In summary, the work station should be anthropometrically matched to the worker, stress should be minimized and muscle activity minimized. A backrest for the lumbar spine, a foot rest to incline the feet, an intermediate level height of chair all are biomechanically sound concepts for sitting. This latter is particularly useful in situa-

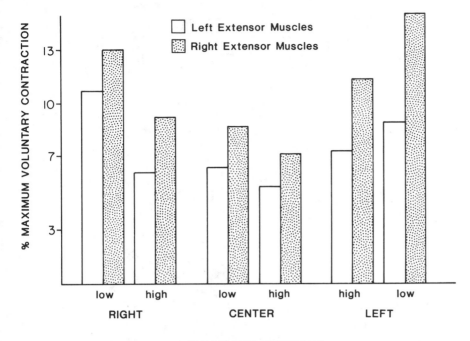

Fig. 12-6. *Muscle action potentials recorded during computer workstation performance. Differences between muscle tension were noted when document was placed equidistant to right and to left. Eye dominance and functional scoliosis, among other factors, may account for such differences. (Adapted from Nancy Hamilton, dissertation, Neck tension and effect of document placement, University of Illinois at Urbana-Champaign.)*

tions requiring changes between sitting and standing, since the thigh and trunk are positioned to form a favorable hip angle. (See Fig. 12-7.) The footrest in Fig. 12-7 was designed to relieve pressure on the thighs and to exercise/relax the feet. Note the center has a swivel surface and the rollers act to massage the feet.

RANGE OF MOTION (ROM)

Normal ROM charts have been published by numerous investigators since the 1920's. As has been mentioned elsewhere in this book, individual differences are so great that these charts should be used as guides only. Persons who have less than normal ROM for a specific task will undoubtedly have difficulty performing that task. Although it is relatively easy to increase ROM, this is not the case with link lengths.

Above all, it must be remembered that range of motion is joint specific, and right- and left specific. Normal range in one joint does not guarantee normal range in another. Refer to figure 12-8 as an application of normal range of reach at a sitting work station.

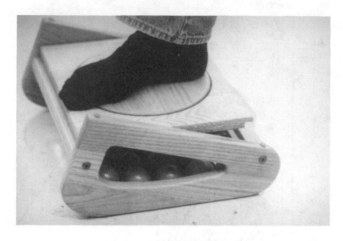

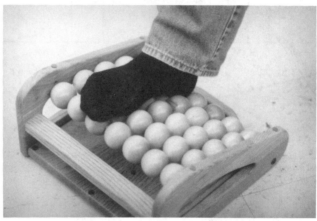

Fig. 12-7. *Foot rest that also functions as an exercise and massage device for the feet. (Courtesy of R&R)*

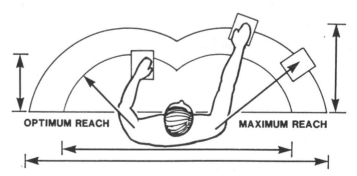

OPTIMUM REACH   MAXIMUM REACH

Fig. 12-8. *Normal reach distance for a visual display unit (VDU) workstation are identified as maximum reach and optimum reach. Determine the dimensions for your personal anthropometrically correct workstation by measuring your arm length, biacromial width, and chest width. Calculate optimum reach as 65% of your maximum reach. (Adapted from Ericsson)*

390

STRENGTH MEASUREMENTS

The evaluation of muscular strength is vital for all physical occupations, especially lifting and handling jobs. There are four types of strength evaluations commonly used by the biomechanics expert: whole-body static strength, localized static strength, whole-body dynamic strength, and localized dynamic strength. Although general strength tests can be performed, a more viable evaluation is to simulate the posture or dynamics of the occupational task and test appropriately. This is suggested because the positioning of the joint and the links of the body affect the ability to produce force. The strength of the worker is dependent upon the position of the link system at the instant of application of the force. Refer to Fig. 12-9. As the angle of pull of the muscle changes, the effective moment arm changes. Therefore, the longest moment arm for the biceps bracchi will be at the 90 degree angle at the elbow. The worker is most effective, and less susceptible to fatigue at this position.

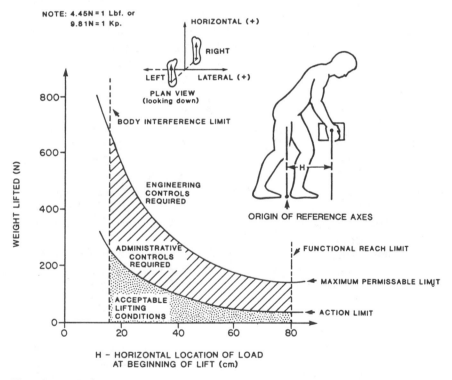

Fig. 12-9. *The action limit and maximum permissible limit for lifting loads from the floor from different locations in front of body. The equation for determining these limits is AL = (HF)(VF)(DF)(FF), where these are the discounting factors for horizontal and vertical starting distances, vertical distance of lift and frequency of lift. 3AL = MPL. (Reprinted with permission from Chaffin and Andersson p. 13.)*

OCCUPATIONAL BIOMECHANICS   **391**

NON-AUTOMATED MATERIALS HANDLING LIMITS

Pushing, pulling, lifting, and carrying objects without the aid of automation accounts for almost 90% of the industrial overexertion claims made for lower back pain. Although automation will reduce the number of workers performing these handling tasks, many tasks will not be automated in the foreseeable future. Thus, the strength requirements of the task must be evaluated with respect to such factors as frequency and duration of tasks, weight and dimensions of the object handled, and the geometry of the workplace.

The National Institute for Occupational Safety and Health (NIOSH) has published recommendations for lifting and has specified two levels of hazards. These levels are the action limit (AL) at which 75% of women and 99% of men can perform safely, and the maximum permissible limit (MPL) at which only 25% of men and less than 1% of women can perform without hazard. The MPL is equal to 3 AL. Anything above these limits requires engineering controls, not human lifting strength.

What are these limits and how were they determined? The setting of limits was the result of a pooling of research literature and experts working from four perspectives:

1. Epidemiology of musculoskeletal injury.
2. Biomechanical concepts.
3. Physiological considerations.
4. Psychophysical (muscular strength) lifting limits.

The determinants of limits for symmetrical lifting tasks of moderate-sized loads under favorable conditions, that is, adequate friction, posture, and gripping were identified as initial position of load, distance to be moved, and frequency of lift. In addition, the strength and the reach of the lilfter and the load were considered. The equation

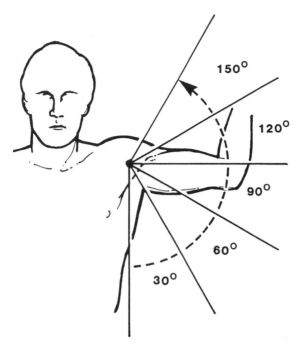

Fig. 12-10. *Shoulder abduction strength related to shoulder abduction angle. Strength drastically decreases at the 150 degree angle of abduction. At the other positions strength is at least 80% of maximum occurring at the 30 degree angle. (Modified from Stobbe, 1982.)*

for determining these limits can be found in the NIOSH guide. The values for lifting various weights at different horizontal locations on the floor to a height of 60 cm on an infrequent basis (once every five minutes) are depicted in Fig. 12-9. The horizontal location of the load at the beginning of the lift is the most important determinant of limit.

There are no values for asymmetrical lifting tasks, but the factors identified in symmetrical lifting tasks can be used as a starting point for biomechanical evaluation of risk of injury during asymmetrical lifting tasks. Posture and frictional forces probably will need to be included in the equation to determine lifting limits. Strength capabilities appear to decrease approximately 20% with asymmetric posture. Positioning of the feet and avoidance of twisting require further study.

MINI-LAB LEARNING EXPERIENCES

Investigate the strength capabilities at different arm positions by attaching a strap to the arm above or below the elbow, depending upon the test, and connecting the other end to a spring scale. Compare your data with that of other persons or appropriate data in tables.

OCCUPATIONAL BIOMECHANICS   **393**

1. Test shoulder abduction strength with strap above elbow. Shoulder strength in abduction as the arm moves from angles of 30 to 150 degrees was reported by Stobbe and is shown in figure 12-10.
2. Test forearm flexion strength with strap at wrist. Forearm flexion pulls from mid-center, 45 degrees to the side, and at the horizontal have been graphically displayed by Chaffin and appear in Fig. 12-11. Which position of the forearm is the strongest?
3. Test arm flexion strength with strap at wrist. Maintain a constant angle at the elbow. What is the relationship of flexion angle to strength? Compare your data with that of fatigue with respect to holding time in the various positions. Measure holding time and compare performances.

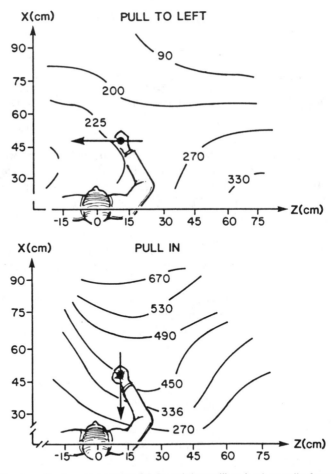

Fig. 12-11. *Arm flexion strength pattern when pulling horizontally from mid-center and 45 degree side positions. (Adapted from Chaffin and Andersson).*

394   *THE BIOMECHANICS OF HUMAN MOVEMENT*

TOOL USE AND DESIGN

Carpel tunnel syndrome and its cumulative trauma disorders have become prevalent among workers using hand tools on a continuous basis. The radial or ulnar nerve, artery, or the tendons are traumatized through repeated movements, pressures, or extremes in positioning of the hand and fingers.

Since grip span is related to grip strength, tools need to be designed to fit the anthropometry of the hand. Average maximum-grip strength is achieved at a span of 5-8 cm. If, however, a single tool shaft is held, the diameter should be approximately 4 cm. The most important factor, however, is to maintain the hand coplanar with the forearm. Thus, there will be little impingement on the tissues crossing the wrist. (See Fig. 12-12.) The ability to produce grip strength can be tested using an adjustable hand dynamometer. Place the dynamometer in the hand, and grip it with the hand in a neutral position, flexed, extended, ulnarly deviated, and radially deviated, and compare the scores. Experiment also with adjusting the span of the dynamometer handle.

VIBRATIONS

Investigation of effects of vibration upon the body segments and tissues is the final area of concern in occupational biomechanics. The human body is modeled as a dynamic mechanical system of springs, attenuators, links, and masses as shown in Fig. 12-13. The resulting resonant-frequency levels vary among body parts as shown when vibrations of 100 Hz or less are applied to the body as a whole. Think of the body being analogous to jello set in a bowl that is shaken. Stretch reflexes, muscle fatigue, and organ muscle contractions have been documented as responses due to whole-body vibrations. Precise effects upon the nervous system are largely unknown. Psychological stress reactions as well as reductions in consciousness, however, have been noted.

Low-back problems have been attributed to whole-body vibrations experienced by tractor, bus, and truck drivers. Segmental vibrations have been known to cause sudden blockage of circulation of blood, most notably Reynaud's syndrome, in which precision movements are impaired and tactile sensitivity is reduced.

Limits of tolerance to vibrations and standards for occupations in which vibrations are a component of the environment have been summarized by Chaffin and Andersson. They also report that vibration studies represent an important challenge to future biomechanists.

KINETIC MODELING

Kinematic models could be and are used in occupational biomechanics, and such models are described in other chapters. Kinematic

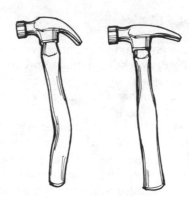

Fig. 12-12. *A, Hammer handle orientation to reduce carpal tunnel syndrome possibility. Hand and forearm are aligned (coplanar). B, Regular handle and ulnar deviation of downswing.*

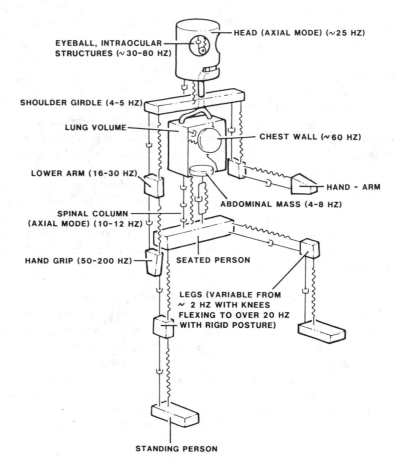

Fig. 12-13. *Mechanical system representing the human body subjected to vertical vibration. Note the highest vibration frequencies are the hand grip, chest wall, and eyeball. (Adapted from Chaffin and Andersson's adaption from Rasmussen et al., 1982.)*

models are most useful as templates to compare individual performances, including performances on work tasks. Forces acting on the worker, however, are not treated in kinematic models. The primary purpose of kinetic modeling is to understand the stresses to the human body in order to determine risk of injury. Although any part of the body or the total body can be modeled, there are six common sites of interest in occupational biomechanics: (1) lumbar spine, (2) elbow, (3) hand, (4) knee, (5) hip, and (6) shoulder. The whole body usually is modeled for investigations of stresses at the lumbar spine, hip, and knee. One-link models may be adequate for modeling the hand, and one-, two-, or three-link models are used for investigations of stresses at the elbow and shoulder.

As outlined in Chapter 4, the simplest modeling is the planar static single-link model. In the job-related situation, the hand carrying a load is one of the simplest models to depict. Figure 12-14 is the representation of this model, with the configured drawing and the free-body diagram.

Note that in figure 12-14B, the arm is considered to be a rigid single link with the shoulder the site of reaction. The bony structure transmits the weight of the load directly to the shoulder. If muscles of the arm and hand are weak and the load is heavy, the load is borne through the bony structure of the arm to the shoulder and the worker will feel the pull at the shoulder and possibly feel a post-ache in the muscles crossing the shoulder. Note also that the free-body diagram has the vectors drawn to scale, and either drawn parallel side-by-side or in one vertical line. Thus, it is evident that the sum of the forces equals zero and the system is in equilibrium. There is no upward or downward movement of the load or the shoulder. Muscle force prevents the shoulder from dislocating. If a FBD is drawn only of the

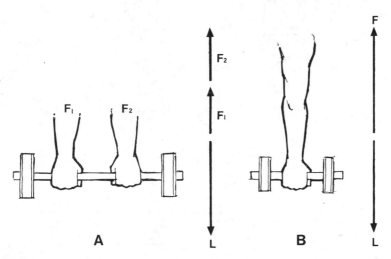

Fig. 12-14. *Load held in one hand and load held in two hands. Free body diagrams are depicted to left of situation. F, muscular force; L, load to be lifted or held.*

OCCUPATIONAL BIOMECHANICS

internal forces at the shoulder, the weight of load would be drawn downward and the muscle force would be drawn upward. This represents an internal action-reaction situation.

The advantage of holding a load in two hands is depicted in Fig. 12-14A. Each arm has a reaction of half the weight of the load; therefore, muscle effort would be half that of the previous load situation.

In the preceding examples, there were no moments of force (torques). Rarely does this condition exist in occupational tasks. Joint angles usually are not at 180 degrees (or 0 degrees depending upon one's perspective). Therefore, the adjacent body segments are not aligned in a straight line. No consideration also was allotted to the weight of the body segment. The joints of the body must always support the weight of the segment or segments that are distal with respect to the support reaction. For example, during standing the hand-segment weight is distal to the wrist, the forearm plus hand is distal to the elbow, and the total upper extremity are distal to the shoulder. The

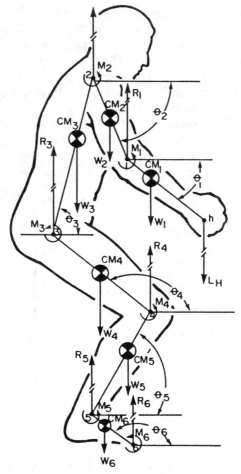

Fig. 12-15. *Six-link free body diagram of forces and moments in sagittal plane in quasi-static position during lifting.*

total body reaction will be at the joints of the foot-ankle system. (See Fig. 12-15.)

Note that the body segment weights act at the center of mass of the segment or system of segments (one link). If the support for the body changes, the reactions due to body segment weights will change accordingly.

MOMENTS OF FORCE (TORQUES)

Static equilibrium also requires that the sum of all moments equal zero to prevent rotation from occurring. A moment is superimposed upon the reaction forces due to segmental weights acting at the joints. This moment is created by the body segment weight acting at a distance from the joint. There is no moment if the body segment weight acts through the joint.

Calculation of moments of force is important in the assessment of the many postures of work, for example, standing and pulling a lever that is above eye level and working at a desk. To determine the direction of the moments (clockwise or counterclockwise), imagine the force of gravity acting through the body segment and causing a rotation about the joint. Draw the moment as a curved vector in the direction of possible rotation. Reverse direction for the reactive moment of force (torque) at the joint. As posture changes, the moment values change.

MINI-LAB LEARNING EXPERIENCES

Calculate the moments at the hip in three work positions, utilizing your anthropometric data, your length of body segments and your body weight. What are the two ways to obtain the reaction force at your hip joint? Which posture results in the greatest moment of force at your hip? (See Fig. 12-16.)

Estimating the moments and reactive forces at the joints is one method of estimating the relative magnitude of muscular activity required to maintain the integrity of the joint. In static situations, the muscles must produce forces equal in magnitude but opposite in direction to the moments of force and reactive forces at the joint to maintain equilibrium. Thus, the greater these reactive moments of forces, the greater the muscle force requirement. During non-static situations, the role of muscles in producing the movement (concentric contraction) and regulating lengthening of the muscle (eccentric contraction) can be ascertained. Dynamic situations, however, are more complex since dynamic forces (ma and Iα) must be included in the model. The actual concept of modeling is no different. The sum of the forces and moments will be equal to zero if these dynamic forces are included in the equation.

OCCUPATIONAL BIOMECHANICS   **399**

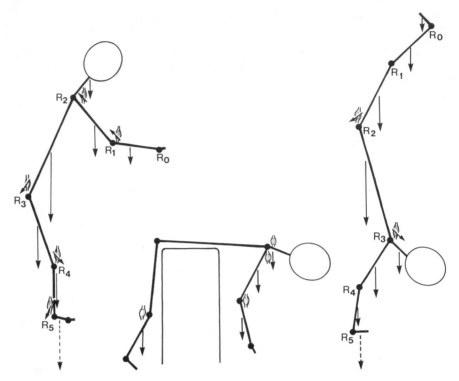

Fig. 12-16. *A, Free body diagram of forces due to weight of segments only minus the moments. Muscle forces depicted with line of pull indicated, but not magnitudes. The open link system (upper extremities) act as third class systems, whereas the lower body must be considered as first class balancing systems since this part of the body is a closed linkage. B, Free body diagram of reaction forces due to weight of segments minus the body parts supported by the external object (fender of automobile). C, Free body diagram of reaction forces due to weight of segments only minus the moments. Body is supported from hands.*

A general rule of biomechanics is that an analysis should be conducted as if the body were stationary. Then keep as is, the forces and moments caused by the movement. Use it as a multiplier to increase or decrease the moments and forces at the joints. If the acceleration doubles, the reaction at the joint will double. Why is this true?

THREE-DIMENSIONAL MODELING

Complex computer software and sophisticated data collection are required for true three-dimensional modeling. Pseudo-3-D can be conducted relatively inexpensively with two video cameras. The planar images from each camera are analyzed separately and moments and forces estimated for each plane. If values are low with respect to one plane, they can be considered negligible. Thus, some movements can be investigated in single planes (2-D). If, however, an individual has large force values for a work task in which the normative data include only low values, this pseudo-3D has been worthwhile. That individual is at risk, and must be taught to modify the techniques used to perform the task or change jobs.

The modeling of occupational tasks has been the basis for obtaining a wealth of knowledge concerning performance and safety. The greater the information accumulated, however, the more complex becomes the interpretation. For example, based upon research concerning lifting tasks, the compressive stresses were less in the squat-style lift than the stoop-style lift. The shearing forces, however, were greater in the squat style. What does that mean?

ANALYSIS OF WORK TASKS AND EXISTING ENVIRONMENT

Biomechanical analyses of the work station (Fig. 12-17) can be reduced to a four-step process consisting of (1) the historical, (2) use of biomechanical tolerance checklist, (3) analytical process, and (4) projective analysis.

1. Historical: Search of the literature related to the task or the broad category into which the task can be placed is the first step. Injury data, potential problems associated with the task, and findings of researchers in this area are the basis for further analyses. More importantly, this information is useful to determine the direction and factors to be used in an analysis design.
2. Biomechanical Tolerances Checklist: Use the following checklist proposed by Tichauer (1978) to determine obvious changes to be made in the work-task. This checklist consists of 15 prerequisites to biomechanical work tolerance. Five prerequisites are grouped into each of the following three areas: (1) postural correlates, (2) engineering correlates (human being-equipment interface), and (3) kinesiological (anatomical functioning) correlates.

   Biomechanical Tolerances Checklist
   1. Postural Correlates
   Keep elbows down.
   Minimize moments on spine.
   Consider sex differences.
   Optimize skeletal configuration.
   Avoid head movement.
   2. Engineering Correlates
   Avoid compression ischemia.

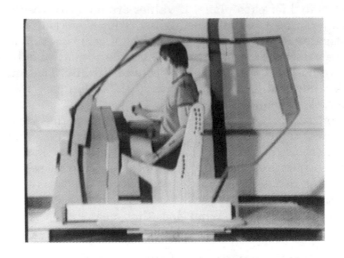

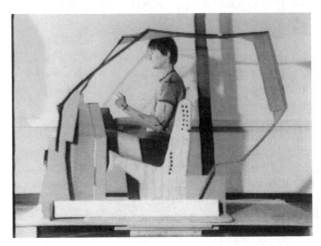

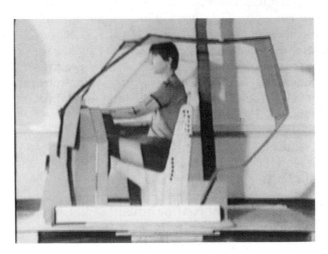

402

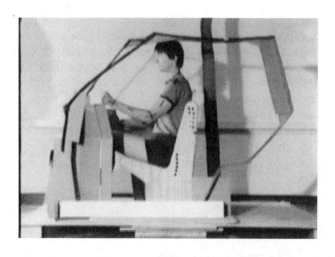

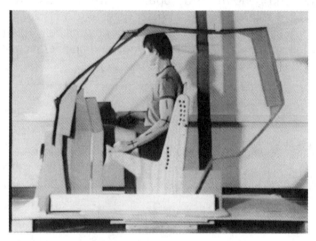

Fig. 12-17. *Video taped sequences of performance at a workstation.*

Avoid critical vibrations.
Avoid stress concentration.
Keep wrist straight.
Individualize chair design.
3. Kinesiological Correlates.
Keep forward reaches short.
Consider working gloves.
Avoid muscular insufficiency.
Avoid straight-line motions.
Avoid antagonist fatigue.
3. Analytical Processes: Although visual analysis utilizing checklists can be performed, such analyses are usually too superficial. It is necessary to obtain a permanent record of per-

formance so that detailed in-depth analysis are possible. The main features of the analysis process include: (1) categorizing the movement patterns, (2) identifying missing correlates, (3) determining the ranges of motion, (4) determining spatial orientation of motions, (5) measuring frequency of performance, (6) estimating forces, loads, and moments of force (torques).

4. Projective Analysis: This final step is an interpretive one. Based upon the data collected in Step 3, the movement analyst postulates the probable trauma sites and types of injury. Modifications in the task then are proposed based upon such postulates.

MINI-LAB LEARNING EXPERIENCES

Select and perform an occupational task and use the biomechanical work tolerance checklist to note any omissions of necessary correlates. Analyze the movement anatomically (planes and lever systems) and kinematically (speeds and accelerations, ROM). Estimate the moments and forces.

REFERENCES

Chaffin, D.B. and Andersson, G. (1984) *Occupational biomechanics,* New York: Wiley-Interscience.
Ergonomic Principles in Office Automation, AB, Sweden, (1983), Ericsson Information Systems.
Hamilton, N. (1986) A Postural Model for the Reduction of Neck Tension. unpublished dissertation, Urbana-Champaign, University of Illinois.
Tichauer, E.R. (1978) *The biomechanical basis of ergonomics: anatomy applied to the design of work situations,* New York: Wiley-Interscience.

13

Biomechanics in the Arts

INTRODUCTION

In the arts, particularly the performing arts, individuals refine techniques and movements to become more efficient as they reproduce patterns in dance, music, theatre, and art which convey their artistry. In these art forms, except for dance, the movement itself is not the product to be evaluated or critiqued. But the artist must be concerned with the biomechanics of movement to a degree very similar to that of an athlete or dancer. Effective movements and postures are the means by which the performer/artist creates the desired artistic expression. Since the show must go on, it becomes critical to the performing artist that injury or medical complications do not disrupt concentration, practice, or performance.

Dancers, musicians, artists, and actors/actresses practice and perform very long hours on a daily, weekly, and lifelong basis. For many, it is a lifelong endeavor, focusing on an art form at an early age with the expectation of many years of active participation. Unlike most sports participants and dancers, who are adolescents or young adults when they attain peak performances, it is not uncommon for a talented musician, artist, or stage performer to reach a peak in middle age and continue actively into the final years of life. As in sport, some individuals choose an art form as a career, but for others, it is an intensely pursued avocation. Specialization begins at a very young age, following progressions of skill development handed down from teacher to teacher—even when that progression is not biomechanically sound. In progressing from beginner to skilled artist, intensity increases, as does time spent in practice and performance. Sometimes as much as 10 hours in one day are spent practicing. Such concentrated, repeated movements lead to overuse syndromes in musicians, artists, and dancers similar to the problems of the weekend athlete whose activity is also compressed into a short time period. As one easel artist suggested, his brush arm took as much punishment as that of a major league pitcher (Rowes, 1986).

Dedication to improved technique, and thus performance, has sometimes been carried to such extremes as to be detrimental. Pianist Robert Schumann rigged a weighted pulley system attached to the ceiling to strengthen his fourth finger. As a result, he permanently damaged his hands because he was not aware of the anatomical constraints of finger extensor tendons, which prevent the fourth finger from working independently (Ortmann, 1962).

To convey their ideas, artists must sometimes perform under very difficult conditions. Frequently, stage and movie actors assume contorted postures or wear heavy costumes, headgear, and make-up to convey their ideas. Consider Jose Ferrer in the role of French artist, Toulouse-Lautrec. He performed for long hours with his lower leg strapped to his thigh to portray the artist, whose legs were deformed due to the bone-growth disruption in the long bones of the leg. Mime artists count on the success of their illusion to produce an image of a real event. Marcel Marceau performs a magnificent sequence of walking against the wind. To do this, he assumes a very awkward body position for a person not leaning into an actual wind force. The illusion is complete because he is able to maintain his center of mass aligned over his base of support in the absence of the actual gale force. To lose balance destroys the illusion, yet, in the absence of an actual force, muscles must contract in tense, uncomfortable patterns.

Participants and teachers of an art form share similar concerns: At what age, for instance, should one begin to dance en pointe? Are there physical characteristics that facilitate technique, or do they contraindicate successful performance, for example, dental problems that hinder the playing of wind instruments? What is the most efficient way to perform or to develop techniques? How can postural tensions be reduced during practice and performance? Which muscle groups control the required movements. How can injury be avoided—especially injury severe enough to stop performance? The latter concern is one typically given consideration only after a medical problem arises.

As opposed to athletes who are accustomed to physical training and the body's need for strengthening and stretching of muscles, artists rarely consider the consequences or needs of their body in practicing or performance. For example, take the case of a high school cymbalist whose marching band practiced 22 hours over a 7-day period. The young musician complained of painful shoulders much like the bicipital groove, biceps tendon pain experienced by swimmers— a clear case of overuse without appropriate conditioning or rest periods (Huddleston & Pratt, 1983; Lubell, 1987).

Recognition of the special needs of the artistic community has resulted in a new medical specialty, arts medicine, which is growing rapidly, as did sports medicine in the last decade. The Miller Health

Care Institute for the Performing Arts, located in Manhattan just a few blocks from sites where dancers, musicians, and actors perform nightly, is an example of the new medical centers devoted to the problems of performing artists (Rowes, 1986, Van Horn, 1987). The institute uses a team approach combining the efforts of physician/orthopedist, laryngologist, physical therapist, and artist to resolve physically debilitating problems. In an effort to keep the artist performing and active, the team analyzes movements as carefully as a teacher/coach, seeking to identify the cause of painful or stiff movements. As a result of their work with artists, Miller clinicians have suggested that a performing artist must engage in warming up, muscular strengthening, and stretching regimes similar to those of athletes. Biomechanists have consulted concerning safety, injury prevention, technique, and conditioning for the artist, dancer and actor. Biomechanical analysis of movements used by artists is as valuable to the performing artist as it is to the person participating in a sport or performing a routine occupational task.

BIOMECHANICAL PRINCIPLES FOR ARTISTS

The following principles are some of the basic ones described in Chapter 5, restated and reemphasized for their importance to the analysis of artists' movement.

Stability

The body is stable when the center of gravity is maintained over the base of support. The intersection of the line of gravity with the center of the base of support yields the greatest stability. Intersection of the line of gravity near the edge of the base lessens stability but facilitates mobility. Decreasing the size of the base of support or increasing the height of the center of gravity will decrease stability. Postures that align body segments and external implements over the base of support provide stability with less muscle fatigue.

Inertia

The body will continue in a state of rest or uniform motion unless acted upon by a force sufficient to disturb this state. Segments or implements can be efficiently maintained in a state of motion when a small force is required to maintain that motion.

Acceleration

The acceleration of the body is directly proportional to the force imparted to it, in the same direction as the force and inversely proportional to its mass.

Leverage

Shorter levers rotate faster. When moving a long lever or implement, apply the force as far as possible from the center of rotation to produce greater muscular control of that implement.

Friction

(Friction is the ease of one surface moving on another surface.) The amount of friction depends upon the nature of the surfaces and the forces pressing them together.

Force Development

To maximize force, apply that force directly in line with the center of mass and in the direction of desired movement. When possible, use large muscles to initiate actions and follow sequentially with segments of decreasing mass. Implements and objects concentrated close to the body's center of gravity can be moved or controlled using less force than when objects are held further away.

Force Absorption

The velocity of the body should be slowed gradually overtime, especially during landings. The area of the absorption should be as large as possible.

THE DANCER

Dance is an art form which uses the body as its instrument of expression. It differs from sport since it is not concerned with movement as a means of performing some feat, such as scoring points, but rather with the artistic intent and expressive quality of the movement. It is an arrangement of patterns in space and time, which requires varying degrees of force to perform. The properties of movement that a dancer must consider include moving through space using locomotor patterns such as walking, running, jumping, and hopping or moving within a personal space using non-locomotor movements. The dancer is concerned with initiating and terminating actions, airborne moves, balances, turns, extensions of the limbs, spatial relationships, rhythmic patterns, force, and energy—all performed with efficiency, fluidity, and artistic expression.

Many forms of dance have evolved throughout history and in different geographical locations. Today, training in ballet is very fashionable, especially for the young female, and aerobic dance is one of the most popular activities for women who are interested in physical fitness. Since the major emphasis in aerobic dance is placed on exercises and cardiovascular fitness rather than as an art form, aerobic dance is included in Chapter 10.

Breakdancing, which captured the fancy of male teenagers in

particular, seems to be slowly decreasing in mass appeal. These and other popular forms of dance have unique and specific performance characteristics. All dance forms, however, are based on the same biomechanical principles as general movement and sports. The expert dancer and/or choreographer will learn about biomechanical principles and apply them artistically without losing the aesthetic qualities of the dance.

Dance Injuries

In recent years, an increasing amount of attention has been directed toward dance injuries. To excel, the young dancer today is forced to train longer and harder, and begins training early in life. The dancer may sustain a variety of injuries caused by technique problems, the dancer's physique, the dance environment, or a combination of these. Because of the complex relationship of these three factors, a problem in one area may be magnified and ultimately lead to injury.

The most common sites of dance injuries are in the lower extremities. Feet, ankles, knees, shins, hips, and lower back are customary sites of problems. Chronic rather than acute injuries are more common in most dance forms, with the exception of breakdancing. In breakdancing, the injuries are often comparable to the orthopedic injuries that occur in unsupervised athletic situations (Norman, 1984). Many dancers strive to continue despite injuries, but early detection and proper care is very important to successful rehabilitation. An injury may not be debilitating to the general population, but for the dancer, it may mean giving up a life-long dream.

The effective and efficient use of the body is important and incorrect biomechanical performance of dance technique may provoke a dance injury. Turnout of the legs is used in the performance of many dance forms. Dancers strive for perfect turnout, which requires that the feet and knees face directly sideward at 180 degrees. The amount of turnout is influenced by bony, ligamentous, and musculotendinous factors. Careful static stretching and early training may serve to increase the amount of turnout. Some dancers show greater external rotation at the hip joint during passive examination than when they actually dance. Optimum turnout for a given body structure will result if the dancer has adequate strength in the deep external rotators and adductor muscles of the hip joint and uses appropriate muscle activation patterns. Some dancers try to achieve a better turnout than they are capable of correctly performing by forcing the feet beyond the natural line in the turnout from the hip. They often assume the perfect turned-out position while the lower legs are flexed, and then straighten the legs and attempt to adjust alignment from the floor upward. This faulty technique is generally accompanied by pronating the feet excessively, by "screwing (twisting) the knees" and/or by hyperextension of the back—all of which may cause a myriad of dance injuries if continued over time.

Foot pronation is important to shock absorption of the body. The subtalar joint, just below the ankle, has a primary function in transmitting the various forces from the foot to the leg and defines the way in which the foot pronates in reaction to these forces. In excessive pronation, the subtalar joint allows the heel (calcaneus) to evert, and the talus is forced to internally rotate and to plantarflex; the foot collapses and the arch rolls in upon itself (Fig. 13-1).

Internal rotation of the lower leg is caused by the transfer of the rotational force of the talus through the ankle joint to the lower tibia and fibula. A significant shearing force at the knee and a tendency to pull the patellar tendon internally, directing the patella (knee-cap) off its normal track, is due to the leg rotating internally at a faster speed than the thigh. The undersurface and surrounding tissues of the patella thus become inflamed, producing "dancer's knee." Stress fractures to the outside of the ankle joint may also develop due to torque forces relative to the internally rotating talus. The plantarflexion of the talus produces a greater collapsing effect on the foot. This collapse places considerable strain on the many tissues (muscles and fascia) on the bottom of the foot and is a common cause of arch and heel pain. The collapsing of the foot also provides excessive strain to the tibialis posterior muscle, which overworks, attempting to "hold up the arch." This strain may cause pain, identified as a shin splint, in the dancer (Kravitz, 1987).

Screwing of the knee in the attempt to improve turnout uses the iliotibial band to gain further external rotation of the tibia at the knee. The patellar attachments of the iliotibial band pull the patella into an abnormal position while being subjected to large compressive forces generated during a plie. These strains often lead to medial knee pain (Teitz, 1987).

Increasing the hyperextension or lumbar lordosis of the back to increase turnout may allow increased external rotation of the hip by

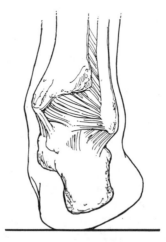

Fig. 13-1. *Excessive pronation with calcaneal eversion (rearfoot view.)*

decreasing the tension on the iliofemoral ligament. This results, however, in undue strain on the lumbar spine, which repeated over time, may cause low back pain. Low back pain may also be caused by other technical errors such as forcing the spine into a hyperextended position (Fig. 13-2) or by externally rotating the hip to achieve the desired height of the back leg in the arabesque position. Incorrect lifting and lifting of excessive loads, as in partnering, is another primary cause of low back pain (Kelly, 1987).

The Dancer's Physique

The structure and physical condition of the body, the dancer's instrument of expression, is an important consideration for a person selecting dance as an avocation or a profession. The novice dancer should be aware of the limitations of an unconditioned body and choose dance activities carefully. A child should not be allowed to progress to the use of pointe shoes until 11 or 12 years of age, when approximately three years of serious ballet technique study have prepared the foot and body for the additional stresses of pointe work.

If a person is interested in dance as a career, rigorous training is necessary, and overuse injuries may be aggravated by an unsuitable physique. A preferred physique for those who wish a professional career in ballet is described as follows. The ballet dancer's body should have extraordinary ligamentous flexibility, especially in the knee and hip, to be able to assume the turned-out ballet positions and leg extensions typical of ballet technique. Total body alignment and symmetrical muscular balance between anterior and posterior lower limbs are also important. The ankle should not be too mobile or too stiff, and toes should be round and of medium size, with the first two toes of equal length. Foot arches should not be flat nor too high, but should be capable of development through flexibility and strengthening exercises.

Muscular balance, including balance of strength, flexibility, and

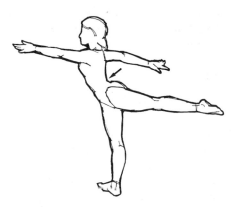

Fig. 13-2. *Strain on lumbar spine due to hyperextension. How can this be avoided? What other dance activities and daily living skills perpetuate this posture?*

BIOMECHANICS IN THE ARTS 411

endurance of opposing muscle groups, is an important physical consideration for dancers. Muscular imbalance, or an unequal capacity for contraction and/or stretch of the agonistic and antagonistic muscle groups, may be structural or caused by consistent patterns of mis use or overuse. A snapping or "clicking" hip may occur with hip flexion, with hip abduction, or in the supporting leg when balancing on one leg. A muscular imbalance causes the snapping sensation as the tendons slide over the greater trochanter, or the iliofemoral ligament slides over the femoral head. Other common muscular imbalances in dance include tightness of the hip flexors, the lateral snapping hip, the anterior snapping hip, increased pelvic inclination, imbalance between the inward and outward rotators of the hip joint, imbalance of strength between the flexors and the extensors of the torso, pectoralis minor syndrome, and neck and shoulder tension. If left uncorrected, almost every muscular imbalance will result in some type of pain. Often in muscular imbalances, the agonist may be tight, but the pain may occur in the antagonist. Corrective exercises may help relieve the imbalance, and thus the pain, if both agonist and antagonist are lengthened and strengthened through developmental exercises (Fitt, 1987).

Dance Environment

The environment in which a dancer performs also contributes to injuries—particularly the construction of dance shoes and dance floors. In ballet, shoes have not changed much since the 18th century. Generally, dance shoes have no cushioning, no shock absorbent material or design features, and no space for orthotics. Pointe shoes have a stiffly constructed box to enclose the front of the foot, which is padded with lamb's wool or other cushioning material. Footgear is also designed especially for aerobic dancing. There are two areas of concern about dance floors—hardness and amount of friction. Most dancers feel that a suspended floor is important for absorption and resiliency. The correct amount of friction with the floor is important to prevent slips and falls, and yet permit the dancer to perform turns with ease. Rosin is often used by dancers to increase friction. Too much friction, however, may also be dangerous.

Results of Biomechanical Research

Biomechanical research in dance is in its infancy. High-speed photography and electromyography are the most frequently used tools in the biomechanical study of dance. Cinematography has been used to compare the filmed performance of specific dance steps to that described in the dance literature. It has also proved to be valuable in unveiling the hidden worlds of the dancer. Since many dance movements are performed rapidly, the naked eye may be duped into thinking (seeing) the body doing something other than what is actually occurring. Based upon analysis of high-speed film it was found that subjects began the rotation for the tour jete on takeoff rather than as commonly thought, during the flight component. The head and upper body began rotating before the supporting leg left the floor (Hinson et al., 1977–78). Other researchers have shown that dancers did not retain their original turn-out throughout the preparatory phase of the sissonne ourverte. The change in turn-out (Fig. 13-3) was not noticeable through observation, and was not realized by the dancers (Brink, 1987).

Electromyography is another technique which has been used in dance research. Researchers demonstrated that different dancers had their own unique patterns of muscle useage in the performance of the grand battement devant, even though the dancers had many years of standardized drilling in the performance of the battement (Ryman and Ranney, 1978).

Other research tools used in biomechanical dance research include pressure transducers, isokinetic dynamometer, and the Leighton flexometer. Pressure transducers have been used to study the relative pressures on the toes in pointe shoes. It was found that the great toe always bore the most pressure and pressure on the second toe varied with the toe length and the shoe padding. An everted position in relevé (Fig. 13-4) was the cause of increased pressures in the meta-

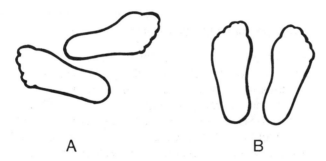

Fig. 13-3. *Position of feet (a) start and (b) end of sissonne.*

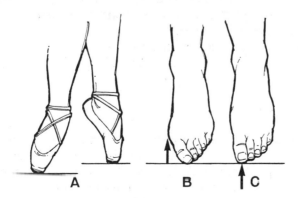

Fig. 13-4. *Relevé en pointe with eversion (a), shear pressure at metatarsal-phalangeal joint (b), and normal pressure en pointe (c).*

tarsal phalangeal joint (Teitz, Harrington & Wiley, 1985). An isokinetic dynamometer was used to measure nonspecific peak torques of female and male dancers who were then compared to other athletes. Male dancers had similar characteristics to other male athletes, but female dancers were lower in relative force production than other female athletes (Kirkendall et al., 1984).

Physiological profiles of dancers have been studied. Cardiovascular response was measured using a modified Balke treadmill protocol; endurance was assessed using an isokinetic dynamometer, and flexibility was measured by a Leighton flexometer. The results of the study were as follows: ballet dancers possessed aerobic fitness levels higher than the general population of the same age and sex, but lower than that of endurance athletes. Female dancers had strong lower-extremity musculature, but relatively weak upper-extremity muscles, and they had a remarkable degree of flexibility (Micheli, 1984).

There is an increasing interest in the area of biomechanical research in dance. As research tools become more sophisticated and the artistic world of dance is influenced by this scientific high technology, many questions currently raised may be studied from the biomechanical perspective to identify safe, effective, and efficient dance technique.

MINI-LAB LEARNING EXPERIENCES

1. Describe three balance positions used in dance, and discuss how the principles of stability influence them.
2. Why does the dancer keep the center of gravity slightly more forward while using a walk movement than in a normal walk?
3. What technique skills does a dancer use in the absorption of the weight of the body on landing from a jump?
4. How can a person being lifted by a partner assist in the lifting process?
5. The body is accelerated in jumps and leaps in dance. What forces cause these accelerations, and what would be considered as the mass?
6. How does rosin on dance shoes increase friction?

THE MUSICIAN

Vocal and instrumental musicians use muscles to control air flow, embouchure, fingering, bowing, and slide manipulation, as well as posture while performing. As they work to perfect techniques handed down from one generation of musicians to another, it is important that they protect themselves against the constant bodily abuse of rapid, repeated actions performed with considerable strength and precision—movements that do not fit a "natural" pattern. Introduction to music as an art form occurs at a very early age, and it is not uncommon for a musician to remain active very late in life. Fox example, classical guitarist Andre Segovia performed well into his 90's. Small discomforts that serve as a warning of overuse are frequently ignored because practice and performance is not inhibited. In perfecting the fingering of a difficult passage, the pianist or guitarist rarely considers the possibilities of carpal tunnel syndrome, nor does the violinist relate to temporomandibular dysfunctions caused by tightly pressing the violin between the chin and shoulder.

Instrumental and vocal musicians search for efficiency in controlling airflow as well as the neuromuscular control of the facial muscles and lips, the arm and the fingers. Several researchers have approached technique improvement by contrasting professional musicians with a student or novice group. Ortmann (1961), an early pioneer in applying science to music performance, focused on the movement patterns of pianists in coordinating the fingers and arms for weight transfer, vertical and lateral arm movements, and finger stroking required to play staccato, legato, portamento, octave tremelos, arpeggios, cadenzas, etc. He demonstrated clearly that greater vertical arm motion was required in playing fortissimo than pianissimo, that volume increased relative to the number of body segments (finger, hand, forearm, arm, and trunk) utilized, and that faster passages were played with less vertical action and increased use of the elbow in pulling the hand away from middle C.

Sieber (1967), Polnaur (1964) Morasky, Reynolds and Clarke (1981) utilized electromyography to identify bow and finger control in string players. Lammers (1983) focused upon the neuromuscular control of the slide in all seven positions of the slide trombone. Henderson (1942), White (1972) and White and Basmajian (1973) clarified the muscular pattern of the lips in controlling trumpet embouchure. Although White (1972) was also interested in mouthpiece pressure, it was Froelich (1987) who refined the instrumentation and protocol to effectively identify direct (normal) and shear forces applied to the trombone mouthpiece. He found direct pressures higher in trombonists playing in the high registers or playing fortissimo. A high note played loudly used three times the force of a low note played softly (571 vs 1875 grams). As the first researcher to consider mouthpiece shear force, Froelich suggested greater shear force was used to perform fortissimo and at higher pitches; however, he also noted more force was used to perform low pitches than to perform the middle pitches. He also suggested that less shear force seemed to identify a better quality of sound.

In controlling their technical performance, most musicians also manipulate cumbersome instruments which encourage awkward postures or positions because of the nature of the instrument or the cramped orchestra pit in which the musician must perform. Typically, the number of musicians exceeds the space requirements, for comfortable playing, and instruments may be held in an awkward position, or musicians must sit with leg and hip imbalances due to sharing a music stand or difficulty in manipulating a bow or slide while keeping both the conductor and music clearly in view.

Control of the instrument itself or the arms in moving to produce sound frequently leads to problems of the upper extremities and/or low back. Silverstople (1983), Fry (1986), and Elbaum (1986) note that musicians suffer from upper limb overuse syndromes. Flute, double-bass, guitar, violin, and cello are particularly problematic instruments for musicians ages 17–24, who have the highest incidence of back pain. Sex differences exist only in relation to those instruments which are predominantly played by males, e.g., double-bass (Silverstople, 1983).

Note the pianist in Fig. 13-5 whose upper body is totally tense in playing a chord. If it is not the final chord that ends the musical selection, it would be impossible to reposition the hands on keys in the upper register. This is similar to the fencer who commits totally to the thrust, without considering the possibility of being parried. Playing from an erect posture allows the pianist to use a slight body lean to play notes in the upper register (Fig. 13-6) while remaining prepared to move to another keyboard position. If only the arms are moved to play high octave chords (Fig. 13-7) the pianist would quickly fatigue the muscles of the back and shoulder. Sitting erect at the piano (Fig. 13-8) and using a bench height that maintains the lower arm parallel to the keyboard is the posture which produces the least tension in the shoulders and upper back. The pianist in Fig. 13-9 collapses the spine which produces fatigue in the back and shoulder muscles. To alleviate this discomfort, the pianist retracts the shoulders, allows the pelvis to tilt forward, and sits (Fig. 13-10) with a hyperextended lumbar spine to relieve tensions—a position conducive to producing low back pain.

Playing style for the violin changed from being held against the chest to the virtuoso technique of Paganini. As a result of the violin being fixed at the chin, considerable fatigue and pain occurred in the bow arm and lower back. Sieber (1969) studied the violin bowing arm in an effort to identify problems unique to its use. A recent Swedish invention of a different form of support for the violin was developed to minimize spine problems. Gamba leg has been described among musicians who attempted to play the gamba (an old-time, violin-type instrument), and who suffered overuse syndrome of the leg as a result of holding the instrument securely against the chest by using leg pressure (Howard, 1982). Of those under age 25 who play the violin, 75% suffer back pain (Silverstople, 1983), which suggests that, at an age when musicians are increasing practice and performance time, back injury is prevalent. Biofeedback during practice has been utilized to help string and woodwind musicians reduce unnecessary tensions (Levee, Cohen and Rickles, 1976, Levine and Irvine, 1984, Morasky, Reynolds and Clarke, 1981).

Double-bass and cello players may suffer targets for back prob-

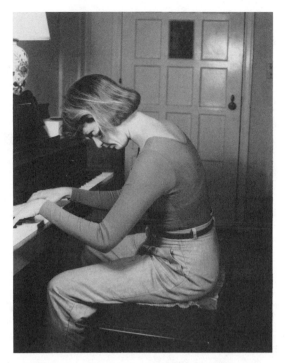

Fig. 13-5. *Pianist striking chord with total upper body tension.*

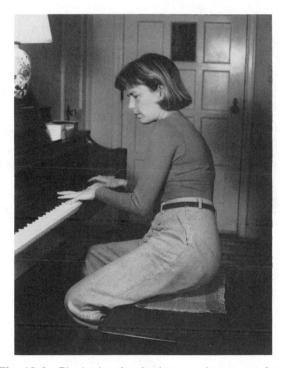

Fig. 13-6. *Pianist leaning body toward upper register.*

417

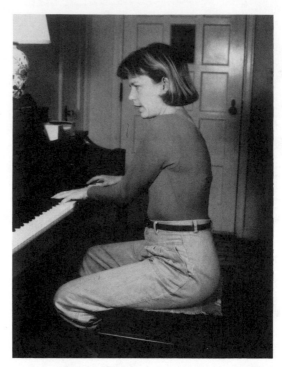

Fig. 13-7. *Pianist moving only the arms toward upper register.*

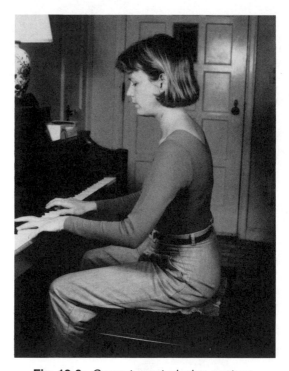

Fig. 13-8. *Correct erect playing posture.*

418

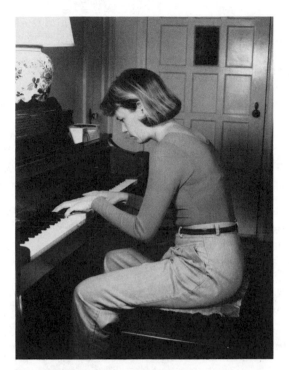

Fig. 13-9. *Playing keys with a collapsed spine posture.*

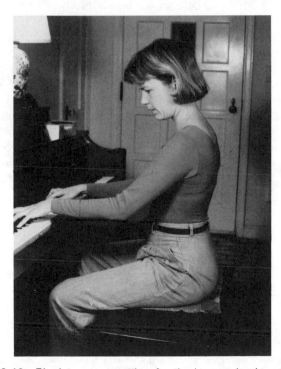

Fig. 13-10. *Pianist compensating for tired upper back muscles.*

419

lems because of the instrument's massive size, and the functioning of the instrument as a long lever. Considerable effort has been directed toward improving posture of double-bass players as well as their facility for manipulating the large implement through variations in chair height and music stand placement. Guitarists also have problems related to the imbalanced positioning of their instrument during play (Silverstople, 1983).

In singers and wind instrumentalists, abdominal control of breathing is critical. In novices, serious back problems are related to lack of abdominal strength and the inability to control the pelvis during standing and seated playing. It is important that, even during practice, these musicians maintain a balanced, erect posture to facilitate their breathing and performance. Although a relatively lightweight instrument, the flute forces an imbalanced posture because the performer must sit or stand with arms directed to the right side of the body, away from the body center. This posture leads to back difficulties; therefore, flutists are encouraged to execute movements toward the opposite side of the body or to perform relaxation exercises during resting passages (See Fig. 13-11).

Pianists and drummers are especially susceptible to overuse injuries of the hands. Fry (1986) noted that among injured pianists, the problem was not a simple acute attack of pain. Nearly half had experienced symptoms for a period of one to five years, and one fifth had suffered longer. As might be expected the site of pain was predominantly the hand/wrist and all levels of the spine. Leading with a flexed hand in a fast upward run of the piano (Fig. 13-12) is more damaging than leading with the elbow and maintaining the wrist as an extension of the forearm (Fig. 13-13). Drummers, because they use the sticks almost as if they were weapons, suffer not only from chronic hand problems but may also develop calluses around the nerve which require surgical removal (Lubell 1987; Van Horn, 1987).

Contrasts between differing levels of instrumental musicians have indicated that professionals generally play more efficiently (with less muscular activity) and control the mouthpiece and bow with less force. In the bowing arm, Sieber (1969) found greater muscular activity among

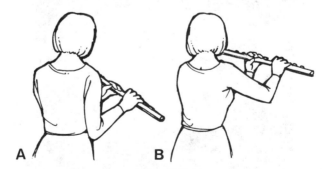

Fig. 13-11. *Playing the flute (a) using the hip for support and (b) holding the flute correctly.*

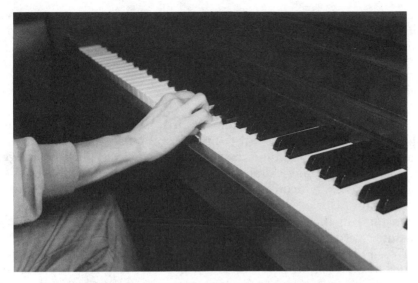

Fig. 13-12. *Scale run with wrist leading a radially flexed hand.*

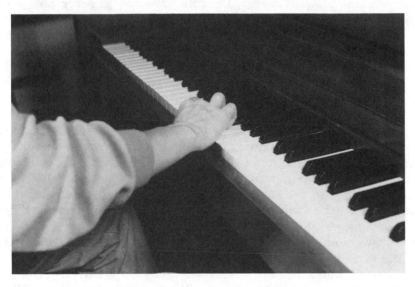

Fig. 13-13. *Run played with elbow leading and the hand wrist aligned.*

the student violinists when compared with professionals. Lammers (1983) identified professional trombonists as moving the slide more quickly to position with less muscular activity thus allowing greater time for controlling tonal qualities. Froelich (1987) described professional trombonists as using less direct pressure as well as shear force against the mouthpiece. White (1972) identified that muscular activity in the lips of trumpet players was equally divided between the top and bottom lips in professionals, but more weighted toward the top lip in beginners. Froelich (1987) supported this finding in trombonists, suggesting that shear force was detrimental to the quality of the tone produced.

OTHER ARTISTS

The stage performer is often required to manipulate heavy implements, remain in distorted positions, and rehearse for long hours. Consider the role of Albin in the show "La Cage aux Folles." For eight shows a week for more than a year, Walter Charles maneuvered in high-heel shoes, which caused his calf muscles to knot up, resulting in a painful Achilles tendon. This was in addition to the risk of falling downstairs in the unaccustomed footwear. As a result of an ankle fracture, Katharine Hepburn was forced to play her role in *A Matter of Gravity* from a wheelchair. Because of the complexity of the make-up for *Elephant Man,* the actor was trapped for long hours behind the heavy debris configured to resemble the physical change in the man he portrayed. In *Creeps,* actors produced the effect of moving as if they had cerebral palsy. However, the role gave rise to aches and pains and reactivated old injuries, until physicians and physical therapists, serving as medical choreographers, identified problematic repeated movements and worked with the actors to find a safer way to produce the same effect (Rowes, 1986).

Historically, people maneuvered flags, banners, and weapons. Film and theatrical performances require that these implements be handled safely and efficiently in a confined space. Stage fights of all types must be carefully choreographed to prevent unnecessary injury to the adversaries or the surrounding cast. Movements of flags and banners must be carefully practiced to minimize the low back pain associated with balancing a long, weighty lever. Tree trimmers who use a saw blade attached to the end of a long pole also have back pain; thus, back pain is not an unusual reward for controlling banners and flags.

Because of the hazardous actions executed in movies and television shows, stunt men and women have become important performers. In the early stages of a career, an actor or actress may be asked to perform all stunts without a stand-in; however, when the economic value to the movie or show changes, the star is replaced in any dangerous action. The replacement is usually a stunt athlete, who is an expert at absorbing force in a very short time, with the aid of various shock-absorbing materials, such as mats and pits. When the hero is thrown from a second-story window, the stunt man takes the fall, landing on shock-absorbing materials not seen by the audience. In sports, we see similar force absorption in the flexing of legs and trunk or the use of a special pit in landing. A beginning judo lesson includes the practice of various techniques for landing safely.

Art medicine clinics also note complaints from professional visual artists, who have a high incidence of low back, neck, and shoulder complaints. Solutions were found through a video analysis of the artist at work. A fifteen-minute video revealed biomechanical factors which contributed to these musculoskeletal complaints (Chang, Bejjani, and Chyan, 1986). The angle of the neck and trunk flexion, as well as angular velocities of the trunk and limbs were significantly higher among males. As might be expected, artists working on fine detail showed less variation in back and neck flexion than did artists who made larger brush movements. Calculated muscle tensions were several times greater than those of the neutral body position. When painting for long hours, the artist's arm might well feel as fatigued as that of a baseball pitcher (Rowes, 1986).

TRENDS AND GUIDELINES

Sophisticated technological tools can and have been used for more stringent scientific analysis of artists movement patterns. When used by a team of concerned individuals from several professional groups, the risks to performance can be reduced, and movement efficiency enhanced. A three-year program of biyearly screening of dancers at the University of California, Irvine has resulted in reducing the number of alignment problems. More dancers are visiting the trainer or kinesiologist as soon as a problem develops, and the number of debilitating injuries has been reduced. The medical team at Irvine includes an athletic trainer, an orthopedic surgeon, an expert in evaluating feet for pointe work, and a kinesiologist, who work closely in monitoring and advising dancers (Plastino, 1987). Similar teams have reported positive results with artists at the Miller Health Care Institute for the Performing Arts in New York (Rowes, 1986; Van Horn, 1987). Early screening to identify functional anatomical or postural alignment problems also plays a role in the development of technique in children. Because of their skeletal immaturity, elementary-age children might be encouraged to play trumpet, rather than tuba, and ballet dancers encouraged to wait until they are older to begin pointe work.

Because artists need a healthy body to perform, they are encouraged to enter into a conditioning and warm-up routine not unlike that of an elite athlete. All artists are encouraged to warm up their bodies and the active body parts, their hands, arms, and shoulder area, before engaging in their art form. Strength development of important muscle groups is encouraged even to the extent of suggesting that dancers might train with external weights (Plastino, 1987). Dancers also need to stretch the agonist and antagonist muscles to facilite greater range of motion in all planes. To meet the needs for long periods of technique practice, artists should begin work very gradually after a prolonged layoff. With a better understanding of the anatomical, biomechanical, and physiological aspects of controlling fingers or bowing arm, and the limitations of the body, artists can expect to be more successful in preventing injurious conditions that result from overuse or faculty technique. They will also be able to pace their work, cope with fatigue, and perform more effectively.

MINI-LAB LEARNING EXPERIENCES

1. Assume the correct position of the flute player in Fig. 13-11, using a ruler or stick for the flute. Try both seated and standing variations in positions of spine and feet and different size and direction of your supporting base. Identify the best position for lengthy practice periods.
2. Sit at a piano striking a key or chord, using the weight of the finger, finger and hand, adding additional segments until finger, hand, forearm, arm, and trunk are involved. What action produces the loudest sound, the best staccato, the fastest tremelo? How is production of a loud tone similar to throwing a ball for distance?
3. Play a piano chord in the low registers for a maximum sound. Can you move quickly to play a chord in the high register of the piano? What makes it easier to move? What movement concepts are similar to a fencer lunging for a point and returning to en guarde or retreat?
4. Hold a canoe paddle as if it were a flag in a parade. Experiment with different angles from vertical to horizontal. Which is easiest and which hardest to control? Try different hand positions. Which gives greatest control of the flag?
5. What suggestions could you give a comedian for taking a pratfall (landing on the seat and/or back) on stage? How is this force dissipation similar to sliding in baseball?

MINI-LAB LEARNING EXPERIENCES

A basic movement pattern in the arts may be performed in different ways to create different effects. For example, a drummer may toss and control the sticks between beats on the drum without change of the underlying rhythmic pattern. Dancers can perform leaps in various ways to create different aesthetic qualities.

Compare the two leaps in Fig. 13-14, describing and measuring the differences. Hypothesize what the goals were for each dancer.

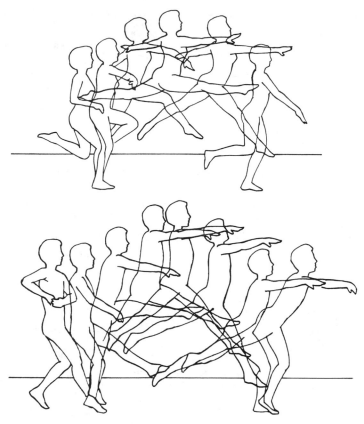

Fig. 13-14. *Two styles of leaps executed for two different purposes. Analyze the height, distance traveled and pertinent limb movements that differentiate the two performances. (Courtesy of Ray Garcelon.) Scale = 25:1.*

REFERENCES

Brink, C. (1987). Cinematographic analysis of the sissonne ouverte in female dancers. Unpublished doctoral dissertation, University of Minnesota, Minneapolis.

Chang, W., Bejjani, F. J., & Chyan, D. (1986). Biomechanical basis of musculoskeletal disorders among visual artists. In Bejjani, F. J. (Ed.) *Proceedings of North American Congress on Biomechanics.*

Elbaum, L. (1986). Muscularskeletal problems of instrumental musicians. *Journal of Orthopaedic and Sport Physical Therapy, 8*(6), 285–287.

Fitt, S. S. (1987). Corrective exercises for two muscular imbalances: Tight hip flexors and pectoralis minor syndrome. *JOHPERD, 58*(5), 45–48.

Froelich, J. P. (1987). Mouthpiece forces during trombone performances. Unpublished doctoral dissertation, University of Minnesota, Minneapolis.

Fry, H. J. H. (1986). Overuse syndrome of the upper limb in musicians. *The Medical Journal of Australia, 144,* 182–183, 185.

Henderson, H. W. (1942). An experimental study of trumpet embouchure. *Journal of the Acoustical Society of America, 13,* 58–64.

Hinson, M., Buckman, S., Tate, J. & Sherrill, C. (1977). The grand jete en tournant entrelace (Tour Jete): An analysis through motion photography. *Dance Research Journal CORD, 10*(1), 9–13.

Howard, P. L. (1982). Gamba leg. *New England Journal of Medicine, 306*(18), 1115.

Huddleston, C. B. & Pratt, S. M. (1983). Cymbal player's shoulder. *New England Journal of Medicine, 309*(23), 1402.

Irvine, J. K. & LeVine, W. R. (1981). The use of biofeedback to reduce left hand tension for string players. *American String Teacher, 31,* 10–32.

Kelly, E. (1987). The dancer's back. *JOHPERD, 58*(5), 41–44.

BIOMECHANICS IN THE ARTS **425**

Kirkendall, D. T., Bergfeld, J. A., Calabrese, L., Lomabrdo, J. A., Street, G., Weiker, G. G. (1984). Isokinetic characteristics of ballet dancers and the response to a season of ballet training. *The Journal of Orthopedic and Sports Physical Therapy*, 5(4)207–211.

Kravits, S. R. (1987). Basic concepts of biomechanics relating the foot and ankle to overuse injuries *JOHPERD*, 58(5), 31–33.

Lammers, M. E. (1983). An electromyographic examination of selected muscles in the right arm during trombone performance. Unpublished doctoral dissertation, University of Minnesota, Minneapolis.

Levee, J. R., Cohen, M. J. & Rickles, W. H. (1976). Electromyographic biofeedback for relief of tension in the facial and throat muscles of a woodwind musician. *Biofeedback and Self-Regulation* 1(1), 113–130.

Levine, W. R. & Irvine, J. K. (1984). In vivo EMG biofeedback in violin and violin pedagogy. *Biofeedback and Self-Regulation*, 9(2), 161–168.

Lubell, A. (1987). Physicians get in tune with performing artists. *Physician and Sportsmedicine* 15(6), 246–256.

Micheli, L. J. (1984). Physiologic profiles of female professional ballerinas. *Clinics in Sports Medicine*, 3(1), 199–209.

Morasky, R. L., Reynolds, C. & Clarke, G. (1981). Using biofeedback to reduce left arm extension EMG of string players during musical performance. *Biofeedback Self-Regulation*, 6(4), 565–572.

Norman, D. O. & Grodin, M. A. (1984). Injuries from break dancing. *American Family Physician*, 30(4), 109–112.

Ortmann, O. (1962). *The physiological mechanics of piano technique*. New York: E. P. Dutton & Co., Inc.

Plastino, J. G. (1987). The University dancer physical screening. *JOHPERD*, 58(5), 49–50.

Polnauer, F. & Marks, M. (1964). *Senso-motor study and its application to violin playing*. Urbana, Illinois: American String Teachers Association.

Rowes, B. (1986). To deal with their special needs, painters and performers can turn to a new specialty! Arts medicine. *People Magazine*, 26(21), 101.

Ryman, R. S. & Ranney, D. A. (1978). A preliminary investigation of two variations of the Grand Battement Devant. *Dance Research Journal, CORD*, 11(1), 2–11.

Sieber, R. E. (1969). Contraction-movement patterns of violin performers. Unpublished doctoral dissertation, Indiana University, Bloomington.

Silverstolpe, L. (1983). Ergonomic problems amongst musicians. Lecture Fimm-Congress, Zurich, Sept. 10.

Teitz, C. C. (1987). Patellofemoral pain in dancers. *JOPHERD*, 58(5), 34–36.

Teitz, C. C., Harrington, R. M. & Wiley, H. (1985). Pressures on the foot in pointe shoes. *Foot and Ankle*, 5(5), 216–221.

Van Horn, R. (1987). Music medicine: The Miller Health Care Institute. *Modern Drummer*, 28–31, 100–105.

White, E. R. (1972). Electromyographic potentials of selected facial muscles and labial mouthpiece pressure measurement in the embouchure of trumpet players. Unpublished doctoral dissertation. Columbia University, New York City.

White, E. R. & Basmajian, J. V. (1973). Electromyography of lip muscles and their role in trumpet playing. *Journal of Applied Physiology*, 35(6), 892–897.

Part IV   Sports Biomechanics

Essential concepts for teaching, coaching, prevention of injury, enhancing performance, and training in sports

14

Catching, Falling, and Landing

MECHANICS OF STOPPING MOVING OBJECTS

Among the motor skills that human beings perform is stopping a moving object. The object may be external, such as a ball, or it may be the performer's own body, as in landing from a height. The pattern of joint action varies with the situation, but in all situations, the mechanical principles are the same.

When stopping an action if the stop is skillfully made, the momentum of the moving object is decreased gradually by joint actions. These actions are such that the object is permitted to continue its motion as its velocity is gradually decreased. If the object is contacted with the hands and the arms extended to meet it, the joint actions are those of a pulling pattern, usually extension of the upper arm and flexion of the forearm. Although the joint actions in pulling and stopping are the same, the source of energy differs. The momentum of the oncoming object moves the segments in the direction in which the object was moving; at the same time, muscular effort resists that motion. As the upper arm is extended by the force of the object, the shoulder flexors resist; as the forearm is flexed, the elbow extensors resists. In pulling, the object to be moved resists while shoulder extensors and elbow flexors contract. Thus the muscular tension is greater during pulling than catching. Likewise, when the body lands from a height, the momentum of the center of gravity tends to cause flexion at the ankle, knee, and hip joints. These actions are resisted by the extensor muscles at the joints.

Catching, falling, and landing are specialized cases of impact, or collision. They represent the impacting of a living body with another living body or with an external inanimate object. There was little or no consideration given to reducing risk of injury.

The basic mechanical principles involved in stopping a moving object or one's own moving body in action are based on the effective and efficient manner of dissipating the kinetic energy of the moving body without injury to the performer. The kinetic energy ($\frac{1}{2}$ mV^2) of an object can be reduced to zero or to other safe limits by the following methods:

1. Using as great a surface area as possible in catching or landing.
2. Using as great a distance as possible. This may be accomplished through movement of body parts, deformation of body parts, or moving the entire body.
3. Using as great a mass as possible in catching or landing.
4. Regulating the position of one's center of gravity for dynamic control. For example, in falling, the person is able to continue movement of the body into a controlled rolling action that terminates in a stance, rather than lose equilibrium, which causes the body to tumble several revolutions and in uncontrolled directions, terminating in an upside-down position.
5. Using materials other than the human body to perform steps 1 to 4.

CATCHING

Catching is the act of reducing the momentum of an object in flight to the point of zero or near-zero velocity and retaining possession of it at least momentarily. This is accomplished by using the hands, body, feet and auxiliary pieces of equipment. The momentum of the object is transferred to the receiving mechanism. When an object is light in weight and traveling slowly, a human being can easily stop it. However, if the object is heavy or is traveling at great speed or both, the transfer of momentum must be gradual to prevent injury to the hands or other parts of the body and to allow the receiver to control the object once in possession of it.

When one part or parts of the body, such as the hands, are held rigid at the moment that a fast-moving object comes in contact with it, they must absorb the full force of the impact. In sports, the momentum of an object being caught is decreased by increasing the distance at which it is caught; this process is known as giving, or recoiling, with the object until it is traveling slowly enough to be controlled accurately.

If the object to be caught is heavy, such as a large medicine ball, or is traveling unusually fast, such as a fastball thrown by a baseball pitcher, to dissipate its momentum over a long distance may be difficult and will take more time than can be allotted during the process of playing a particular game. The more practical procedure is to increase the mass (inertia) of the stopping mechanism and decrease the distance over which it travels. For example, the baseball catcher dissipates the momentum of the ball thrown by the pitcher by placing the body directly in front of the path of the oncoming ball. He assumes a stance whereby the feet are placed in a stride position with the legs flexed and the center of gravity low; this is the best posture in which to recoil from the force (momentum of the ball), and at the same time offering as much of the body to absorb the momentum of the ball as possible.

The receiver must be careful not to make unnecessary body motions when running to receive an object. Unnecessary up-and-down movements such as raising and lowering the center of gravity and thereby moving the head and eyes up and down through a vertical plane, may cause the receiver to lose track of the flight path of the object. Outstretching the arms while running may cause receivers to slow down because they are not using the arms properly in the run and also they are projecting the center of gravity too far forward. It also may tense the arms and cause them to drop the ball.

A ball is not caught with the fingers; rather, it is received first against the middle of the palm of the hand (made into the form of a cup), and then the fingers close around it, preventing it from escaping. If it is caught against the rigid heel of the hand, it is likely to rebound too quickly from the hand and may also cause injury.

The effective catcher (receiver in any sport or endeavor) has loose, flexible hands to catch the object and to dissipate its momentum gradually. Correct body posture is also essential. Placing the hands in the best possible position is another requirement for success. For example, a ball traveling at a height below the waist is caught with the fingers pointing downward. In all instances, the hands are placed so that they have a basketlike quality. Seldom does a skilled performer not make use of two hands, even though the actual catch is made with one hand. The object (such as a ball) may rebound out of one hand if the momentum is not properly dissipated. The use of both hands aids in trapping the object.

Large objects thrown with great speed, such as a football (which is also thrown with a spin), are caught and then quickly cradled; that is, the receiver pins the football against the body as soon as possible to prevent its escape because of the reaction. If the arms do not have to be extended fully for the catch, the receiver, in this instance, should not do so. In the flexed position, the arm muscles can withstand the force of the impact with no chance for injury, since the impact will elicit further flexion.

When the gloves or mitts are used to catch fast-moving objects, two principles can be considered. The first principle is to allow some part other than the human body to absorb the force of impact, which can be considered as having a certain amount of either kinetic energy or momentum. The second principle is that of dissipating the force through a distance. The use of catcher's, fielder's, and first-base mitts and gloves is based on these principles (Fig. 14-1).

The material comprising the mitt usually deforms. Thus the ball embeds in the mitt and dissipates its force (energy) both through a

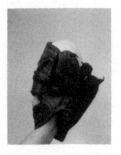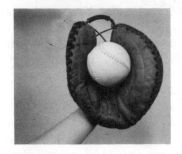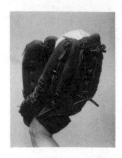

Fig. 14-1. *Catching a softball with three different mitts. Note the differences in moment arms (ball to wrist) among the three ball-mitt systems. Which one has the greatest extension of the hand? This represents the system with the longest moment arm and therefore the mitt absorbing the energy of the ball through a greater distance than the other two mitts. Which mitt appears to have the greatest amount of material to absorb the energy of the ball through material deformation?*

large surface area and increased distance. The first-base mitt functions more on the principle of increasing the distance through which the mitt moves, thus dissipating the kinetic energy of the ball. The distal end of the mitt, and thus the ball, will move approximately 15 cm after initial contact and then, because of its movement of force, cause the hand to move. Then the elbow, shoulder, and other joint angles of the body will change. The fielder's glove incorporates certain features of each of the previously-mentioned mitts.

The quantification of what actually happens during catching may be described by use of the following example: cradling a lacrosse ball in a lacrosse stick (Fig. 14-2). When the ball strikes the lacrosse basket, the materials of ball and basket deform, but only the deformation of the basket can be seen. These deformations are not sufficient to prevent rebounding of the ball. Thus the movement of the stick and arms must be performed in the direction of the ball flight.

If the flight velocity of the ball had been 20 m/sec before impact, its kinetic energy would be $\frac{1}{2} mV^2$, or 48 Nm, or joules (based on a ball weight of 2.4 N; which is 0.5 lb). Both deformation of the basket and the reactive forces caused by the lengthening and narrowing of the basket opening reduce the kinetic energy of the ball as much as 90%. Thus the ball velocity for rebounding may be no more than 5 m/sec. Movement of the arms and stick adds mass to the moving ball system and reduces the ball velocity to 0.2 m/sec, based on the conservation-of-momentum principle. Observation of the performance indicates that a distance of 0.6 m is required to reduce the velocity of the ball and arms to zero.

During the game of lacrosse a catching distance of 0.6 m requires too much time and places the ball and stick in an unsatisfactory position. An alternate method of catching involves the cradling, or rotation, of the stick about its longitudinal axis, which causes the ball to rebound from one side of the basket to the other. Thus linear dis-

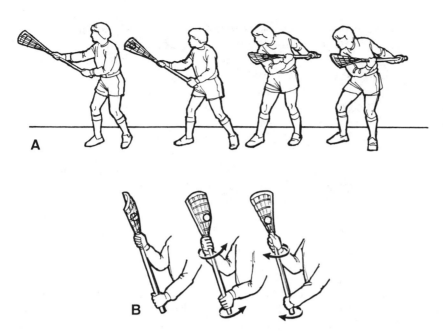

Fig. 14-2. *Catching (A), and cradling (B) techniques used in lacrosse to dissipate kinetic energy of the ball. In A, the person reaches forward toward the ball and during the catch moves the stick in the direction of the ball flight. In B, the ball is caught with a rotational movement of the stick, thereby assuming the momentum of the ball. The ball is then oscillated between the sides of the basket until it comes to rest or is thrown.*

placement is replaced by rotational displacement for the dissipation of the kinetic energy of the ball.

In most sports situations, the momentum gained during the catch may be used in starting the next movement. If the next action is to be a throw, the ball is drawn back during the catch in preparation for throwing. Whenever possible, the receiver should move the body into position for the next action as the catch is made, to reduce still further the time required for the complete movement. In addition, the momentum of the ball (since it seldom comes to a complete rest but usually continues in a small angular path as the arm is moved to throw) may be used in moving the ball in the new direction.

FALLING

Correctly-performed falling involves a gradual reduction in the momentum of the body when it comes in contact with the floor, ground, or other surface. Four general principles and techniques of protection in falling may be listed:

1. In the sit-down-and-roll technique, the center of gravity is lowered, and the action in falling is such that the weight of the body is distributed over large area. If the fall is vertical, the

CATCHING, FALLING, AND LANDING **433**

momentum should be transferred from vertical to horizontal as soon as possible to reduce the force of the fall.

2. The body projections of the body must be protected by using the fleshy parts as striking surfaces.
3. Extended levers offer a greater potential range of motion than do flexed ones. Therefore when the legs or arms strike the surface in falling, they should be prepared for the contact by being placed in near extension. Care must be taken to avoid hyperextension, which causes the joint to be rigid and to resist flexion of the limb. With the joint at an angle slightly less than 180 degrees, the force of the fall can then be taken by a gradual flexion of the legs or arms.
4. If, during a fall, the landing is made on the feet, the person must bring the center of body weight to a position above the feet, in order to utilize the shock-absorbing action of the ankles, knees, and hips.

The recovery from a stumble is mainly reflexive. Both the righting reflex and equilibrium reactions (which are instinctive) are activated. As the toe trips over an obstacle and the body starts to fall forward, reflex and equilibrium reactions are initiated. Normally the head and trunk are extended to counteract the forward momentum. The arms are often abducted to assist in regaining balance.

A person who starts to fall to the right side, for example, usually elevates and abducts the arms and extends the forearms (with arms out to the sides). The body is shifted to the left to help check the momentum to the right. The side of the buttocks is offered as the landing surface. The legs are flexed to decrease the force of the blow and to lower the center of gravity so that the distance of the fall is reduced. A rotation of the trunk may take place so that the momentum of the fall is dissipated in two directions—opposite and to the rear. Protective extension of the arms is often used to help dissipate the momentum of the fall. This action, however, has proved dangerous when the forearm has gone into hyperextension. Gymnasts, dancers, and others must be cautioned not to use the rigidly extended arm to attempt to stop a fall.

LANDING

Landing is a type of fall that is both controlled and expected and that enables the performer to strike a surface without incurring injury to the body parts if possible. Landings occur in many activities of life, from the mild ones of foot landings during walking to the landings of ski jumpers, sky divers, and pole vaulters. When a body falls, its vertical force, kinetic energy, and momentum are directly related to the distance through which it falls. Since the rate of falling is 9.8 m/sec^2, the velocity of the body increases exponentially, not linearly, as the height of fall increases. Therefore, landing on a rigid, rather nondeformable material is dangerous from heights of 3 m or more. If the landing is headfirst, the result is often death, except for the very young. In the sports arena, specialized landing surfaces are required for high jumping, pole vaulting, long jumping, and certain gymnastics events. When a landing cannot be made with the feet, the fleshy part of the thighs, hips, and shoulders are preferred landings areas. These parts are the primary landing sites in judo. For ectomorphic persons, however, no area of the body may have sufficient "padding" for a safe landing, even with landing mats. In such instances, the landing should be with the feet unless protective equipment is worn.

Kneepads are common in the sports of volleyball, basketball, football, skateboarding, and soccer. Shin guards are recommended for field hockey and soccer. Thigh pads are used in softball, baseball, and football. It is recommended that hip or thigh protection be used for gymnasts performing on the uneven parallel bars. Padding of the bars may be an alternative to padding the human body. The higher the skill level, the greater the forces are apt to be; however, the lower the skill level, the more it is likely that there will be uncontrolled landings.

In activities in which the landing is the terminal point in the movement pattern, such as in high jumping and pole vaulting, the landing surface is padded, rather than the performer. Both the pole vaulting and landing pits are above ground to decrease the falling height, and therefore the final velocity, of the performer at landing. The pits are made so that the penetration by the performer into the landing pit is approximately half the depth of the landing pit at the time the performer reaches zero velocity. This distance allows a safe, low rebound from the pit.

Since the vertical drop in long jumping is much less than in pole vaulting or high jumping, and since the landing is on the feet, an elevated landing pit is not needed. A sand pit in which the body can penetrate from 10 to 30 cm into the sand is adequate for safety. In fact, the long jump pit is slightly below the level of the takeoff board.

During recent years, the public has shown a concern for reducing the injury rate in sports. Manufacturers have produced more and better protective devices to be worn by the performer or on which the performance takes place. Sometimes there are conflicting problems in the manufacturing of a product that must be designed not only to improve safety but also to improve performance. Often an improvement in safety alters the performance capabilities or prevents the attainment of a satisfactory performance. For example, shoulder pads restrict the ability of football line players to raise the arms above shoulder height. Original tumbling mat design and construction allowed the impact forces to be absorbed at landing but prevented the execution of a second tumbling movement directly from landing. As new materials were developed, mats with an elastic component were constructed. These mats not only attenuated the energy of landing but gave a "spring" to the performer. As skill levels in tumbling improve and more complex stunts at greater heights are executed, the mats may no longer be safe, or the safe mats of today may limit the acquisition of certain skill, especially for Olympic-caliber performers.

A similar inadequacy of sports equipment has been noted with respect to jogging. Many persons, estimated in the millions, are jogging several miles on concrete sidewalks and paved streets, and competing in long-distance races on similar terrain. Jogging shoes were not originally designed with the shock attentuation qualities necessary for such conditions. Research that identifies the impact forces and the sites of impact is now helping manufacturers to design safe shoes for jogging.

The Committee on Sports Facilities and Equipment of the American Society for Testing Materials is the standards-setting body in the United States that studies the safety and performance of the equipment and facilities used in sports. Teachers and coaches can help the committee to identify problems and can provide the following information:

1. What types of injuries occur in a specific activity?
2. What landing surfaces and protective devices are in use when injuries occur?
3. Which products are unsatisfactory?
4. What is the nature of the performance in which injuries occur—for example, falling from a height, rotary movements, or absorbing forces?

IS PROTECTIVE EQUIPMENT REQUIRED?

The following questions may be posed by the movement analyst:

1. Does the force of the collision approach or exceed human tolerances?
2. Does collision occur frequently?
3. Is there a high rate of injury for this collision?

If the answer is yes to any of these questions, protective equipment should be considered.

Selection of adequate protective equipment should be based on the following criteria:

1. Protective equipment must fit the anatomy of all performers. Quite often protective equipment is designed for the average person and is unsatisfactory for some persons.
2. Protective equipment must allow freedom of movement. For example, shoulder pads used in football sometimes restrict the movement of the players to the detriment of performance.
3. Protective equipment must attenuate the "excess" force. Analysis of the protective equipment after hours or seasons of use should be made to check attenuation characteristics.

Persons with physical impairments and those with muscular weaknesses may need some type of protective equipment for activities of daily living. The tolerances of their body tissues may be much lower than those of the athletic population. In particular, the frictional forces may cause injury to hand of persons with these impairments but may have no effect on hands of athletes. Anatomic considerations, again, are of vital concern to the movement analyst in identifying the forces and level of safety of movement patterns.

MINI-LAB LEARNING EXPERIENCES

1. Rank the kinetic energy (KE) of the following falling bodies (vertical direction) and the approaching objects (horizontal direction), using the formula $KE = \frac{1}{2} mV^2$.
   a. Adult, 588 N, jumping from a bus step, 1 m above ground.
   b. Diver, 490 N, diving from a 3-m board.
   c. Ball, 19.6 N, traveling 10 m/sec.
   d. Ball, 9.8 N, traveling 30 m/sec.
   e. Long jumper, 588 N, with center of gravity 2 m above ground.
   f. Pole vaulter, 534 N, clearing a 5-m bar with a 1.5-m landing pit.
   List one or more factors of methods useful in dissipating the kinetic energy of these moving parts.
2. Observe persons catching two medicine balls of different weights. Describe the effectiveness of the action in response to both a moderate speed of flight and a fast speed of flight.
3. Catch a softball in the following manner:
   a. With "board hands," remaining stiff and letting the ball rebound.
   b. With hands.
   c. With forearms and abdomen.
   d. With hands and under conditions of increasing speed of flight until the ball "stings" at impact.
   e. With a mitt and at increasing speeds (greater than those used in step d).

REFERENCES

Annual Book of Standards—Section 15 Vol. 15.07 End Use Products (1986). American Society for Testing and Materials.

Coleman, J., Adrian, M., Yamamoto, H. (1984); "The Teaching of Mechanics of Jump Landings." In *Second National Symposium on Teaching Kinesiology and Biomechanics in Sports*, Shapiro, R. (Ed.). NIV, Dekalb.

Doherty, J. K. (1964); *Modern track and field*, Englewood Cliffs, NJ: Prentice-Hall, Inc.

Hodgson, V. R., and Thomas, L. M. (1973); Biomechanical study of football head impacts using a human head model, final report, Detroit, National Operating Committee on Standards for Athletic Equipment.

Too, D. Adrian, M. (1987); "Relationship of Lumbar Curvature and Landing Surface to Ground Reaction Forces during Gymnastic Landing." In *Biomechanics in Sports III & IV*, Terauds, J., Gowitzke, B., Holt, L. Academic Publishers: DelMar, CA.

CATCHING, FALLING, AND LANDING　　　　　　　　**437**

15
Running

INTRODUCTION

Running is a modification of walking and differs from the latter in significant aspects. First, during one phase in running, neither foot is in contact with the ground; second, at no period are both feet in contact with the ground. Although these distinctions necessitate difference in joint action, the same joints and segments are used in running as in walking. Differences in joint degrees and timing of actions can be anticipated. Since only one foot is on the ground at one time, and both feet are off the ground at one time, it is possible to run relatively smoothly with one leg shorter than the other, whereas in walking, this same condition would cause a limp. In addition, once speed in running has been developed, the force of the forward momentum is greater and contributes more to forward movement of the body than during walking. The action of the swinging leg in running is greater in amplitude and velocity and is likely to contribute the most to the forward movement of the body.

Running is a bipedal, three-dimensional action, just as is walking. All the determinants of walking are prominent in running. Pelvic rotation, pelvic tilt, lateral motion of the pelvis, flexion at the knee, foot and ankle motion, and knee motion all are present to a greater degree in running than in walking. In addition, there are greater flexion and extension of the legs and arms resulting in a wider range of motion. Thus, running requires greater lengthening of muscles and greater flexibility at the joints than does walking. The faster the run, the greater the change in movement range. A major difference is that, whereas in walking there is an overlapping of the stance phases, in running there is an overlapping of the swing phase.

Often the factors that are important in speed running are considered less important in distance running. Proper mechanical positions and speed are essential to a sprinter, whereas, physiological endurance, efficiency, and pace are all important to a distance runner. In races involving both speed and endurance, the ability to utilize proper mechanics and to have sufficient endurance is paramount. There is some use of both factors by the sprinter and the distance runner: (1) Some element of endurance is necessary in a longer sprint race, and (2) At the end of a distance race, the distance runner may need to become a sprinter and use correct mechanics to win the race.

Minor differences in postures and movement patterns have been identified in runners competing in races of varying lengths. For example, four runners are shown in Fig. 15-1 at the midsupport position. Number 1 is a sprinter and 400 m runner; number 2, an 800 m runner; number 3, a 1500 m runner; and number 4, a marathon runner. The runners have certain postural similarities and differences. The trunk angle is nearly perpendicular in all runners; the knee angle of the lead leg is higher with the sprinter and lowest with the marathon runner. The arms are moved vigorously and with more amplitude the shorter the distance if the runner is running at regular speeds. This is similar to that reported by Slocum and James.

It is believed that the mechanics of running have an effect on efficiency of performance. One measure of energy cost in running relates to the rise and fall of the center of gravity (COG). A sprinter produces a pronounced rise and fall while a distance runner exhibits a more even COG path. A distance runner may delay the onset of fatigue by maintaining a smooth, even, compact stride. Momentum is more constant, since fluctuation of force is a change in momentum. In turn, more energy is required. It may be possible to delay the onset of fatigue by maintaining effective mechanical positions such as a proper knee lift and an upright trunk.

In distance running, the less body weight carried during the run, the more effective the runner. Height varies among individuals who are successful. Excessive height could be detrimental because of wind resistance, and most distance runners are at or below the population

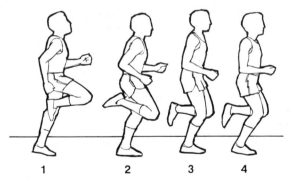

Fig. 15-1. *Four runners are shown, each in the mid-support position. In order from left to right they are: a sprinter and 400 m runner; 2, a 800 meter runner; 3, a 1500 meter runner; 4, a marathon. The runners have certain postural similarities and differences. The trunk angle is nearly perpendicular in all runners; the knee angle of the lead leg is higher with the sprinter and lowest with the marathon runner. The arms are more vigorous and with more amplitude the shorter the distance if running at regular speed. (Similar to that reported by Slocum and Bowerman.)*

mean for height. Extremely short (several inches below the mean) individuals would have difficulty when a long stride is needed. Again, a light body weight (with low body fat) would be advantageous in distance running for the short individual, especially the runner with slow-twitch muscle fibers. In speed running, fast-twitch muscle fibers are essential to be a champion.

STEP AND STRIDE

Since there is disagreement among some scholars in defining step and stride, a definition of each will be given here. A "step" is that part of the running action which commences at the moment when either foot terminates contact with the ground and continues until the opposite foot contacts the surface, whereas a "stride" consists of two steps during which there is a period of support and a period of flight. A "stride" is identified by the termination of contact of a foot with the ground through the next contact of this same foot—thus, the involvement of two steps.

GENERAL MECHANICS OF RUNNING

Stride Length

Many authors (such as Hoffman, Teeple and Sparks) have shown that there is a positive relationship between step or stride length and running velocity. It must be kept in mind that speed of the run equals stride length times stride frequency. If a short-legged runner desires a fast pace, this runner will have to take more strides per unit of time than a longer-legged runner, whose stride should be longer. A combination of long stride and high frequency is an indication of a fast runner, all other things being equal. Explosive push-off and flexibility help determine stride length. On the other hand, a runner desiring to run a long distance will run with a short stride and will depend on pace and low stride frequency to conserve energy.

In most instances, leg length is associated with body height. The taller person usually has longer legs and therefore should be able to take a longer stride than a shorter person. In addition, a positive relationship exists between the force exhibited by the legs at push off and length of stride. Furthermore, if there is a minimum amount of braking force at the foot down position, the runner can move faster in a forward direction.

Speed runners use the longest stride of all the runners. The stride length is approximately 4.87 m (16 ft) for men and 3.65 to 4.26 m (12 to 14 ft) for women. The top female sprinters have a step frequency of 4.48 steps per second, and the male sprinters, 5 steps per second. (Use double these values for stride frequency.)

It has been reported that initial increases in speed by an experienced runner is a result of increased stride length (SL). After a stride of optimum length has been attained, further increase in speed becomes a matter of increasing stride frequency (SF). A formula to have in mind in evaluating running is speed $= SL \times SF$. It must also be kept in mind, however, that excessive increase in SL may bring about a decrease in SF.

Arm Action

The main purpose of the arm action in running is to counterbalance the off-center thrust of the legs. The arms of the fast runner move in opposition to the legs and are 180 degrees out of phase with the adjacent leg, as in walking. However, as the speed increases, the arms move more rapidly in a flexed to partially extended position. The arms move toward the midline of the body in the forward position and then to the rear, with the hands seldom going beyond the hips (See Fig. 15-1.)

Aristotle (384–322 B.C.), who has been called the father of kinesiology, was able to observe arm action and its contribution to the running motion. More than three centuries before Christ, Aristotle wrote:

> The animal that moves makes its change of position by pressing against that which is beneath it. Hence, athletes jump farther if they have the weights in their hands than if they have not, and runners run faster if they swing their arms, for in extension of the arms there is a kind of leaning upon the hands and wrists.

The path of the center of the body during the running stride has been studied by Beck. The subjects, 12 boys ages 6 through 12 years and representing the first 6 grades, were selected from their classmates as having the better time scorers in a 27.4 m (30 yd) run. Beck found that, regardless of the runner's age, all paths were wavelike, reaching the high point, shortly after the body became airborne. After the high point the center of gravity moved downward through the next foot contact and for a short time afterward. The next rise began while the foot was in contact with the ground and continued through the takeoff, and the cycle was then repeated. With increased age, there was an increase in the horizontal and vertical distances traveled by the center of gravity during each stride, and the stride also became longer. With age, the percentage of the total stride time represented by foot contact decreased, and, of course, that of flight time increased. The horizontal velocity of the center of gravity also increased with age; for the flight phase, however, the percentage of the horizontal velocity decreased, and for the support phase it increased.

Center of Gravity

The rise and fall of the center of gravity is greater in running than in walking (5 to 6.3 cm (2 to 2.5 in)), but the amount of force against the ground is nearly the same for running and walking, approximately two times body weight. (See Fig. 15-2.) Slow or unskilled jogging may produce greater vertical forces than running and may impose undue stress on some of the internal organs.

The jarring effect of jogging can be reduced by using rubberized or foam insoles, which reduce the friction and vertical force to the body. They have a cushioning effect of up to 20% to 30% more than a regular shoe and can be a hope to many who jog, including elderly persons.

Speed/Tension

To prevent tension from occurring in the arms and neck, the runner must learn to run explosively but in a semi-relaxed manner; that is, the runner tries to run as fast as possible without unduly contracting the arm and neck muscles or other muscles extraneous to the action. This is termed differential relaxation. Runners use some of the following strategies to reduce tension: (1) Relax the hands by closing the fingers without clinching the fist. During distance running, the hands are held very loosely. (2) Relax the jaw by keeping the mouth open and the jaw loose.

Tension usually begins in the neck, jaw, and arms and then proceeds to the torso and finally to the legs. As a result of extraneous tension, the legs may rotate so much externally that the stride of the sprint runner is decreased considerably and the speed is reduced.

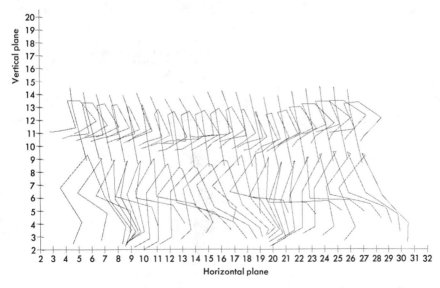

Fig. 15-2. *Computer printout of line segment tracings of film of marathon runner. Note short stride and small lift of body's center of gravity. (Prepared by James Richards)*

Foot Position

The contact of the runner's foot with the ground at foot strike is slightly different from that of the walker's foot, the degree of difference depending on the velocity of the run (Fig. 15-3). At high speed, the contact is first made on the lateral edge of the ball of the foot. The heel is lowered, and a controversy exists as to whether it actually touches the ground. In middle-distance running, the first contact is made with the rear part of the foot. In the case of slower speed or distance running, the heel does come down so that the foot is flat on the ground at contact. In very slow running, the heel strikes the ground first. The body weight moves forward after foot contact, as in walking. However, the contact time of the foot in running is much shorter than in walking, being slightly less than 0.01 second for speed runners and greater for other runners, depending on their body velocity. In walking, it is plus-or-minus 1.0 second, depending on speed.

In reviewing publications on the direction of foot movement immediately before contact, Fortney found that authors did not agree on the direction but also, that in most cases, they did not make clear whether they referred to movement with reference to a fixed point in space or to a fixed point in the body. In studying film of eight elementary school boys whose runs were photographed when they were in the second grade and again in each of the three following years, Fortney found that the heel moved forward with reference to a fixed point in space and that there was no apparent difference between runners classified as good and those classified as poor. However, she found that the heel moved backward with reference to a point within the body (the knee). Since the forward movement of the total body was greater than the backward movement caused by flexion at the knee

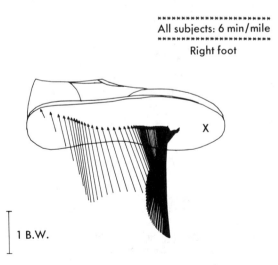

All subjects: 6 min/mile

Right foot

1 B.W.

Fig. 15-3. *Computer graphics of magnitude and direction of force vectors acting on shoe during running. (Courtesy Penn State University Biomechanics Laboratory.)*

and extension at the hip, the foot moved forward immediately before contact.

Other findings by Fortney are used to point out differences between the skilled and the unskilled runners: 1) at the beginning of the flight phase, the skilled runners had greater flexion in the leading limb at the knee and the hip, the latter bringing the thigh closer to the front horizontal; 2) at the beginning of the contact phase, the skilled runners had greater flexion at the knee of the rear limb, bringing the heel closer to the buttock.

Knee Action

During speed running, the knee lift (thigh flexion) should reach nearly the level of the hip, and the rear "kickup" of the foot (flexion of leg during swing phase) should again be nearing the horizontal. Knee lift and rear kickup are not as pronounced in the distance runs.

The position whereby the heel is moved high and just to the edge of the buttocks during the running cycle is an advantage. The radius of rotation is decreased as the heel moves high and closer to the edge of the buttocks. This position is a characteristic of a fast runner.

Flexion at the knee occurs at foot down, and extension occurs as the toe-off movement takes place. There is some disagreement regarding the amount of extension present as the foot leaves the ground. Apparently, with the world's top sprinters, complete extension does not occur, because of the short time the foot is in contact with the ground (support time). Some researchers have found an increase in flexion at foot down concomitant with an increase in running velocity.

Braking Force

It has been hypothesized that if the foot of a runner is moving backward as it strikes the ground with a negative velocity equal to the positive velocity of the center of gravity moving forward, the braking force would be zero. It is known that faster runners show a greater negative foot velocity than do slower runners. It appears that this diminution of the braking force aids in speed running. Most researchers agree that if the foot at foot strike is directly under the center of gravity, the braking force is reduced to a minimum.

Hip Action

Considerable rotation at the hip occurs during the sprint action, whereas much less occurs during long-distance running. The former motion results in a long stride and facilitates the development of greater stride frequencies. The reverse is desired in long-distance running.

Support and Nonsupport Time

It has been found that as the speed of running increases, the nonsupport time increases and the support time decreases. Most researchers have found that the respective times may be close to 50% for each. With distance runners, the ratio may be reversed. World-class sprinters show an increased nonsupport time (52% nonsupport and 48% support). It is just the opposite in the fatigue situation; the more fatigued the runner, the more time is spent in support.

Trunk Angle

The trunk angle, or upper body lean, during running has been a subject of debate for some time. Body lean is intertwined with acceleration, forward lean occurring during acceleration, backward lean occurring during deceleration. There is some agreement that after the initial starting distance, which is 13.71 to 28.28 m (15 to 20 yd) in sprinting, there need be very little lean or inclination. Many coaches are now advocating an almost upright position after an optimum running posture is attained.

It is known that sprinters do not accelerate after running 54.8 to 64.0 m (60 to 70 yd, 6 seconds) from the start. They just try to maintain a constant velocity as long thereafter as possible. On the other hand, distance runners set a pace and may accelerate at times to obtain a better position among the other runners or to relieve monotony or tension. In the latter instance, they may lean forward to increase velocity, and then as they assume a more even pace, they become more upright.

Usually the researchers find a trunk lean of 5 to 7 degrees forward during sprint running. A few have even found a trunk lean a few degrees to the rear. In distance running, the trunk lean is about the same as in sprinting. Depending on the wind or air resistance, the lean may be greater or less than upright. The important factor is that muscle effort should not be used to maintain body lean, and the respiratory muscles must be free to function.

It has been said by some that the sprinter inclines the trunk more than does the long-distance runner. Slocum and James question whether any skilled runner, regardless of the distance of the run, inclines the trunk forward beyond the vertical after the acceleration of the start. They also maintain that there is a backward tilting of the pelvis accompanied by flexion of the spine and that this "flat-backed" position increases the ability to rotate the thigh laterally. (Lateral rotation of the thigh is needed to place the foot in the desired direction as the pelvis is rotated forward over the supporting hip.) The lower-limb actions of a sprinter and distance runner are the same in general appearance, but there are differences in detail. The sprinter has greater thigh flexion in the swinging limb and thus raises the flexed knee higher; the stride is also longer, there are more strides per second, and a smaller area of the foot contacts the ground. Other investigators (Sparks, for example) found trunk inclination to be 2 to 4 degrees forward of the vertical.

TYPES OF TERRAIN

Curve Running

Running a curve is relatively easy at a slow pace. As velocity is increased, the runner must make certain accommodations to negotiate the curved path effectively. For example, the center of gravity is moved laterally to the inside of the track oval (body lean toward curb), and a wider base of support is achieved with the feet spaced somewhat apart to give better balance. The runner may accelerate part of the way on the straightways, but must run under control at the initial entrance onto the curve; then the runner may accelerate on the curve. These accommodations are necessary because of centrifugal force. To overcome this force, the runner initially pushes outward with the feet and leans the body toward the inside to reduce the radius of rotation and increase the lateral ground reaction forces; otherwise the runner would be forced toward the outside and would not be able to run the curve effectively. The greater the velocity of the runner, the greater will be the lean.

Grade Running

Henson studied six cross-country male runners while they were running on a treadmill at 15 combinations of speed and grade. He found that when increasing speed on a downhill slope, the runner should do so primarily by increasing the length of his stride. This results in a more bounding type of movement but makes greater use of the pull of gravity as the runner moves farther down the hill with each stride as the flight phase becomes greater. The muscle contractions would be primarily eccentric opposing the pull of gravity, which do not require the same amount of energy as concentric contractions which dominate when running on the level or uphill. Also, because fewer strides per minute are required in this bounding type of movement, the limbs are not required to oscillate as rapidly nor as frequently; thus, additional energy is saved in accelerating and decelerating the limbs. When running up a long incline, the runner should shorten each stride and lean into the hill slightly, slowing the pace to avoid producing excessive oxygen debt. These techniques should aid the novice runner in making the most efficient adjustment to a hilly cross-country and result in maximum improvement of performance (Henson, 1976).

ANALYSIS OF JOINT ACTIONS

Joint Actions of Supporting Limb

In Fig. 15-4 are shown the angles of the lower limb measured on film of a male Olympic competitor as he neared the finish line in the

1500 m race. The time per frame for this film is based on the speed, which is assumed to be approximately 64 frames/second. The support phase was therefore approximately 0.075 second. The runner landed with full foot contact, and the foot flexed immediately and continued to do so for 0.03 second. This action would be caused by the forward momentum of the body and consequent rotation at the ankle joint. At 0.03 second, extension at the ankle begins, the forward momentum cannot now rotate the body around the ankle joint, and its force must act at the metatarsal joints. This action continues to the takeoff. Extension at the ankle, as the foot (except for the toes) is lifted, moves the leg backward and upward from the positions to which it would be carried solely by the metarsophalangeal action. The leg flexes at contact, easing the force of impact as the foot touches the ground. During the final 0.045 second, there is extension at the knee, carrying forward the entire body except the supporting leg and foot. This action is due to contraction of the knee extensors and the forward momentum of the body. Flexion at the hip joint occurs at impact, followed by extension to maintain the angle of inclination of the trunk.

It is interesting to compare the joint actions of the skilled runner

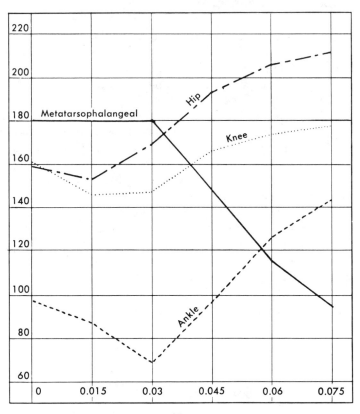

Fig. 15-4. *Joint actions of supporting limb of male Olympic contestant during foot contact in running. Time in seconds is shown at bottom; angles between body segments are shown in degrees at left.*

with those of a college woman who had no special training in running. The joint actions of the woman as she ran at her top speed are shown in Fig. 15-5. The pattern of action is the same for the two runners; that is, the direction of joint angle change is the same. The differences are in speed of action and in range and are shown in Table 15-1. Compare the information in Figs. 15-4 and 15-5. Except for the metatarsophalangeal joints, the range of movement for the man is greater, especially at the knee and hip joints. The speed of the man's actions is also greater at all joints; in particular, at the knee, the difference is more than 8.8 times as great. Further comparisons can be made of the angles of inclination.

Joint Actions of Swinging Limb

The joint actions of the swinging limb can be visualized from the positions shown in Figs. 15-6 and 15-7. The differences in segmental inclinations of both supporting and swinging limbs are shown. The ensuing description is of the runner in Fig. 15-7. In the takeoff, the rear limb is about to leave the ground, and the swing will begin with the hip and knee at 180 degrees. During the period of no contact, this limb will reach the position of the rear limb shown at contact. During this time, which for the 1500 m male runner equals the support phase, the runner has not yet brought the thigh in line with the trunk, but the lower leg has flexed through almost 120 degrees, bringing the

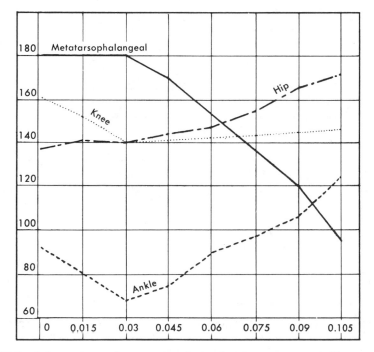

Fig. 15-5. *Joint actions of supporting limb of college woman (with no special training in running) during foot contact in running.*

Table 15-1. *Comparison of joint actions of trained and untrained adults. Note the least favorable actions.*

Joint Action	Trained			Untrained		
	Range	Time	Velocity (degrees/sec)	Range	Time	Velocity (degrees/sec)
Metatarsophalangeal extension	86	0.045	1911	85	0.075	1133
Ankle extension	73	0.045	1622	56	0.075	746
Knee extension	32	0.045	711	6	0.075	80
Hip extension	59	0.06	983	32	0.075	426

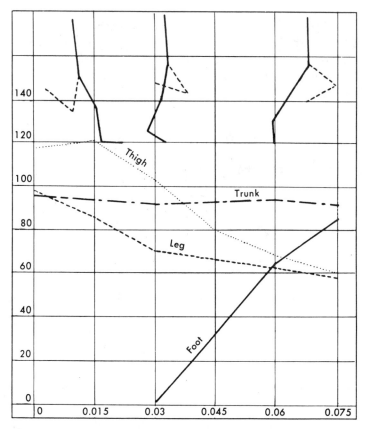

Fig. 15-6. *Segmental inclinations of supporting limb of male Olympic contestant during foot contact in running. Time is in seconds at bottom. Angles between body segments are shown in degrees at left.*

450

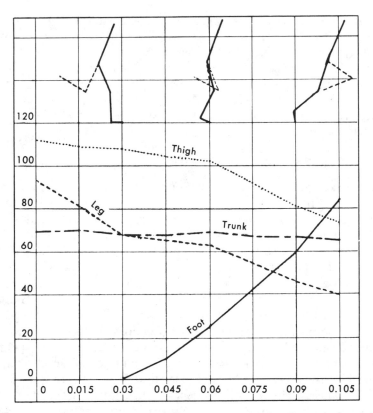

Fig. 15-7. *Segmental inclinations of supporting limb of college woman with no special training in running. Time in seconds and angles between body segment are shown on left.*

heel to hip level. At contact, the runner flexes rapidly at the hip, bringing the thigh in line with the trunk and then up toward the front horizontal at takeoff. During the first two-thirds of support, the swinging lower leg flexes, bringing it closer to the thigh. This moves the center of gravity of the limb toward the fulcrum (the hip) and facilitates its flexion. The speed with which the thigh and lower leg are swung forward and upward (closer to the front horizontal) during contact adds to the projecting force. Observation of a vigorous kick will show that the swinging limb can move the whole body forward. (One film of an expert football punter shows that the body is moved forward more than 0.6 m (2 ft) with no observable action in the supporting limb.) According to Fenn and Fortney, better runners, bring the thigh closer to the horizontal at takeoff.

From the position at takeoff, the leading limb during flight prepares for contact by extension at the hip, thus lowering the entire limb, and the lower leg is extended, thus increasing the length of the stride. In other film observations, some runners have been seen to flex at the knees just before contact. This action moves the foot back under the body and may decrease the possible backward push on contact, but it does decrease braking force and enables the runner to move the leg rapidly forward. In many cases, the forward movement of the total body is greater than the backward movement of the foot because of flexion at the knee. This seems to be advantageous, since this action rotates the distal end of the leg backward. As foot contact is made, flexion at the ankle rotates the proximal end of the leg forward. Thus the direction of leg rotation before contact is continued after the foot is placed on the ground.

Angles of Inclination of Supporting Limb

The graphs in Figs. 15-6 and 15-7 show that to understand movement in running, one must consider both angles at the joint and inclination angles of body segments. The inclination of the trunk of both runners remain at an almost constant angle during foot contact, and yet the angle at the hip joint (which moves the trunk) increased 59 degrees in the man and 32 degrees in the woman (Table 15-1). In both runners, thigh inclination has equalled hip action. Foot inclination is the same for both runners, approximately 85 degrees; leg inclinations differ, indicating a difference in ankle action. During foot rise, the man's leg inclines 12 degrees and the woman's more than twice that amount. If the man is using better running mechanics, the primary cause of the woman's lesser performance may be the small range of extension at the ankle. Do her extensor muscles lack strength, or does the reflex for foot flexion fail to respond with sufficient strength? Leg inclination could explain the difference in thigh inclination. That of the woman is less. Greater thigh inclination combined with her leg inclination could be too much for balance. These possible causes of lesser performance have been suggested; their validity requires further testing. Thus values and limitations of film analysis can be seen.

Additional Joint Actions

It was noticed in reviewing the film (Fig. 15-8) of the male runner that the pelvis rotates to a greater degree in running than it does in walking. When the thighs are separated, the pelvis is rotated on the supporting femur. As one thigh is swung forward, the pelvis rotates forward on the same side, adding length to the step. Thus, part of the males' greater speed in running is due to an increase in the length of stride.

It can be seen that the arms swing in opposition to the legs. They aid in maintaining a forward position of the upper trunk, which would otherwise tend to face in the same direction as does the pelvis. The arm swing also affects the center of gravity of the whole body. At takeoff, one arm is raised to the front and the other to the back. These positions raise the center of gravity of the total body, which reaches its highest point at takeoff. Shortly after contact, when the thighs are parallel, the arms are at the side of the body, with the forearms approaching extension. The arms now tend to lower the center of gravity

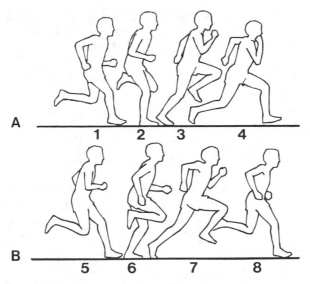

Fig. 15-8. *Sprinter in action. Reading from top left to bottom right the sequence is described as follows: 1, Foot strike on outside border of foot near ball. 2, Foot-down position with foot completely flat. (Some sprinters show heel not touching surface.). 3, Toes almost ready to leave surface (#7 supporting foot's toes just touching surface). 4, Both feet are off ground (nonsupport). 5, Rear foot lift (also see #s 1 and 8). 6, Knee lift in front, almost complete. 7, High knee lift and long stride potential. 8, Foot strike as seen in #1.*

of the entire body, which reaches its lowest point at this time. Modern sprinters are de-emphasizing the backward extended movements of the forearms for a more rapid arm movement forward. This seems to be associated with increased leg action.

TRACK STARTS AND INITIAL SPRINTING PHASE

In most running races, it is desirable to move the body forward as rapidly as possible from the start. This is especially important in sprints, and most investigators have found that the start is faster when executed from a crouching position rather than a standing position. A crouch start places the runner (sprinter) in a position to move the COG rapidly well ahead of the feet. The runner must then accelerate very rapidly or fall. In the longer races, the runner, usually uses a standing start because rapid acceleration at the start is not necessary.

It has been found through experience that the start is faster if blocks are provided for the backward push; they, too, increase the amount of push that can be directed horizontally. A noted coach has increased the height of the front block to decrease the amount of backward movement of the front foot and thus decreased the time that the foot pushes against the block.

As the runner takes the crouching position, hands, feet, and rear knee are in contact with the supporting surface, with the rear foot supporting little of the body weight. The distance between the hands and the forward foot is short enough to force the spine to flex (arch). The value of this flexion will be shown later.

In the "get set" position, which precedes the actual start, the rear knee is raised from the surface until the rear leg is inclined some 25 to 30 degrees as measured from the front. (However, some runners completely extend the rear leg.) Both thighs are moved upward and forward by extension at the knee, thereby moving the trunk and the center of gravity farther forward. At the same time, the spine flexes more; the head is held at the same height that it had in the first position.

As the trunk is raised, the rear foot pushes by sudden knee extensor action which moves the thigh forward. As viewed with film, the feet are moved slightly backward preceding the push. This push is of short duration because the limb must be moved forward quickly for the first step. Before the rear foot has left the block, leg extension at the front knee begins, moving the front thigh forward. Both knee actions are examples of reversed muscle action and are the primary sources of power for putting the body into motion. The leg of the front foot keeps a fairly constant inclination, adjusting its position to the movement of the foot. The trunk, which has been inclined slightly above the horizontal during the push of the rear foot, is raised somewhat as the rear foot is moved forward for the first step. Since the center of gravity is ahead of the supporting front foot, gravity will rotate the foot about the metatarsophalangeal joints. In general, the action is that described in the discussion on mechanics of the stepping pattern.

The first five or six steps after the push differ from the steps of the run. There is only a short period in which both feet are off the surface. Because the center of gravity is so far ahead of the takeoff foot, little upward projection is given to it, and the succeeding step must be taken quickly to prevent it from falling below the desired line of flight. After the first step the trunk is gradually raised, thus increasing the amount of upward direction given to the center of gravity. With this change, the steps can be gradually lengthened to equal those which will be used in the sprint stride.

During the striding action of the lower limbs, the arms move in opposition to them. The upper arms are moved by shoulder joint muscles, and the forearms are held in approximately 90 degrees of flexion to shorten the moment arm of the shoulder levers.

At the starting signal, the contacting segments leave the surface in sequence. According to Bresnahan, who observed 28 trained sprinters, all right-handed, the order of breaking contact in all subjects was left hand, right hand, right foot, left foot. The average time between the signal and the left-hand break was 0.172 second and between the signal and the left-foot break 0.443 second. Bresnaham also observed one left-handed sprinter in whom the breaking order was reversed—right hand first and right foot last.

As the hands are raised, the spine extends, counteracting the pull of gravity on the upper trunk while the lower trunk is supported by the feet. As the spine extends, it moves the head and the center of gravity forward. In looking at film of this action the view is reminded of Gray's statement: "By arching and extending its back, a galloping dog greatly increases the power and length of its stride."

The forces made against starting blocks by runners using the crouching starts are shown in Fig. 15-9. In the crouching start, note

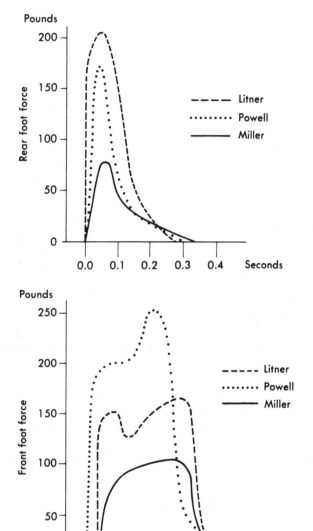

Fig. 15-9. *Starting block force-time curves for three runners using the crouching start. Note similarity among the rear foot impulse. Note differences in front foot impulse.*

that the front foot, in most instances, exerts force over a longer time but for less maximum force. (The impulse is greater for the front foot since impulse force is integrated over the time.)

The effect of foot-spacing on velocity in sprints was studied by Sigerseth and Grinaker. The subjects were 28 male college physical education majors. In the crouching start, the feet were separated 10, 19, or 28 inches, and times were checked at 10, 20, 30, 40 and 50 yards. At every distance, the time for the 19-inch start was the lowest, but the records were statistically significant only when the means for the 19- and 28-inch starts were compared for the 10, 20, 30 and 50 yards.

Sprint Starting Mechanics

The following are certain starting mechanics agreed on by investigators Barlow and Cooper:

1. Block spacings vary from 27.9 to 38.1 cm (11 to 15 in.), partially according to leg length. This arrangement enables the sprinter to attain a fast start.
2. In the set position, the front knee joint angle should be near 90 degrees, since the sprinter remains longest over this leg before leaving the blocks.
3. The rear leg is near extension (varying from 140 to 170 degrees) to react to the gun signal as soon as possible and to apply nearly maximum thrust.
4. The head of the sprinter is relaxed. It is the first body part to move the body in the desired direction.
5. A sprinter usually takes about 0.11 second to react to the gun.
6. The time of exit of the rear foot from the rear block (mean time, 0.270 second) was less than Morris found for untrained sprinters (mean time, 0.343 second).
7. The mean time spent in the blocks by the front foot was 0.446 second.
8. The greatest horizontal force against the blocks was exerted by the rear foot. However, the front foot generates slightly less force over a longer time, producing greater impulse.
9. The first step by the best sprinter off the blocks was longer and closer to the ground.

Overstriding and Understriding

Recent studies (Cavanagh and Williams; Clarke et al.) have been conducted on overstriding and understriding. In overstriding, "a 10% increase in stride length resulted in an increased peak shank deceleration (leg shock) upon landing," (Messier, Franke, and Rejeski, p. 276). Overstriding results in increased cardiorespiratory demands (Cavanagh and Williams, 1982). It would appear that overstriding mechanically causes increased tension and some malfunction of the rhythmic contraction of leg and even arm muscles. If the stride is decreased, there is less peak shank deceleration. Deshon and Nelson (1964) found that, in sprint overstriding, there was a decreased angle at touchdown. This, in turn, results in greater braking force. There is deceleration at foot, forefoot, or heel. If the foot decelerates, the only way the runner can maintain constant velocity is to increase the forces at toe off. This coupled with increased braking force would call for the expenditure of increased energy. The runner who runs correctly from a biomechanical standpoint should not be required to overcome inertia at every step.

Understriding results in the lead foot being placed almost under the runners's center of gravity. Thus, the center of gravity of the runner is not elevated vertically as much and the flight time is reduced. Advantageously, there is a decrease in braking force at heel strike when understriding. Cavanagh and Williams found that understriding was more efficient than overstriding. However, Messire, Franke, and Rejeski found that a small decrease in stride length did not adversely affect a runner's performance. On the other hand, they discovered that a large reduction in stride length did.

Running Economy

Style, technique, training, and age affect the amount of energy expended in running. Obviously, the longer the distance of the run, the more important the conservation of energy becomes. Extraneous movements add to the cost. Even the excess use of the arms in a long distance run may exact a toll. There is argument as to optimum stride length and frequency. If 148 cm is the stride length of a given runner, a shift of −5 to +10 cm will change the energy output. Pugh's data (as reported by Best and Bartlett) on comparing track and treadmill running in relation to energy are as follows:

1. There was a marathon-pace difference of 7 to 8% at the middle distance pace.
2. There was 20% decrease in energy cost during drafting. Also, they reported one author got a decrease in energy cost due to clothing changes and a hair cut.

Optimum stride length and frequency changed slightly (4%) when the arms were held across the chest. When the trunk movement was over emphasized, there was 16% change. Also, there were changes when the legs were lifted higher than in normal running.

No difference was found in VO^2 between running on the ball of the foot and having the heel planted first.

Length of stride in speed running is dependent on several factors: (1) It is positively correlated with the ratio of leg length to body height; (2) it is directly proportional to the amount of force extended to propel the body into the air during push off; and (3) it is inversely proportional to the amount of braking force at touchdown.

It is known that experienced runners tend to use running strides that are near to their optimum stride. From a mechanical viewpoint, after years of experience, these runners have found, through trial and error, the most relaxing stride without reducing their momentum. Their measuring stick is in the preconceived cost in energy output and their times in races. Experimenting with a measured length of stride probably would be advocated.

Fatigue Effects

In middle-distance running, Sparks found the following:

1. The best runners depend on their ability to consume and use oxygen efficiently. These same top runners supply more energy by the aerobic system and therefore produce less oxygen debt.
2. The better runners are more airborne during the race; that is, they are in the air slightly longer than on the ground. The reverse often happens as they become fatigued.
3. As the stress of the run becomes greater toward the end of the race, the stride often is shortened, and to keep up the pace the runner increases the stride frequency. The center of gravity is lowered, and the knee lift (leg flexion) is decreased as fatigue sets in.

In distance running, the same mechanical effects from fatigue can and often do occur. Stress tolerance and ability to consume and use oxygen efficiently may delay or even prevent the occurrence of mechanical faults. A strobe picture of a runner in action (Fig. 15-10) includes the leg and arm action in one plane clearly. The outward rotation of the foot is also depicted.

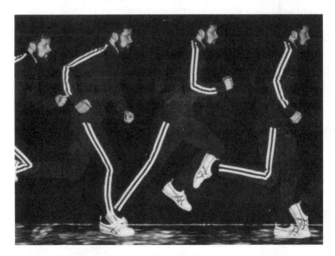

Fig. 15-10. *Strobe photograph, taken at 300 flashes per minute (50 per second). Foot, arm, and leg action are seen clearly in their sequential relationships. (Courtesy of Phillip L, Henson, Biomechancis Laboratory, Indiana University)*

Several investigators have found that a fatigued runner exhibits most of the following:

1. Lower center of gravity of the body during air phase.
2. Greater forward body lean.
3. Lateral extension of the arms.
4. Decreased leg lift.
5. Shorter strides.
6. Decreased step frequency.
7. Wider base of support, with the legs rotated laterally (externally).

FORCES AND ANATOMICAL ADJUSTMENTS

Mann (1982) has stated that in running, as regards the vertical force curve, the initial contact of the running foot on the ground is approximately 150% to 200% of body weight, forward shear force is about 50% of body weight and medial shear force is about 10% of body weight. At contact of the foot with the ground, there is rapid extension at the hip and knee and further dorsiflexion at the ankle. There is also pronation of the foot and internal rotation which occurs throughout the lower limb. This, in turn, causes eversion of the calcaneous, which unlocks the transverse tarsal joint bringing about flexibility with the entire foot. Adduction at the hip is also happening. It is easy to see this is a coordinated effort as the muscles that cross the hip, knee, and ankle joints help maintain stability of those joints.

The swing leg is flexed during the rapid extension of the stance leg. This is coordinated and related occurrence. The absorption of force at impact lasts for 50% of the stance phase with the continuous dorsiflexion at the ankle joint and flexion at the knee joint. Upon passing the stance leg (the supporting mechanism) the swinging leg causes the center of gravity to move again in front of the stance foot. Then external rotation occurs in the pelvis. This rotation is caused by the swinging leg which rotates the stance leg pelvis by activation of the adductor muscles. The center of gravity is lowest during the stance phase just before the extension at the knee joint and plantar flexion at the ankle joint takes place. At this time, the leg is also being abducted. The vertical force at the time of midstance is 250% to 300% of body weight with the aft shear force approximately 60% of body weight. Most of the muscles cease to fire during the last third of the stance phase. Probably this is because the center of gravity has gone beyond the stance leg foot. Therefore, the forward propulsion of the body is caused by the swinging leg and arm motion.

Active peak flexion at the hip occurs during the latter part of the swing phase. No forces are active against the foot after it leaves the ground.

During the last fourth of the swing phase, many of the muscles become more active, namely, the hip extensors and hamstrings, the quadriceps about the knee, and the posterior calf muscles in preparation for the initial contact with the ground.

Pronation of the foot at initial contact is one way the body (part) helps in decreasing the force. Also, the whole foot and ankle enter into the action. There is eversion of the subtalar joint as pronation of the foot takes place. The eversion brings rotation of the tibia, the greater the eversion, the more rotation. In walking, it is normally 6 degrees to 9 degrees. Usually runners exhibit greater than 9 degrees.

SPEED AND EFFICIENCY

In sprinting, the runner attains maximum velocity at 60–70 meters from the starting position. The fastest reaction time in leaving the blocks is an asset, provided the sprinter has fast leg speed.

It must be kept in mind that short sprinters tend to start fast but reach maximum acceleration first. Also, they usually have difficulty maintaining top speed in a sprint race. In a recent 20.46 second 200-meter dash, the top sprinter had a speed of 9 strides the last 20 meters. The less time it takes for each stride, the faster the runner. However, the very best runners are able to maintain a fast speed longer. Sprinters pump their arms but use very little shoulder movement, whereas distance runners use less arm action and more shoulder twist.

In walking, the energy absorption period in which one second elapses is from heel strike to heel strike. In running, the runner decreases the time the foot is on the ground up to 0.2 seconds (200 ms.). The events occurring during the stance phase in running happen three times or more faster during sprint running. This points out the necessity of being mechanically correct and efficiently sound to run at top speed.

Dillman discusses the mechanical aspects of running that affect the effective utilization of human resources in distance running. Since it is impossible to run at top speed for any great length of time or long distance, the distance runner must conserve energy. The velocity of a competent distance runner ranges from 4.5 to 6.5 meters per second (m/s) which is from 10–14.6 miles per hour. Contrast this with the velocity of a sprinter, which is 21–23 miles per hour.

The average horizontal velocity of a skilled runner is 5.2 m/s. A runner at this speed in a six-mile race would have an elapsed time of 30 minutes. Dillman calls running "a series of projections that results in translation of the body over the running surface," and states: "Running speed can be varied by manipulating both the impulse of the thrust force and the frequency of application."

To conserve energy, the distance runner must run at a relatively constant pace (stride frequencies) through most of the race. Most top runners do vary their stride lengths, which, in turn, affects their speed. They also have less knee lift and less arm action than sprinters.

RACEWALKING

Racewalking is a specialized walking technique, usually found in a competitive situation in which the walker comes very close to running. The speed of the movement is faster than that of brisk walking. (The heart-rate attainment is often the same as in running at average speeds.) The distances raced are usually 20 and 50 kilometers. There is an attempt to have the walking action continuous, as much as possible.

The interaction of the ground and the push-off, including the reaction of the walker to these forces, are factors in executing the walking technique. The knee moves first, and then the ankle follows in the action. The knee joint has a velocity of 7 m plus per second. To be classified as a legal walking action, as Cairns stated, "the forward foot of the walker must make contact before the rear foot leaves the ground, and the supporting leg must be straight in the vertically upright position." These are the constraints as contained in the rules. (See Fig. 15-11.)

Analysis of the Racewalking Act

Racewalking is a heel and foot action with the outside edge of the heel contacting the ground first. As the body weight moves forward, it is slightly on the outside edge of the foot. Then the toes of the rear foot push the foot off the ground, and the body continues forward.

The walk should be direct, or as straight as possible, to conserve

RUNNING   **461**

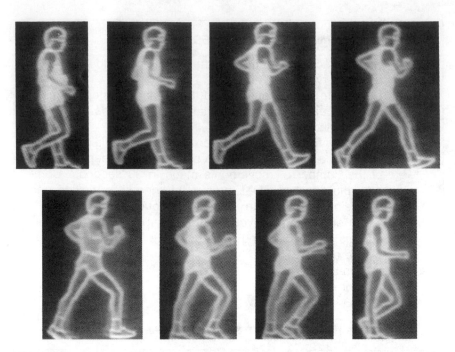

Fig. 15-11. *Race walking sequences taken from videotapes produced from biomechanics research at European Championships.*

energy. The center of mass should move vertically as little as possible. After the heel contacts the surface, the forward leg is straightened immediately. It remains so until the push off from the back leg commences. The straightened leg and the hip rotation help to keep the center of mass from rising too drastically.

Overstriding expends unnecessary energy. A beginner should start with using short strides. As the speed of the walk increases, the length of stride will increase. The forward leg moves the pelvic area on that side forward. The forward and backward movement is accomplished without too much twisting so as not to interfere with the rapid and lengthening action of the legs.

The trunk is held upright with the head kept vertical. Any large degree of head-forward inclination affects the stride length. The upper body is erect and some lean forward occurs, putting the center of mass ahead of the push-off foot. A backward lean will cause shortening of the stride and may cause back problems to develop.

The racewalker reaches maximum velocity sooner than in running. The faster the striding rate, the faster the walker will move. As the support phase decreases, the recovery phase increases. At landing or striking of the lead foot and in transversion or conversion, the center of mass remains higher and doesn't go up and down as much as in running.

The arms remain flexed and are moved in synchronization with the leg action. The arms move just across the midline of the body at sternum level. The arms remain near the body, not laterally away from it, as they are "pumped" vigorously. On the backswing of the arms, the elbow may be raised vertically near shoulder level. The hands are relaxed, passing back and forward near the pelvic region.

As the speed of the walk increases, the arms move faster to counterbalance the action of the lower body. This vigorous action of the arms is similar to the arm action in running, but of lesser amplitude.

MINI-LAB LEARNING EXPERIENCES

Compare racewalking and walking using films, EMG, dynamography, and other instrumentation.

Murray et al. compared racewalkers from a temporal and angular perspective, and racewalkers and fast walkers using conventional or normal style. The racewalkers had longer strides than the walkers and faster rates, with the stance and swing times approximately equal. Other comparisons were:

1. The racewalkers had increased dorsiflexion at heelstrike.
2. The racewalkers had increased hyperextension at the knee in midstance.
3. There was increase flexion at the knee and hip during the leg swing by the racewalkers.
4. Increased pelvic rotation by the racewalkers took place.

Cairns et al. found similar results in comparing gaits of walkers and racewalkers in the following: stride lengths, cadence, stance time, swing time, peak ankle dorsiflexion, knee extension at midstance, peak hip flexion, peak pelvic displacement in all three planes, and peak vertical, anterior, and medial components of the ground reaction force. There was considerable difference in these values between the racewalkers and fast walkers.

Cairns stated:

The seemingly exaggerated angular motions of racewalking are necessary to attain increased velocities within the rules of racewalking and to modulate the excursions of the center of mass. The increased vertical and anterior components of the ground reaction forces are related to the increased propulsive forces associated with increased stride length and velocity in racewalking. The increased medial component of the ground reaction force seems to be a compensatory force related to lateral pelvic shifting. There is a support and recovery phase, as is present in conventional walking.

Table 15-2. *Racewalking Data*

horizontal velocity of arms	2–6 meters per second
vertical velocity of arms	.5–2 meters per second
angular velocity of upper arms	8 radians per second
angular velocity of forearm	9 radians per second
angular velocity of thigh	12–13 radians per second
angular velocity of lower leg	15 radians per second
linear velocity center of gravity	4.1–4.3 m/second, 20 K race
	3.7–3.8 m/second, 50 K race
stride length	220–260 cm, 20 K race
	220–240 cm, 50 K race
linear velocity of knee	7 meters per second
linear velocity of ankle	9 meters per second

In reviewing the film of the European Track and Field Championships of 1983, researchers found that the racewalker's center of gravity is shifted 3 to 6 cm as the pelvis is rotated. This is a minimum shift and considered to be the newest trend in racewalking techniques. Previously, the pelvic rotation, and consequently the center of gravity shift, was more exaggerated to produce a long stride. The minimum shift has been found to permit the walker to increase the leg velocity and yet attain a long stride.

The arm actions are an integral part of the walking technique. The arms are moved very vigorously in synchronization with the leg movements. Kinematic data are listed in Table 15-2. Note the high vertical velocities of the arms and the ratio of ankle speed to speed of the racewalker (center of gravity data).

The decrease in pelvic turn enables the walker to increase leg velocity. The emphasis is on economy of effort and relaxation during certain phases. Fast leg action should be executed with a minimum elevation of the center of gravity.

Table 15-3. *Means of selected variables which differentiate between two performances of race walkers.*

Variable	Performance Group 1	Performance Group 2
Velocity (m/s)	3.13	4.07
Stance Time (s)	.40	.40
Stance Time/Swing Time Ratio	1.14	.89
Anterior GRF (x bw)	.29	.39
Stride Length (m)	2.17	2.56
Leg Length (m)	80.06	83.82
Max Knee Extension (deg)	184.00	190.00

THE BIOMECHANICS OF HUMAN MOVEMENT

Cairns, using the best performers, found the following mean values: velocity, 4.07 m/sec; stride length, 2.56 meters; stance time, .40 sec; stance and swing time, .89 sec. (Table 15-3). She summarized the results of her study by stating, "It is evident from this investigation that increased stride length, an increased anterior component of the ground reaction force, and a stance time/swing time ratio which approaches 1.00 are characteristic of increased velocity and better performance times in racewalking."

REFERENCES

Abbot, R. R. (1985) Cinematographic analysis of the techniques of hurdling 57, *Encyclopedia of Physical Education, Fitness and Sports,* Cureton, T. (Ed.). Reston, VA: AAHPERD.

Adrian, M. and Kreighbaum, E. (1971) Physical and mechanical characteristics of distance runners during competition, Third International Seminar on Biomechanics, Rome.

Barlow, D. A. and J. M. Cooper (1972) Mechanical Considerations in Sprint Start, *Athletic Asia* 2:27, Aug.

Bates, B. T. and Haven, B. H. (1973) An analysis of the mechanics of highly skilled female runners. In Bleustein, J. L., editor: *Mechanics and sport,* New York: American Society of Mechanical Engineers.

Beck, M. C. (1965) The Path of the Center of Gravity During Running in Boys Grades One to Six, dissertation, U. of Wisconsin.

Bresnahan, G. T. (1934) A study of the movement pattern in starting the race from a crouch position, *Res. Q. Am. Assoc. Health Phys. Educ.* 5(1) (supp.):5.

Cairns, M. A., R. G. Burdett, J. C. Pissiotta and S. R. Simon (1986); A Biomechanical Analysis of Racewalking, *Medicine and Science in Sports and Exercise.*

Cairns, M. (1987) Contribution of Kinematic Variables to Racewalking Velocity. *Proceedings of ISBS Biomechanics in Sports III & IV,* Editors Juris Terands, Barbars A. Gowitzke and Lawrence Holt, Del Mar, CA: Academic Publishers.

Cavanagh, P. R. and K. R. Williams (1982) The Effect of Stride Length Variations on 02 Uptake During Distance Running. *Medicine and Science in Sports and Exercise,* 14:30–35.

Clarke, T. E., L. Cooper, D. Clark and C. Hamill (1983) The Effect of Varied Stride Rate and Length Upon Shank Deceleration During Ground Contact in Running. *Medicine and Science in Sports and Exercise,* 15–170.

Deshon, D. E. and R. C. Nelson (1964) A Cinematographical Analysis of Sprint Running, *Res. Q.* 35:451–455.

Dillman, C. (1984) Distance Running, *Biomechanics of Running,* Ed. Cureton, *Encyclopedia of Physical Education,* 1984. Reston, VA: AAHPERD.

Dintiman, G. B. (1974) Research Tells the Coach About Sprinting (pamphlet). Washington, DC: AAHPER.

Fenn, W. O. (1930) Work Against Gravity and Work Due to Velocity Changes in Running, *Am. J. Physiol.* 93:433.

Fenton, R. M. (1987) *Racewalking Ground Reaction Forces,* Editors Juris Terands et al., Del Mar, CA: Academic Press.

Fortney, V. (1963) Trends and Traits in the Action of the Swinging Leg in Running, thesis, University of Wisconsin.

Gray, J. (1960) *How Animals Move,* London: Cambridge University Press.

Henson, P. L. (1976) Pace and grade related to the oxygen and energy requirements, and the mechanics of treadmill running, doctoral dissertation, Indiana University.

Hoffman, K. (1972) Stride length and frequency in female sprinters, *Track Tech.* 48:1522.

Hubbard, A. W. (1939) Experimental analysis of running and of certain fundamental differences between trained and untrained runners, *Res. Q. Am. Assoc. Health Phys. Educ.* 10(3):28.

James, S. L. and Brubaker, C. E. (1972) Running mechanics, *J.A.M.A.* 221:1014–1016.

Jensen, C. R. and Fisher, A. G. (1979) *Scientific basis of athletic conditioning,* Philadelphia: Lea & Febiger.

Mann, R. (1982) Biomechanics of Running, *Am. Academy of Orthopedic Surgeons, Symposium of the Foot and Leg in Running Sports,* Ed. Robert P. Mack, St. Louis: C. V. Mosby.

Messier, S. P., W. D. Franke, and W. J. Rejaski (1986) Effects of Altered Lengths on Ratings of Perceived Exertion During Running, *Research Quarterly for Exercise and Sport,* Vol. 57, No. 4, Dec.

Morris, H. H. (1971) The effects of starting block length, angle, and position upon sprint performance, doctoral dissertation, Indiana University, November.

Murray, M. P., et al. Kinematics and Electromyographic Patterns of Olympic Racewalkers, *American Journal of Sports Medicine* 11(2), 68–74.

Phillips, S. J. and J. L. Jensen, Kinematics of Racewalking, Ed. Juris Terands, et al.; *Proceedings of Sports Medicine,* Del Mar, CA: Academic Publishers.

Rienzo, J. D. (1983) *Hurdles, Track and Field Quarterly Rev.,* Summer.

Sigerseth, P. O. and Grinaker, V. F. (1962) Effect of foot spacing on velocity in sprints, *Res. W. Am. Assoc. Health Phys. Educ.* 33599.

Slocum, D. B. and Bowerman, W. (1962) The biomechanics of running, *Clin. Orthop.* 23:39.

Slocum, D. B. and S. L. James (1968) Biomechanics of Running, *JAMA*, 205:721–728.

Sparks, K. E. (1974) Physiological and Mechanical Alternations Due to Fatigue While Performing a Four-Minute Mile, Unpublished paper, Indiana University.

Teeple, J. B. (1968) A Biomechanical Analysis of Running Patterns of College Women, Master's thesis, Pennsylvania State University, December.

Track and Field Quarterly Review, Vol. 80, Summer, 1980.

Ward, P. (1973) An analysis of kinetic and kinematic factors of the standup and the preferred crouch starting techniques with respect to sprint performance, doctoral dissertation, Indiana University, August.

16
Jumping

INTRODUCTION

Jumping is one of the fundamental movements made by children after learning to walk and run. It is practiced by many of them to some degree at least until the teenage years and is a highly specialized activity of a few adults, such as Olympic competitors.

There are several kinds of jumps, such as the standing long jump, standing vertical jump, long jump, high jump, and pole vault, as well as certain specialized jumps made in games and contests.

Jumping is a projection of the body into the air by means of a force made by the feet or hands against a surface. Often the jump is made after a run, and the takeoff may be made from either one foot or two feet.

The ability to project the body at an optimum angle at the takeoff is one of the factors determining the distance or height of the jump. Takeoff speed is another factor involved in the quality of jumps. Usually the force multiplied by the time of application ($F \times t$ = Impulse) determines the longest or highest jump. The best jumpers have the greatest impulse. In addition, they apply the force in the shortest time but have greater vertical force than the poorer jumpers.

Whenever a run precedes the jump, there is a problem of redirecting some of the horizontal velocity into vertical velocity. Inevitably, there is some sacrifice of one in an attempt to optimize the other.

The path of the jumper who is in the air is that of a parabola, except in a purely vertical jump. The crossing of a bar or a landing for distance involves manipulating the center of gravity to gain advantages in its placement in the body or outside the body.

There is a rotational component connected with the takeoff in jumping. Most researchers (such as Bedi) consider the rotational component to be in a forward direction. Either using this force or counteracting it may aid the jumper.

A one-foot takeoff provides the greatest forward momentum at takeoff but is the hardest to control in relation to timing a hit while the jumper is in the air, such as in a block in basketball. For distance, such as in the long jump, or height, such as in the high jump, the one-foot takeoff after a run is preferred.

The moving of the arms and legs while the jumper is in flight (airborne) does not add to the distance covered nor to the height of the center of gravity of the body. However, movement of the center of gravity within the body or outside of it can be accomplished by moving the body parts. Many of the leg, trunk, and arm movements are made for balance purposes, or to project the center of gravity vertically or horizontally within the path prescribed.

If the airborne jumper moves a part of the body in one direction, another part will move in the opposite direction. For example, movement of the head and upper torso forward and downward (clockwise) causes the feet and lower body to move upward and forward (counterclockwise). This action-reaction principle may be an asset or a liability, depending on its use. In addition, the timing of one movement to cause reaction in another is crucial to performance. One arm moving clockwise too soon may cause the performer's other arm to move counterclockwise, striking a crossbar and nullifying an otherwise effective action.

STANDING JUMPS (PUSHING OFF WITH BOTH FEET)

Standing Long Jump

The standing broad jump is most frequently used in schools and colleges as one measure of motor ability and physical or motor fitness. It is a modification of the walking step—a modification that low-level performers frequently do not achieve effectively. These performers take off from one foot when they attempt to take off from both. This is a reflex, or inherent, reaction to maintain balance.

Joint Actions in Takeoff Phase. The following analysis of the mechanics of the jump is based on a film of a 12-year-old girl whose score ranks above the ninety-fifth percentile in a nationwise sampling of girls 12 to 17 years of age. The discussion is based on graphs of joint angles and segmental inclinations shown in Figs. 16-1 and 16-2. The lines in the illustrations begin at the time that the heels leave the ground and show that the propelling actions occur in slightly more than 0.25 second from raising of the heel until the final thrust is made. For the first 0.18 second, as the foot is raised from the floor, no action (or very little) occurs at the ankle joint, except for the slight flexion and immediate recovery at 0.09 seconds. This lack of extension at the ankle is noteworthy, since many authors attribute rising on the toes to extension at the ankle. These graphs, like many others, show that as the center of gravity of the body is moved downward by gravitational force, the foot rotating at the metatarsophalangeal joint is moved in an upward direction. This occurs only when the ankle extensors prevent flexion at the ankle. This apparent paradox—movement in

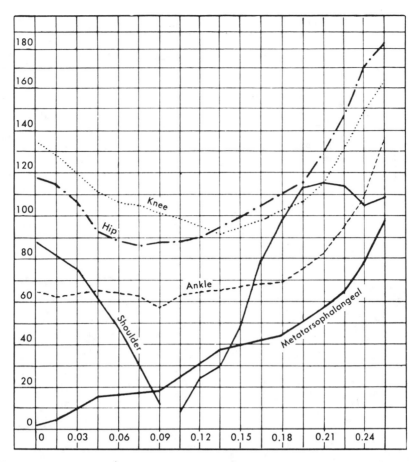

Fig. 16-1. *Joint actions during the propulsive phase of the standing long jump of a highly skilled 12 year-old girl. Time in seconds is shown at bottom with 0.24 second point being the instant of takeoff; angles between body segments are shown in degrees at left. For all angles, the downward direction of lines represents flexion and upward slopes represent extension. Note nearly constant angle at the ankle during the majority of the jump. During the last 0.18 seconds prior to takeoff, the extension at most joints increases rapidly.*

an upward direction because of gravitational force—was also noted in connection with teeterboard action.

Once the leg has reached the desired angle of inclination, extension at the ankle parallels extension at the metatarsophalangeal joint from 0.135 to 0.21 second (Fig. 16-1), and by this means the inclination of the leg is kept almost constant (Fig. 16-2). In the final 0.03 second, extension at the ankle exceeds action at the metatarsophalangeal joint, and the leg is raised 10 degrees, adding to the upward thrust.

The lower leg flexes for the first 0.135 second, carrying the thigh downward and backward in reference to the knee. However, from 0.06 to 0.135 second, the thigh is not inclined backward with reference to

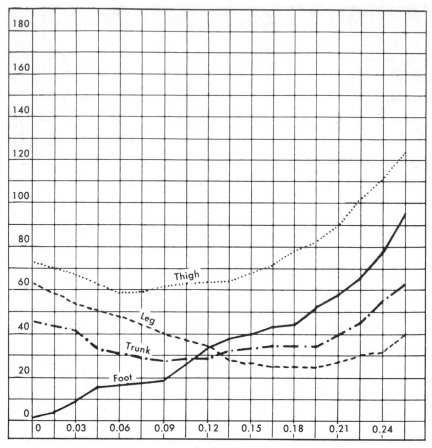

Fig. 16-2. *Angles of inclination of body segments during the propulsive phase of the standing long jump of a highly skilled 12 year-old girl (same as figure 16-1). The propulsive phase begins at time zero and takeoff occurs at 0.24 second. The angles are in degrees. Note the foot consistently changes it angle of inclination starting with a zero position (horizontal) and moving to the vertical position prior to takeoff.*

the horizontal because the forward inclination of the leg at this time exceeds flexion at the knee. At 0.21 second, the thigh reaches the vertical, and after this point all limb actions increase in speed. Up to 0.21 second, thigh extension has lifted the thigh and the torso against gravitational pull; after that time, both thigh extension and gravity are applying force in a downward direction. All joints (metatarsophalangeal, ankle, knee and hip) react to this change in gravitational pull; all rotations at these joints increase in speed. Here is an example of the marvelous capacity of a living organism to adjust to a situation; one can be assured that these adjustments are not voluntarily controlled. The nervous system reacts to balance and to the speed of the thigh; guided by the intended action, it provides the necessary movements at the joints.

The shoulder measures shown in Fig. 16-1 are those of the angle formed by lines drawn through the upper arms and the trunk. As the heels leave the ground, the arms are back of the trunk at an angle of 88 degrees. They are moved downward by flexion at the shoulder, pass the trunk between 0.09 and 0.105 second, and reach the height of their swing just before the thighs reach the vertical.

In this swing, the arm movement affects the position of the center of gravity of the entire body, tending to move it forward and downward until the arms pass the trunk and then forward and upward.

In studying the standing long jump of 20 boys (five each at ages 7, 10, 13, and 16 years) who were selected as average jumpers, Roy found that the peak angular velocities at the knee, ankle, and metatarsophalangeal joints reached maximum values at takeoff, except for one 10-year-old boy whose maximal velocity at the knee occurred 0.07 second before takeoff. Using measures derived from film and a force platform, Roy concluded, "Kinematics of jumping are well established by the beginning of school age and remain essentially constant through mid-adolescence for average performers."

Factors Affecting the Distance of the Jump. The standing long jump is customarily measured from the toes at takeoff to where the heels touch the ground in landing. This distance is determined by four factors: (1) the distance to which the center of gravity of the body is carried forward by the lean at takeoff, (2) the horizontal distance through which the center of gravity is projected during flight, (3) the distance beyond the center of gravity that the heels reach on landing, and (4) the time spend on the takeoff surface. Felton compared these factors as shown in the performances of five high-scoring college women, whose jumps averaged 2.19 m (86.22 in) and of five low-scoring ones whose jumps averaged 1.08 m (42.78 in). At the time of takeoff, the centers of gravity of the high-scoring group averaged .78 m (30.62 in) in front of their toes; for the low-scoring group the average distance was 45.9 cm (18.74 in). The heels of the high scorers landed 14.1 cm (5.56 in) ahead of the center of gravity, and the heels of the low scores 9.14 cm (3.6 in) ahead. The degree to which the center of gravity is in front of the toes at takeoff is affected mainly by the degree of knee extension. The 12-year-old girl whose angular kinematics were shown in Fig. 16-1 reached an extension at the knee of 164 degrees. In Felton's comparison of high-scoring and low-scoring women, the average extension at the knee were 165.7 and 141 degrees, respectively. The degree of extension may be due to the balance mechanism. The strength of the ankle extensors could also influence the amount of lean, for the tension in these muscles must move or hold all parts of the body above the ankle joint.

The position of the thigh at landing is the determining factor in the length of the reach with the heel. The more closely the thigh approaches the horizontal, the longer the reach. When the thigh is nearly horizontal on landing, the legs are almost vertical. This landing position enables the body momentum to carry the center of gravity over the stationary feet. In a running long jump, the horizontal velocity during flight is greater, and the legs can reach farther without the likelihood of the body's falling back of the contact point. The horizontal position of the thighs changes the position of the center of gravity and permits the point to approach closer to the ground before the landing contact is made. This increases the time of flight, adds to the horizontal distance gained during flight, and facilitates forward rotation of the body at the ankle, thus decreasing the possibility of falling backward. Observation of hundreds of films of children by Glassow has shown that the position of the thighs at landing is a distinguishing feature between high-scoring and low-scoring long jumpers.

The flight adds the greatest proportion to the distance of the jump. The range of flight is determined by the angle and speed of the projection (velocity).

Measures of Velocity and Distance. A measure of the velocity of the center of gravity is rarely made; yet this is the most valid evaluation of the force developed in the takeoff. Halverson found an average velocity in the jump of kindergarten children to be between 1.8 and 2.1 m/sec (6 and 7 ft/sec), and the highest was 2.52 m/sec (8.28 ft/sec). Felton calculated the mean velocity of five high-scoring college women to be 2.47 m/sec (8.11 ft/sec) and that of five low-scoring women to be 1.72 m/sec (5.66 ft/sec). The highest velocity was 2.81 m/sec to be 1.72 m/sec (9.22 ft/sec) and the lowest 1.53 m/sec (5.02 ft/sec). With horizontal and vertical scores from Roy's study, projection velocities of the center of gravity were calculated to be 2.72 m/sec (8.9 ft/sec) for age 7 years, and 3.04 m (10.0 ft) for age 10 years, 3.20 m (10.5 ft) for age 13 years, and 3.93 m (12.9 ft) for age 16 years. The increase from age to age was due to greater horizontal velocity, whereas vertical velocity changed little, indicating that with age the center of gravity is lowered at takeoff.

Different scores for various age groups are fairly common. For example, in unpublished scores for elementary-school boys found in studies at the University of Wisconsin, the first-grade boys averaged 1.16 m (46 in), and the eighth-grade boys averaged 1.93 m (76 in). The scores for intervening grades fell between these; the score for each grade was higher than that for the grade below it. The shorter time spend on the takeoff surface, exhibited by the best performers, varied from 0.24 to 0.29 second.

Standing Jump for Height

The standing jump for height is widely used as a test item, and its successful performance adds to playing ability in many sports. Sargent was the first to propose the jump for height as a measure of motor ability. In 1921, he said, "I want to share what seems to me the simplest and most effective of all tests of physical ability with the other fools who are looking for one." Since that time many investigators have found that Sargent jump test, or the "jump and reach," a valuable item in a test battery. For games in which an attempt is made to catch or to strike a high ball, the ability to jump is an asset. The receiver of a forward pass in football, the infielder and outfielder in baseball, the spiker in volleyball, and the basketball player who attempts to tip a ball toward the basket or to a teammate will play more effectively if they can add to their reach by a jump for height.

Henson, Turner, and LaCourse have developed a predictive test of explosive power to be used in predicting power for track and field athletes. Those with the highest scores are to be considered potentially outstanding prospects for sprints, hurdles and field events. Success is predicted for women who jump more than two feet vertically and almost nine feet horizontally. Similarly, men who can jump almost three feet vertically and more than eleven feet horizontally probably will score well in sprints, hurdles and field events. (See Table 16-1.)

Table 16-1. *Test for determining potential for track and field athletes: Sprinters, hurdlers, throwers and jumpers. (From Philip Henson, Paul Turner and Mike Lacourse. Paper presented to Tac Olympic Development Committee. 1986)*

FILE NAME:	BROWN		
VARIABLES:	VJ		
	SLJ	N = 98	Men
	AGE		

VARIABLE: LOW	HIGH	MEAN (in inches)	STD DEV
5. VJ 14.00	(N = 97): 34.00	26.0928	3.3004
6. SLJ 80.00	(N = 97): 127.00	106.6804	8.8881
13. AGE 18.00	(N = 97): 23.00	19.4536	1.3151

FILE NAME:	SMITH		
VARIABLES:	VJ		
	SLJ	N = 37	Women
	AGE		

VARIABLE: LOW	HIGH	MEAN (in inches)	STD DEV
5. VJ 15.00	(N = 37): 26.00	20.2973	2.8271
6. SLJ 70.50	(N = 37): 104.00	90.1554	8.5591
13. AGE 18.00	(N = 37): 22.00	19.3243	1.3345

* VJ   Vertical Jump
* SLJ   Standing Long Jump

Hudson (1987) found the following interesting information as a result of studying the vertical jump:

1. In the crouch or preparatory position the muscle-connective tissue system is "stretched" in eccentric tension, or more specifically, elastic energy is stored. She stated that if the eccentric contraction is followed immediately by concentric contraction, some of the stored elastic energy is re-used during the concentric contraction. This seems to imply that the crouch should be followed as soon as possible by the jump.

2. The two groups (male and female) used as subjects jumped approximately 23% of their height and crouched 17% of their height.

3. The mean angle at the knee for the two groups was slightly less than 90 degrees at maximum crouch and the start of the movement upward took 0.25 second, just as they left the ground to move upward in the propulsive phase.

4. The angle at maximum flexion at the knee, but not hip or ankle, was related to the use of stored energy.

5. Those subjects having faster extension time used more stored energy.

6. The ability to integrate the downward movement of the legs and to integrate the movement of the arms were related to use of stored elastic energy.

7. The more skilled performers were able to execute the upward propulsion in 100 ms less than the less skilled performers.

8. The more skilled performers crouched to a 96-degree angle at the knee, whereas, the less skilled performers flexed 12 degrees beyond 90 degrees.

9. The center of gravity descended 25 cm for the more skilled performers and 34 cm for the less skilled ones.

10. The takeoff velocity of the more skilled performers was higher than the less skilled subjects. Coordination and integration of the body segments coupled with rapid contraction and a smaller range of motion seemed to characterize the more skilled performers.

11. She stated, "The skilled jumpers had very brief timing lags between adjacent segments at both the start and the end of the propulsive phase of the jump."

12. Hudson said it was more important to time the pattern of movement correctly than it was to have the action move from proximal to distal.

13. She also found it was more important to have a "synchronization between the trunk and thigh" than "between the thigh and shank."

14. If the purpose of the vertical jump is to gain greater height, the range of motion in the preparatory position should be slightly more than 90 degrees and full extension of the body.

Based upon a comparison of joint actions in the standing long jump and the jump for height of the same performer, only minor differences in the action at the knee, hip, and shoulder exist. These common actions are much like those in Fig. 16-3. The action at the ankle joint is an important difference in the direction of the two projections. In the first third of the time between raising of the heel and final thrust, flexion at the ankle of one skilled performer (a college woman) was 10 degrees in the standing long jump and 5 degrees in the jump for height. Since flexion at the ankle carries the center of gravity of the body forward and thereby increases the effect of gravitational pull (which pulls the feet, except for the toes, from the floor), the difference in the metatarsophalangeal angle at this time (15 degrees and 5 degrees) is to be expected. Beyond this point, the extension occurred at the same rate until the final thrust, when the action in the jump for height exceeded that in the jump for distance. The first reached an extension of 134 degrees and the second an extension of 123 degrees. The leg in the first was closer to the vertical with reference to the ankle. Since the foot in the first third of the projecting time had been lifted farther from the floor in the long jump, gravitational action was greater, and the foot rose more rapidly. At the final thrust in the long jump, the foot was at an angle of 78 degrees with the horizontal (measured from the back) and in the high jump at an angle of 44 degrees.

Since the inclination of any segment affects the inclination of all segments above it, in spite of the similarities of proximal joint actions in the two jumps the difference in foot inclinations results in differences in inclination of the remaining segments. In the observed actions, the inclinations (measured from the front and with those in the jump for height given first) were as follows: leg, 91 degrees and 44 degrees; thigh, 102 degrees and 60 degrees; and trunk, 80 degrees and 37 degrees in the standing long jump, gravitational force adds to the final push; in the high jump, it adds little or nothing. Without the aid of gravity, the velocity in the jump for height therefore is slower than for the standing long jump.

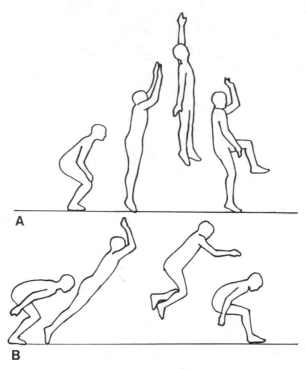

Fig. 16-3. *Film contourograms of a standing long jump and standing vertical jump. Note, from a qualitative perspective, that there are differences in body lean. Actual measurement of these differences will be more valuable. Likewise the apparent differences in arm flexion needs to be quantified. One will then see that the apparent differences are illusions since the arm orientation to the trunk is similar for the two jumps. The orientation in space is the difference. Quantitatively compare these two performances.*

Racing Dive

The racing dive is an excellent example of the action of the lower limbs described previously in the discussion of mechanics of the stepping pattern. However, in this skill, the projection force is directed almost horizontally, with little in the vertical direction. Therefore the directing segment, the leg, will be close to the horizontal in the force-producing phase.

The diver stands at the edge of the pool with feet separated to bring them in line with the hips for an effective push. The eyes are looking downward and forward at approximately 45 degrees. Next, flexion of spine and head and forward raising of the arms with reference to the feet have moved the body's center of gravity forward, resulting in flexion at the ankle. The flexion is possible because the ankle extensor muscles have permitted it by a lengthening contraction. The importance of streamlining is evident as the body readies itself to become a projectile in the air. The path of the center of gravity is determined at takeoff. The conservation of energy law could apply here (that is, energy can be neither created nor destroyed); thus the change is from potential to kinetic energy, resulting in the transfer of momentum, which is in fact the basic mechanical principle applied to the windup start technique (Fig. 16-4A).

One of the newer racing start techniques is the grab start, whereby the swimmer holds onto the starting platform until the gun is fired and enters the water sooner than when using the windup start and at a lower angle. The swimmer gains in execution because the swimming action was started sooner. (See Fig. 16-4B).

Ankle extensors are contracting with sufficient force to prevent flexion at that joint; now gravitational force rotates the entire body around a fulcrum that is the point of contact between the feet and the edge of the pool. In addition, preparation has been made for the final application of force. The arms have moved backward; flexion occurs at the knees; the hip angles are at increased flexion, bringing the trunk close to the thighs; and the spine has flexed. The last action, like that described in the crouching start for running races, prepares for spinal extension, which will add to the power and distance of the body's flight.

Note that the change of inclination of the legs is due to changes in foot inclination, not to changes at the ankle joint. Application of initial force is delayed until the legs are at, or close to, the desired direction. The beginning of the force-producing phase is seen—forward movement of the arms, facilitated by slight flexion at the elbow, spinal extension, and beginning extension at the knee. The knees and ankles have extended vigorously. In the last-named action, since the feet no longer support the body weight, extension at the ankle is a result of movement of the feet; however, extension at the knee because the feet resist a horizontal push, is due to reversed muscle action and the thighs move instead of the shank. During the forward,

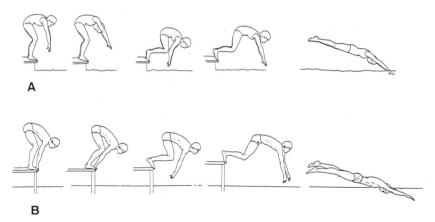

Fig. 16-4. *Two types of racing dives used in swimming competition. A, windup start dive of national champion. B, grab start dive of collegiate swimmer. Note the similar angle of the thigh, shank, and foot prior to pushoff. What differences can be noted between the two divers? (cue: angle of entry)*

JUMPING 477

downward movement of the thighs, trunk inclination will be maintained close to the horizontal by extension at the hip, a direction technique.

Then head flexion can be seen affecting the position of the center of gravity within the body. Gravitational force will respond by changing the inclination of the entire body. The upper part will incline downward and the lower part upward. At entry, the inclination of the body is approximately 20 degrees; because this angle is small, the dive will be shallow, and forward momentum will be much greater than the downward momentum. The diver will glide until the momentum is equal to that of swimming speed.

The major propelling forces are extension at the knee, gravitational pull, and the final thrust from the feet and toes. The time spent on the starting surface is less for the better performers in relation to the time of entry.

A newer racing dive is a deep one. It is dangerous for unskilled to use in shallow water.

RUNNING JUMPS (SINGLE-FOOT PUSH)

Running Long Jump

The running long jump is a modification of the running stride. The differences can be seen by comparing the line representations shown in Fig. 16-5 with those in Fig. 15-6. On contact the center of gravity in the jump is seen to be farther back than it is in the run. After contact the jumper relies on the momentum of the run to carry the body mass forward with flexion at the ankle joint of the takeoff foot.

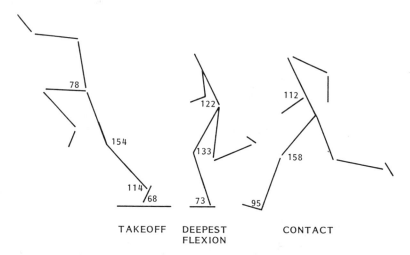

TAKEOFF   DEEPEST   CONTACT
                 FLEXION

Fig. 16-5. *The final step and takeoff of the running long jump. The numbers represent the angles (in degrees) at the joints during contact, deepest flexion at the knee, and at takeoff.*

Adjustments to bring the center of gravity of segments closer to the fulcrum (the contact point) are made by flexion at the knee and hip in the supporting limb and by flexion at the hip in the swinging limb. As the supporting limb reaches the point of deepest leg flexion, ankle extensors prevent further flexion at that joint, and the pattern described for walking, running, and the standing long jump follows; that is, the heel is raised from the ground. At deepest leg flexion, the center of gravity is almost over the foot and will be moved forward rapidly by extension at the knee of the supporting leg, flexion of the swinging limb, and flexion of both arms.

No action occurs at the ankle joint as the foot begins to rise; extension at the ankle begins as the center of gravity passes the metatarsophalangeal joints, but the range of this extension is approximately slightly more than half of that at the metatarsophalangeal joint and therefore the leg is inclined downward by foot action.

The takeoff shown in Fig. 16-5 shows that the force of the joint actions will be directed upward more than forward. This has been found to be 3.6 G's (3.6 times the performer's weight). If the jumper has not lost the momentum of the run, there will be a forward component acting on the body mass, and the resulting angle of projection will be between the horizontal and that suggested by the takeoff position. In the depicted jumper, it was calculated to be 33 degrees. Bunn reported that Jesse Owens' angle of projection was between 25 and 26 degrees. Findings from recent studies show the takeoff angle to be even less, around 17 degrees for world-class jumpers. This low angle indicates that the jumper is not able to transfer his horizontal velocity into a vertical thrust. His jump reflects reliance to a great degree on horizontal velocity. Angles of much less than 45 degrees are essential for maximal distance, since the center of gravity at landing is lower than at the beginning of flight and increased vertical projection greatly reduces the horizontal speed. Minimuzation of the angular momentum is one of the reasons for the long standing jump of more than 29 feet by Beamon.

The movement in the air by the arms and legs is for balance and to counteract the forward rotation produced at the time of takeoff. The arms and legs each produce a secondary axis of rotation, which causes the body as a whole to rotate backward around the center of gravity. This places the body in a better landing position by extending the lower limbs ahead of the path of the center of gravity to increase the measured distance of the jump.

The reach on landing can be longer than in the standing long jump. A horizontal position of the thighs and a greater degree of extension at the knee will add to the measured distance. The trunk is hyperextended at midpoint in the flight and is then flexed to prepare for projecting the center of gravity forward at landing. If flexion at the ankle occurs immediately on contact, the horizontal component of the velocity of projection will carry the body mass forward past the feet. Flexion at the hip, to raise the thighs before landing, will also incline the trunk, bringing the center of gravity forward. By swinging forward, the arms can assist in carrying the body over the landing contact. The legs are flexed to absorb the shock as landing is completed.

The flight of the center of gravity cannot be altered after the takeoff. The path is determined by the angle and speed of projection and by gravitational force once the body is in the air. The only aids to distance that can be made during flight are positioning of the thighs and legs for the reach and of the trunk and arms for carrying the center of gravity forward on landing.

Bedi, investigating the long jumps of medium skilled performers, concluded the following:

1. The jumpers in their run up to the board averaged 8.1 m/sec (26.6 ft/sec), with the best performers running the fastest.
2. The vertical force averaged 4133.64 N (930 lb), with the best jumpers exceeding this amount by more than 441 N (100 lb) of force.
3. The braking force was 3036.04 N (683 lb) on the average.
4. The largest impulses (force multiplied by time) were recorded by the best jumpers.
5. The best long jumper spent 0.11 to 0.12 second on the board, whereas the poorest jumper spent 0.13 to 0.14 second.
6. The jumpers all had a forward rotation at the takeoff, with a large horizontal braking force contributing to this rotational component.

Bedi believes that to jump farther, the performers need to reduce the horizontal braking force at takeoff. This to minimizes the forward rotation and maintains horizontal velocity. To achieve this, other researchers have noted that jumpers adjust their last 6–8 steps of the approach. They visually perceive the best step placement for an effective and legal takeoff.

Triple Jump

The actions of a triple jumper are also that of a long jumper (Bedi, 1975), especially at the instant of the final takeoff. The triple jump involves more than a true jump. Once the triple jump was called the hop, step, and jump, which is more descriptive because it incompasses three movements: The approach, aside from the run up, utilized in the modern period, might be described as a hop, a bound, and a jump.

Whereas in the long jump (discussed previously), there is one flight period, in the triple jump, there are three flight periods. Couple these with not one, but three, takeoffs and three landings, and this event is an intriguing one to study. (See Fig. 16-6 from World Championships.)

The ratio of the distance of the three movements might be nearly even in the immediate future. Yoon found the ratio to be 7:6:7 for

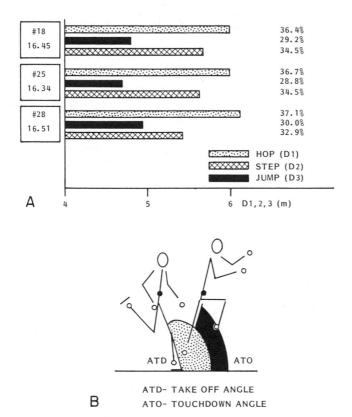

A

B

ATD– TAKE OFF ANGLE
ATO– TOUCHDOWN ANGLE

Fig. 16-6. *Data from triple jump athletes competing at the European Cup, 1987. A, Percent of contribution to distance jumped. All three athletes jumped approximately 16.5 meters. B, Angle of touchdown and takeoff for each of the three propulsive phases. The angle was measured as the angle through the estimated center of gravity of the body with respect to the horizontal in the triple jump. (Courtesy of Petra Sushanka, Charles University Prague).*

the hop, step, and jump, respectively. Many coaches are proposing a 36:30:34 ratio.

The triple jump is a beautiful motion when it is executed by an outstanding competitor. The rhythmic sounds made by the performer could be recorded and used by the beginner to facilitate improvement.

Some comments on the performance in this event are as follows:

1. The initial takeoff in the triple jump is at a lower angle than in the long jump. Descriptive terms might be low, higher, and highest for the three phases, in that order. The takeoff angle at each stage is 8 to 12 degrees.
2. There is a continuous compromise being made between horizontal speed and vertical lift, and the angle of takeoff is considerably lower than in the long jump.
3. The movements must be executed so that the movement is as nearly continuous as possible. The momentum of the jumper

must not be decreased too much at each takeoff position; that is, the braking forces must be minimized.

4. There is a forceful downward extension at the hip, knee, and ankle joints of the takeoff leg at each position.
5. The center of gravity is maintained in front of the takeoff foot at the takeoff position.
6. The torso of the jumper is essentially an erect one so that the landing leg can be extended and the force of the foot against the ground can be exerted somewhat vertically.
7. The arms move laterally, backward and then forward together to provide a transfer of momentum from one movement to another and to help in maintaining horizontal momentum.
8. The landing foot first moves forward and then backward to ensure that the foot is moving backward faster than the body's center of gravity is moving forward. This enables the jumper to move to the next phase.
9. The landing shock is attenuated by the flexion at the hip, knees, and ankles. The arms move forward in extension, and the torso's forward lean (flexion) enables the jumper to fall forward at landing.

Running High Jump

The takeoff for the running high jump is in the flop-style like that for the running long jump. (Most world-class high jumpers use the flop-style.) The principal difference is that the COG is projected at a much greater angle at takeoff in the high jump. This is accomplished by taking a longer penultimate step which lowers the COG just before takeoff. The takeoff foot is then planted in front of the COG which helps to convert the horizontal momentum into vertical lift. Much as in the long jump, the high jumper should strive to take a quick last step, although the step will still be considerably in front of the COG. As was shown in the description of the standing jump for height, the inclination of the foot will affect the inclinations of all other segments. As in the standing jump for height, actions at the ankle and hip serve to maintain the desired direction. The final force is derived from running momentum, from extension at the knee, and from the forceful swing of the free lower limb and the arms. Segmental inclinations of the foot, leg, thigh, and trunk are closer to the vertical and takeoff than in the long jump.

The flop-style high jump utilizes a curved approach, which allows centrifugal force to be exerted at the instant of takeoff. This centrifugal force helps in (1) providing a lifting component at the time of takeoff, (2) providing a horizontal component to carry the jumper into the pit, and (3) providing rotation to help the athlete rotate around the crossbar for optimum bar clearance.

The height of the center of gravity at takeoff is important. If a jumper is 1.82 m (6 ft.) tall, the center of gravity in the normal standing position, according to Palmer's formula, would be 1.036 m (40.65 in) above the soles of the feet. In rising to the tip of the toes at takeoff, the jumper could raise the COG 17.78 cm (7 in). The position of the elevated arms and the swinging leg could add another 20.32 cm (8 in), bringing the position of the COG 1.41 m (55.65 in) above the ground at takeoff. How high would and could the velocity of the jump carry the center of gravity to enable the jumper to clear the bar at 2.28 m (7.5 ft)? If a superior jumper could raise the COG another 0.76 m (30 in), the attained height would be slightly over 2.13 m (7 ft). Additional height is gained by manipulation of the body segments, which allows the COG to pass almost under the bar.

One researcher has stated the belief that the requirements for world-record high jumping are the following (with the latter the more important):

1. Long legs, high center of gravity.
2. Enough speed and strength at takeoff to give an upward thrust of considerable magnitude.

The Fosbury flop style is shown in Fig. 16-7. The ease of execution and high lift of the hips (center of gravity) possibly make this style mechanically best. (See Hay for greater detail.) The flop-style performer usually develops and utilizes greater horizontal velocity than other jumpers.

Ward has shown that force, action, and time aspects can be synchronized as shown in Fig. 16-8. Such a study involves using a force

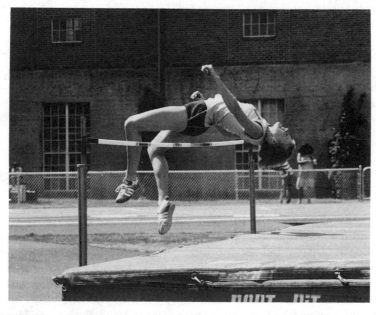

Fig. 16-7. *Flop style of high jumping. (Courtesy of Sports Information, Washington State University.)*

JUMPING

483

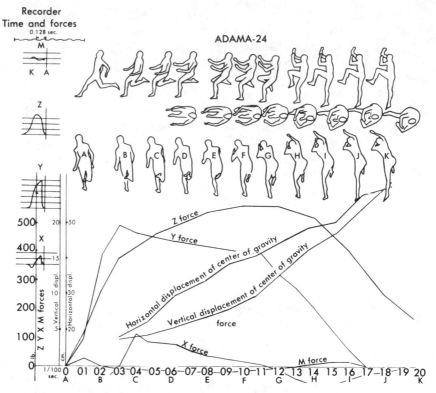

Fig. 16-8. *Force-action-time relationships during propulsive extension of takeoff leg for straddle roll type high jumper. Contourograms of three planar views are synchronized in time with force platform recordings and calculated displacement plots of the center of gravity. (From Ward, R. D. An investigation into the use of computer integration of kinematics, kinetics, and cinematography data in motion analysis. Dissertation, Indiana University, 1971.)*

plate, three cameras, and an oscillograph recording device. The jumper shown here is a straddle roller. The shortest time on the ground at takeoff (0.15 sec) and the most vertical thrust (4 g) have been recorded for the best jumper.

Pole Vault

In the running high and long jumps, the momentum of the run rotates the body over the supporting foot. The foot and lower limb serve much the same function as the pole does in the vault. During the run, the pole is carried by the front arm in medial rotation, and the shoulder is adducted with some flexion. The elbow is flexed, and the forearm is pronated. In the rear arm, there is some extension at the shoulder and the arm is also flexed at the elbow (Fig. 16-9). A horizontal velocity is imparted to the pole by the run, and since the pole is raised upward and pointed downward in the final step, it will be rotated upward and forward, after contact with the box, by the horizontal velocity.

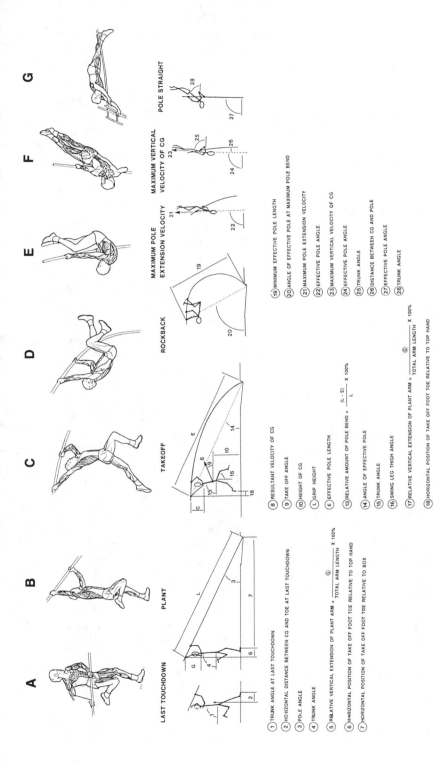

Fig. 16-9. Sequential contourogram-muscle tracings of pole-vaulter during approach, pole plant, takeoff, rockback, pullup, inverted pushup, and release. List the primary muscles acting at each of these phases as shown. Estimate the position of the center of gravity of the body and determine its distance to the pole. How do the movements of the arms and legs and the position of the center of gravity influence muscle contraction? (Reprinted with permission of National Strength and Conditioning Association Journal Vol. 9, No. 2, April/May, 1987. Railsback, D. "The Pole Vault," pp. 5–8 and 78–80.) B, Line segment tracings and key kinematic/kinetic variables to measure with respect to the major phases of pole vaulting. (Courtesy of P. McGinnis)

485

At the plant of the pole in the box, the right hand is placed as high above the head as possible and should be directly over the left foot. The horizontal velocity at plant and the height of the right hand are the two single most important preparations for a successful vault. The right arm is laterally rotated and flexed at the shoulder. There is extension at the elbow. The left arm has flexion at the shoulder and some at the elbow (C). The left hand is open and then closed, momentarily releasing the pole and then regrasping it. The tracings in Fig. 16-9 were taken from a film in which the performer used a glass pole.

As the pole is placed on the ground and the final thrust is made by extension of the thigh and plantar flexion of the foot of the supporting limb, the left forearm is extended and the arm is flexed at the shoulder. The right forearm extends to retain the grasp on the pole as it rebounds from its compressed position. Note that the hands are spaced well apart. Assisting the thrust of the lower limb is the rapid upward movement of the pole and of the swinging right lower limb.

At takeoff the supporting leg, according to Ganslen, is inclined 78 degrees, and since the trunk remains vertical, the thrust of the supporting joints can be assumed to be close to the vertical. As the pole rotates upward around its ground contact, the body rotates around the hand contact on the pole. The body rotation will be faster than that of the pole, and as the extended body passes the pole, its speed of rotation will be increased by flexion at the hips and knees.

For elevation of the lower part of the body above the hands, first there is flexion at the hips and the knees (Fig. 16-9), then the knee position decreases the amount of force needed to flex the legs by moving the center of gravity of the lower limbs closer to the fulcrum (the hip joints). As the thighs approach the vertical, extension at the knees occurs to bring the legs in line with the thighs. The body's center of gravity is now close to the pole so that the vaulter is able to take greater advantage of the pole action. In F, the trunk has begun to rotate to the left; pelvic rotation will follow, and the right leg will scissor over the left. As the jumper's center of gravity passes the pole, the pulling is converted into a pushing movement, which is achieved by flexion at the shoulder and extension at the elbow. This action is completed in one continuous movement, and the left hand is released from the pole first. The forearms are pronated as the release of each is accomplished. To project the legs as high as possible, the vaulter should keep the chin down toward the chest in preparing to go over the bar. The movement of the lower limbs downward after crossing the bar raises the trunk and arms. Elevating the arms still higher helps keep them from striking the bar as they go over. The vaulter must be sure to wait until the pole has almost reached the vertical position before executing the pull up.

The higher the vaulter places the hands on the pole at the start, the faster the run will be, and the steeper the parabola of the path of the center of gravity in flight, the higher the vault should be.

Barlow, using rather elaborate electronic equipment, including force plates, special slow-motion camera, force transducers, recording oscillograph, and necessary accessories, was able to secure kinematic and kinetic parameters of the pole vaulting of top performers. These data were analyzed by a computer and digitizing system.

Some of his findings were as follows:

Kinematic Factors

1. The last stride of all vaulters was shorter than the preceding stride.
2. The second-to-last stride was longer than either the third to last or the last stride.
3. The best vaulter (who was of world class) took longer strides throughout, than did any of the other subjects, and shortened his last stride the least.
4. All pole plants of those who vaulted 4.87 m (16 ft) or higher were initiated in 0.423 second (mean time), compared with 0.408 second for the pole plants of those who vaulted less than 4.87 m.
5. Considerable deceleration over the final three strides occurred for those who vaulted less than 4.87 m.
6. The best vaulter accelerated longer in the run and decelerated less during the final strides.
7. Those who vaulted over 4.87 m. attained a maximal velocity of 8.83 m/sec (28.97 ft/sec) during the second-to-last stride, whereas those who vaulted less than 4.87 m attained a maximal velocity of 8.30 m/sec (27.26 ft/sec) under the same conditions.
8. The average takeoff angle for the center-of-gravity projection of all vaulters was 21.9 degrees.
9. The angle of takeoff tended to increase as the height of the crossbar was elevated.
10. When the pole was perpendicular, the top vaulters had no vertical acceleration, and the poorer ones had negative vertical velocity.

Kinetic Factors

1. The average time on the force plate (of the takeoff foot) was 0.122 second.
2. The fastest time was 0.116 second for the top vaulter.
3. The peak vertical striking force at takeoff was an average magnitude of 3635.8 N (819 lb).
4. The top performers attained greater vertical force at takeoff than did those who were poorer vaulters.

5. The top vaulters supplied greater braking impulse at takeoff.
6. The vertical extension force tended to increase with the increased height of the crossbar.

What meaning can be derived from these data? We now know that the pole vaulter, in fact, does jump at the takeoff, attempts to generate considerable vertical force, and runs at close to top sprinting speed. Finally, by studying such data, we may find distinguishing factors characteristic of the better vaulters. McGinnis has done this.

Hurdling

The high hurdler is a runner who vaults a series of hurdles. The run must be slightly modified on the approach to each hurdle. There is flexion and abduction at the shoulders and the scapulae are elevated (Fig. 16-10). As the body's center of gravity is moved forward by the momentum of the run, the heel is raised (B to D). At the same time, the knee of the supporting limb extends. Considerable flexion at the hip of the lead limb takes place as the limb is swung forward with the leg extended. (Most hurdlers attempt to prevent the leg from extending into a locked knee position.) The skilled hurdler flexes the neck as well as the trunk so that the center of gravity will not go too high over the hurdle and contact with the ground will be made sooner.

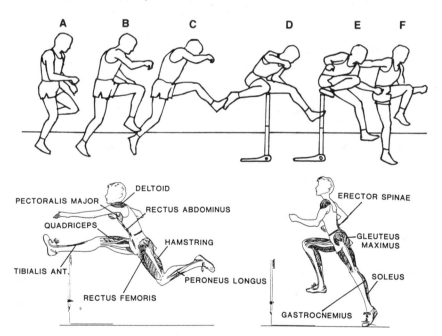

Fig. 16-10. *Sequence of contourograms of hurdler and takeoff and flight phase of one hurdler, with muscles highlighted. What are the major differences in kinematics of the two hurdlers? Which muscles contract for takeoff, but not flight action, and which muscles contract at both times? (Courtesy National Strength and Conditioning Association Journal Vol. 8, No. 6, 1986. McFarlane, B. "High Performance Hurdling—the Women's 100 m Hurdles," p. 4–13.)*

The high point of the parabola should occur in front of the hurdle. Thus, the athlete is actually on the way down when crossing the hurdle. This helps in spending as short a time as possible off the ground and prevents "floating" the hurdle. Note that the hurdler starts flexion of the trunk and neck before leaving the ground (C). The rear leg (D) is brought forward by flexion at the hip. As the thigh is moved forward, it is abducted and rotated medially, bringing the flexed leg close to the horizontal (D and E). At the same time that the trail leg is being brought forward, the arm on the same side is driven forcefully to the rear. This creates an action-reaction situation and assists in bringing the trail leg through quickly and back down into a sprinting position.

After the hurdle is cleared, the lead thigh extends to lower the foot, and the leg flexes, thus moving the foot backward with reference to the knee (E and F) and decreasing the possibility of backward push at contact. The rear thigh, after the hurdle is cleared, adducts and rotates laterally (F) to bring the foot in line for the next step. After contact, body momentum helps to extend the supporting limb.

The hurdler attempts to raise the center of gravity only high enough to clear the hurdle. Likewise, an attempt is made to get the lead leg down as soon as possible so that the feet are in contact with the ground and the hurdler is able to run rapidly to the next hurdle. This involves an action-reaction phenomenon in that as the hip flexes, it aids in balance when the thigh is extended. The reason is that the extension of the thigh creates the action-reaction and brings about an extension of the trunk.

Steeplechase

The steeplechase is a type of endurance run coupled with a hurdling and jumping action. The mechanics used in running 3000 m are similar to those used in any run of that distance. However, scaling five hurdles or obstacles over each 400 meters, with one located just before the water barrier, puts considerable emphasis on the endurance factor. Many performers in the past have jumped on top of the barrier and then attempted to clear the water area. The other four hurdles are jumped over, or the performer leaps on top of the barrier and then jumps into a running stride. The water jump is the one discussed here.

Many authors contend that a fast approach and rapid mount (if this is used), followed by a smooth takeoff, are the ingredients for success in this event. Formerly the steeplechaser usually tried to maximize the horizontal displacement and minimize vertical displacement. The jumper usually landed about 0.60 m (2 ft) from the forward edge of the water area in a stride position and accelerated from a flexed front leg (which reduces the body's moment of inertia) out the water as rapidly as possible. A runner from the University of Wisconsin recently introduced a new technique whereby he jumps the water hurdle (rather than mount the barrier and then jump into the water) and lands just beyond the middle of the water hazard. He landed sooner and was out of the water sooner than his opponents. His technique bears more scrutiny and research.

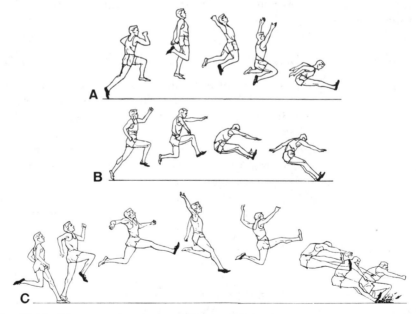

Fig. 16-11. *Three commonly used styles of flight during the long jump. B, The sail is a held position requiring strong flexor muscles crossing the hip. A, the hang is a held upright posture requiring rapid flexion at the hip at the appropriate time for a reach at landing. C, the hitch kick is a dynamic movement simulating running more nearly than the other styles.*

REFERENCES

Barlow, D. A. (1983) Kinematic and kinetic factors involved in pole vaulting, doctoral dissertation, Indiana University, August.

Bedi, J. F. (1975) Angular momentum in the long jump, dissertation, Indiana University, May.

Bunn, J. W. (1955) Scientific principles of coaching, Englewood Cliffs, NJ: Prentice-Hall.

Chistyakov, U. (1966) The run of a high jumper, *Track and Field,* No. 8, Dec.

Doherty, K. (1972) High jump—transition phase—skill and form, *Track and Field Quarterly Rev.* 71:234–236.

Doherty, K. (1984) *Track and Field,* Swarthmore, PA: TAFMOP Publishers.

Elsheikh, M. (1975) A three-dimensional model of the ideal technique in the broad jump, doctoral dissertation, Washington State University.

Felton, E. (1960) A kinesiological comparison of good and poor performers in the standing broad jump, thesis, University of Wisconsin.

Ganslen, R. V. (1941) Mechanics of the pole vault, *Athletic J.* 21:20.

Ganslen, R. V. (1970) *Mechanics of pole vault,* ed. 7, Denton, TX: R. V. Ganslen, Publisher.

Ganslen, R. V. (1985) Triple jump, *Encyclopedia of Physical Education, Fitness and Sports:* Cureton, T. K., (Ed), Reston, VA: AAHPERD.

Ganslen, R. V. (1985) Mechanics of the pole vault, *Encyclopedia of Physical Education, Fitness and Sports:* Cureton, T. K., (Ed), Reston, VA: AAHPERD.

Gros, H. J. (1984) Computerized analysis of the pole vault utilizing biomechanics, cinematography and direct force measurements, unpublished dissertation, University of Alberta, Edmonton, Canada.

Halverson, L. (1958) A comparison of the performance of kindergarten children in the takeoff phase of the standing broad jump, dissertation, University of Wisconsin.

Hay, J. G. (1973) Technique—ultimate in high jump style (forward dive style), *Athletic Journal,* March.

Holmes, D. (1985) High jumping—various styles, *Encyclopedia of Physical Education, Fitness and Sports:* Cureton, T. K., (Ed), Reston, VA: AAHPERD.

Hudson, J. L. (1987) What goes up, unpublished paper presented to AAHPERD National Convention.

Isom, J., et al. (1981) The flop and other topics on high jumping by other authors, *Track and Field Quarterly,* Rev. Winter.

McGinnis, P. (1986) Pole vault report, USOC/TAC Sports Science Project.

Pepin, G. (1976) The long jump, *Track and Field Q. Rev.* 76:Fall.

Ramey, M. (1976) A matter of projection: the long jump, *Track and Field Q. Rev.* 76:13, Fall.

Roy, B. (1971) Kinematics and kinetics of the standing long jump in seven, ten, thirteen and sixteen year old boys, dissertation, University of Wisconsin.

Sargent, D. (1921) Physical test of a man, *Am. Phys. Educ. Rev.* 26:188.

Steben, R. E. (1978) *Track and Field: an administrative approach to the science of coaching,* New York: John Wiley & Sons.

Steben, R. S. (1985) Factors related to success in the pole vault, *Encyclopedia of Physical Education, Fitness and Sports:* Cureton, T. K., (Ed), Reston, VA: AAHPERD.

Ward, R. D. (1971) An investigation into the use of computer integration of kinematics, kinetics, and cinematography data in motion analysis, dissertation, Indiana University.

Yoon, P. T. E. (1970) The triple jump, Wilt, F. and Ecker, T., editors, *International Track and Field Coaching Encyclopedia,* West Nyack, New York: Parker Publishing Co.

17

Biomechanics of Throwing

Throwing includes a rapid acceleration of the trunk and arm segments, usually after a step and just before release of an object. Sometimes it involves a summation of the velocities of the body parts, all adding up to a crescendo at the time of release. At other times, some body parts are moved for positional purposes to allow for the freedom of the body parts engaged in the primary action. In addition, an axis (pivotal point, fulcrum) around which the body rotates as the throwing action takes place is established so that the movement is effective.

ACCELERATION

Throwing a lightweight object such as a ball usually consists of accumulated accelerations of successive segments, especially of the upper extremity. This movement can be labeled concurrent motion; that is, all successive limbs move in the same direction. The result is much greater contraction of the large muscles, such as the pectoralis major and the latissimus dorsi (which are actually arm muscles, in terms of action, even though they are located on the thorax and back). They attach to the humerus in the bicipital groove.

This type of high-velocity throwing calls for greater contractile length of the muscles of the throwing arm than of some of the lower-extremity muscles. The reason is that many of the arm muscles are biarticular in nature; that is, they usually move two joints in the same direction at the same time. This factor calls for proper timing of the action so that the thrower is able to be consistent. A slight error in any part of the movement is accentuated at the time of release. If accuracy rather than velocity is the objective, then the thrower uses the least number of segments possible. The pattern in such a case may be quite different because only a few segments are involved.

493

The movements involved in a high-velocity throw are as follows: (Adapted from Gaul, 1968).

1. The center of gravity shifts backward and then is displaced forward.
2. The performer steps forward with the leg opposite the throwing arm.
3. The upper portion of the body is flexed after being extended (first acceleration).
4. The trunk rotates about its longitudinal axis to pull the throwing arm forward (second acceleration).
5. The scapula moves forward over the back (torso), as much as 15.24 cm (6 in) or more. This is one key to the ability to throw efficiently. A large scapula is considered an asset in high-velocity throwing.
6. The humerus acts in conjunction with the scapula as the former flexes on the latter over a range of 90 degrees.
7. The humerus rotates internally around its long axis up to 90 degrees (another major acceleration). Just as the throw of an object is near the release point, there is some retraction of recoil in the shoulder area.
8. The extension at the wrist at the end of the backward motion of the arm and the flexion at release together add another acceleration. (There is some controversy regarding this statement. Some researchers contend that there is no acceleration involved in the extension of the wrist and that the situation is only positional. Also, to speak of the "cocking," or flexing, and then extending at the wrist is misleading. It is the hand that does most of the movement, not the wrist.)
9. The fingers are extended first and then flexed to add a final acceleration.

AXES OF ROTATION

There are four axes (fulcrums or pivotal points) of rotation often involved in high-velocity throws. They are the planted foot on the opposite side of the throwing arm, the hip opposite the throwing arm, the spine, and the shoulder of the throwing arm. The body as a whole rotates about one axis—namely, the foot—whereas the other body parts rotate about various axes such as a joint or joints. In the so-called overhand throw, the throwing arm begins the action from an extended-arm position with the hand pointing downward. The arm moves in an angular path to the rear and upward. From this rearward, fully-extended position, the arm translates upward and backward. Then the arm flexes and moves forward at the elbow to increase the angular motion, after which it extends laterally before release takes place. This latter action gives the opportunity for centrifugal force to be applied. The lateral body lean in the opposite direction enables the arm to be extended upward (Fig. 17-1). The nonthrowing hand moves backward, assisting in the torso rotation and arm motion. Almost all throwing action has some or all of these segmental movements. Small, light objects are released in a plane lying parallel to the body and tangential to the movement. Heavy objects, such as in a shot put, are released in front of the body; otherwise, injury to the elbow would occur frequently. These objects are linked to the length of the moment arms.

The function of the arm in a throwing situation is to position the hand for the throwing action and to help develop efficient velocity of the hand. (The object is released with the same velocity that the hand has accumulated.)

For a better understanding of the upper limb complex and the amazing action that occurs during the throwing action, it seems appropriate to mention some anatomic and biomedical aspects.

A total of 28 bones in the arm-shoulder area are used in the whip-rack, flail-like action occurring during throwing. The scapula, humerus, radius, and ulna, proximal row of carpals, distal row of carpals, metacarpals, and finally the phalanges are involved. In addition, the clavicle serves as a strut supporting the whole arm during the act of throwing.

The astounding thing about the shoulder girdle complex is its lack of stability, which results in great freedom of motion. In the upper swing of the arm, the great range of movement is further enhanced by the broken hook structure involving the clavicle, acromion process,

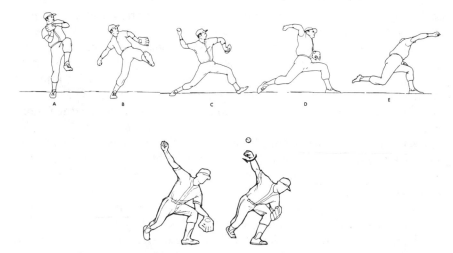

Fig. 17-1. *A high-velocity throw is characterized by a step forward, counter rotation and forward rotation of the trunk and lateral and medial rotation of the arm. Note at the termination of the throw there is pronounced lateral body lean and pronation of the forearm.*

BIOMECHANICS OF THROWING   **495**

top of glenoid fossa, and coracoid process. Furthermore, the scapula moves on the clavicle, and the clavicle moves on the sternum. The shallow depth of the glenoid fossa pushes the humerus farther away from the center of the joint, promoting still more freedom of motion. The joint then has to rely on the rotator cuff muscles—the subscapularis, supraspinatus, infraspinatus, and teres major—as well as on other shoulder girdle muscles to preserve its integrity.

The spins and swings of the arm about its long axis, whereby acceleration is produced from a small radius of gyration, enable the arm to have great spinning motion. Its motion has been compared to that of a jackhammer.

The main muscles of the arm and adjacent region involved in throwing, as determined by electromyography, are the pectoralis major, latissimus dorsi, deltoid, trapezius, serratus anterior (magnus), rhomboids, and levator scapulae. The muscles acting on the scapula function as a force couple: One group produces an upward rotation, and another causes a downward rotation. This is similar to the action of a revolving door. The longer in length the scapula, the farther down the muscles attach, creating the possibility of a large force—hence one of the reasons tall persons can throw at the rate of 160.90 kmph (100 mph), whereas smaller persons throw at slower speeds.

There is usually a proximal-to-distal action of the segments during throwing. This means that the heavier parts initiate the movement, and the distal, lighter segments benefit by transfer of momentum and also are easier to move at the crucial point of release.

The hand is designed so that the grasping aspect is utilized in throwing. For example, there is opposition of the thumb, which is used only during the early stages of the throwing motion but is not evident at the release of lightweight objects. The skin of the hand on the palmar side is tight for grasping and flexibility, but on the back the skin is loose. The skin creases of the fingers are not located only over the joints, but are on either side, allowing for greater flexibility. A natural pocket is formed by the thenar and hypothenar muscles and the metacarpals, and there is an increased angle of application of the profundus and superficilis when they are lifted upward to produce more effort.

All forceful throws from almost any position are characterized by medial rotation of the humerus and pronation of the forearm and hand (Fig. 17-2). The radius of movement of the forearm ranges from long to short to long, which gives the arm the longest moment arm and raises the possibility that the radius and the moment arm will be the same length. A throw of high velocity is likely to be the result.

It is possible for the thrower in certain situations to have lost contact with the ground and to be airborne before releasing the object. This is true in both shot putting and discus throwing. The object has by this time accumulated its own momentum and will continue unimpeded on its course, even though a foot is not anchored to the ground.

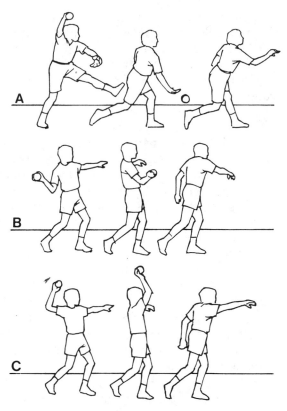

Fig. 17-2. *Evidence of pronation of the forearm during the underarm (A), side-arm (B), and overarm (C) throwing patterns.*

THROWING PATTERNS

Mechanics of Underarm Pattern

The underarm pattern is most frequently seen in skills that project an object by a throw. Its outstanding characteristic is movement of the arm, usually with extension at the elbow, by action at the shoulder. At the height of the backswing, the arm is approximately at shoulder height; during the force-producing phase the arm is moved rapidly downward, and at release or impact it reaches a position that is usually parallel with or slightly beyond the line of the trunk.

The lever of this arm action includes the bones of the upper arm and forearm, the wrist and hand, and, in the throw, the portion of the phalanges up to the center of gravity of the projectile. If an implement is used, all the phalanges will be included, in addition to the length of the implement from grasp to point of impact. The resistance arm includes the same rigid masses as does the entire lever; the fulcrum is in the shoulder joint. The length of the moment arm at the time that the object is started on its flight will be the distance from the proximal end of the humerus to the point of impact or the center of gravity of the projectile. This line will be perpendicular to the axis and to the line of the applied force (Principle of Perpendicularity).

Various levers can be added to this primary action to increase the amount of applied force. Among the most common is that which moves the pelvis by rotation at the hip joint. This lever will include the pelvis, the spine, the right side of the shoulder girdle, and the rigid masses included in the shoulder-action lever. (This description and that which follows refer to a right-handed performer.) The resistance arm will include the same masses as does the entire lever. At release or impact the length of the moment arm will be the distance from the axis (a line passing through the hip joint about which the trunk is rotating) to the point of release or impact. This line, perpendicular to the axis and to the direction of applied force, can be changed in length by the positions of the trunk and the arm. If the trunk is flexed to the right, the moment arm will be lengthened; if the trunk flexed to the left, the moment arm will be shortened. If the arm is abducted, the moment arm will be lengthened. In some underarm patterns that have been studied, although pelvic rotation occurred during the force-producing phase, it was not found to occur at the time of application of force. Thus, if the linear velocities of moment arms acting at release or impact are determined and if the velocity of pelvic rotation is not one of them, pelvic rotation makes no direct contribution to the force at that time. Most likely its contribution, made before the final phase, is reflected in the actions at the other joints.

Pelvic rotation is facilitated by a transfer of weight of the total body. In the preparatory phase the weight is transferred to the right foot, and the pelvis is rotated to the right; rotation can be more than 90 degrees from the intended direction of flight of the projectile. This range of rotation is not possible unless the weight is taken from the left foot. Pelvic rotation facilitates arm action. As the pelvis turns, it carries the torso with it until it, too, is at right angles to the intended line of flight. As the arm is raised upward and backward, it is abducting, instead of extending, as it would be if the torso were facing forward. The shoulder joint's abduction range is greater than its hyperextension range, and according to present knowledge, a segment can be moved faster if its range of motion is increased.

While the weight is on the right foot, the left foot can be lifted in preparation for a forward step. No evidence is available to indicate the most advantageous length of this step. Studies do show that good performers take longer steps than those who are less skilled and that the length of the step is a feature that distinguishes between good and poor performers. As the forward step is taken, some forward movement of the whole body occurs. This adds to the force that can be imparted to the projectile, but compared to that developed by trunk, spine and arm action this force is small. The step alone is not an important factor in increasing force; the step, however, facilitates increased range of trunk and arm action. Thus the step is important.

Rotation of the spine can add another lever to the pattern. In comparison to other possible levers that may be a part of the pattern, the spine makes a small contribution. Although the action occurs in many vertebral joints, the fulcrum can be considered to be located at the level of the sternoclavicular joint. The lever will include the right clavicle and the masses included in the shoulder lever; the resistance arm will include the masses of the entire lever. The length of the moment arm will be the perpendicular distance from the axis; it will pass through the upper spine to the point of release or impact. The length of the moment arm can be altered by changes of trunk or arm position, as described for the moment arm of pelvic rotation.

An important lever acts at the wrist joint, because the wrist can be the fastest of the acting joints and because the length of the moment arm can be greatly increased by an implement. For the throw, the lever arm and the resistance arm include the bones of the hand and fingers to the center of gravity of the projectile; for the strike, they include the bones of the hand and fingers and the implement, if one is used, to the point of impact. In a throw, depending on the size of the hand, the moment arm from the wrist to the center of gravity of the projectile could be 7.6 to 10.1 cm (3 to 4 in) in a child and 20.3 and 22.8 cm (8 to 9 in) in an adult.

The levers described in the preceding paragraphs, acting at shoulder hip, spine, and wrist, are those most commonly used in a variety of underarm patterns. Whether more than one is used in the pattern will depend on the demands of the situation. Movements from the shoulder axis will always be used, since it is the basis for the underarm classification. It is possible that in some situations movements about other joints can be used efficiently, but such additions will not change the classification.

Mechanics of Overarm Pattern

The overarm, like the underarm, pattern is commonly used in throws and strikes. Its distinguishing feature is action that rotates the humerus laterally during the preparatory phase and medially during the force-producing phase. Persons who cannot readily visualize these actions may be helped by going through the following movements: Hold the upper arm at the side in such a position that, when the forearm is flexed 90 degrees, the forearm will be horizontal and pointing directly forward. (If you don't remember anatomical terminology, review Chapter 3.) Keeping the upper arm at the side, move the forearm to the right 90 degrees in the transverse plane; the forearm will now point directly to the side. The joint action that brought about this change in the position of the forearm was lateral rotation of the humerus. If the forearm is now moved back to the original position, the action involved is medial rotation of the humerus.

These rotations at the shoulder can be made while the upper arm is in many positions. One position frequently used is described as follows: With elbow extended, abduct the entire arm 90 degrees to the horizontal. Adjust the position of the upper arm so that when the arm is flexed 90 degrees at the elbow, the forearm will point directly forward. Move the forearm until it points directly upward. This will be accomplished by 90 degrees of lateral rotation of the humerus. Lower the forearm until it again points forward; it has been moved to this position by 90 degrees of medial rotation at the shoulder joint. This rotation of the humerus is the outstanding characteristic of the overarm pattern; this bone is usually abducted in the force-producing phase.

Feltner and Dapena calculated the resultant joint forces and torques at the shoulder and elbow joints in baseball pitching throughout the entire motion. They found that as the forward step came in contact with the ground, there was a horizontal adduction torque at the shoulder joint and the shoulder was externally occurring at the same time. As the upper arm began to rotate internally, (they stated this was 30 ms before release of the ball), it was still in a state of external rotation at the time of release of the ball.

Present observations suggest that next to hand flexion, medial rotation of the humerus is the fastest action of the upper limb. Apparently there is a limit to the speed with which each body segment can be rotated. Because the moment arm of humeral medial rotation can be longer than that acting at the wrist joint, its linear velocity and therefore its contribution to the force imparted to a projectile can be greater than those contributed by action at the wrist (hand movement).

With respect to lateral and medial rotation of the humerus, the axis passes through both the shoulder and elbow joints and the length of the humerus, whereas in the other actions at the shoulder the axis passes through only the shoulder joint, humerus. The length of the moment arm in the rotating actions (lateral and medial) is the distance from the axis to the point of release or of impact. The line representing this distance must be perpendicular to the axis and also to the line of applied force. The moment arm will be longest when the forearm is perpendicular to the humerus; when the forearm is flexed either more or less than 90 degrees, the moment arm will be shorter.

With the forearm extended (but not locked), medial and lateral rotation can be used effectively when an implement is held in the hand. If the arm is held at the side, the elbow extended, and a tennis racket held in the hand so that it is at right angles to the arm, the racket can be moved through 180 degrees in the transverse plane. In this action, pronation and supination of the forearm will add to the range and the speed as the humerus is rotated.

Other levers that are commonly combined with arm action in the overarm pattern are the same as those described for the underarm pattern; they are brought into action by pelvic and spinal rotation and hand flexion. Their resistance arms will be those described for the underarm pattern. The lengths of the moment arms for pelvic and spinal rotation are likely to be longer in the overarm than in the underarm pattern because the humerus is usually abducted.

According to Tarbell, the variety of types of the overarm pattern that the upper limb can perform is characteristic of the versatility of this section of the body. This limb can apply great force and also act with extreme precision. In part, this is due to the structure of the connection with the trunk. The humerus is connected to the freely movable scapula. The humeral head, which is almost half a sphere, fits into a cup of cartilage attached to the inner surface of the fossa on the upper distal section of the scapula. This attachment permits flexion, extension, and abduction of the humerus and the antagonistic actions. Variations are increased by movements of the scapula, which has no direct connection with the trunk. The scapula and clavicle are a functioning part of the upper limb and take part in practically all movements of the humerus, not adding to strength of action, but, rather, increasing range and versatility.

Mechanics of Sidearm Pattern

The sidearm pattern, like the underarm and overarm ones, is generally used in throws and strikes. Unlike the previous two patterns, the distinguishing feature of the sidearm pattern is not the type of shoulder action but the lack or limitation of action at this joint. The main action in the sidearm pattern is pelvic rotation, with the arm held fairly stable in an abducted position. The lever and the resistance arm for this action include the segments described for it for the underarm pattern. The moment arm for the pelvic lever can be one of the longest found in common throwing activities. It extends from the axis passing through the left hip (for right-handed performers) to the line of applied force and includes the width of the pelvis, often the length of the whole arm, and part of the hand. The length of the moment arm is increased by the length of any implement that is used. With a tennis racket or a baseball bat, the length of the moment arm could be 1.828 m (6 ft) or more in an adult. Other actions that are commonly combined with pelvic rotation in this pattern are spinal rotation, hand flexion, and often a small range of arm adduction.

Another outstanding feature of the sidearm pattern is the plane in which the movements are made (that is, the transverse); many movements of the underarm and overarm patterns are made in the sagittal plane or the diagonal plane.

The basic sidearm pattern, in which the shoulder and elbow joints are fixed, is rarely used in throwing light objects. Only when heavy objects are projected and in young, inexperienced children is the basic pattern likely to be observed. In a study of the sidearm and overarm throwing patterns of a highly skilled man and woman, the preliminary parts of the movements were found to be much alike. The differences were seen to be in the position of the arm and the degree and timing of extension at the elbow. The arm in the sidearm pattern was close to the horizontal as rotation at the hip began, and the forearm was more fully extended at release. These arm positions would lengthen the moment arms at pelvic and spinal levels and shorten the moment arm for shoulder rotation. The pelvic action in both subjects contributed a greater proportion of the velocity in the sidearm throw than it did in the overarm pattern. The ball velocity for the man's sidearm throw was 3.657 m/sec (120 ft/sec), and, for the women's, 2.73 m/sec (89 ft/sec).

Continued study of the so-called sidearm throws of skilled performers has shown so much similarity with the overarm throw, especially those in which medial rotation of the humerus is followed by forearm extension, that some students have questioned classifying them as different patterns. Other observers believe that a distinguishing feature in the sidearm throw is a circular arm movement preceding release and that this is never seen in the overarm throw. Such observers say that the throw with the circular pattern should not be classified with the overarm throw. The overarm and sidearm patterns may be primarily diagonal patterns with difficult directions of trunk lateral flexion. The sidearm includes a lean of the trunk toward the throwing arm; whereas an opposite lean occurs during overarm throwing.

MINI-LAB LEARNING EXPERIENCES

1. Put up a target and have class members throw at it, using underarm, overarm, and sidearm patterns, and using only the arm segment. Record the differences.
2. Bring to the laboratory pictures of all types of throwing actions, preferably in sequence. Note segmental action.
3. Have a skilled performer demonstrate and explain his or her throwing action. Evaluate the statements with respect to what was demonstrated.
4. Contrast poor and skilled performances in a throwing action.

BIOMECHANICS OF SELECTED THROWING SKILLS

A number of analyses of selected throwing skills involving sidearm, underarm and overarm patterns are presented here. There has been no attempt to include all the movements; only a representative sample is discussed. In the sidearm example, only the discus throw is presented; however, many striking patterns utilize sidearm actions.

Sidearm Throw—Discus

The discus throw is a type of sidearm throwing action. This throwing movement is used because it enables the thrower to attain the greatest possible distance. Factors influencing the flight pattern are height, velocity at release, and angle at release. In addition, the discus in flight is subject to aerodynamic factors and angle of attack (air resistance), which influence the distance traveled.

The velocity of the released spinning discus accomplished by top performers is 24.38 m/sec (80 ft/sec) or more, and the angle of release is approximately 35 degrees. The angle of attack, about 15 degrees, is the angle of the plane of the discus and the relative wind. The discus is thrown with a slight tilt so that the lift factor is greater than the drag factor. (See Chapter 6 for more information on lift and drag.) A head wind coming toward the performer at an angle of 45 degrees from the right (with a right-handed competitor) is the most advantageous wind, in terms of direction, for top performers.

If the radius of the throwing arm is long (externally extended) and coincides with the moment arm, great velocity is generated at release. Furthermore, the throwing arm is extended downward at the start of the spin and then is extended laterally and upward, utilizing centrifugal force at release.

The discus throw is an excellent example of the basic sidearm pattern, to which has been added a preparatory movement of the entire body. In the area (a ring with a diameter of 2.5 m (8 ft 2.5 in)) within which the body is permitted to move, the progression includes total rotation of the body one and one-half times, as well as movement from the back to the front of the space. Some of the world's best performers use all of the ring, starting well to the back and ending with the final step at the front of the ring. Some performers are now using two full turns.

The first step is taken with the left foot, which is moved toward the front of the ring and placed in line with the right foot. As the steps continue, they resemble those of a sprinter more than do those shown in Fig. 17-3. As the turns are made, the legs are flexed, and the right arm is held fairly close to the side, with the discus dragging behind.

These actions lower the center of gravity of the body and aid in balance. The arm position also moves the center of gravity of the rotating body closer to its axis and enables it to turn with greater speed. The speed of rotation during the stepping should accelerate and be as fast as possible and still allow the performer to maintain balance. The general concept is that the thrower moves slowly during the first turn, accelerates during the step phase and explodes into the throwing action.

On the final step, the right arm is abducted, lengthening the moment arm of the pelvic lever, which can also be increased if the discus

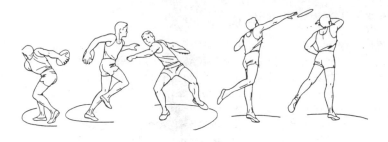

BUGAR 66.94M

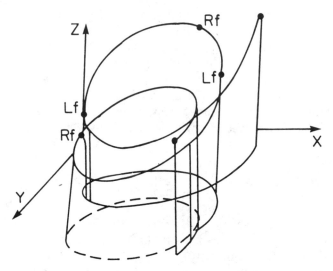

Fig. 17-3. *The discus throw is characterized primarily by rotary movements. The discus is kept close to the body during the initial turn and is abducted and the forearm extends prior to release. Often release velocity is limited by the angular momentum that can be developed and controlled during the body spins. The helical path is depicted three dimensionally for Bulgar during the World Cup, Helsinki. (The latter reprinted from Scientific Report 1st World Junior Championships, Athens 1986, P. Susanka, P. Bruggemann, Tsarouchas.)*

is held as close to the end of the fingers as possible and is still controlled. Adduction of the arm at release will start the flight well beyond the front of the ring. Hand action in the final phase can be added to impart more velocity. The discus is released by rolling it off the index finger with the thumb providing the control.

Gregor et al., studying the 1984 Olympic winners and placers of the discus throw for both men and women, found some very interesting results. Height, angle, and velocity of the discus and the throw's trunk angle were measured, using film data. They found little difference between men and women (women throw a smaller discus) in regard to the kinematics of the throw. There were, however, anthropometric differences which influenced the kinematics. The higher

Table 17-1. *Kinematic Data for Olympian Discus Throwers.*

	Speed of discus	Height of release	Distance between feet	Trunk angle at release	Release angle from ground	Distance of throw
males						
Ht = 1.73 m	24.8 m/s	1.73 m	.80 m	97.4 deg/sec	35.6 deg	65.6 m
females						
Ht = 1.48 m	25.0 m/s	1.48 m	.85 m	97.5 deg/sec	34.7 deg	63.5 m

standing height of the men meant that the release of the discus was at a higher arm position than that of the women. A comparison of these performances can be made by studying Table 17-1.

Gregor et al. mentioned that the release velocity and the release height are the two most important variables in determining distance of throw. Many other investigators support these latter comments.

MINI-LAB LEARNING EXPERIENCES

1. Estimate the moment arm with the discus close to the shoulder and at intermediate positions until fully extended. What is the potential for injury, loss of control and for learning the correct action for beginners?
2. Obtain two or more frisbees of different size, weight, and/ or materials. Using a sidearm throwing pattern, compare the flight patterns of the frisbee and the arm, hand, trunk and leg movements of the throw. Rather than merely "eye-balling" these throws, videotape several trials and analyze the throws using stop-action playback of the tape.
3. Investigate the aerodynamic characteristics of the frisbees (and relate to the discus) by analyzing the frisbee 10 degrees, 20 degrees and 30 degrees, always performing a horizontal throw.

Underarm Patterns—Softball Pitching, Hammer Throw, Bowling, Curling

Pitching Underarm. In the basic underhand pattern, the joints about which levers rotate in the direction of the throw normally occur in the following sequence: hip (rotation), spine (rotation), shoulder (adduction and flexion), and wrist (flexion). As the trunk is rotated backward, the arm is raised to the rear in a combined abducting and extending action; as the arm is moved forward, it is kept in the sagittal plane by a combination of adduction and flexion at the shoulder. The underarm throw and pitch are much alike in joint and lever actions. The moment arm lengths for this form of throwing were previously described. However, observers will find many individual modifications of the basic joint actions.

Normally, the first forward movement is a step with the left foot (right-handed pitcher). This necessitates first putting the weight on the right foot, facilitates pelvic rotation over the support, carries the left side of the pelvis forward, and increases the length of the step. As the left foot contacts the ground, the right arm usually reaches a horizontal position and is ready to begin its forward swing. For most effective action the upper torso would, at this time, be facing to the right with the shoulders in line with the direction of the throw. Unskilled performers often fail to take advantage of this position. Instead, they tend to keep the upper torso facing the direction of the throw and thereby decrease both hip and spinal actions, sometimes with complete loss of the latter. The major forward movement of the body is made as the left foot moves forward; there is rarely a slide on the left foot such as in bowling. At the time of release, forward movement of the body contributes little to the force of the throw. A 3-D skilled women's fast-pitch underarm throw is shown in Fig. 17-4.

Note the lengths of the step for each and compare the step length to the leg length of the respective pitcher. The lead foot moves directly forward toward the batter. Study carefully the similarities with the computer-generated views. Which figures are more interesting, and how much information is included in each? Differences in arcs for a change-up and fastball are depicted in Fig. 17-5.

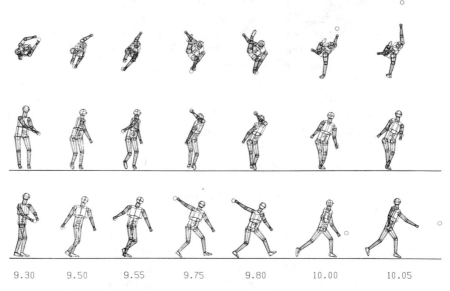

| 9.30 | 9.50 | 9.55 | 9.75 | 9.80 | 10.00 | 10.05 |

Fig. 17-4. *The action of the slingshot style of fastpitch softball is displayed as 3-D computer generated contourograms. Note the nonplanar path of the arm at the height of the swing and the speed at the lowest part of the arc. Note the differences in action of the lead leg between this particular pitcher and that of the overarm pitcher in figure 17-1.*

506   *THE BIOMECHANICS OF HUMAN MOVEMENT*

At release, the contributing joint actions are left hip (rotation), right shoulder and wrist (flexion), and left ankle (flexion). The increasing speed of the ball can be seen in the line segment illustration. Medial rotation of the humerus and supination of the forearm will impart rotation to the ball. Based upon film observations, men frequently flex at the elbow and use either lateral or medial rotation of the humerus to develop speed. In doing so, they decrease the amount of flexion at the shoulder. Present information does not indicate whether rotation of the humerus develops more speed than does greater flexion at the shoulder with the forearm extended.

Measurements of the basic pattern provide insight into the potential contributions of each lever. Observations were made of the film of a skilled college woman pitcher. The measurements were made for two frames, including that showing the release; the time for all limb actions except the hand was 0.03 second. The action at the wrist occurred in less than the time of one frame, and the time of this action was calculated to be 0.008 second. In the measurements given in Table 17-2, the range is expressed in degrees, the angular velocity in degrees per second, the moment arm length in centimeters (feet), and the linear velocity in meters (feet) per second.

The sum of the velocities is 21.5 m/sec (70.59 ft/sec); the ball velocity in the film was measured at 21.4 m/sec (70.26 ft/sec). Using the sum of the linear velocities as the total, one finds the contributions of limb segments rotating about the following joint (expressed in percentages), to be as follows: hip, 14.3 spine, 7.9; shoulder, 45.3; wrist, 32.4. Arm flexion at the shoulder is the major contributor. Hand

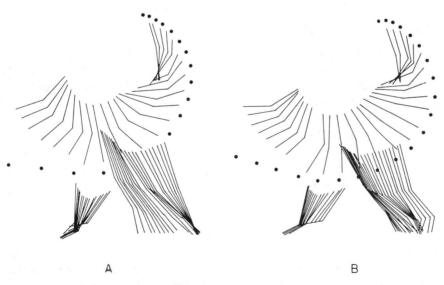

A   B

Fig. 17-5. *Line segment tracings of A) fast pitch and B) change-up. (Courtesy of Mary Boedigheimer.)*

Table 17-2. *Lever Contributions to Ball Velocity in Underarm Throw (Pitch)*

	Range (degrees)	Angular velocity (degrees/sec)	Moment arm length		Linear velocity	
			cm	ft	m/sec	ft/sec
Hip rotation	12	400	44.7	1.45	3.08	10.12
Spinal rotation	6	200	48.7	1.60	1.70	5.59
Shoulder flexion	22	733	76.2	2.50	9.74	31.98
Wrist flexion	30	3750	10.6	0.35	6.97	22.90

flexion about the wrist in the throw with the lighter ball is more forceful than in bowling.

Velocity measures of ball projections are not commonly made; however, they are a more valid measure of the force imparted by body levers than is a measure of distance. In measures made under the supervision of Glassow, two male pitchers on softball teams had velocities of 32.91 and 33.22 m/sec (108 and 109 ft/sec); two women majors in physical education threw balls at 19.81 and 19.50 m/sec (65 and 64 ft/sec); and a teenage girl, an outstanding pitcher in a city softball league, delivered a ball at 24.68 m/sec (81 ft/sec). In addition, Joan Joyce, once the outstanding fast pitcher for women's softball, is reported to have thrown a ball at approximately 193 kmph (120 mph).

MINI-LAB LEARNING EXPERIENCES

Time the speed of a pitched softball in the following situations:

1. Legal slow-pitch softball (ball must have an upward arch).
2. Legal fast-pitch fastball
   a) windmill style
   b) sling shot style
   c) figure 8 style

Compare results. State the mechanical principles as you explain results.

Hammer Throw. The hammer throw is an underarm, two-handed throw unique in that a weight of 7.25 kg (16 lb) is attached to a wire string 117 to 121 cm in length. This increases greatly the arm length of the thrower. This sport is one of the few such activities in which centrifugal force is exceptionally high. Thus a relatively lightweight object such as a hammer can be propelled into the air rather easily by utilizing this force.

There are two or three twisting actions of the hammer around the body prior to the actual true turns about the circle. These preliminary moves are done so the thrower gets a feel of the hammer in relation to the body. Then the hammer thrower executes the three or four turns about the circle, advancing slightly from rear to the front.

Two factors stand out as being important in gaining velocity at release and consequently greater distance in the throw: a long turning radius and an increased turning speed. Black (1981) has made this statement:

> In an analysis of the Munich competition, we found that the top throw by A. Bondarchuk of the USSR of 247' 8" (75.48 m) was achieved with a turning interval of 1.51 seconds. A further breakdown shows the increased body speed from one turn to the next.

The hammer is released at 26+ m/sec by the top throwers. Thus a decrease in turning time increases the final distance, provided that all other factors are held constant.

The thrower must keep in balance and control, gradually accelerating the hammer during the turns. There is torque between the upper and lower portions of the body. In a sense, the hammer thrower hangs onto, or some say against, the hammer as velocity increases. The thrower makes three or four turns about the circle before the hammer is released, as stated previously.

There is an orbit, or path, established by the thrower turning about the circle and a high and a low point of the hammer's path. A right-handed thrower flexes the right arm and then extends it to regain a tighter hold on the handle. The left arm is kept straight (extended) throughout the movement. During this acceleration phase, the plane of the hammer is relatively level. Any additional force, such as a pull inward, will decrease the radius and also prevent pelvic rotation (causing the hip to lead the movement).

As the thrower winds the hammer about the body, the center of rotation being the right shoulder, the degrees of rotation change from a low point of 280 to 290 degrees to a maximum of 320 to 325 degrees. These windups, or sweeps, have to be done with no loss of balance and with increased velocity of the hammer.

A "sit-and-stretch" action helps the shoulders relax and thus increase the radius. Doherty has stated that for every inch gained in radius, there is a possibility for a 6-foot gain in distance. The flexing at the knees helps increase the length of the radius and also aids in maintaining balance by lowering the center of gravity.

The period of maximum acceleration is during the hammer's descent. The thrower at this time "sits" vigorously and thus increases the centrifugal pull. The "sit" is necessary to keep the center of gravity over the feet, especially the left heel (for a right-handed thrower). Usually the left foot stays in contact with the circle area throughout the turns.

As the thrower moves about the hammer ring, he attempts to increase the time of double support of the feet and to decrease that of single support. It has been shown that the hammer acceleration occurs only during the double-support period. Double support is referred to as the "power" aspect and single support as the "gliding" phase.

The thrower must turn fast enough to stay ahead of the rotating hammer as he turns. Failure to do so causes a decline in acceleration, especially during the second and third turns.

To increase the torque in the body, whereby there is a twist between the upper and lower portions, the thrower rotates the hips ahead of the shoulders during the turns. The hip lead with respect to the hammer is anywhere from 45 to 90 degrees.

The height of release is governed by the physique of the thrower and the position of the hammer. The angle of release is considered to have the greatest influence on the distance of the throw. It is a result of the application of the horizontal and vertical forces at the moment of release. The best release angle for distance is between 42 and 44 degrees, since the hammer is released at shoulder height.

Two force couples act in the hammer throw. The first one is the outward, centrifugal pull of the hammer, which is countered by the inward, centripetal force exerted by the thrower. The latter involves the pulling of the thrower's weight through the center of mass downward. This force is opposed by the pushing of the ground upward against the thrower's feet. More centripetal force is needed to counteract the centrifugal pull as the speed of the turns increases. The Russians have conducted experiments measuring the strain on the handle of the hammer during the throwing action. Hwang and Adrian also measured the strain in the wire.

Within each wind and turn, the force increases and decreases, but it consistently increases from the first wind to the last turn. The maximum force at release was measured to be 1400–2000 N, and was positively related to the distance of the throw.

Using Schultz's Mathematical Model, the muscle forces and compression on the lumbar spine were estimated. The basic theory underlying this modeling approach was that only the muscles that are necessary to contract would do so; the other muscles would relax. Each contraction composite would produce precisely the required force to produce or oppose the force measured on the hammer. This means that each muscle contributes according to its estimated line of pull and estimated cross-sectional area. These concepts are based upon the Optimization Theory: Every force is optimum.

Estimated stress to the lumbar spin (L3) was calculated and found to be greater than forces occurring during lifting tasks as used in various occupations. The latter also were estimated through modeling via the Optimization Theory. Such modeling has value on predicting risk of injury or levels of physical conditioning to prepare for high level sports competition.

Relaxation of the shoulders helps increase the radius. There is a position of the central axis of rotation within the hammer-athlete-lever system. To keep the system stabilized, the athlete must center the base of the axis over the left heel, thus increasing the smoothness of execution. The left heel is not only the center of rotation but the axis of the lever system.

Dapena has made a technical study, including calculations of center of mass of the thrower, the hammer, and hammer-thrower system. He found that the up-and-down motions of the center of mass of the thrower was ahead of the hammer by about a third of a cycle, and this made it possible for the upward "vertical acceleration of hammer-thrower system to almost coincide with the double-support phases." In the horizontal direction, the center of mass of the hammer and the thrower in their rotations were out of harmony by about half a spin.

Hwang and Adrian also reported on the kinematics of the hammer. Regarding the displacement of the hammer head, they found the pattern to be neither symmetrical or purely circular. There was a continuous changing of the shape and slope of the eliptical pattern as the turns occurred. (See Fig. 17-6)

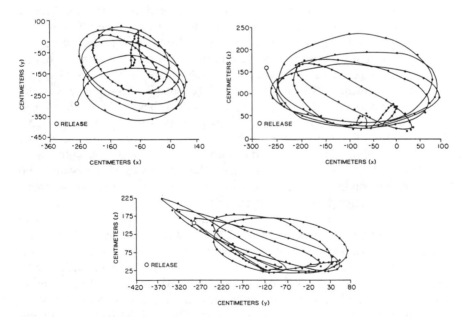

Fig. 17-6. *Three planar views of the path of the hammer during the hammer throw event. Note especially the change in the slope of the path as seen in the frontal view (90 degrees to path of throw). The open circle denotes the release point. (Reprinted from Biomechanics, proceedings of the Olympic Scientific Congress, 1986. Microfilms Publishers.)*

Bowling. Among the least complex of the underarm patterns is the bowling delivery. Obviously, the major contribution to the velocity of the ball is the force derived from arm action. It is also apparent that rotation at the hip and spine about the vertical axis will be limited, since the bowler tends to keep the upper torso facing the lane, and the weight of the ball will limit hand action.

Although each bowler's performance differs in detail from that of others, a general idea of the contribution of each acting lever can be gained from the following analysis. From a film showing the delivery of a male physical education major, observations disclosed that at the time of release, spinal rotation and flexion at the shoulder occurred, but there was no rotation at the hip or flexion at the wrist. An unexpected action was flexion at the elbow.

To determine the contribution of each acting joint, researchers made the following measurements for the two frames preceding release: (1) the range of action of each joint (Table 17-3A), and (2) the time during which this action occurred. The time per frame was 0.0158 second, and for 2 frames was 0.0316 second, or approximately 64 frames/sec. The length of each moment arm at the time of release was measured from a side view. These moment arms were (1) from shoulder to center of the ball), (2) for the elbow (from each elbow to center of the ball), and (3), for the spine (a horizontal line from the upper spine to a vertical line passing through the center of the ball).

The sum of the linear velocities of the three levers is 7.8 m/sec (25.60 ft/sec). The velocity of the ball as it moved away from the hand was measured and calculated at 8.8 m/sec (29.11 ft/sec). The difference may be attributed to a contributing factor not included in the analysis or errors made in measurement. The former was true, based upon further study of the films, the torso moved forward during the two frames because of sliding on the left foot and flexion at the left ankle. The distance that the shoulder moved forward was measured as 44 mm (0.144 ft). The linear velocity of this movement would be 1.4 m/sec (4.56 ft/sec). The summed velocities were now 1.4 m/sec (30.16 ft/sec), or 0.32 m (1.05 ft) more than the measured velocity of the ball. The discrepancy is less than the 1.07 m (3.51 ft) before the forward movement of the body was observed; however, better techniques are needed to provide greater accuracy.

The film of a highly skilled woman bowler, whose season's average score in three leagues was 182, was studied by Anhalt; results are shown in Table 17-3B. Measurements were made from a side view.

As shown, the moving levers at release were the shoulder-arm, elbow-forearm, and wrist-hand. The sum of their linear velocities is 6.64 m/sec (21.81 ft/sec). The body was moving forward at the same time at a rate of 1.4 m/sec (4.72 ft/sec). This, added to the lever velocities, totals 8.08 m/sec (26.53 ft/sec). The measured velocity of the ball in the film was 8.15 m/sec (26.74 ft/sec) after release. The degree to which the summed velocities agree with the ball velocity indicates the accuracy of the measurements.

Table 17-3-A. *Lever Contributions to Ball Velocity in Bowling**

	Range (degrees)	Angular velocity (degrees/sec)	Moment arm length cm	ft	Linear velocity m/sec	ft/sec
Shoulder	14	443	74.67	2.45	5.770	18.94
Spine	6	190	31.69	1.04	1.050	3.45
Elbow	4	127	44.20	1.45	0.978	3.21

*Skilled man bowler.

Table 17-3-B. *Lever Contributions to Ball Velocity in Bowling**

	Range (degrees)	Angular velocity (degrees/sec)	Moment arm length cm	ft	Linear velocity m/sec	ft/sec
Shoulder	12	400.00	75.59	2.480	5.27	17.31
Elbow	2	66.66	46.63	1.530	0.54	1.78
Wrist	11	366.66	12.95	0.425	0.83	2.72

*Skilled woman bowler.

Increased velocity of the ball should be a goal for beginning bowlers; observations have not been extensive enough to set such goals with confidence. Casady and Liba recommend that women bowlers should impart a velocity to the ball that would send it from the foul line to the head pin in 2.50 to 2.75 seconds (7.31 to 6.67 m/sec (24 to 21.9 ft/sec)), and men bowlers in 2.0 to 2.5 seconds (9.14 to 7.31 m/sec (30 to 24 ft/sec)). How much speed must a bowler impart to the bowling ball? Review Table 17-4 in which data are listed from randomly selected league bowlers. Since the expert does not deliver the ball with the greatest possible velocity but only with enough to make

Table 17-4. *Ball Velocities and Time to Travel the Length of a Bowling Alley (60 feet) of League Bowlers.*

	Ball velocity	Time of ball (sec)
men (+190)	8.65 m/sec (28.38 ft/sec)	2.11
women (+180)	8.61 (28.26)	2.12
men (150–160)	8.8 (29.12)	2.06
women (120–130)	7.29 (23.94)	2.50

BIOMECHANICS OF THROWING   513

effective impact with the pins, the velocity of the highly skilled performer is one that the beginner can attain.

Both the man and the woman whose bowling delivery was studied derived over 60% of their velocity from the lever acting at the shoulder joint. The bowler should strive to use this action effectively. It is frequently said that the arm should reach the horizontal at the height of the backswing. Shoulder hyperextension, when the body is erect, will not carry the arm to this height. By flexing at the hips, therefore, the bowler inclines the trunk forward. In this position, although the range of shoulder hyperextension is not increased, the arm, depending on the degree of trunk inclination, can approach, reach, or pass the horizontal. Widule found in the groups that she observed, that the upper arms reached the following positions: skilled men, 185 degrees; average men, 180 degrees; skilled women, 199 degrees; average women, 163 degrees. (The horizontal is represented by 180 degrees; more than that means higher than the horizontal.) Inclinations measured from the horizontal of the trunk for these groups were 35 degrees for skilled men, 51 degrees for average men, 41 degrees for skilled women, and 54 degrees for average women. (If the trunk were erect, the inclination from the horizontal would be 90 degrees; the greater the forward inclination of the trunk, the smaller the inclination measure.) The height of the arm on the backswing depends on the degree of trunk inclination and the degree of hyperextension at the shoulder joint. At the height of the backswing, Widule found the following hyperextension measures: skilled men, 40 degrees; average men, 52 degrees; skilled women, 59 degrees; and average women, 37 degrees. (The greater the measure, the greater the degree of hyperextension).

The length of the bowler's arm will also affect the linear velocity of that lever. In the measurements shown in Table 17-3, had the moment arm for arm flexion been 0.67 m (2.2 ft) instead of 0.74 m (2.45 ft), and had the angular velocity been the same (443 degrees/sec), the linear velocity would have been 5.18 m/sec (17.01 ft/sec). A difference of 7.62 cm (3 in) in length decreased the velocity almost 0.60 m/sec (2 ft/sec).

The strength of grip has been shown by two researchers (Curtis and Sabol) to be related to the speed of the swing. The nervous system evidently controls the speed, limiting it to the ability to hold the ball as it moves through the backward and forward arcs. The difference in grip strength of grip enables men to use a heavier ball than women usually use.

The contribution of the approach steps is not entirely shown in the forward movement of the torso at the time of release. As the ball is moved backward past the right leg by the arm, the approach steps are moving it forward. In the film study, the ball was observed to move forward faster than it moved backward, so that during the backswing the ball was moving forward. This may be more easily visualized when compared to a person walking toward the rear of a railway car as the train moves forward. The person is walking backward but moving forward. As the bowling swing begins its downward, forward action, the ball already has a forward velocity, and the body levers add to this, rather than beginning from a zero velocity. The velocity of the approach increases with each step; the speed of the steps is usually kept constant, but the length of each increases over that of the preceding one.

If the velocity derived from the body levers is to be fully used, there should be no downward direction in the ball's movement as it touches the floor. The arm should be a degree or two past the perpendicular at release, even if this means that the ball is released a few centimeters above the alley. The impact with the floor from this height will be slight and will be decreased by the roll given to the ball at release. Widule found that the upper arm had passed the perpendicular at release and also that the arm was flexing at the ball release. This action not only raises the ball slightly but adds to the velocity. (See Table 17-4).

The analysis of the swing thus far has dealt with factors affecting the speed of the ball. The direction given to the ball is an important factor in the number of pins knocked down. In the distance that the ball travels from release to the pins, approximately 18 m (60 ft), a slight deviation from the exact line to the point of aim can result in marked deviation as pin contact is made. For every 0.25 degree deviation the ball will miss the point of aim by approximately 7.62 cm (3 in). A variation of 1 degree in direction would miss the point of aim by 30 cm (12 in); a ball started at the midpoint of the alley, if it deviated by 2 degrees from a perpendicular to the foul line, would end up in the gutter. Since slight deviations in direction have this marked effect on point of contact, the bowler must give careful attention to factors affecting accuracy.

Among these factors is the point at which the ball crosses the foul line. The starting position should be carefully determined with reference to this line, and the approach should be consistently straightforward. From the point on the foul line, the ball should be directed along the selected line of direction. That line should be clearly visualized, and the arm should swing along this line even after the ball is released. (For additional details on achieving accuracy, see Casady and Liba.)

MINI-LAB LEARNING EXPERIENCES

1. Time the speeds of balls by bowlers of different skill levels. Explain reasons for differences.
2. Compare speeds of balls bowled from a stationary position, one step approach, 3-step, and 5-step approach. Explain results.

Overarm Patterns—Football Passing, Baseball Pitching, Shot Put and Javelin

When great speed and control are desired in a throw, often the overarm pattern is used. This uses the two joint actions that appear to have the highest speeds: flexion at the wrist and medial rotation at the shoulder. The sequence of joint actions can be seen in the football pass (Fig. 17-7) and in the baseball pitch (Fig. 17-1). Both show the step forward with the left foot, pelvic and spinal rotation, and medial rotation of the humerus. Apparently, less hand action occurs with the football throw than with the baseball pitch, which explains the greater velocity obtained with the smaller ball. Note in both series of pictures that, as the torso is rotated forward by pelvic and spinal actions, the humerus is rotated laterally. This timing is an important feature of complex movement patterns. The slower joints begin their forward movement as the faster more distal joints complete their backswings. No appreciable pause between the backswing and forward swing of these faster-moving joints is necessary. The muscles responsible for the forward swing can begin contraction to stop the

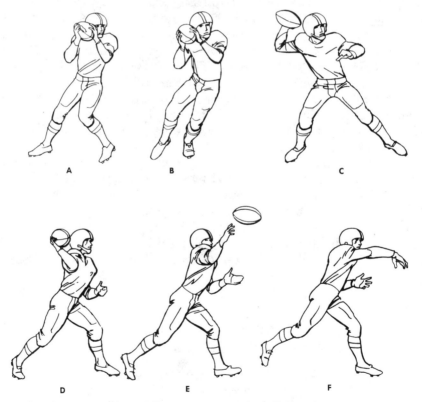

Fig. 17-7. *The football pass utilizes the typical lever systems of the overarm throwing pattern. Note the lateral and medial rotation of the humerus. Note the differences in step length compared to a baseball pitch. What other differences are there between a baseball pitch and football pass?*

backswing. The combination of backward movement and beginning contraction stretches the tendons and connective tissue in the muscles, and thus the forward movement can be more forceful.

Note that in both throws the forearm extended somewhat before the ball was released, shortening the moment arm for shoulder medial rotation. Apparently, then, this action develops its greatest linear velocity before release, and this velocity must be used by the joints acting at release. However, forearm extension lengthens the moment arms for the pelvic and spinal levers and adds to the linear speeds of these levers at release. In both performances the right foot, as it supports the body weight during the backswing, is placed at right angles to the direction of the ball flight, which permits a greater range of pelvic rotation at the right hip.

Figure 17-8 shows the path of the wrist in two throwing actions. The release of the ball by the pitcher is at the height of the movement at the wrist, but the football passer, because of the spin that must be imparted to the ball, releases it when the hand is moving downward.

A physical education major, in analyzing his own football passes, measured the ball velocity as 18 m/sec (60 ft/sec) immediately before release. Humeral medial rotation contributed 62%, spinal rotation 35%, and hand flexion 3%. He had no rotation at the hip during the release phase.

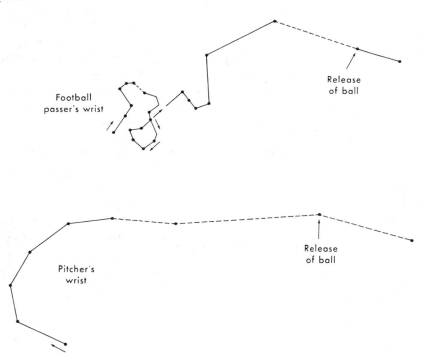

Fig. 17-8. *Path of wrist (traced from movie film) of two throwers, one in football and one in baseball. Note that the football thrower releases the ball after maximum height of the wrist has been reached, but the pitcher releases the ball at maximum height.*

BIOMECHANICS OF THROWING 517

Film study of the overarm baseball throw of a skilled man (a major league player) and a highly skilled woman was useful in determining contributions of the four levers of the pattern and also of individual adjustments in it. See Table 17-5.

The time in which the limbs moved through the given range was 0.025 second for the man, except for the hand, for which the time was 0.007 second. For the woman, the time was 0.028 second except for the hand, for which the time was 0.008 second. The high linear velocity for hand flexion shown in Table 17-4 has been questioned by later research, and the basis on which it was determined may be of interest to those who study film. Note that in the table the time for the measured range for the hand is less than for the other joints. In the frame before release, the angle at the wrist was measured; in the next frame, the ball had been released and the wrist angle had changed. The change was assumed to have occurred during the time that the camera shutter was closed, and this time, rather than the frames per second, was used to determine the velocity at the wrist joint. If this procedure is acceptable, the time cannot be longer than shutter time, and it could be less; in that case the angular velocity would be greater than was reported.

The sum of the linear velocities for the man is 39.50 m/sec (129.6 ft/sec); the ball velocity measured on the film was 39.90 m/sec (130.9 ft/sec). For the woman, the sum of the linear velocities is 30.11 m/ sec (98.8 ft/sec); the measured film velocity was 29.24 m/sec (95.93 ft/sec).

The hand action in both performers is the greatest contributor to the linear velocity; the hip ranks second and shoulder last. Both performers extended at the elbow just before release, thus shortening the length of the moment arm of the shoulder lever.

In a study of the moment arm lengths in the overarm throws of high school girls, the highest velocities were found to be developed by the girls who had the longest moment arms for the hip rotation levers

Table 17-5. *Lever Contributions to Ball Velocity in Overarm Throw*

	Range (degrees)	Angular velocity (degrees/sec)	Moment arm		Linear velocity	
			cm	ft	m/sec	ft/sec
Man						
Hip rotation	20.6	824	64.6	2.12	9.29	30.5
Spinal rotation	9.6	384	83.8	2.75	5.60	18.4
Shoulder rotation	38.5	1540	8.2	0.27	2.22	7.3
Wrist flexion	60.0	8571	14.9	0.49	22.34	73.3
Woman						
Hip rotation	20.6	735	70.7	2.32	9.08	29.8
Spinal rotation	20.9	746	67.7	2.21	8.77	28.8
Shoulder rotation	29.0	1036	10.6	0.35	1.92	6.3
Wrist flexion	42.0	5250	11.2	0.37	10.33	33.9

and consequently the shortest moment arms for the shoulder medial rotation levers.

The tabulation of moment arm lengths shows that, for the man, the moment arm for the hip is shorter than that for the spine. This is due to a leaning to the left so far that the upper spine is to the left of the hip joint at release. The lateral flexion may be the cause of the small range of movement in the spine.

Certain limitations should be remembered regarding these reported contributions of limb actions to the velocity of an overarm projected ball. In each case, the measurements are those made for one subject and were taken during the release phase, so that they do not indicate contributions made in earlier phases. Furthermore, cinematographic methods have improved since the reported observations were made; accuracy of the earlier methods of measuring limb actions may have unacceptable levels of error. The doubtful measures are included here as an illustration of a procedure that can be followed with refined techniques to determine the contributions of the body levers to ball velocity.

The earliest most detailed and extensive study of joint actions in the overarm throw was reported by Atwater, who observed action in three planes, using side, overhead, and rear camera views. She included 15 subjects to provide opportunity for comparison: five skilled college men and women, and five average college women. Her observations include not only the release phase but also the 400 msec preceding the release. For the skilled groups, that time period encompassed almost all the overarm pattern, including the backswing; for the average women, only the later stages of the backswing occurred in the selected time. Displacement of the ball was measured in three planes, and the three velocities determined were combined algebraically into one "resultant velocity." Measured joint actions were related to ball displacement on the basis of observation and logic; moment arms and linear contributions of joint actions were not studied.

In observing displacement of the ball before its release from the hand, Atwater found that although the movement is primarily forward, vertical and lateral movement occur also. None of the subjects accelerated the ball continually, but all accelerated rapidly shortly before release, the men as much as 457.20 to 609.6 m/sec^2 (1000 ft/sec^2); skilled women, 304.80 m/sec^2 (1000 ft/sec^2); and average women, 121.92 m/sec^2 (400 ft/sec^2). (See Fig. 17-9.)

In comparing limb actions, Atwater found that all skilled subjects used essentially the same actions but that the range and speed were generally greater for the subjects who had the fastest ball velocities at release. Some of these differences can be seen in Fig. 17-9, which represents positions at times of approximately 0.070 and 0.025 second before release of the ball and 0.005 second after release. Note that in the lowest tracing for each subject the ball is behind the hand and that this distance is greatest for the skilled man and least for the average women. Differences in ball position at this time can be at-

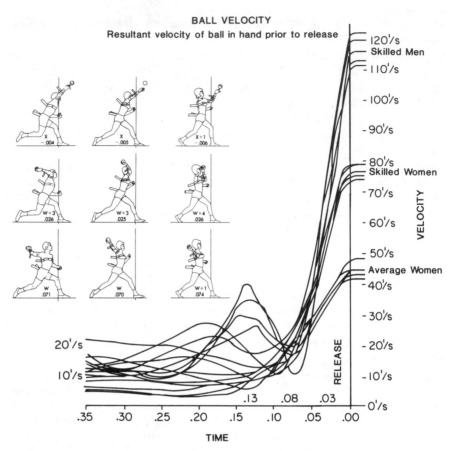

Fig. 17-9. *A, Tracings from movie film of skilled man (left); skilled woman (middle); and woman with average skill (right) at the end of backswing, 25 ms prior to release, and immediately after release. Qualitatively assess the differences in step length, counter rotation, lateral rotation of the humerus and extension to the arm. B, Resultant velocities, calculated from displacements measured from side, rear, and overhead views. (From Atwater, A. E., Movement characteristics of the overarm throw, dissertation, University of Wisconsin, 1970)*

tributed largely to trunk position; the trunk of the skilled man is not yet facing slightly beyond that direction. To reach the positions shown in the top tracings the man's trunk moves through a greater range than do those of the women, and its rotation must therefore be at a faster angular velocity. Note also that the forearm of the average women is flexed 50 to 60 degrees at release, whereas those of the skilled performers are almost completely extended.

The differences in length of stride are not as clearly seen. Atwater reports considerable differences in the average stride length for the three groups: that of the skilled men was 1.18 m (3.87 ft); that of the skilled women was 15.8 cm (0.52 ft) shorter, and that of the average women 47.8 cm (1.57 ft) shorter than that of the men. A similar finding related to stride is reported by Ekern, who studied the overarm throw of boys and girls selected as the better throwers from second, fourth, and sixth grades. Within that group, she found that the better throwers, whose projected balls were fastest, took longer steps.

Fisk, in a review of the data in his study "The Dynamic Function of Selected Muscles of the Forearm: an Electromyographical and Cinematographical Investigation" made the following comments:

> Analysis was made of electromygraphical data obtained from 12 subjects in the study. A great deal of individual variety in the function of the four muscles (identified in Fig. 17-10) during the performance of the overhand straight throw and the overhand curved throw was found. Conclusions drawn from the study indicate that the electrical response generated in the muscles took place during the final movements of the "laying back of the arm," just prior to when the elbow begins its forward movement and the hand assumes its "cocked position." Once the forward movement of the arm begins, the flexors diminish electrical activity. All four muscles were more active during the throws with spin than during the straight throws; therefore, it is assumed that greater muscular effort was required to perform the throws with spin. The onset of the maximal action potential response occurred earlier and endured longer for the throws with spin, and occurred earlier and endured longer among the experienced performers. The contribution of the pronator teres muscle still remains partially unsettled; however, this muscle contributed to the spin imparted to the ball at release when the throws with spin were performed. (Fisk, 1976).

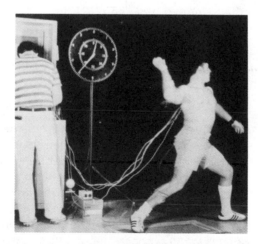

Fig. 17-10. *Electromyographic instrumentation used to study muscular involvement during overarm throwing. In-dwelling fine wire electrodes were located in the lateral head of the triceps brachii, in the flexors carpi ulnaris and radialis, and pronator teres muscles. The step has been taken and the rear foot has exerted force against a force plate embedded in the floor.*

BIOMECHANICS OF THROWING   **521**

The velocities of balls projected by the overhand throw have been measured more frequently than those of any other movement pattern. Among the reported velocities are the following:

1. Bob Feller's pitch, measured in 1946: 44.19 m/sec (145 ft/sec).
2. The throw of the winner of a city-wide contest in Philadelphia, an 18-year-old high school boy: 39.62 m/sec (130 ft/sec).
3. The mean velocity for 911 college women, reported in 1964: 13.59 m/sec (44.6 ft/sec); and for 1072 college women, reported in 1965: 12.95 m/sec (42.5 ft/sec).
4. The mean velocity of a group of high school girls, measured at the University of Wisconsin in 1959: 17.19 m/sec (56.4 ft/sec); highest velocity in the group: 27.64 m/sec (90.7 ft/sec).
5. Mean velocities for boys and girls, collected during 1956 through 1961 (with the mean velocities for intervening grades progressively higher):
   a. First-grade girls: 8.53 m/sec (28 ft/sec)
   b. Eighth-grade girls: 16.45 m/sec (54 ft/sec)
   c. First-grade boys: 10.66 m/sec (35 ft/sec)
   d. Eighth-grade boys: 22.86 m/sec (75 ft/sec).
6. Individual pitching velocities of seven men varsity pitchers (Slater-Hammel and Andres):
   a. For fast balls: 26.19 to 37.18 m/sec (86 to 122 ft/sec)
   b. For curve balls: 22.86 to 32.91 m/sec (75 to 108 ft/sec)
7. The mean velocity for 80 high school boys, reported in 1966: 20.84 m/sec (68.4 ft/sec).
8. Standards selected after personal observation and study of available data by Atwater in 1970 (see also data shown in Fig. 17-9)
   a. For skilled women: a range of 21.33 to 24.38 m/sec (70 to 80 ft/sec)
   b. For average women: 12.19 to 15.24 m/sec (40 to 50 ft/sec).
   c. For skilled men: 30.48 to 36.57 m/sec (100 to 120 ft/sec).

FACTORS AFFECTING BALL FLIGHT

Most objects are thrown (released) with a topspin. The human being can release an object with the greatest velocity (because of the final position of the fingers) if the object is spinning. If the object is light in weight, there would be lateral deflection as it progresses toward its destination. Watts explains this curve phenomena by stating that it involves a boundary layer of thin fluid (air) that is very near the object. The air moves around the front half of the object, say a ball. This involves creation of a separation point, a downstream, called the wake, which occurs away from the front of a ball. The flow of air over the ball is equal in speed to the velocity of the ball. The pressure in the wake region (drag) is lower than the pressure on the front of the ball. This tends to slow the object. If the wake is not symmetrical, the flow of air is redirected off the rear of the ball, causing deflection. It is clear that a baseball can be made to curve or rise or fall in regard to its normal parabolic path. However, this is only possible if the force generated to spin the ball is large enough. Watts reports an investigator (Briggs) found that in baseball, pitchers rotated the ball 7 to 16 times (revolutions) on the throw to home plate.

Putting something on the ball, such as petroleum jelly, saliva, and sweat drops, reduces the spin. The knuckle ball thrown with the first knuckle of the throwing fingers has a similar effect. The effect of scuffing up the ball causes the ball to spin toward the roughened area. This is an illegal pitch but has been used.

MINI-LAB LEARNING EXPERIENCES

1. Throw a football, rugby ball, baseball and/or other ball, differing in size, weight, and shape. Identify the types of spin easily imparted to each ball and the type of throwing pattern naturally used.
2. View video of each of above to determine the similarities and differences in the action.

Shot Put

Shot putting is a modification of the throwing action (see Nebel). It is a combination of overarm throwing and pushing because the shot cannot be thrown as in many high-velocity throws (Fig. 17-11), since the rules state that the put must be initiated from in front of the neck and above the shoulder. This results in a push put instead of a true throw.

Dessureault found the following in his kinematic and kinetic study of poor and world-class shot-putters:

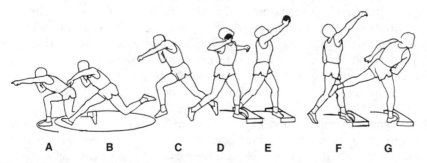

    A   B   C   D   E   F   G

Fig. 17-11. *The height of the shot put at the start, at final step, and at release should be of increasing values. For example, in this performance the initial position is half as high at the release position. Measure it to compare. The athlete should utilize the complete diameter of the circle, does he? Note in the final two figures the momentum of the body has been dissipated by changing the supporting foot.*

BIOMECHANICS OF THROWING   **523**

1. The entire action lasted 2.16 mean seconds.
2. The best shot putters extended their bodies farther outside the rear of the circle and flexed at the right knee more before beginning the move across the circle.
3. The shot putters' mean displacement of the center of gravity was 1.52+ m (5+ ft) during the action.
4. The path of the shot followed a linear and slightly upward direction by the best performers and dropped nearly vertically during part of the movement by the poorer performers.
5. The angle of release for the best performers was 38 to 41 degrees and was as low as 27 degrees for the poorer performers.
6. The majority of shot putters lost contact with the ground and became airborne at release.
7. All performers had greater horizontal than vertical velocity at release.
8. The shot was released at a linear velocity of 13.52 m/sec (44.36 ft/sec) for the best performer; other velocities were less, the slowest being 9.14 m/sec (30 ft/sec).
9. The superior performers were in contact with the ground for a shorter time after the glide. (Mean time for all subjects was 0.296 second in the vertical plane and 0.287 second in the horizontal plane.)
10. There was a mean value of 2781.4 kg (613.2 lb) of peak vertical thrust by the supporting foot, and a mean value of 1337.9 N (301 lb) by the front foot.

The shot putter faces to the rear, as seen in Fig. 17-11A, in preparation for moving across the ring. The weight is on the right foot. From position A, the performer hops on the right foot to place it in the position shown in C. This action gives a forward movement to the shot, which should be used by adding to it the final lever actions (C to E). Flexion at the knee (C) is important for development of force. As the left foot makes ground contact (D to E), the torso can be moved rapidly upward by extension of the rear (right) thigh, and as the left foot takes the weight, the pelvis can rotate on the left limb. These two actions can accelerate the movement of the shot. Note that the upper arm is abducted to the horizontal in D; this position lengthens the moment arm for the lever moving at the left hip.

In the last phase of trunk rotation, adduction, and flexion at the shoulder, move the upper arm forward and upward. At the same time, the forearm extends, moving the forearm forward and counteracting the upward movement of the upper arm. Final impetus is given by hand flexion. Although all these levers contribute to the force developed, as does the initial glide, the major contributor is the pelvic lever. The actions occurring from E to G are made to maintain balance.

Because the velocity of the shot is much slower than that of many objects that people project, and because its release point is higher than the landing point, the projection angle should be less than 45 degrees, above the horizontal, as indicated by Dessureault's findings (reported previously).

Instead of a glide across the ring, many of the world's best shot putters are utilizing a spinning action similar to that used by the discus throwers to attain higher velocity rates at release. A kinematic and kinetic study of this new method should be made to determine its potential and actual advantages and disadvantages.

MINI-LAB LEARNING EXPERIENCES

1. View videotape to analyze the shot-put action.
2. Observe two shot putters having great differences in throwing distance to ascertain the reasons for the disparity in performance.
3. Obtain a film of the new spinning action throw and analyze it for possible differences in velocity and distance.
4. Construct a physique for an ideal shot putter. Do so within the limits of the body as we know it now, and construct a physique that transcends our current physical/anatomical structure.

Javelin Throw

The javelin throw is similar to other types of overarm throwing actions in which the throwing objective is distance.

The shape of the javelin is unique as a throwing implement in that it is long and light weight.

The 1987 NCAA rule book includes the following standards for the javelin:

	Length		Weight
	Minimum	Maximum	
Women	2.20 m (7′ 2.78 in.)	2.30 m (7′ 5.459 in.)	600 GM (1 lb, 5.16 oz.)
Men	2.60 m (8′ 6.375 in.)	2.70 m (8′ 10.250 in.)	800 GM (1 lb, 12.25 oz.)

A wide throwing stance is utilized just before release, and the body is projected into the air and follows in the direction of the javelin after release.

The purpose of the run up to the throwing area is to gain body momentum. The extreme stretching of the arm-throwing muscles facilitates the throwing motion. The various axes of rotation—namely, the opposite hip, the spine, and the shoulder—increase the radius and moment arm at release (Fig. 17-12).

The angle of projection of the javelin is determined by the height of release above the ground, air resistance, the direction of the wind, and the velocity of the javelin at release. The javelin has aerodynamic qualities and is released at a lower angle than might be anticipated. Although some javelin throwers release the javelin at an angle of 42 to 50 degrees, the best throwers in the world release at about 30 degrees.

The javelin thrower attempts to release the javelin with as much velocity as possible (27.43 to 30.48 m/sec (90 to 100 ft/sec)). The thrower often goes into the air one step before release. Horizontal momentum is created during the run, and a braking force occurs at release, causing the momentum of the run to be transferred to the arm and to the javelin.

The run is executed at a controlled speed and involves an acceleration in its last stages. Before the last step is taken, the body weight is on the right foot; with the penultimate step, the pelvis rotates at the right hip, adding to the length of the step. As the weight is shifted to the left foot, the humerus is rotated medially and the forearm is flexed. The final force, added to the forward movement of the body, is derived from pelvic and spinal rotation, medial rotation and slight adduction of the humerus, and flexion of the hand.

Note the position of the pectoralis major in Fig. 17-12. This muscle is well suited for medial rotation of the humerus. In addition, the action of the latissimus dorsi should be visualized here, since it, too, is a medial rotator and its contraction would lower the humerus and pull it backward. The latter two actions are prevented from occurring

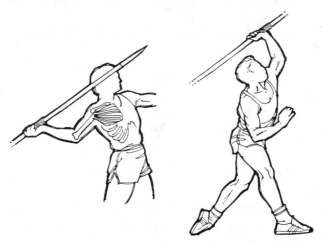

Fig. 17-12. *A, Initial and final position of preparatory phase and initial and final position of delivery phase of the javelin throw. The pectoralis major is the primary muscle initiating the arm action in the delivery phase. B, illustration of Detlef Michel of Germany, winning the first I.A.A.F. World Championship in Helsinki, Finland, 1983. First lefthanded thrower to win a major international meet. Note the position of the non-throwing foot and throwing leg.*

526 *THE BIOMECHANICS OF HUMAN MOVEMENT*

by the pectoralis major. Acting together, these two muscles are excellent rotators of the arm. Note that in the javelin throw the elbow is not fully extended during the final thrust, and the moment arm for medial rotation at the shoulder is almost a maximal length. In this skill, medial rotation of the humerus is a greater contributor than is hand flexion.

The release of the throw is crucial, not only because of its length and low weight, but because of the effect the wind may have on its flight. Injury to the shoulder and arm muscles often occurs because of the position of each during or prior to release. There is a large torque at the humerus.

Usually, there is no true parabolic flight path to the thrown javelin. This is due in part to the lightness of the object, the air resistance, the pull of gravity, and other factors to be discussed later.

There are certain rules to follow, such as the thrower must stay within the lane markers in the runup, must stay behind the scratch line in the follow-through, the point of the thrown javelin must land first, and the discus-type spin of the body is prohibited. In addition, the javelin must meet the standards set by the governing bodies relative to its shape, and particularly in reference to the location of its center of gravity.

Certain factors stand out in regard to javelin performance. There are lift and drag components while the javelin is air-borne. Lift is the component of the total air force on the javelin perpendicular (normal) to the direction of the air flow. Drag is the component of the total air force on the javelin parallel to the direction of the air flow.

The lift on the javelin in flight is not as influential as the angle of attack which is the acute angle between the long axis of the javelin and the direction of the air flow. The angle of attack is in the vertical aspects; the positive angle is with the tip up and the negative angle with the tip down. When the angle of attack during the flight is small, the lift of the javelin is not optimum, and conversely if the angle of attack is too great, the javelin stalls in the air and lands short of the obtainable distance. The new javelins have a larger diameter in the rear position. This contour of the javelin is called planform.

The attitude angle is the acute angle between the long axis of the javelin and the horizontal. When the javelin's front point is above the horizontal as at the release, the attitude angle is positive, and if the point is below the horizontal, it is negative. In order to have a fair throw, the javelin must land with a negative attitude angle (Terauds, p. 19). If there is head wind, the attitude angle at release should be reduced; if there is a tail wind, the angle should be increased.

The center of pressure on the javelin is the point at which it is in balance. This varies with the angle of attack and the amount of rotation along its long axis. Terauds has stated that there are 16–24 revolutions per second for top performers. This helps stabilize the javelin in flight.

The magnus effect is present when a javelin is airborne. It is the force produced that is perpendicular to the motion of its long axis in flight (Fig. 17-13).

The moment of inertia of the javelin is the sum of the mass of the javelin times the distance between the mass and the javelin's axis of rotation squared.

The grip is important to the execution of the throw. The thumb and middle finger grip just behind the cord or binding appears to be the best for most throwers. The thrower can get rotation on the javelin (its long axis) by pushing against the cord as the javelin is released. There is also rotation about the short axis of the javelin among some javelin throwers:

The javelin thrower usually takes 10–12 strides prior to release. A cross-over step is used to enable the performer to have the feet in front of the upper part of the body. This enables the thrower to land on the front foot, so the throw can be executed effectively. About 5 strides from the scratch line, the javelin is started back toward a throwing position. The runner-thrower moves the legs rapidly just prior to the release at about 6' in height. It takes a javelin thrower about 6 steps to recover and not go over the restraining line.

In the final analysis, the most important aspect in throwing the javelin is the release velocity. All other aspects have their influence, but only in contributing to the final action. Most throwers have strong, but short levers (especially arms). Strength is essential. The acceleration of the throwing arm and hand is crucial to high release values.

Komi and Mero conducted a study of performances of both men and women finalists in the javelin throw at the 1984 Los Angeles Olympic Games. They found that the men had the highest release velocity, 29.12 m/sec, and that there was a strong positive relationship between the release velocity and the distance attained. However, with the women the release velocity in spite of a wide range in dis-

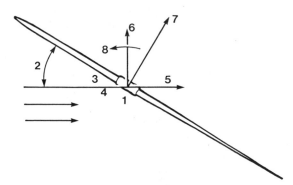

Fig. 17-13. *The javelin in flight is subjected to environmental forces and motion forces which negate the usual parabolic flight of balls. The javelin is revolving about its long axis during flight and the javelin flight will be affected by the following: 1. axial force, 2, angle of attack, 3, center of gravity, 4, center of pressure, 5, drag, 6, lift, 7, normal force, and 8, pitching moment.*

THE BIOMECHANICS OF HUMAN MOVEMENT

tance attained (55 m+ to 69 m+) was relatively close. Both the men and women had high impact loading with the last foot to contact the ground, which was of short duration (0.0325). They also had high velocity of flexion at the knee.

MINI-LAB LEARNING EXPERIENCES

Compare (From Fig. 17-14) the mechanics of throwing the javelin from a wheelchair and from a running approach.

Best and Bartlett (ISBS Conference, Athens, 1987) investigated the characteristics of the javelin used by women and reported smaller lift, drag, and pitch coefficients than for the men's javelin. Lift/drag ratio was also smaller for the women's javelin in comparison with the men's javelin. The center of pressure of the women's javelin was behind the center of gravity. The men's had a constant site for the center of pressure and the women's did not. They predicted that the ballistic range of the women's javelin is 3–4% shorter than the men's. They also stated that the release speed is the greater determinant of range than is the runup or delivery angle.

The transverse moment of inertia is such that wind effect is negligible on flight, though tail wind is best wind direction for performance. There were no data on release speed of women's javelin throw-

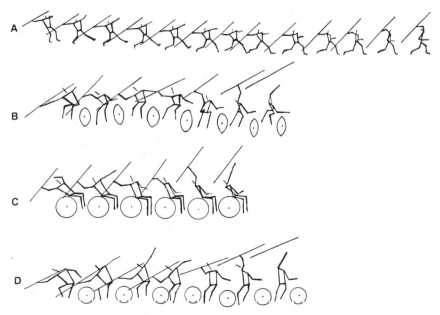

Fig. 17-14. *Line segment tracings of performances of throwing a javelin with a run-up and from wheel chairs. Compare the performances.*

BIOMECHANICS OF THROWING 529

ing. Gyration of the javelin will reduce the total amount of pitch. Optimum conditions to produce greatest distance, for the women were: 78 m/sec, 35 degree angle of release, 0.8 angle of attack and -20 degree/sec pitch rate. The men's optimum conditions for javelin thrown at same speed and same release angle are $-.28$ angle of attack and -8.3 degree/sec pitch rate. The javelin, however, will not have reduced range until a wide variation from the optimum occurs.

MINI-LAB LEARNING EXPERIENCES

1. Top performers in all the sports analyzed in this chapter should perform before the class, and the members should analyze the action through observation.
2. Analyze film, slides, or photographs of as many throwing actions as possible.
3. Calculate the velocities and accelerations of a throwing action similar to the procedudre used in this chapter.
4. Ask a coach of a throwing activity to present ideas on performance of a skill. Evaluate these ideas in a biomechanical framework.

The Curling Delivery

Many skills are required to successfully make shots and score points in the game of curling. Of particular importance is the delivery of the curling rock. The performance objectives of the delivery action are target accuracy (hitting the broom) and weight control (imparting the required momentum to the rock). Based upon results of a study conducted in 1982, Bothwell-Myers identified the importance and specific roles that each of the seven phases of the delivery action has in propelling the rock and curler forward, toward a target. (See Fig. 17-15).

Stance. The stationary positioning of the curler in the hack (foot hold) prior to the delivery. The functions of the stance phase are target viewing, alignment of the body and rock with target, and positioning of the hack foot (right foot for right handed curlers) for balance and leg drive leverage. (See Fig. 17-15A)

Backswing. The delivery motion, backward, from the point the rock loses contact with the ice to the maximum vertical displacement of the rock (top of the swing). The functions of the backswing are positioning of the body, body levers, and rock for the production of forward motion and controlling the weight of the shot. The height of the backswing serves only to position the rock and body for the generation of momentum (predominately rock momentum). Thus, the height of the backswing reflects the amount of rock momentum that the curler can control and comfortably integrate into the delivery, rather than the called for weight of the shot. Actions in the backswing in-

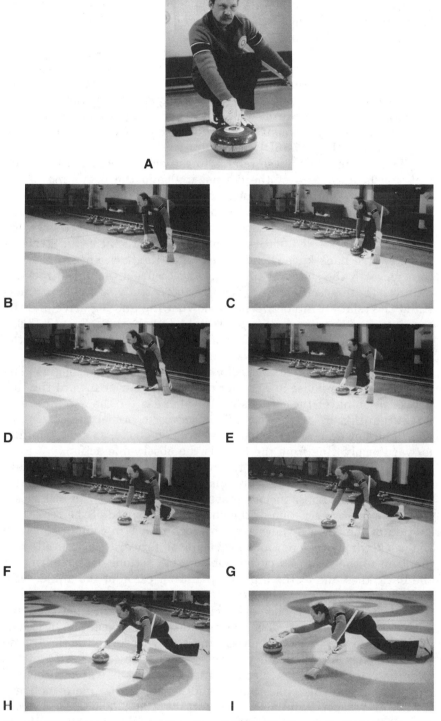

Fig. 17-15. *The sequence of a curling delivery. A, stance; B, C, backswing; D, downswing; E, transition; F, G, leg drive; H, glide; I, release.*

clude a slight forward motion of the rock and body to help overcome the inertia of the stone; elevation of the body from the stance position; backward pull or swing of the rock; and counterbalancing movement of the broom and sliding foot (Fig. 17-15, B and C).

Downswing. The downswing or forward swing begins at the top of the backswing and ends when the rock contacts the ice surface. The function of this phase is the production of rock and centre of mass momentum, but predominately rock momentum. Actions in the downswing include forward swing of the throwing arm and rock, body fall forward, and placement of the sliding foot forward to receive the body's weight. (Fig. 17-15D)

Transition. This phase relates to the actions occurring between rock touch down (end of the downswing) and the beginning of leg drive—i.e. extension of the hack knee. The function of this phase is the conversion of angular rock momentum to linear rock momentum. Actions include rock touchdown (initial contact of the rock with the ice surface), rock soled (entire running edge of rock contracts the ice surface), and hack knee flexion. Flexion at the hack knee appears to coincide with the soling of the rock, and occurs after initial rock-ice contact. These specific events require more study to further understand the relationship between the downswing and leg drive and the conversion of angular motion to straight line motion. (Fig. 17-15E)

Fall Forward. This consists of the forward displacement of the curler's center of mass or forward lean of the curler which occurs as the rock touches the ice and before hack leg extension begins. The functions of this phase are acceleration of the curler toward the target, positioning of the curler's center of mass for the acceptance of force from the leg drive action. This serves to propel the curler forward and upward, but primarily forward. The body, as a unit, falling forward or pivoting from the hack is the observable action.

Leg Drive. Extension at the hack knee, after the forward fall, that results in the forward propulsion of the curler from the hack. Functions of this phase include propulsion of the curler and rock closer to the target, acceleration of the curler to the speed of the rock, regulation of the release velocity of the rock either in conjunction with the backswing or alone, and provision of forward (horizontal) momentum to the rock and curler. Observable actions are extension at the hack knee and at the hip, and plantar flexion of the ankle. (Fig. 17-15E and F.)

Glide or Slide. If the curler is propelled forward from the hack with sufficient momentum, a gliding phase is observed. The functions of this phase are to bring the rock and curler closer to the target and to correct for the weight of the rock by adjusting the length of the slide and, therefore, the release point. The body is extended behind the rock during this phase and is sliding along the line of delivery toward the target. A number of important weight and accuracy control mechanisms are active during this phase (Fig. 17-15H)

Release. The function of the release is to impart a clockwise or counterclockwise rotation to the rock. (Fig. 17-15I)

Determinants of Success. Identification of the primary function of a specific action is an essential step in movement analysis. Grouping actions by function can further assist the coach with fault identification and correction. The actions observed in the delivery motion can be categorized into three functional groups:

1. Actions that generate momentum; that is, those actions which serve to propel the rock and curler out of the hack toward the target. Key actions which serve this function are (a) angular acceleration of the rock during the downswing which contributes to rock momentum, (b) the smooth soling of the rock during the transition phase which contributes to the maintenance of rock momentum, (c) angular acceleration of the curler during the forward fall, (d) hip, knee, and ankle flexion during leg drive, which contributes to rock and curler momentum, and (e) trunk flexion, shoulder and elbow extension during the glide phase, which contribute to rock momentum.

2. Actions that correct or adjust the amount of rock momentum (weight control mechanisms). Examples of observed weight control actions which result in braking are (a) lengthening the slide, causing deceleration of the rock and curler, (b) lifting the trunk during the slide, which shifts the curler's weight backwards producing a drag, (c) shifting body weight to the broom or rock during the slide, and (d) flexing the throwing elbow during the slide to pull back on the rock, thereby decelerating it. Actions which may result in enhancing momentum are (a) increasing the height of the backswing, (b) increasing the angular acceleration of the rock and throwing arm during the downswing, (c) falling forward faster by flexing the hack knee, and (d) increasing leg drive propulsion by more complete and forceful extension of the hack leg.

3. Actions that contribute to target accuracy. These actions include (a) body alignment in the stance, (b) "straight back" displacement of the rock during the backswing, (c) balancing and counterbalancing actions of the throwing arm, broom arm, and sliding foot, (d) flat footed sliding position, (e) elongated position of the body behind the rock during the sliding phase, and (f) lengthening the slide, thereby bringing the rock closer to the target before release.

The pattern of acquisition of momentum (i.e. horizontal velocity) for the delivery of the rock and the forward propulsion of the curler is as follows: (a) at the end of the downswing phase, approximately 90% of the final release velocity of the rock had been acquired, compared to approximately 35% of the final release velocity of the center of mass (curler); (b) at the end of the forward fall phase, the rock and centre of mass velocity had both been increased by approximately 20%; (c) at the end of the leg drive phase, the rock velocity had been augmented again by approximately 20%; the centre of mass velocity had been increased by 55% or more; and (d) at the end of the glide phase (slide), the rock velocity had been diminished by between 12% and 26%. The rock decelerated more than the curler during the slide for a given type of shot.

Based upon these results, the downswing (forward swing) phase contributes most to the acquisition of rock momentum; the forward fall phase contributes equally to the rock and curler momentum; the leg drive phase contributes most to the acquisition of curler momentum; the slide phase contributes to deceleration of the rock and center of mass for both draw shots and takeout shots. That is, the rock is decelerated more than the curler during the slide. Also, the rock is decelerated more for draws than for takeouts during the slide.

It should be noted that there appears to be a close association between curler and rock during the downswing phase which is not present during the other phases of the delivery. In fact, during the leg drive and slide, the rock and curler are essentially acting independently or in a more complex manner not yet identified.

Weight control mechanisms in curling were investigated by looking at force production during the delivery. For comparative purposes, the total force required to produce the known release velocity of the rock and curler was estimated and then compared to the force which was actually generated for the shot. For takeouts, approximately seven times more rock force was generated than required; for draws, approximately ten times more rock force was generated than required. Why such inefficiency? Possibly excessive momentum is generated to overcome the retarding effect of sliding friction during the slide phase. In a practical sense, it is possible that the curler makes a "rough" assessment of the momentum that must be generated during the downswing, forward fall and leg drive phases, (i.e. weight) and then "fine tunes" or corrects the momentum during the slide.

REFERENCES

Adrian, M. and Enberg, M. L. (1971) Sequential timing of three overhand patterns, *Kinesiology Review*, Widule, C. J., editor, Reston, VA: AAHPERD.

Allman, W. F. (1980) *Pitching, Science* #82, October.

Annarino, A. A. (1973) *Bowling, individualized instructional program*, Englewood Cliffs, NJ: Prentice-Hall.

Ariel, B. C. (1973) Computerized biomechanics analysis of the world's best shot putters. *Track and Field Quarterly Rev.*, Dec.

Atwater, A. E. (1970) Movement characteristics of the overarm throw: a kinematic analysis of men and women performers, thesis, University of Wisconsin.

Bartlett, R. M. (1983) A cinematographic analysis of an international javelin thrower, *Athletic Coach*, Sept.

Bothwell-Myers, C. (1982). Kinematic characteristics of the curling delivery. *Dissertation Abstracts International*, 43, 3840A. (University Microfilms No. DA 8308845)

Black, I. (1980) Hammer Throw, *Track and Field Quarterly* Rev. 80, 27–28.

Brodie, J. and Houston, J. D. (1974) *The open field*, San Francisco: Houghton Mifflin.

Broer, M. and Houtz, S. J. (1967) *Patterns of muscular activity in selected sport skills; an electromyographic study*, Springfield, IL: Charles C. Thomas, Publisher.

Brown, G., editor (1979) *Football, a collection of articles,* Danbury, CT: Arno Press.

Casady, D. and Liba, M. (1968) *Beginning bowling,* ed. 2, Belmont, CA: Wadsworth Publishing.

Cole, S. S. (1977) Design, construction and testing of a bowling machine for biomechanical research utilization, doctoral dissertation, Indiana University.

Dapena, J. (1986) A kinematic study of center of mass motions in the hammer. *J. Biomechanics,* **19**(2):147–158. Pergamon Press, (printed in Great Britain).

Dessureault, J. (1976) Selected kinetics and kinematic factors involved in shot putting, doctoral dissertation, Indiana University.

Doherty, J. K. (1976) Track and Field Omnibus, 2nd ed., Los Altos, CA: Tofnews.

Feltner, M. and Dapena, J. (1986) Dynamics of the shoulder and elbow joints of the throwing arm during a baseball pitch, *Journal of Biomechanics,* **19**(2):147–158.

Fox, E. C. (1984) *Team cohesion, ability and coaches leadership effectiveness as predictors of success in women's intercollegiate softball,* Microform Publications, University of Oregon.

Gregor, R. J. and Pink, M. (1985) Biomechanical analysis of a world record javelin throw. *International Journal of Sport Biomechanics,* Human Kinetics Publisher, 1-73-77.

Grinfelds, V(1980). *Complete book of bowling, right down your alley,* West Point, NY: Leisure Press.

Gregor, R. J., Whiting, W. C. and McCoy, R. W. (1985) Kinematic analysis of Olympic discus throwers, *International Journal of Sport Biomechanics,* **1**:131–138, Human Kinetics Publishers, Inc.

Hwang, I. and Adrian, M. (1986) Biomechanics of hammer throwing. In the *Proceedings of the 1984 Olympic Scientific Congress,* Adrian, M. and Deutsch, H., editors: University of Oregon, Microfilm Publications.

Javver, Jess (1986) The throws, 2nd ed., *Track and Field News,* Box 296, Los Altos, CA.

Kneer, M. E. and McCord, C. L. (1976) Softball: slow and fast pitch, Dubuque, IA: W. C. Brown Co.

Komi, P. and Mero, A. (1985) Biomechanical analysis of Olympic javelin throwers, *International Journal of Sport Biomechanics,* **1**(2):, Champaign, IL, May, Human Kinetics Publishers.

Knox, D. (1977) The effect of stride on the velocity of the softball pitch, unpublished master's thesis, California State University, Long Beach.

Reiff, G. (1971) What research tells the coach about baseball, Reston, VA: AAHPERD.

Sanders, J. A. (1976) A practical application of the segmental method of analysis to determine throwing ability, doctoral dissertation, Indiana University.

Schwartz, G. (1983) Two major obstacles to effective discus throwing, *Track and Field Quarterly Review* **83**(1):25.

Scott, T. M. (1985) *Bowling everyone,* Winston-Salem, NC: Hunter Textbooks.

Selin, C. (1959) An analysis of the aerodynamics of pitched baseballs, *Research Quarterly* **30**, May.

Sing, R. (1988) *The dynamics of the javelin throw,* Cherry Hill, NJ: Reynolds Publishers.

Tarbell, T. (1971) Some mechanical aspects of the overarm throw. In Cooper, J. M., editor, *Proceedings of the Committee on Institutional Cooperation Symposium on Biomechanics,* Chicago: The Athletic Institute.

Terauds, J. (1985) *Biomechanics of the javelin throw,* Del Mar, CA: Academic Publishers.

Terauds, J. (1978) Technical analysis of the discus, *Scholastic Coach,* **47**(8):98.

Uebel, R. (1986) *The effects of varied weighted implements on the kinematics of the shotput,* University of Oregon, Microform Publications.

Watts, R. C. (1985) The kinematics of baseballs, yearbook of science and the future, *Encyclopaedia Britannica,* Chicago.

Woicik, M. (1983) The discus throw, *Track and Field Quarterly Review.*

Zollinger, R. L. (1973) Mechanical analysis of windmill fast pitch in women's softball, *Research Quarterly* **44**:290–300.

18

Selected Striking and Kicking Skills

Striking is the act of one object hitting another. For example, it may involve moving the hand or foot (in soccer, sometimes the head) in the striking action, as in throwing, or an extension of the arm, such as a bat or a racquet, may be used. This latter type of implement will increase the radius of motion. The run or step made before an object is contacted increases the momentum of the foot or hand at contact because of transfer of momentum from a part to the whole.

Striking an object at rest, such as a golf ball or a soccer ball that is stationary, is somewhat different from striking a moving object, such as a baseball. Counteracting the momentum of a ball traveling at 144.81 kmph (90 mph) means that the mass times velocity of the bat must be greater than the velocity of the ball times its mass.

The stationary object must be struck with a force of sufficient magnitude to overcome its inertia. This involves the application of Newton's first law of motion. In addition, attaining of the maximum distance or maximum velocity in the flight of the struck object can be ensured if the striking implement contacts the object at a point tangential to the swing and through the center of gravity of the object. The takeoff angle of the struck object must be high enough to achieve maximum distance of flight if distance is the objective. Some of the struck objects have aerodynamic qualities, and the resistance to flight or form drag is increased. The dimples in a golf ball help a golfer attain a greater distance in a drive. Both the number and depth of the dimples influence the distance of the flight. Why is this so? Use the information in Chapter 5 to answer this question.

The spinning ball traversing in the air is confronted with the so-called Magnus effect. For example, catchers in baseball know that a pop fly struck into the air behind home plate will curve toward the stands on the way up and toward the infield on the way down. Consequently, to avoid missing the catch on the ball's return to the ground, they station themselves with their back toward the infield. In this position, a catcher who slightly misjudges the flight path can block the ball with the body and then catch it. Likewise, a spinning baseball, hit to the outfield along or near the foul line on either side of the field, will curve toward the outside. Outfielders know this and play the ball accordingly.

Based on the research done with the use of cinematography, the velocity of a badminton racquet, a tennis racquet, a baseball bat, and other striking implements decreases slightly at contact. In addition, there is a short period when the object struck is compressed, sometimes to as much as half its normal shape, before it rebounds. Furthermore, there is a period when the object struck adheres to the striking implement's surface before rebounding from it. The type of surface, the velocity of the implement, the type of object and the material of the object determine the degree of compression.

There are other considerations that should be mentioned in relation to the striking action. For example, vibration of a compound pendulum occurs in various striking actions. If a bat is suspended from one end, its parts will vibrate at different rates. In a sense, pendulums of different lengths are involved, since the weight is distributed along the length of the bat.

Particles of the bat will vibrate more slowly near one end than elsewhere. A particle that will vibrate at the same rate as the undivided bat is located at the center of oscillation. The real length of the bat swinging as a pendulum is thought of as the distance between the center of suspension and the center of oscillation, comparable to center of gravity.

If the bat is struck at its center of oscillation with a sledge as it is suspended, it will swing evenly and without shocking or jarring the hands. If the bat is struck at any other point along its length, it will not vibrate smoothly, and will therefore sting the hands of the striker. This center of oscillation is identical with the center of percussion, which is that point along a suspended object where a blow to it produces the least detrimental effect. A ball can be hit with more velocity if it is struck at the center of percussion, called the "sweet spot" by performers. The location of the center of percussion varies according to the length and composition of the bat. The same is true with tennis racquets and other striking implements.

It has been found that a baseball hit with a metal bat rebounds at a faster velocity than one hit with a wooden bat. This is due to the flexibility of the metal bat.

BASEBALL AND SOFTBALL BATTING

The objective in baseball/softball batting is to use a bat to strike a ball thrown with varying velocities by a pitcher. The softball batter has a smaller range of motion in the swing than the baseball batter.

The softball pitcher is closer to the batter and often throws with greater velocity.

The bat is cylindrical in shape, and the ball is small and usually spinning as it is struck, making effective striking action difficult. The Magnus effect has influence, through air resistance, on the thrown and struck ball's flight. The stance of the batter and subsequent mechanical actions made by the batter determine the ability to hit the ball in a consistent manner.

The path of the center of gravity of an unskilled batter may show a drop of as much as 15.2 to 20.3 cm (6 to 8 in.) during the swing. None of the skilled batters show a drop of more than 7.62 cm (3 in.). The skilled batters also turn their heads more to face toward the pitcher, to enable them to see the ball longer. The long radius and long moment arm aid the batter in achieving high bat velocity. Unskilled batters often pull the handle of the bat toward their bodies as they swing, reducing the length of the radius; skilled batters extend their arms.

There is some "hitch," or backward movement, of the batter's arms before they move slightly downward and forward. Depending on the height of the thrown ball, the path of the bat may follow the body's center of gravity or move downward and upward.

The rapid extension of the arms just before or as the step toward the pitcher is taken increases the speed of the end of the bat. Not only are the radius of swing increased and the moment arm lengthened, but centrifugal force comes into play to aid in bat velocity. The bat swing time has been calculated by Breen to take 0.19 to 0.23 second for the top hitters and 0.28 second for the poorer hitters, as calculated from the time the bat started movement toward the ball until contact with the ball was made.

During the swing, the body weight of the above-average batter shifts forward, moving the center of gravity forward. The shoulder turn causes the batter to be facing the pitcher as the ball is contacted. The rear foot is in plantar flexion, with only the toes touching the ground. Approximately 75% of the body weight is forward at the time of contact.

The head is held relatively stationary during the action. The eyes follow the ball until it is within 0.914 to 1.52 m (3 to 5 ft) of the plate. This is called "looking the ball into the catcher's glove," but in reality the eyes do not quite accomplish this task.

Hubbard found that batters reacted to the initial flight of the ball in 0.24 to 0.28 seconds. Breen found that the skilled batters started their swing when the ball reached half the distance to the plate, and that unskilled batters started their swing sooner, or before the ball reached half the distance to the plate.

The action used in batting normally is started from a position in which the performer has assumed a relatively wide base of support. Usually the stance is such that the feet are approximately 43.2 cm (17 in) part. The step is 25.4 cm (10 in) as the ball approaches the plate (Fig. 18-1). The weight is mainly on the right foot (for right-handed batters), which is at right angles to the intended flight of the ball to permit freedom of pelvic rotation at the right hip. As the weight is transferred to the left foot, the pelvis is rotated at the left hip, turning through 90 degrees. The bat is moved forward in the transverse plane first by the turning of the torso and finally by action at the wrists. A slight movement at the shoulder joints takes the upper arms forward and away from the trunk. The main contributing levers are those acting at the hip and wrist joints; the lengths of the moment arms for these levers have been greatly lengthened by the bat. Strong muscles acting at the wrist are important because they must hold the bat in the horizontal position, resisting gravitational pull, and move it with great speed in the final force-producing phase.

Note that the head is turned to the left to focus on the approaching ball. As the torso turns to the left, the head does not turn with it but remains facing toward the ball. Many coaches believe that if the batter's head moves to the left as the bat is swung, the left shoulder will be elevated, thus changing the path of the bat and reducing the possibility of contacting the ball. A tonic neck reflex may also act to interfere with the swing.

After studying film, Breen concluded the following:

1. The center of gravity of the body follows a relatively level plane, thus indicating a level swinging of the bat.
2. Hitters are able to adjust their heads to a position from which they can obtain a better look at the flight of the ball for any given pitch.
3. The leading forearm tends to straighten immediately as the bat is swung toward the ball, immediately moving the end of the bat and resulting in faster bat speed.

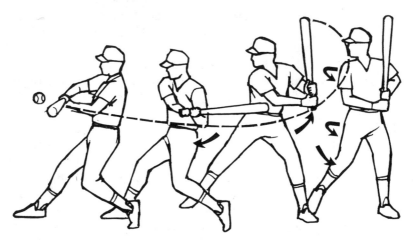

Fig. 18-1. *Body rotation and hip action during batting. The sequence is leg step with rotation at the femur to open the hips, then pelvic rotation which provides the momentum for the upper spine rotation and then the arm swing.*

4. The length of the stride is the same for all pitches for any single skilled hitter.
5. The body is flexed in the direction of the flight of the ball after contact has been made, thus putting the weight on the front foot.

Contact of the ball with the bat is most effective if made at the center of percussion. If the baseball batter undercuts the ball slightly, (if too much of the ball is undercut, it will pop up) the distance the ball will carry will be increased significantly by as much as 50 feet. Additionally, by undercutting, the number of revolutions of the ball may increase by 1,000–2,000 rpms. Undercutting and getting backspin results in a lifting force. Backspin without undercutting is almost impossible since the coefficient of friction between a wood bat and a baseball is low. A sticky substance, such as pine tar, placed on the bat would increase the coefficient of friction. There is, however, a restriction on the amount of the surface of bat that can be covered with friction enhancing substances (Watts).

RACQUET SPORTS

Tennis, badminton, racquetball, and squash involve the use of an implement that has strings to "catch the ball" and propel it back in the relative direction from which it came. This catching, of course, cannot be seen because the ball or shuttlecock are in contact with the strings for only a few milliseconds. Through the analysis of high-speed film, however, researchers have been able to identify the amount of depression of the ball and the deflection of the strings as well as deflection of the racquet frame itself during the contact of tennis balls. A novice experimenter will be able to see this depression if the strings are loose and the racquet frame is very weak and fatigued. The speed of the ball and the shuttlecock leaving the racquet strings are influenced by string tension, the size of the racquet head, the shape of the racquet head, the materials from which the racquet head has been made, and the type of material used for the strings, as well as the site of ball/racquet contact. In the non-racquet sport, table tennis, the surface of the paddle also has a significant influence upon the flight of the ball. Sandpaper paddles, rubber-covered paddles, cork paddles, and other materials have been used to influence the ball rebound and ball spin.

The weight of the racquet, length of racquet and the size of the grip with respect to the hand size and muscular strength of the player all influence the development of speed. The badminton racquet is lightest and can be swung fastest of the four racquets; tennis is heaviest and will be swung at the slowest speed. The difference in momentum, however, may be negligible. Linear momentum is what needs to be developed in order to provide the force to impact the ball or shuttlecock. Since the shuttlecock is very light in weight, the mo-

mentum that is necessary to counteract the momentum of the shuttlecock is not great or need not be great.

MINI-LAB LEARNING EXPERIENCES

Weigh a shuttlecock, tennis ball, and racquetball, and squash
ball. Next weigh the four racquets. Assume the racquetball is traveling one hundred and forty feet per second, the squash ball is
traveling one hundred and eighty feet per second, the tennis ball
is traveling one hundred and twenty-five feet per second, and the
badminton shuttlecock is traveling one hundred and eighty feet per
second. Calculate the momentum of each ball. Calculate the momentum of the racquet, assuming the racquet is traveling half the
speed of the shuttlecock before impact.

Discuss the law of conservation of momentum during a collision. Discuss the effect of the strings upon the object's velocity
after rebound.

Stroke Mechanics in Racquet Sports

It is evident that the same general principles utilized for throwing are also utilized in the stroking skills of racquet sports. The objects are hit in a rather horizontal stroking pattern, a high-to-low
stroking pattern, a low-to-high stroking pattern, and backhand and
forehand stroking patterns. The player will use the legs either to take
a step, to obtain rotation at the trunk, and to push from the ground.
The step will create linear momentum to facilitate the angular momentum of the torso. Pelvic of lower trunk rotation occurs usually
prior to an upper body rotation. The armstroke then lags behind and
begins with an upper arm movement, then a forearm movement, and
lastly a hand movement. Independent action of the hand and of the
forearm are more common in badminton and racquetball than in tennis and squash, however, the action at the hand is very common in
squash as well. In all cases, the action is a sequential kinematic link
system, in which each body part develops a force and therefore forms
a kinetic chain, in which the forces are summated. This summation
provides the linear velocity to the head of the racquet, and thus the
ball or shuttlecock can be hit with a high velocity.

In the following section, selected strokes in the various racquet
sports, as well as table tennis will be described. Since information
from one sport can be transferred with slight or no modifications to
the other racquet sports, basic principles applicable to all racquet sports
will be listed.

Principle 1. To create maximum force, a follow-through is necessary. The follow-through assures that maximum velocity will occur
at the time of impact. The deceleration of the racquet then will not

occur until well after the ball or shuttlecock has left the strings. The follow-through also is a protective mechanism to prevent too rapid reduction of momentum to zero.

Principle 2. The player has very little control on how long the ball or shuttlecock will remain on the strings. The duration of impact is governed by the type and tension of strings and compressability of the ball and shuttlecock head.

Principle 3. String tension is parabolically related to control and ball velocity. Loose tension in the strings will decrease velocity up to an optimum point; ball velocity will increase with increase in string tension. With further increased tension on the strings, the ball velocity decreases. The greater the string tension, the shorter the racquet/ball contact time. A probable explanation for this phenomenon is that the strings and the ball deform, and, thus, energy is absorbed and then given back to the ball in instances where string tension is lower. To impart spin, the ball is hit outward and upward for topspin, forward and downward for backspin. Topspin is rarely used in squash; but is commonly utilized in tennis.

Principle 4. Acceleration rates of the hand, forearm, and upper-arm create stress and possible trauma to the wrist, elbow, and shoulder in racquet sports. Strength training of supporting structures will be required to protect against these acceleration forces.

Tennis

With respect to technique, there are several general concepts of value to players. These have been paraphrased from the writings of Groppel.

The fewer the body segments used, the less chance for error. Therefore, a minimum number of segments should be used during the toss of the ball for the service. When lobbing or merely meeting the ball at the net for a volley, a minimum of body movement will also achieve greater effectiveness and more accurate ball placement. A player should not jump into ground strokes but, rather, remain on the ground to create a ground reaction force to be transferred to the angular momentum of the racquet. If there is a jump, it should occur near the instant of contact. This will mean that the push is being utilized in the stroke. The idea that one should always turn with the side to the net when hitting ground strokes is not true. In many cases, there may be inadequate time to take the turn with the body; the ball may be coming so fast that there is no necessity to add to the momentum of the ball in the return stroke. Additionally, one might want to utilize another movement pattern in order to return the ball very quickly. This pattern is the open-stance forehand. A sidestep is taken to create the angular rotation at the hip. The trunk rotation, therefore, can be extremely effective for forehand drives. A two-hand backhand drive is as effective, with respect to reach, as is the one-hand drive. It is fairly common practice now to teach the two-hand backhand, since it is a simple segmental link in keeping with the principles identified in gymnastics. There would be a two-link system composed of (1) the trunk rotation and (2) the arm swing. With the one-hand backhand, the trunk is rotating, one arm is swinging, and the second arm is a third link in a three-link system. Greater speed and control and less fatigue probably are advantages with the two-hand backhand drive as compared with the one-hand backhand drive.

MINI-LAB LEARNING EXPERIENCES

Identify the active muscles in Fig. 18-2. Contrast this stroke to that of batting.

Tennis Serve

The tennis serve is an overarm type of striking movement. At the beginning, the trunk is rotated to the right (in a right-handed player) with the weight shifted to the rear foot. Note in Fig. 18-3, as in football passing and overarm pitching, that the right foot is placed at a right angle to the intended flight of the ball. This placement and the flexion at the left knee and lifting of the left heel permit greater rotation of the pelvis at the right hip joint. From full extension the right arm is abducted and laterally rotated, and the forearm is flexed. At the peak of the backward movement, the back is hyperextended with the hand extended. Note the continuation of the head of the racquet downward as the player's body moves forward. As the player moves the racquet toward the ball, the right arm is medially rotated and the forearm is extended. The trunk and pelvis are rotated to the left.

The tilting at the torso to the left, which is due to abduction at the left hip, is frequently seen when height of reach is desired. This

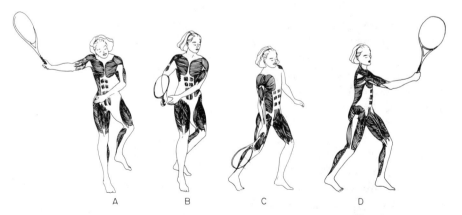

| A | B | C | D |

Fig. 18-2. *The muscles involved in the forehand drive in tennis. Identify the role each group of muscles has during the respective phases of this stroke.*

THE BIOMECHANICS OF HUMAN MOVEMENT

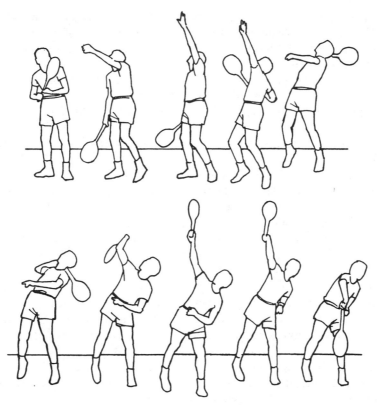

Fig. 18-3. *The tennis service as viewed by the receiver. Note trunk lean and rotation, lateral and medial rotation of the humerus, and other similarities with the basic overarm pattern of throwing. What major differences exist between the tennis service and the overarm pitch? (See figure 17-1.)*

raises the right shoulder girdle and increases the length of the moment arm for spinal rotation.

In the tennis serve, medial rotation of the humerus is a major contributor to the speed of the racquet. However, as in the overhand throw, this action makes its major contribution before the impact phase. The humerus is laterally rotated, close to 90 degrees. Here medial rotation imparts speed to the racquet. Next the forearm extends to achieve height. Also during this time the hand makes its contribution by flexing. Except for the position of the upper arm, the tennis serve and the overhand pitch are much alike. The moment arm for hand action is lengthened by the racquet, and here, as in the golf swing, hand action will be of major importance. Plagenhoef states that racquet speed is no more important than firmness of grip.

The velocity of the ball and the height of impact will determine the angle at which it should be directed to clear the net and to land in the service court. Gonzales, whose serve was measured electrically at 50 m/sec (164 ft/sec), is reported to have the fastest of measured serves. Kramer's serve was measured as 46.6 m/sec (153 ft/sec). These

STRIKING AND KICKING SKILLS 545

velocities will permit the ball to be directed below the horizontal. Stan Smith's serve has been reported to travel at the rate of approximately 60.6 m/sec (199 ft/sec). Some of the younger current international players exceed this speed.

A beginning player, before attempting to direct the ball downward, should develop such a velocity in the serve that when the ball is projected horizontally, it will clear the net and land in the service court. If the impact is 2.4 m (8 ft) above the ground and the projection is horizontal, gravitational force will bring the ball to the ground in 0.704 seconds (solve for $8 = 16.1\ t^2$).

In this time, the horizontally directed ball must travel approximately 17.6 m (58 ft); its velocity would be $0.704\ x = 17.6$ m or $x = 25$ m/sec (82.4 ft/sec). If the impact were 12.2 m (41 ft) from the net, the ball would clear the net in 0.485 second, and gravity will have moved it downward 1.15 m (3.79 ft). Thus the net is cleared by 37 cm (1.21 ft). It is evident that a beginning player should develop a velocity of at least 24.4 m/sec (80 ft/sec) before attempting to direct the ball downward, unless the height of impact is considerably more than 2.4 m. The average tennis player can develop this velocity.

A velocity of 30.5 m/sec (100 ft/sec) has been measured in the better tennis players among college women. If impacted at a height of 2.4 m and directed downward at an angle 3 degrees below the horizontal, the ball will clear the net by 10.6 cm (4.2 in). That angle allows little margin for error and shows the importance of the height of impact.

These calculations were made without consideration of air and wind resistance and ball spin. If a player were able to develop a ball velocity well over 30.5 m/sec, the stroke should impart spin to the ball. Plagenhoef reports that five men whose serves he studied had ball velocities of approximately 44.5 m/sec (146 ft/sec), or 160 kmph (100 mph). For these projections, the racquets were moving at approximately 36.5 to 37.8 m/sec (120 to 124 ft/sec), showing that, as reported for golf, the ball can move with greater speed than does the striking implement. This phenomenon is a result of the duration of force application (Impulse = Ft), or the work (Fd) on the ball while the ball and the racquet strings are in contact with each other.

Smith did a comparative study of the kinematic and kinetic parameters of the flat and slice serves in tennis and found the following:

1. The mean backswing time in the serve was 1.62 seconds and composed 92% of the serving time.
2. The temporal analysis revealed that the mean total serving time was approximately 1.74 seconds.
3. The center of gravity of the racquet reached a mean linear velocity of 33.6 m/sec (84+ ft/sec), with the flat serve being slightly faster.
4. The mean ball velocity for the flat serve was 43.8 m/sec (143.9 ft/sec) and for the slice serve 40.5 m/sec (133 ft/sec).

5. The mean angle of projection was different for each serve: 6.67 degrees for the flat serve and 8.00 degrees for the slice serve.
6. The ball was tossed approximately 0.76 m (2.5 ft) before contact was made with the racquet.
7. In the kinetic analysis, the vertical peak force, corrected for body weight, was 480 N (108.2 lb) for the flat serve (2.79 N per kilogram of body weight) and 521.8 N (117.4 lb) for the slice serve (3.05 N per kilogram of body weight).
8. The peak force of the swing before racquet contact with the ball occurred at 0.046 second for the flat serve and 0.051 second for the slice serve.

Much research has been conducted on the design of tennis racquets, and the following information has been acquired.

1. Larger headed racquets tend to dampen the vibration of impact as vibration travels into the hand. This is usually because the moment of inertia of the racquet head is increased. Therefore, eccentric strikes of the racquet will not cause rotation of the racquet as much as they do with the smaller sized racquet heads.
2. There is a lower predominance of "tennis elbow" occurring from midsized racquet heads than for oversized racquets. Clinical research data were collected by Nirschl to substantiate this. Again, the cause may be because of the greater sweetspot in the oversized racquet.
3. Graphite appears to dampen the vibration impact more than does wood and metal.
4. Changing the center of percussion in racquet design and identifying power spots has led to more effective tennis racquets.

Badminton

Badminton is a game that challenges one's reflexes and demands the most precise timing. This is particularly true due to the uniqueness of the flight of the shuttlecock. The shuttlecock's weight and shape is affected by air resistance which reduces the velocity rapidly. This necessitates timing that is quite different from striking a ball. The shuttle's flight does not follow a true parabolic curve.

Since the shuttle can travel faster (214.8 mph) or slower (almost zero mph) than almost any struck object and can be played with a variety of spins and slices, the possible flight trajectories outnumber those in other racquet sports.

Badminton is the only racquet sport in which the struck object is not allowed to bounce; therefore, an opponent has only a short time to prepare for the return.

The player must develop footwork (Fig. 18-4) which allows him or her to recover immediately and return to a center court position

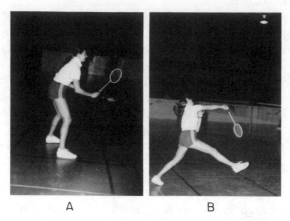

A   B

Fig. 18-4. *A, The basic defensive position (ready or preparatory position) is typical of many sports positions. The anti-gravity muscles are contracting to support the trunk and thighs in their semiflexed positions. B, Attack movements can require large ranges of motion which could result in unbalanced positions. Note the extreme inward rotation of the striking arm and large movement of the ipsilateral leg. From such a position the badminton player must quickly return to position A.*

in a minimum amount of time. Many strokes are executed while the player is airborne.

The racquet and the shuttlecock are both very lightweight; therefore, great force can be produced by increasing the acceleration. Because the shuttlecock is so light, there is a minimum deceleration of the racquet at contact. The key to a powerful smash as stated by Gowitzke and Waddell is to increase "optimum ranges of movement coupled with precise timing with a series of purposeful joint actions" in order to achieve maximum racquet acceleration (Newton's second law: $F = ma$).

An understanding of badminton strokes should be approached with respect to the similarity of fundamental throwing motions to the strokes. Some underhand strokes (See Fig. 18-5A) include: serves, redrops at the net, underhand clears, and defensive blocking actions. The deep singles serve best follows the mechanical principles of a basic underhand pattern. The stroke that best fits the mechanical principles of a sidearm pattern is the drive (forehand or backhand) (Fig. 18-5B). The overhead strokes include drops, clears, and smashes hit from forehand, backhand, and round-the-head positions. The most powerful badminton stroke is the overhead forehand smash (See Fig. 18-5C).

There are many similarities when comparing the baseball and javelin throws or the volleyball and tennis serves to the overhead badminton smash. All of these sport actions follow the basic mechanics of a high-velocity overarm pattern. Since the smash is the most powerful technique of all the strokes, it will be described in more detail.

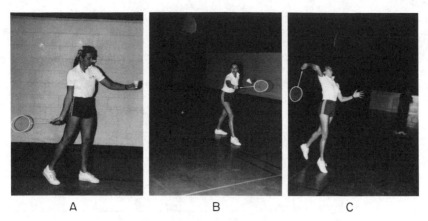

A   B   C

Fig. 18-5. *The three basic underarm patterns are prevalent in badminton. A, The underhand serve in badminton has similarities to the underhand throw, however, the distance between the feet is shorter and the trunk remains more erect. Because of the aerodynamic characteristics of the shuttlecock, the height of the badminton net, and the distance to be served other differences also can be noted between the two skills. B, The backhand stroke in badminton is similar to the drive in tennis. C, The smash, drop, and clear are basic overarm patterns with the characteristic lateral rotation of the humerus that occurs in the baseball pitch. Badminton players attempt to initiate all the overarm patterns from this basic position to deceive the opponent. (Original photos by Bob Clay.)*

Other strokes can be analyzed using information found in other literature, including chapters in this book.

ELEMENTS THAT ASSIST IN POWER DEVELOPMENT

Summation of Forces

Following Newton's first law, the larger muscles contract first to overcome the inertia of the body. The principle of summation of forces dictates that the larger, more proximal body segment leads the movement pattern, followed by the smaller, more distal segments. (Refer to Table 18-1, time-phase relationships chart.) The main contributing levers are medial rotation of the upper arm and pronation of the forearm. Lateral flexion of the trunk aids in this lever action. The radius of movement of the forearm should be long-short-long. More than 50% of the force comes from this lever action while airborne. Since 1980, almost all the skilled players, even the very tall, jump to hit smashes, clears, and drops. They come out of the backcourt and jump in the air with a scissors-kick action as the stroke is being played. Short players tend to use a "cheerleaders arched" action. All the top level players also jump to strike the shuttle early at the net. The resultant speeds attained during the badminton smash have been reported by numerous researchers, some of which are tabulated in Table 18-2.

STRIKING AND KICKING SKILLS   **549**

Table 18-1. *Time-phase relationships of the badminton overhead forehand smash. Gowitzke and Waddel have shown that the characteristic features of a badminton stroke, from backswing to follow-through take place in less than 0.1 second, and can only be revealed when data are sampled at frequencies of 0.01 second or less. Note the nonsignificant action at the wrist and the significant radio-ulnar pronation, humeral medial rotation and flexion at the elbow all being initiated at less than 0.02 seconds prior to shuttlecock contact.*

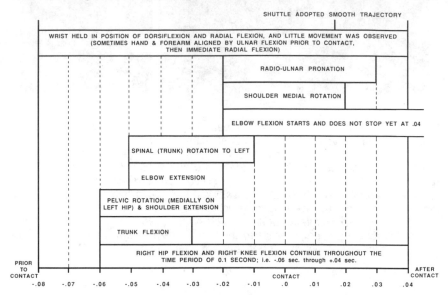

Continuous Loop

There is no hesitation at the end of the backswing. The movement should continue to follow as each joint action continues the kinetic chain. When the objective is power, the backswing should be timed to loop into the forward swing. The acceleration of the racquet will reach its maximum velocity at or near the reversal of direction enabling a greater velocity at the forward swing. Gowitzke and Waddell suggest that "techniques of getting the racquet back early and waiting for the shuttle should be discouraged for the advanced player." Although as a timing technique this is successful, speed will not be effectively produced. Relearning the smash will be required to improve beyond a mediocre smash level.

Increase ROM

A four-sequence portrayal of the badminton smash propulsive phase is depicted in Fig. 18-6.

Preparatory Phase
Basic Biomechanical Principles:

1. Place muscles on stretch.
2. Position for largest range of motion.

Table 18-2. *Comparison of forehand badminton smash velocities as reported by researchers. These speeds can shatter nonsafety eyeglasses and cause bruises, as well as prevent the opponent from being able to respond quickly enough to execute a successful stroke.*

Study identified by author	m/s	ft/sec	km/hr	mi/hr*
Adrian-Enberg (reported in ft/sec)	56.0	183.6	201.6	125.2
Poole (reported in ft/sec)**				
Subject A	42.1	138.2	151.6	94.2
B	30.1	98.8	108.4	67.4
C	21.1	69.2	76.0	47.2
D	26.6	87.2	95.8	59.5
Gowitzke-Waddell				
Subject 1	80.0	262.5	288.0	179.0
2	55.7	182.7	200.5	124.6
3	65.4	214.6	235.4	146.3
4	72.7	238.5	261.7	162.6
5	83.1	272.6	299.2	185.9
6	71.0	232.9	255.6	158.8
7	76.7	251.6	276.1	171.5
8	96.0	315.0	345.6	214.8
Mean of eight subjects	74.9	245.7	269.6	167.5
Hussey				
Subject 1	60.8	199.5	218.9	135.9
2	58.8	193	211.7	131.5
3	63	206.8	226.9	140.9
4	59	193.6	212.4	131.9
5	61.7	202.4	222.1	137.9
6	59	193.6	212.4	131.9
Mean of eight subjects	60.4	198.2	217.4	135

* Abbreviations: m/s: meters per second
                    ft/sec: feet per second
                    km/hr: kilometers per hour
                    mi/hr: miles per hour

** Poole totalled the velocities of elbow, wrist and racket head to attain a "final velocity".

3. The "ready" position for a forehand overhead smash should be a semi-squat balanced position with the racquet held waist to shoulder height in front of the body. The hand in radial flexion is ready to whip up and back at the appropriate time.

4. The knee and hip angles of both lower extremities should show some degree of flexion as the racquet is drawn backward.

5. The shoulder of the hitting arm should be drawn backward by a combination of lateral rotation at the hip joint of the non-racquet side and rotation of the trunk and intervertebral joints.

6. The non-hitting arm should be raised and the hand should be pointed at the shuttle to aid in trunk rotation (force couple), shoulder leverage, and better body balance.

7. The trunk should show some degree of hyperextension at the conclusion of the backswing.

8. The elbow should be drawn back initially by a combination of lateral rotation at the hip joint of the non-racquet side and rotation of the trunk and intervertebral joints. Horizontal ab-

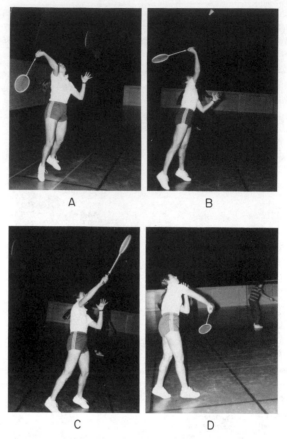

Fig. 18-6. *The propulsive phase of the badminton smash. Note the extreme rotation of the upper arm and the pronation of the forearm. It is no wonder that badminton players hypertrophy the forearm muscles.*

    duction at the shoulder joint also brings the elbow into proper position.

  9. The racquet face should be seen from a side view and the edge should be seen from a back view. The racquet head is well below the wrist and hand.

 10. The racquet head should circle backward and then downward by a combination of previously described movements and by lateral flexion at the shoulder joint, supination of the forearm and dorsiflexion and radial flexion at the wrist joint.

 11. Gowitzke and Waddell observed that "the hand stayed in one place as though it were the center of rotation for these movements."

Basic Biomechanical Principles: Because the badminton player uses a continuous motion to move from the backswing to the forward swing, it is extremely difficult to depict a precise point in time when the backswing ends and the forward swing beings. Gowitzke and Waddell stated that "the lower extremities have started to move forward while the racquet head is still being drawn backward." The force-producing phase is considered to be when all joint actions are moving in the "hitting direction." In this phase:

1. The feet should be well-balanced over the base of support and relatively close together prior to the airborne takeoff.
2. The position of the lower extremities will vary according to court position and ability. The more skilled the player and the deeper the position on the court, the more pronounced the forward leg split should be. This extreme forward stride position aids in achieving better body balance while airborne and recovering to the midcourt position.
3. The trunk should medially rotate over the forward leg at the hip joint as the intervertebral joints are still counter-rotating backwards.
4. The spinal rotation should reverse to a forward motion and the trunk should rotate toward the forward leg while the elbow is still moving backwards.
5. Spinal rotation should continue as the joints of the upper extremity reach the limits of their range so that it gives the impression of the body "moving out from under the arm" with the hand staying almost motionless in space behind the head, according to Gowitzke and Waddell.
6. The upper arm should be extremely abducted with the elbow held high.
7. The racquet should be thrown forward and upward as the player stretches the body up to make contact with the shuttle in front of the body.
8. The hitting arm should be slightly flexed, but near 180 degrees just prior to contact.
9. Medial rotation at the shoulder and forearm pronation are the major force-producing components. The hand should roll through the shuttle in a position of radial flexion. (The frying pan grip is discouraged because it allows one to play "patminton" as opposed to badminton.)

Follow-Through Phase
Basic Biomechanical Principles:

1. The racquet head should continue to move forward and downward until the racquet shaft is in a vertical position below the hand level and in front of the body. The edge of the racquet should point toward the body.
2. After contacting the shuttle, the racquet reaches the above position by continuing forearm flexion, maximum pronation of the forearm, and radial flexion of the hand.
3. Spinal rotation and arm adduction pull the hitting arm down and across the body to complete the follow-through.

STRIKING AND KICKING SKILLS 553

Backhand Overhead Smash

The mechanics of the backhand smash are a reversal of the forehand smash. The forearm is markedly flexed, the force producing motions are lateral rotation at the shoulder and supination of the forearm. Each body segment moves through its full range of motion. The racquet face should be seen in full from a side view after the follow-through.

Round-the-Head-Smash

The mechanics of the round-the-head smash are similar to the forehand smash, however, there is a considerable amount of lateral flexion of the trunk. The trunk should remain parallel to the diagonal of the court in a position to throw (hit) as opposed to squaring off to the net before the forward swing. This will help reduce the errors of hitting the shuttle wide of the sideline. There is a side split of the legs instead of the forward split to return to the ready position.

Many players tend to feel off balance when learning this shot because often the body has been placed in an awkward alignment in trying to hit the shuttle. This occurs due to the lateral flexion of the upper body toward the sideline, and at the same time taking a scissor-kick split step toward the center of the court. A beginner must learn to place the foot of the non-hitting side parallel to the net with the toes directed toward the center of the court. One would almost be in the same position as in a forehand smash except the shuttle would be farther toward the non-racquet side of the body. Laterally flexing and horizontally rotating the trunk are the keys to executing a proper round-the-head smash. The initial foot placement greatly affects the ability to make a powerful stroke and an effective recovery.

Trunk flexibility is crucial to permit the player to reach more shuttles and to execute a quick stroke with deception and power. If the player has trunk flexibility, more shots can be reached with fewer steps, and keeping the body close to the center of the court. This gives the player quick recovery as the trunk flexes laterally toward the shuttle.

The trunk muscles, especially the intercostals, can be injured if a player takes a stance that is square (parallel) to the net prior to contact with the shuttle. This position causes extreme lateral flexion to take place and delay in horizontal rotation of the trunk. Thus, lumbar injuries, especially in the sacroiliac joint, are not uncommon with players using incorrect mechanics.

There is a lack of speed (shuttle rebound or racquet velocity) if a player is off-balance at the moment of impact. Another key is poor footwork, that is, not assuming a stable stance.

The use of the round-the-head smash allows the player to have fewer backhand shots, which tend to be the weakest shot for most players. The player using the forehand shot is in a better position to watch the opponent's readiness prior to contact and during the follow-through. It also permits the performer to have a quicker return to the ready position than when using the backhead.

COACHING PRINCIPLE	BIOMECHANICAL PRINCIPLE
Sit to hit. Be as erect as a fencer.	Dynamic balance is established if hips are positioned on the same vertical line as the shoulders.
Play badminton, not "patminton."	Acceleration of racquet head forward of the wrist will produce required momentum at contact of strings with shuttlecock.

TABLE TENNIS

Table tennis is classified as a striking activity involving all the elements of striking actions, coupled with the slight increase of the length of arm caused by the addition of the paddle. There is a collision of two objects, the paddle and the ball. The ball is much lighter in weight than the paddle. The difference between the momentum of the paddle (the mass of the paddle times its velocity) and of the ball (the mass of the ball times its velocity) determines the direction of the greater momentum. This is an application of the law of conservation of momentum.

The angle of incidence and reflection must also be considered. The angle of reflection is usually greater in connection with spinning balls, which occur, for example, in table tennis. The surface of the paddle, which varies somewhat with the type used, affects the action of the ball. The more irregular the surface, the greater the coefficient of friction, and thus the more spinning action.

As the ball is returned to the table surface by a strike, the ball tends to move at the same speed and in the same direction it assumed after being struck, in accordance with Newton's laws. The table, however, resists the force of the ball and creates an equal and opposite force on the ball. Because of the fricitional component, there is a decrease in the horizontal velocity. There is also some decrease in vertical velocity (V_y) in connection with the coefficient of restitution and in accordance with the momentum of the ball and the striking angle.

The speed and direction of contact of the ball with the paddle determines whether backspin, topspin, or sidespin is the result. If spin is desired, the ball is not struck by the paddle traveling in a completely linear direction. There are often two velocities in connection with top spin. One is the forward velocity in the horizontal direction, and the other is the horizontal velocity in a backward direction as a result of the spin. If the backward horizontal velocity is greater than the forward horizontal velocity, the friction that occurs when the ball strikes the table tends to increase the horizontal velocity. Thus, the table tennis player applies topspin when it is advantageous to have the ball bounce off the table with great horizontal velocity and at a low trajectory.

In certain situations, such as in a smash, the player may try to strike the ball at the center of percussion. This will cause the ball to rebound from the paddle at the greatest velocity and with little or no spin. The opponent's shot should usually be contacted just before the top of the bounce. At this point, the pull of gravity and the vertical momentum are neutralized.

Lopez found that the maximum speed of the ball struck by a defensive player in a backhand stroke was only 12 m/sec (39 ft/sec), compared to the speed of a smash reported to be 18.3 m/sec (60ft/sec) by other investigators. From her comparative study of the backhand stroke of male and female subjects, she drew the following conclusions (Fig. 18-7).

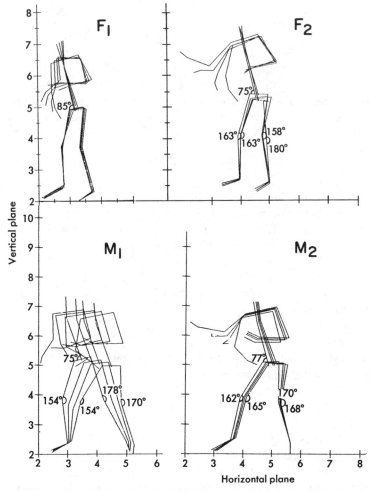

Fig. 18-7. *Computer printout of digitized movie film images of table tennis backhand stroke of male subject (M1, backswing and M2, foreward swing) and female subject (F1, backswing and F2, foreward swing). Note the lesser ranges of motion of body parts for the female subject. (Courtesy Jacqueline Lopez)*

1. The subjects had their legs flexed during the stroke.
2. The backswing of the subjects' paddle was close to the waist.
3. The forward swing of the subjects' paddle was upward and forward across the body.
4. The trunk angle during the stroke was less than 90 degrees.
5. The left arm was flexed and close to the body during the stroke.
6. The subjects stood sideways to the table.

GOLF STROKE

The golf stroke is an underarm striking pattern similar to throwing, with modifications in the arm action. It might be called a reversed underarm pattern, since for the right-handed performer, the left arm is the guiding force, and in the downward swing the left arm action is abduction rather than adduction. The skill also differs from the usual underarm pattern in that both arms are active. (See Fig. 18-8.) Although the right arm does contribute to the force, it is used mainly to support the club except for the hand action. Broer and Houtz have classified this skill as a sidearm pattern. We, however, justify its classification as an underarm pattern on the basis of the move-

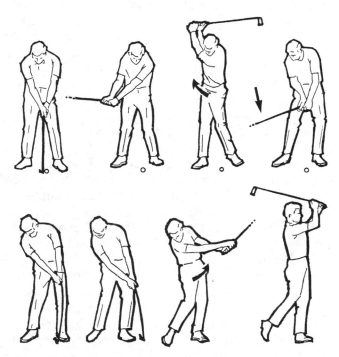

Fig. 18-8. *The golf swing is a two-arm underarm pattern in which the arms move primarily in the frontal plane and the trunk rotates in the transverse plane. Differences in position of the club at the height of the backswing are influenced by strength and anthropometric characteristics of the golfer. Note the characteristic counter rotation and caudal-cephalic summation of forces.*

STRIKING AND KICKING SKILLS

ment of the left arm from a horizontal position above or at shoulder level at the height of the backswing downward to a position parallel with the trunk axis at impact. The observations of Broer and Houtz are that there is greater activity in the muscles of the left arm, supporting their statements that this arm action contributes more force than the right. This concept is subject to debate, as indicated above. The sequence of joint involvement is the usual hip, spine, and shoulder, with the wrist being last. No step is taken, since the feet do not move from the starting position, but the weight shifts to the right foot on the backswing and back to the left foot on the forward swing. This shifting of weight increases the range of hip rotation.

At the height of the backswing, pelvic action is seen to have rotated the pelvis almost 90 degrees and spinal rotation to have turned the upper torso more. As the weight is transferred to the left foot, medial rotation at the left hip turns the pelvis toward the line of ball flight. In the skilled performer, rotation at the hip will begin before the shoulder and wrist have completed the backward movements. As the pelvis rotates forward, it will carry the arms downward. Action at the shoulder begins approximately at the time that the arm has reached the horizontal; action at the wrists will be delayed until the arm approaches the vertical.

The moment arm lengths of hip and spinal levers must be measured from pictures taken with a camera placed in line with the flight of the ball. The moment arms are illustrated in Fig. 18-9. Depending on the length of the club and of the performer's arms and on the amount of spinal flexion, the moment arm length for hip action will be 0.9 to 1.2 m (3 to 4 ft). These factors will also affect the length of the moment arm for spinal action, which will be greater than that for the hip. The angular velocity at the hip and spine will be considerably less than that at the shoulder. A rough approximation of the linear contributions at the acting joints would be 70% at the wrist, 20% at the shoulder, and 5% each at the hip and spine.

Because extreme accuracy is necessary in golf, Cochran and Stobbs recommend that the movement pattern be made as simple as possible; they believe that the important levers are those acting at the shoulder and wrist joints. They state that the difference between skilled and unskilled golfers may lie in the simplicity of action and the ability to generate power in the acting muscles.

Full swings of the various clubs will have the same lever actions and the same proportion of linear contribution to the speed of the club head at the time of impact. In comparing full swings with the driver and with the No. 7 iron as made by five women golfers (handicaps 4, 5, 7, 9, and 12), Brennan found that the same body segment actions were used in the two swings. In the degree of body segment action in the forward swing and backswing, she found only one significant difference in the mean measures. Although the degree of pelvic rotation in the backswing did not differ, with the driver, the pelvis had rotated 7.2 degrees farther at contact than with the iron. The length of the

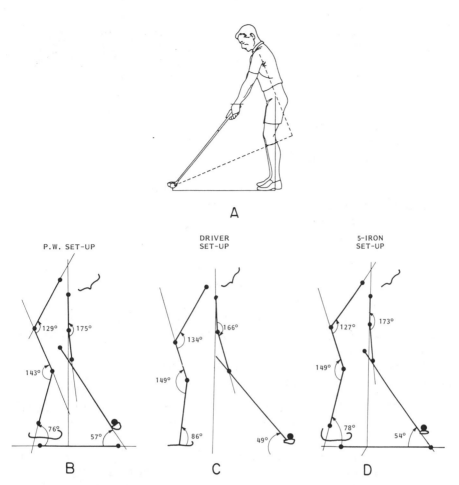

Fig. 18-9. *A, Moment arm lengths in the golf stance are measured as the perpendicular distance from the spinal rotation axis (passing through the forward hip) to the center of the ball. Note how the stance changes for a given golfer when using a pitching wedge (B), 3 iron (C), and driver (D). Construct the moment arms and their lengths to each other ranking them from longest to shortest. Determine percent of change from the longest moment arm. (B, C, and D Courtesy Brian Magerkuth)*

club will affect the length of all moment arms and also the path of the club head; as the club is shortened, the path will become shallower and shorter. Photographs of a No. 2 iron and a wood swung by Bobby Jones show velocities of 40.23 and 43.28 m/sec (132 and 142 ft/sec), respectively, at the time of impact. The shorter distances obtained with shorter clubs result from the lower linear velocities of the lever, as well as from the higher angles of projection.

Lever action in striking activities cannot be evaluated by comparing the summed linear velocities of acting levers to the velocity of the projectile. In throwing, the distal end of each lever is the center of gravity of the object to be projected. As each lever moves, this cen-

STRIKING AND KICKING SKILLS 559

ter of gravity is moved, and at release its velocity equals that of the contribution of the levers. In striking, the projectile is moved by body levers only during the brief period of contact.

The velocity of the golf ball can be greater than that of the club head at impact. Cochran and Stobbs reported that a top golfer can have a club velocity of 272.2 m/sec (880 ft/sec). This is equivalent to 160.9 kmph (100 mph). The subsequent ball velocity will be 362 m/sec (1188 ft/sec). The difference between club velocity and ball velocity is due to the smaller mass of the ball, and to the fact that the ball is flattened on impact, and that during the j0.0005 second of contact the elastic ball pushes away from the club. These authors state that contact time is the same for almost all shots, even that of a putt—always less than 1 ms.

The swing of a skilled golfer is so fast that detailed movement analysis can be made only with some device to aid vision. In the film of a professional golfer, Cochran and Stobbs found the time from the start of the swing to impact to be 0.82 second and that from the start of the downswing to impact to be 0.23 second. The downswing was more than two and one-half times as fast as the backswing. Computer graphics, as depicted in Fig. 18-10, are valuable aids in pattern recognition, changes in velocity, and spatial orientation.

Cooper, et al. studied the kinematic and kinetic aspects of the golf swing and concluded the following:

1. The line of gravity was midway between the two feet at the beginning of the downswing. This means that the force for each foot was the same.
2. The weight shift was such that 75% occurred on the front foot and 25% on the rear at impact (mean shift).

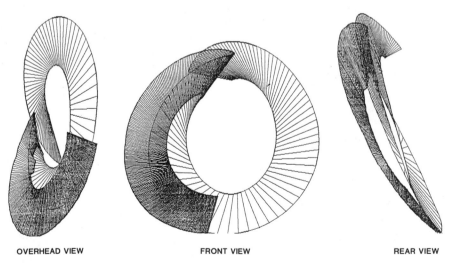

OVERHEAD VIEW   FRONT VIEW   REAR VIEW

Fig. 18-10. *A computer graphics display of three planar views of path of the golf club of a golf swing of an experienced golfer. (Courtesy James Richards)*

3. After impact, there was a continued shift of some weight toward the front foot with most clubs, the greatest being with the high-loft club and the least with the driver.
4. After the impact position was reached, the performers using the highest-numbered club had a force distribution between the feet of approximately 75% on the front foot and 25% on the rear foot. With the driver the weight distribution was approximately equal on each foot.
5. There was some change in the force distribution at the end of the follow-through, in that the shift was almost up to 80% on the front foot with the high-loft club and nearly 70% with the driver.
6. The total vertical force exerted from the downswing to just at or before impact was from 133% of body weight with the high-lofted club to 150% with the driver.
7. The total vertical force decreased with all clubs as impact occurred.
8. The total force exerted in the vertical direction was reduced to 80% of the total body weight, indicating that the centrifugal force of the club had pulled the body upward (Fig. 18-11).

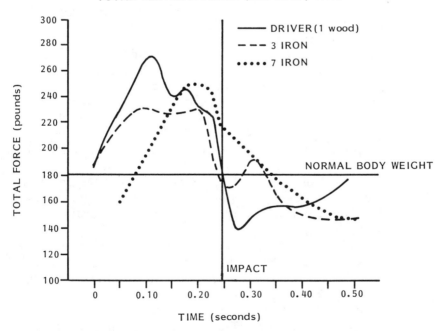

TOTAL VERTICAL FORCE (foot force plates)

Fig. 18-11. *Total vertical force during a golf swing, measured by foot force plates. Note that the force on the plates varies from approximately 1221.06 N (275 lb) during the downswing of the drive to 621.3 N (140 lb) immediately after impact with the ball. Note the unique force-time patterns for the three clubs used by this golfer. Which two patterns are most similar to each other? Why?*

STRIKING AND KICKING SKILLS   **561**

By means of film measures of the swings of an average golfer, a college woman, researchers found the average swing time with a No. 5 iron to be 1.41 seconds and with a No. 9 iron to be 1.34 seconds. The downswings were three times as fast as the backswings. Drives from the tee made by two highly skilled women golfers as they participated in a tournament were measured with a stopwatch and were found to average 0.64 (Berg) and 0.85 (Suggs) second. The swing of a highly skilled college man, measured on film, took 0.77 second; the downswing was twice as fast as the backswing. Films of Bobby Jones showed that the backswing was completed in 70 frames and the downswing in 30 frames. His downswing was two-and-on-third times faster than his backswing.

The Golf Model

Recently, Mann (as reported by Carney 1986), using a special computer, has electronically charted 32 points on the body and seven on the golf club during golf swings of 52 leading male professional golfers. Based on these data, he was able to create an ideal or model golfer. Information concerning the golf swing of the model golfer is as follow:

1. The head remains relatively stationary during the swing and moves no more than 2 inches in any direction.
2. The backswing and the downswing are not identical. It is not a single swing.
3. The hands and the clubhead move on a "warped" path up and down. The hands tend to move on a flatter path than the club head. This range, for the hands, is 10 degrees off the vertical with the driver and 18 degrees for the 9-iron.
4. The top right-handed golfers do not have a straight left arm. Mann states that "the left arm flexes more than 30 degrees at the top of the backswing." He believes amateurs, in attempting to have a straight arm, cause tension to develop in that arm.
5. The "butt" of the club does not point toward the ball at the beginning of the downswing. The top players keep the "butt" end from pointing toward the ball by the natural extension of the arms.
6. The outside-to-inside swing concept is generally not true, but the golfer should feel as if it were true. The hips prevent this from happening. The downswing is outside the backswing.
7. It is impossible strength-wise for a golfer to control the clubhead at ball contact. The proper positioning of the body, grip, and the position of the clubhead are determined early in the downswing.
8. The change in body weight-shift with each club is not correct. There is almost the same weight shift, regardless of the club used. Mann states that "with the driver, weight-shift is 50%

left and 50% right. With the 9-iron the weight-shift is 55% right and 45% left. The ball is positioned within 2.5 inches for all clubs."

9. The concept of one-piece takeaway of the club is only true to a point. "From the address until the hands pass the right pocket, it is virtually a one-piece movement. Arms and trunk turn together. The butt end of the club remains the same distance from the body." To try to keep the club and the body together any more would cause the arms to move away from the body. He contends there is only a small amount of hand flexion (cocking).

10. Most top golfers have similar swings. Shorter golfers have flatter swings than taller golfers. Aside from this, their swings are almost identical. The width of the shoulder, length of arms, and the standing height are among factors that should influence the club lengths.

11. There is basically one swing for all clubs. There is a difference in the backswing because of the length of the clubs. Slight changes in the body positions for the various clubs are due to club lengths.

12. The so-called setup at the beginning often dictates what follows in the swing. Mann states that the setup is 100% of an effective swing.

13. Swing errors, or making compensation for your swing, are as follows: "Stiff-leggedness creates an overly upright swing. Too much leg flexion produces too flat a swing. Weight too far to the left results in a turn centered too far left. Ball position too far to the rear (from driver to 9-iron, only 2.5 inches difference) causes a player to hang back" to the right side.

14. Finally, Mann says the legs initiate the downswing, not the arms. As the hands complete the backswing, the hips and legs have started to move toward the ball. The hips and legs have almost returned to the starting position before the hands have made much movement.

PUTTING

Some golfers contend that 50% of their game depends on skill in putting. Certainly to be a low-handicap golfer, one must be able to putt consistently. Most of the people who study the putting action list the following as important for success in putting:

1. Remain stationary over the ball with only the arms, wrists, and hands moving to make the stroke.
2. Keep the head as stationary as possible, since upward head action shifts the center of gravity, causing a change to take place in the arc of movement of the arms.

3. Keep the body weight evenly distributed over the feet in order to have a firm base and to prevent swaying.
4. The backward takeaway movement of the putter must be close to the ground and executed smoothly. Any extra movement by the golfer's body or arms may interfere with the stroke action.
5. Maintain a firm left side (right-hand putter) with the left hand and left wrist firm. This action coupled with the acceleration of the clubface through the ball, is considered effective putting form. The clubface must strike the ball squarely.

The old adage "Never up, never in" should be kept in mind. Many believe that the golf ball must be struck firmly enough to always reach the hole. If it misses, it should travel past the hole approximately 15 to 20 inches. This means that there was enough velocity imparted to the ball to make it go in the hole provided it was aimed and hit properly.

Other influences must be considered such as the break, grain of the green, spike marks, footprints, wind, and moisture on the greens.

Additional mechanical comments on golfing in general for best performance are listed below:

1. The hands are placed ahead of the ball at address. This enables the club head to contact the ball squarely as the downswing takes place.
2. Too much wrist action is worse than no wrist action. Power hitters use a great deal of "wrist action." If too much is used, it results in a duck hook (closed club head before contact) or in a draw (club head closed during impact).
3. The right forearm moves over the left forearm gradually during the follow-through to enable the arms to extend fully.
4. If the grip is too loose at the top of the backswing, the club centrifugal force will turn the club in the performer's hands, resulting in the club head not meeting the ball at the "sweet spot".
5. The key fingers in the grip for right-handed golfers are the ring and middle fingers. However, all the fingers to an extent must have some feel either of the fingers of the opposite hand or the club. The kinesthetic or tactile aspects of the grip are vital in making a rhythmic (smooth) swing with the club.

MINI-LAB LEARNING EXPERIENCES

1. Have several members of the class demonstrate the golf swing hitting a whiffle ball. Discuss their actions in class. Why do some appear more skilled than others? What parts of the swing can you actually see?
2. a) Construct two pendulums of varying weights and radii and then strike a golf ball or table tennis ball with each

pendulum. Using the Work-Energy and Impulse-Momentum Equations, explain the different results.
    b) Construct a large sling shot and release golf balls at varying angles and velocities. Chart the trajectories and ranges of the balls. State conclusions. Relate to the game of golf.
  3. Observe the stance (setup) with different golf clubs as depicted in Fig. 18-9. Note the relationship of club length to the given body angles.

HANDBALL

Handball involves a type of striking motion which is similar to throwing. The movements are quite varied, depending on the shot desired at the moment. There are overhead, underhand, and sidearm motions. The wall and ceiling hits constitute still other variations. There is even a punch stroke to the ceiling. Most top players use a type of sidearm stroke in most situations. The following principles are especially emphasized in regard to handball strokes:

  1. A nearly stationary head is maintained at the time of contact with the ball to avoid causing the path of the arm swing to change.
  2. The back leg is turned externally so that pelvic rotation takes place as the kill or pass shot is executed. This is especially necessary in sidearm strokes.
  3. The point of contact is tangential to the motion of the arm and is therefore just medial to the inside of the front foot.
  4. The motion is primarily elbow, wrist, and hand action, not a true shoulder swing.
  5. The game as performed by top players is predicated on the execution of a successful serve. This is done with a sidearm motion that causes the ball to attain great velocity at a low angle trajectory striking the wall 1.2 to 1.8 m (4 to 6 ft) above the floor. This angle keeps the opponent from having an easy return shot.

KICKING

The kicking action is a striking pattern used to apply force with the foot. It is a variation of running and thus is a modification of the walking pattern. The kick differs from the walk and the run in that force is applied with the swinging limb rather than with the supporting one. In the final force-producing phase the primary action is extension at the knee. The lever and the resistance arm include the leg and the part of the foot between the ankle and the point of impact. The length of the moment arm is approximately the distance from the knee to the point of impact.

STRIKING AND KICKING SKILLS   **565**

Although little or no action at the hip occurs in the final phase, this joint makes an important contribution in the earlier force-producing phase. As the thigh is swung forward from the hip, it carries the leg and foot with it. During this time the lower leg flexes—an action that moves the foot backward. Based upon film tracings, in spite of this lower leg action, the foot moves forward during this phase. Thigh action in this pattern contributes to the forward movement; in bowling, this action is similar to the contribution of the approach steps, which move the ball forward as the arm is swinging back. The leg, then, will have not only the velocity developed by lower leg extension but also that developed by thigh flexion, even though the latter action does not occur at impact. Immediately after impact, the thigh again flexes and moves the entire limb speedily upward in the follow-through. Unless one has studied this with slow motion film, the pause in thigh action is not likely to be observed. Thigh action is often thought to be continuous, but cannot because of the nature of the quadriceps muscle crossing both the hip and the knee.

Another valuable lever can be added to the kick by pelvic rotation, which can be acting at the time of impact. This lever is used most frequently by performers who have had training in soccer and is effective when the ball is approached diagonally. The lever and the resistance arm of this action include the pelvis, the thigh, the leg, and the part of the foot between the ankle and the point of impact. At impact the length of the transverse moment arm, which is perpendicular to the axis passing through the left hip (if the kick is made with the right foot) and to the line of force, will be approximately equal to the width of the pelvis.

Punting in Football

Researchers of punting skills used in football have shown that the major contributor at the time of impact is the lever action at the knee joint; the lever at the hip joint makes its major contribution before impact. The pattern is illustrated in Fig. 18-12, where from A to B the thigh can be seen to have flexed; from B to C the inclination of the thigh has changed little if any. After C, the thigh flexes rapidly, carrying the entire limb forward and upward.

From 90 degrees of flexion in A, the lower leg extends; it has contacted the ball before C. Impact is likely to be made before the lower leg is fully extended; this and the rapid flexion at the hip after contact protect the knee joint. Rotation of the pelvis can be seen from A to C.

Differences in hip action at the time of impact have been observed. Some performers have no hip action; some have slight flexion, and other have slight extension. Thus it is probable that, at impact, hip action is an adjustment to the position of the ball relative to the supporting foot. If this is true, studies should be made to determine whether a particular position of the supporting foot relative to a sta-

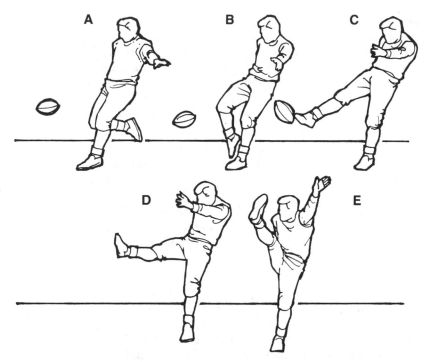

Fig. 18-12. *The football punt. Note backward body inclination to enable the punter to extend further at the hip and knee during the forward swing. The head is relatively stationary through contact with the ball and the supporting leg receives the force of the kicking action.*

tionary ball will result in greater velocity and accuracy. The drop of the ball with reference to the foot should also be studied. Whether the foot is contacting a stationary or a moving ball, the eyes should be focused on it. Therefore, the performer approaching the ball should flex the head and upper spine.

When a step or a run precedes the kick, forward movement of the body can contribute to the force of impact. The placement of the final step differs from that of the running step. In the latter, the leg flexes just before the foot makes contact with the ground, so that the foot is brought more directly under the body's center of gravity; in the kick, the foot is placed well ahead of the body's center of gravity so that the body can be carried forward by flexion at the ankle, thus adding its forward movement to the force. More important is the greater range of pelvic rotation that this foot placement permits.

Similarities in thigh and lower leg actions are reported by Glassow and Mortimer, who studied film of an untrained 9-year-old body punting a ball and of an experienced male player, executing a placekick. The greatest degree of flexion at the knee was the same for the two performers, slightly more than 90 degrees; the rate of extension at the knee at impact was also the same, approximately 1280 degrees per second (22+ radians). The man, whose leg was longer, had a longer moment arm for the lever acting at the knee and, therefore, greater linear velocity for this lever. Flexion at the hip, moving the thigh forward and slightly upward, occurred in both man and boy while the lower leg was flexing. Then the lower leg rapidly extended. Both performers extended the thigh a few degrees just before impact. This action has been observed in several studies; it does not add to the force of impact but is probably an adjustment to the ball position.

Much greater lower leg angular velocity for the kicks of three highly skilled Australian men is reported by Macmillian. These average velocities for each man were 1521.3, 1788.6, and 2008.7 degrees per second immediately before contact. During the same time, the average foot velocity was 23.3 and 23.7 m/sec (76.5 and 77.9 ft/sec). The maximum ball velocities were faster than those of the impacting foot; they were 27.2 and 25.0 m/sec (89.2 and 82 ft/sec). This phenomenon was mentioned in the discussion of golf and tennis in connection with racquet and ball velocity.

The velocity of the force as it strikes the ball, coupled with the angle of release, determines the distance attained. A high vertical velocity and a high angle (60 degrees) bring about a high-lofted kick. Conversely, a high horizontal velocity and a low angle (40 degrees) may cause the ball to reverse a longer distance. A high angle is used with the wind, and a low angle against the wind.

The ball is spinning as it leaves the foot. The reason is that the leg and foot move internally toward the middle of the body on the follow-through. At contact, the foot cuts across the underneath side of the ball, causing the spin. The ball rides on the foot for a few centimeters.

Alexander and Holt found that before contact the superior punter's kicking foot had a linear velocity of 25.3 m/sec (83 ft/sec). The punters in their study struck the football with the kicking leg flexed at the hip, a maximum of 77 degrees. The ball was dropped so that it struck the foot at an angle of 25 degrees across the forepart of the foot to produce the spinning action or spiral during its flight. The foot contacted the ball at approximately 38 cm (15 in) above the ground and rode on the foot. The more horizontal the drop, the more effective the punt.

Barr and Abraham conducted a biomechanical analysis of 22 punts of an outstanding punter using templates with each projected image. They used a Filter-Spline-Filter smoothing scheme for the film data. The punter was described by 21 body points; the ball by two points. Their findings were:

1. On a gross basis, the biomechanical patterns were consistent regardless of the distance attained. The action of the punter's kicking leg was described as that "of a simple rotating limb."
2. The motion patterns of punting were very similar to that of a soccer toe kick.

3. The differences between the farthest and shortest kicks appeared to be in the ankle parameters.
4. Using the ankle point (near the point of contact), they found that the peak resultant velocity occurred just prior to contact with the ball. The longest kicks had resultant peak accelerations in the range of 700–800 ft/s2.
5. What they called the ankle angle (anterior angle between the foot and the lower leg moved quickly toward 180 degrees, varied from 158 to 168 degrees) as the punter contacted the ball and was largest for the longest kicks. This provided a flat, rigid surface for contact.
6. The punter was a shoeless kicker which they contend was an advantage. (See discussion in next section.)
7. The resultant linear velocities and accelerations were only slightly higher for the longest kicks. They believe this is due to the fact that there is greater action in the hip flexors in the longest kicks, yet this is tied to the total limb mechanics of the swinging leg.
8. In the case of the knee joint, maximum angular acceleration occurred just prior to contact, followed by maximum angular velocity at contact.
9. Rotation at the hip was similar in pattern to that at the knee with the maximum acceleration coming prior to maximum velocity.
10. The lower leg was not fully extended at contact (130 degrees) regardless of distance of kick.
11. The acceleration at the hip in punting came prior to acceleration at the knee. They suggest that this means there was a "transfer of power from the upper to the lower leg."
12. Not surprisingly, they found that the resultant ball takeoff velocity after contact was greater than ankle velocity, due to the coefficient of restitution. The ball is compressed when contacted and then regains its original shape. The angle of takeoff of the ball varied from 54 degrees to 40 degrees with a mean average of 50 degrees.

Because of loss of friction, a spiralling ball will go farther into the wind than one punted with an end-over-end turning action. Conversely, an end-over-end punt tends to go farther with the wind than against it. Coaches talk about the ball "turning over" at the height of the flight path. This occurs with a spiralling ball and helps direct the ball less rapidly downward because of lift action of the spinning ball.

The shoeless foot enables the punter to flex the ankle more easily than with a shoe, presents a flatter surface to the ball, and has a peak ankle point velocity just prior to contact. A dominant ankle velocity and a high follow-through results.

Since the kick is initiated after the stepping action by the increase in angular acceleration at the hip and then transferred to the foot, the line from hip to knee and to ankle is extremely critical.

MINI-LAB LEARNING EXPERIENCES

Almost no research exists with respect to the support leg. Observe kickers, place kicks and punters, and the role of the support leg. Discuss your findings.

Soccer Kicking

Soccer kicking is primarily done as an instep striking action. The biarticular muscle action at the hip and knee consists of flexion and extension. Fabian and Whittaker studied the instep kick and recommended that the nonkicking foot be placed alongside the ball. Then the kicking leg should swing forward from the hip, and the lower leg should simultaneously flex so that the heel is well back. When the knee comes in line with the ball and the eye, the lower leg extends. The top of the instep or shoelaces should meet the ball, the toes being extended or pointed downward. The body should be over the ball. The power of the kick comes from the lower leg (knee), not the hip, and is in almost direct relationship to the preparatory flexion at the knee. The muscles of the leg should be relaxed until the kick is started; then the muscles contract strongly until the instep contacts the ball. The toe does not come into contact with the ball. A simple instep kick will have little or no spin and will remain low in flight. See Fig. 18-13 for the critical positions in soccer kicking.

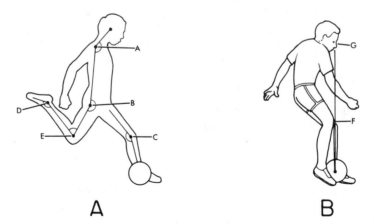

A   B

Fig. 18-13. *The critical positions in soccer kicking are A, The planting of the support foot and the extreme backswing of the kicking leg. The pertinent body angles are labeled. B, The position of the eyes, knee, and foot at the time of striking the ball. The vertical line through the center of ball, outer edge of knee and the eye has been drawn.*

The instep gives the kicker a larger and more stable kicking surface because the whole foot, rather than the toes, is the striking area. Plagenhoef has reported that the side-approach or pivot instep soccer kick produced greater ball velocity than did the straight-ahead approach. He found that the side-approach instep kick produced a ball velocity of 28.9 m/sec (95 ft/sec); whereas the velocity after straight approach with the instep and toe contact was 25 m/sec (82 ft/sec).

If the kicker wishes the ball to have a low trajectory, the nonkicking leg is placed opposite the side center of the ball. If the objective is to elevate the ball, the nonkicking leg is placed 10 to 15 cm (4 to 6 in) to the rear of the ball. The body leans backward so that the hip angle can be 180 degrees at contact. The velocity of the leg swing and the contribution of the pelvic rotation culminates in a resultant force of the magnitude and direction of all the applied forces. The kicked ball's path of flight is the result of the launch angle, the launch velocity, and the aerodynamics of the ball in flight. (Note: launch angle is the same as projection angle.) The angle of inclination of the striking foot and the major axis of the ball and foot also make a contribution.

Abo-Abdo found that the mean linear velocity of the soccer ball was 19.5 m/sec (63.85 ft/sec) and of the kicking ankle 17.6 m/sec (57.86 ft/sec). He supported the concept that the velocity of the ankle and foot depends on the velocity of the thigh and knee and the linear velocity of the body's center of gravity.

Abo-Abdo drew the following conclusions from his study (Table 18-3):

1. From the initial leap through the follow-through, the head-to-trunk angle progressively increased the degree of forward flexion until the kicking foot began descending to the ground. Then the degree of forward flexion decreased. The trunk moved

Table 18-3. *Body angles at the shoulder, hip, knee, ankle, and supporting knee of subject during three phases of soccer instep kicking. Compare the amplitude of the changes at the various joints. Does the soccer kick require extreme ranges of motion at any of these joints? Which one?*

Body angle*	R shoulder	R hip	R knee	R ankle	L knee
At placement of nonkicking foot	137	195	100	121	140
When kicking foot contacted ball	125	160	139	125	121
At highest point of follow-through	112	153	152	115	117

Adapted from Abo-Abdo, H.: A Cinematographic Analysis of the Instep Kick in Soccer, unpublished report, Indiana University, 1979.

* Body angles are expressed in degrees.

R, right; L, left.

STRIKING AND KICKING SKILLS

closer to the ball during the kicking action and was in back of the ball.

2. From the initial leap through the follow-through, the right thigh-to-trunk angle was first greater than 180 degrees (thigh was hyperextended behind the trunk) and less than 180 degrees (thigh was flexed in front of the trunk) as the kicking leg moved forward in the kicking pattern. The forward motion of the kicking leg was started after the leap and before the nonkicking foot touched the ground.

3. As the right foot left the ground on the initial leap, the right thigh-to-foreleg angle began to decrease in size. This flexion continued until after the nonkicking foot had landed; then the foreleg began extending forward for foot contact with the ball and follow-through. As the kicking foot returned to the ground, the degree of flexion increased again.

4. At the time of contact with the ball, the position of the knee of the kicking leg and the focus of the eyes with respect to a vertical line through the center of the ball were as follows: (a) the knee of the kicking leg was in front of the center of the ball and (b) the eyes were focused on the back of the center of the ball.

5. From the initial leap through the follow-through, the foreleg-to-kicking foot angle was one of extension. The angle decreased at the time of contact with the ball, increased immediately after the ball left the foot, and decreased again at the highest point of the follow-through.

6. The placement of the nonkicking foot in relation to the center of the ball was alongside the ball. The nonkicking foot remained in approximately the same position throughout the kicking pattern. In the follow-through movement the heel of the nonkicking foot was not raised off the ground.

7. From the initial leap through the follow-through, the left thigh-to-foreleg angle progressively increased in the degree of flexion until, at the moment before contact, this angle started to extend from the position of the foot at contact until the highest point of the follow-through. Although the increase in flexion at the knee joint of the supporting leg appears to indicate that the center of gravity was lowered throughout the progression of kicking, the reverse was found to be true. The center of gravity was progressively raised throughout the kicking action and reached its highest point just before impact with the ball. This increase occurred because the body was raised by its rotation over the supporting leg, and the increased flexion at the knee joint of the supporting leg was not enough to lower the body's center of gravity before contact. Immediately after contact was made with the ball, the displacement of the center of gravity decreased during the movement from impact to follow-through.

MINI-LAB LEARNING EXPERIENCES

1. Kick a soccer ball and a football at various angles of projection and with spins or end-over-end action. Use moderate force to obtain consistency of kicking effort. Compare results and explain the differences in distances attained and flight patterns.
2. Drop balls from various heights onto different tennis racquets. Note string tension, racquet head size, and other racquet design characteristics. Compare rebound heights and discuss results.
3. Compare flights of indoor, outdoor and competition shuttlecocks.

REFERENCES

Adrian, M. and Enberg, M. (1973) Sequential timing of three overhand patterns, *British Journal of Sports Medicine*, 7.

Adrian, M. and Jack, M. (1980) Characteristics of the badminton smash stroke. In *Proceedings of the National Symposium of the Racquet Sports:* Groppel, J., editor. Urbana-Champaign: Univ. of Illinois.

Alexander, A. and Holt, L. E. (1974) Punting, a cinema-computer analysis, *Scholastic Coach* 43:14, June.

Barr, R. F., Abraham, L. D. (1987) *The punters profile—a biomechanical analysis, SOMA (Engineering for the Human Body),* Baltimore, MD: Williams and Wilkins.

Breen, J. L. (1985) Baseball batting techniques, *Encyclopedia of Physical Education, Fitness and Sports.* Cureton, T. K., (Ed), Reston, VA: AAPHERD.

Breen, J. L. (1967) What makes a good hitter? *JOHPER* 38, April.

Brennan, L. J. (1968) A comparative analysis of the golf drive and seven iron with emphasis on pelvic and spinal rotation, thesis, University of Wisconsin.

Broer, M. And Houtz, S. J. (1967) Patterns of muscular activity in selected sports skills, Springfield, IL: Thomas, C. C.

Cooper, J. M., Bates, B. T., Bedi, J. and Scheuchenzuber, J. (1974) Kinematic and kinetic analysis of the golf swing. In Nelson, R. C. and Morehouse, C. A., editors, *Biomechanics IV*, Baltimore: University Park Press.

Cockran, A. and Stobbs, J. (1968) The search for the perfect swing, Philadelphia: J. B. Lippincott Co.

Cunningham, J. E. (1976) A cinematographic analysis of three selected types of football punts, unpublished doctoral dissertation, Graduate College of Texas A&A.

Fabian, A. H. and Whittaker, T. (1950) *Constructive football*, London: Edward Arnold and Co.

Gowitzke, B. A. and Waddell, D. B. (1977) The contributions of biomechanics in solving problems in badminton stroke production, Conference Proceedings, International Coaching Conference, Malmo, Sweden, pp. 11.

Gowitzke, B. A. and Waddell, D. B. (1979) Technique of badminton stroke production, *Science in Racquet Sports:* Terauds, J., editor, Del Mar, CA: Academic Publishers.

Gowitzke, B. A. and Waddell, D. B. (1979) Qualitative analysis of the badminton forehand smash as performed by international players, *Proceedings: National Symposium of the Racquet Sports:* Groppel, J. L., editor, Urbana-Champaign, University of Illinois, 1–16.

Gowitzke, B. A. (1979) Biomechanical principles applied to badminton stroke production, *Science in Racquet Sports:* Terauds, E. J., editor, Del Mar, CA: Academic Publishers.

Gowitzke, B. A. and Waddell, D. B. (1980) A force platform study of overhand power strokes in badminton, *Proceedings: International Symposium on the effective teaching of racquet sports:* Groppel, J. L., editor, Urbana-Champaign, University of Illinois.

Groppel, J. L., Shin, I. -S., Spotts, J. and Hill, B. (1987) Effects of different string tension patterns and racket motion on tennis racket-ball impact, *International Journal of Sports Biomechanics,* 3(2):142–158, May.

Groppel, J. L., Shin, I. -S. and Welk, G. (1987) The effects of string tension on impact in midsized and oversized tennis rackets. *International Journal of Sports Biomechanics*, 3(1):40–46.

Groppel, J. L. (1986) The biomechanics of tennis. In *The Encyclopedia of Physical Education,* Cureton, T. K., (Ed), Reston, VA: AAHPERD.

Huang, T. C., Roberts, E. M. and Yonn, Y. (1982) Biomechanics of kicking. In *Human Body Dynamics,* Ghista, D. N., editor. Oxford: Claredon Press.

Kermond, J. L. (1977) Biomechanical parameters of punt kicking, master's thesis, Kansas State University.

Klatt, L. A. (1977) Kinematic and temporal characteristics of a successful penalty corner in women's field hockey, doctoral dissertation, Indiana University.

Mand, C. L. (1976) *Handball: Fundamentals*, 2nd ed., Dubuque, IA: W. C. Brown.

Mann, R. (as reported by Robert Carney) (1986) Shattering the swing phase and other teaching myths, *Golf Digest*, July.

McCord, C. (1969) The physics of batting, *Athletic Journal*, December, p. 46.

Plagenhoef, S. (1971) *Patterns of human motion, a cinematographic analysis*, Englewood Cliffs, NJ: Prentice-Hall.

Reilly, T. (1979) What research tells the coach about soccer, Cooper, J. M., Reston, VA: AAHPERD.

Reznik, J. W. (1976) *Championship handball by the experts*, West Point, NY: Leisure Press.

Smith, S. (1979) Comparison of selected kinematic and kinetic parameters associated with flat and slice serves of male intercollegiate tennis players, doctoral dissertation, Indiana University.

Terauds, J., (Ed) (1979) *Science in racquet sports*, Del Mar, CA: Academic Publishers.

Waddell, D. B. and Gowitzke, D. B. (1977) Analysis of overhead badminton power strokes using high speed bi-plane cinematography, Conference Proceedings, International Coaching Conference, Malmo, Sweden.

Waddell, D. B. (1979) *Coaching the power stroke in badminton, Science in Racquet Sports*, Terauds, J., editor, Del Mar, CA: Academic Publishers.

Yessis, M. (1972) *Handball, 2nd ed.*, Dubuque, IA: W. C. Brown.

19
Team Sports

BASKETBALL

Basketball is a multi-dimensional game in that more than one skill is involved. It is a game in which the environment is constantly changing: positions on the court, the size and speed of opponents, the effect of screens, the closeness and distance of the crowd, are all the environmental factors affecting play.

Basketball is connected to other sports in that the fundamental locomotor patterns of running and jumping, along with throwing and other related movements, form the major part of the sport. The physical principles and factors that govern the movements in other activities also prevail here, for example, ground reaction forces, pull of gravity, acceleration, momentum, braking force, path of the center of mass, friction, and lever principles. (See Chapter 5.)

Since basketball is a hand-ball skill, the size of the hand is often a determinate as to the level of accomplishment. For example, most youthful players should have a smaller-than-regulation basketball for learning the skills. Research study findings were the basis for adopting a smaller basketball for women intercollegiate competition. On the average, women were more proficient in ball-handling skills when using the smaller basketball than with the regular basketball. This is not to say a player with small hands can't be a top performer. Other factors may offset the lack of big hands.

SKILLS

The following skills will be discussed in the order listed. They are dribbling, passing, receiving, shooting, jumping and guarding.

Dribbling

Dribbling is the act of applying force against the ball by the hand and causing it to move forward and downward. The pull of gravity and the force exerted by the dribbler determine to an extent the velocity of the ball as it leaves the hand and continues to the floor.

The dribbler must be adept in using both hands since the rules prohibit use of both hands simultaneously. The action moves from one hand to the other and often at different heights depending on the position of the defensive player. The ball rests for a fraction of a second against the hand before it is propelled toward the floor. The inflation of the ball, the resistance quality, of the floor and the height of release are all other factors affecting the velocity and the rebound of the dribbled ball.

Dribbling follows several predetermined principles, including Newton's third law, the law of interaction or the law of action-reaction: "There is for every action an equal and opposite reaction." The dribbled ball follows a curved flight path until it comes in contact with the floor. The floor offers resistance to the ball, and the floor is compressed, but this is an insignificant amount. The ball flattens a considerable amount and then rebounds at an angle into the air. The height of the rebound is determined by the coefficient or restitution which is a value derived from the ratio of rebound velocity to inbound velocity. It is dependent upon the property of both elastic bodies and their ability to regain their original shapes after compression. Theoretically the maximum coefficient would be 1.00. A ball dropped from a height of 6 feet that rebounds 75% of that height or 4.5 feet is considered a "playable" ball. If it rebounds less than that height, it is a "flat" ball and must be pumped with air. One firmer than the 75% is too lively and must be deflated accordingly.

The coefficient of restitution is also involved in a rebound off the glass board or rim. Aside from the inflated condition of the ball, the stiffness or looseness of the rim and backboard affect the rebound.

The dribbler must be moving at approximately the same average horizontal velocity or near to the velocity of the rebounding ball as it returns to the hand. Since the ball rests against the hand for a fraction of a second before being pushed toward the floor, the ball takes on the momentum of the dribbler.

When the dribbler is in a situation where the path toward the basket (goal) is open, several steps may be taken between dribbles and the ball pushed as far forward as deemed appropriate, since running without dribbling is faster than dribbling for 47' (half court). Dean Sempert, basketball coach at Lewis and Clark College, Portland, Oregon, conducted the experiment and reported these results to the authors.

There are certain dribbling techniques which are indicative of a skilled player. They are:

(1) The ability to dribble around an opposing player in a curved path (See Fig. 19-1). This involves the use of centripetal force and overcoming centrifugal force. The dribbler must lean into the circle after setting into a curved path. The player pushes

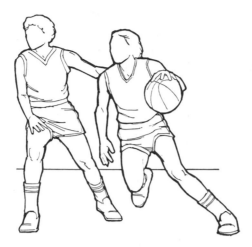

Fig. 19-1. *Dribbling a basketball around an opponent has many of the characteristics of the lean of a skier or surfboard rider described in chapter 5. Note the use of the fingers and their size with respect to the ball.*

with the outside foot toward the outside. This causes the center of gravity to move toward the inside of the curve. The dribbler, upon moving into the curve, accelerates, thus causing the defensive player to be left behind the dribbler.

(2) The behind-the back dribble enables the player to change direction before the opposing player can shift the center of gravity in the new direction soon enough. (See Fig. 19-2.)

Friction, which is the resistance to motion due to the contact of two surfaces moving relative to each other, is involved in this action. The dribbler creates friction when the shoes contact the floor. Then a push in one direction enables the offensive player to move quickly in the opposite direction and move past the defender.

The dribbler protects the ball by placing the body between the ball and the defensive player. It is evident that the dribbler also utilizes friction to a favorable degree in stopping and starting to confuse the opponents.

Passing

Passing is the act of throwing the basketball (which includes bouncing it against the floor) from one player to another, usually done in advancing the ball downcourt.

Passing in basketball is often done with the passer not looking directly at a receiving teammate. In other words, the ball is thrown with deception and frequently not as accurately as when the passer looks directly at the target. Some sacrifice at the expense of accuracy occurs when precise accuracy is not necessary.

There are several types of throws, such as one-hand bounce pass, the two-hand push or chest pass, and the baseball pass.

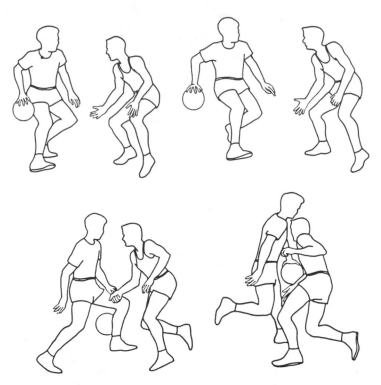

Fig. 19-2. *The behind the back dribble is an example of the necessity for kinesthesis and tactile development since vision can not be used to direct the angle of the bounce. Note the movement to the left of the center of gravity of the guard in response to the position of the ball at the dribblers right side. (Reprinted from Cooper and Seidentop)*

The ball thrown into the air assumes a curved flight path. Gravitational pull causes the ball to descend as it traverses through the air. The effect is barely discernible in short passes, but is easily visible in longer ones. In a case of a ball thrown full court, the passer must throw the ball at approximately a 45 degree angle in order for it to reach a teammate.

Allsen and Ruffner studied the types and frequency of passes used in men's basketball games. They found that the two-hand chest pass was the one most often used (38.6%); the one-hand baseball pass was the next most frequently used (18.6%). The two-hand overhand pass was used 16.6% of the time. Other types of passes were less frequently used. These proportions are still valid today, although different levels of physical condition, age, sex, experience may alter the type of pass used.

An effective passer is one who can pass immediately from the position at which the ball is received. This prevents the opposition from being able to assume a more favorable guarding position in order to intercept the passed ball or prevent it from being passed. Over-the-head and volleyball type passes can be released so quickly the opponents have no opportunity to step into the pathway of the ball in flight. The passer and the guarding opponent wage a constant battle, with the passer having the advantage by being able to determine the direction and the velocity of the ball. In turn, the guard reacts by trying to anticipate and hopes the passer "telegraphs" the direction and speed of the ball.

The "look-away" pass is a pass thrown to a teammate by a passer looking one way and passing another. The look-away pass is effective due to the fact that the defensive players are forced to shift the center of gravity toward the direction of the look and are unable to recover quickly into an effective defensive position.

Most effective passers pass the ball to a teammate so that it arrives near waist height unless a lob pass over an opponent who is fronting a teammate is utilized. A tall player may want to receive a passed ball out in front and at a high position above the head, since a height advantage may be utilized.

The ability to pass on the run is a part of the excellent passer's skills. Also, to pass off the dribble just as the ball bounces up from the floor is an added skill that keeps the defensive player from being too aggressive.

Cooper and Siedentop (p. 39) have listed the following ten principles for skilled passing performance:

1. Successful passers make optimum use of peripheral vision.
2. Except in unusual situations, passes should be executed so the ball is received at waist to chest-high elevation from the floor.
3. Except in unusual situations, passes should be accomplished so the ball is delivered in as nearly a horizontal plane as possible.
   Note: Because of gravity, a horizontal path flight is impossible to attain. However, a pass with too much of an "arched" path is often a dangerous one and is subject to interception.
4. The vulnerable places to pass the ball depends on the foot stance and hand positions of the defensive player. Usually the ball is passed through the following areas: over the shoulder of the down arm, under the raised arm, above the head where the arms are both lowered or extended sideward and between the legs of a wide-feet position.
5. The closer a defensive player is to the passer, the easier it is to pass the ball past the defense.
   Note: This is because the ball can be moved faster than the defensive player can move the hand and arm, since the offensive player moves the hands and arms through a smaller range and knows where the ball will be thrown.
6. A passer must be able to pass the ball as quickly and as forcefully as possible from any receiving position.
7. A definite target spot to pass to should be selected.

Note: Normally, a pass to the side away from the defensive player should be used. If the teammate is much taller or can jump much higher than the defensive player, then the pass may be thrown to a high target, such as hands extended above the head. The receiving player may often come to meet the ball to get away from the defensive player.

8. Leg extension, medial rotation of the arms, and forearm pronation contribute to the force (velocity) when the ball is thrown.
9. The greater the release velocity the ball attains, the more forearm pronation is utilized.
10. The objective is passing is to get the ball to the desired teammate as quickly as possible without telegraphing the path of the ball to the defensive player.

The following should be added to this list:

11. All two-hand passes are actually one-hand in that the dominant hand comes off the ball last.
12. The index and middle fingers are in contact with the ball the longest. Therefore, they give the final impetus to the ball.

There are commonalities in the mechanics of the throwing-pushing action in the execution of the four most used passes. The chest pass, the overhead pass, the baseball pass and the bounce pass will now be analyzed.

Chest Pass. Allsen and Ruffner (pp. 94, 105-107) mentioned that the chest pass is the most common and the most consistent in low turnovers. It is accomplished by the ball being released at or near chest level. The ball is gripped with the fingers spread on the sides of the ball and toward the rear. The thumbs are placed to the rear and parallel to each other. The ball is moved backward in order for the hands to be extended before being flexed. Some would call this action "cocking the wrists", which is not a truly precise statement since the wrist bones move very little. The thumbs come off the ball as the ball moves forward. (The hands at release are behind the ball to apply impetus to it.) The thumbs do not contribute to the forward propulsion but do aid in the gripping of the ball prior to release. (See Fig. 19-3.)

The extending of the hands puts the muscles that control the hand on stretch and thus causes them to contract over a longer distance, generating more force. To increase the velocity of the ball at release, a step forward with the body weight being moved in the direction of the throw is used. When time, however, is a factor, velocity may be sacrificed so that a quick pass can be thrown. Increased velocity may be gained with the arms and hands moving through a wider range of motion, but again this action increases the time and also may telegraph to the defensive players the direction of the pass.

The accurate, relatively long passes are ones with a long follow-through, indicating that great force is generated. The backs of the

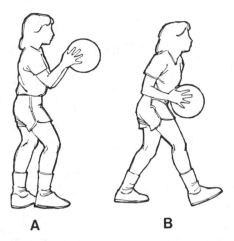

Fig. 19-3. *The chest pass may be executed with a quick, short backswing of arms and hands maintaining the ball at chest level (A) or it may be brought to the pelvic region and circled upward to the chest to increase the distance and speed of the pass.*

hands often end up within six inches of each other because of the pronating action of the forearms and hands.

The follow-through after a short pass is much shorter than after a longer pass. This indicates a reduced velocity, with a small amount of forearm extension and hand flexion and pronation. If the ball is passed with high velocity to a teammate in close proximity, the catch is difficult because the attentuation of the force of the ball is nearly impossible. In this case, "a soft pass often turneth away errors." This would not be true in a long pass and especially a cross-court pass whereby the reverse is true. At best, a cross-court pass is a risky pass.

Overhead Pass. The overhead pass is executed similarly to a chest pass in that there is leg extension, medial rotation, and forearm and hand pronation. Often it is not possible to step forward during the throw, so the velocity at release is generated almost without the transfer of momentum from the step. Most offensive guards out on the court make use of this pass, especially if they are tall and can see over the defensive players.

The ball is held above the head initially, and, as the pass is being executed, the forearms flex and the hands extend, moving the ball backward before it is moved forward to the release position. Strong forearms and hands permit greater release velocity. The same hand and thumb positions are used as in a chest pass. The follow-through is not as pronounced as in the chest pass since the release velocity is not as great and the flight path is usually forward and more downward, taking advantage of gravity.

Bounce Pass. The bounce pass is intended for use in a situation where the ball strikes the floor before the defensive player can intercept it as it goes under the defensive players' arms and rebounds into the arms of a teammate. A "look-away" turn of the head makes the pass more effective.

The beginning of this pass is identical to the chest pass if delivered with two hands. The ball may be released with a back spin which causes the ball to have a higher angle of reflection and reduces its speed due to friction upon impact with the floor. This makes the ball easier to catch.

If top spin is used, the ball bounces off the floor lower, goes a greater distance, and is more difficult to catch. Side spin passes are used occasionally by some passers.

Because the ball velocity at release in a bounce pass must be sufficient to travel downward, impact the floor, and bounce to a teammate, delivery time is increased. More force from the legs, arms, and trunk muscles is needed than in a regular chest pass. The bounce from the floor is not always as accurate as a common chest pass. For these reasons some coaches prefer to limit the use of the bounce pass.

The one-hand bounce pass has many of the same mechanical aspects, except that the ball is released with one hand. Less spin can be imparted to the ball with a quick one-hand release than in other passes and the ball will rebound from the floor at a higher angle because there is less friction.

Baseball Pass. The baseball pass (Fig. 19-4) is usually the type of throw used when the distance to be traversed is equal to or greater than half the court, and the ball must be moved quickly, as well. This usually occurs on a fast break following a defensive rebound, an out-of-bounds situation under the basket from a turnover, or after a successful goal by the offensive team. A strong passer can throw the ball the entire length of the floor. (Sometimes a hook pass is used in such situations, but it has sideward spin, curves in the air, and upon contact with the floor moves in the direction of the spin.)

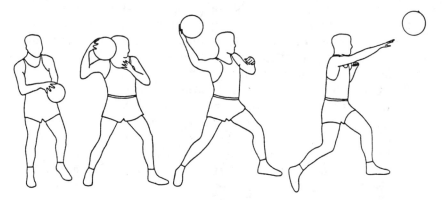

Fig. 19-4. *The baseball pass with a basketball resembles the baseball throw with the classic overarm pattern. Because of the size of ball with respect to the hand size, differences occur with the upper limb movements. Can you describe these differences (refer to figure 17-1 for comparisons.)*

The baseball pass is executed with the ball held low (how low depends on the distance the ball is to be thrown) in one extended hand (right for a right-handed thrower), with the hand behind the ball. The other hand helps support the ball. At the initiation of the throwing action, the fingers of the right hand are spread slightly and face upward. The feet are apart with the left foot slightly in advance of the right. The direction the front foot points helps dictate the direction of the throw. The ball is then moved to the rear, and the forearm is flexed following this action. Next, the ball is moved farther to the rear and behind the right shoulder. When it is possible, a small step by the left foot may be taken prior to the release. The legs may be flexed. The body action may start with the left side slightly rotated to the rear so that as the action takes place the hips may be turned (opened) in the direction of the throw.

The slight step forward with the left foot, the rotation of the hips toward the front, the wide range of the movement of the arm will help to add momentum to the ball as it is released.

The flexion at the elbow occurs prior to the forward movement of the arm with the ball moving above shoulder height. As the arm and hand move forward to begin the release, the forearm extends and moves sideward at shoulder height. The ball is released a slight distance in front of the body. The follow-through will indicate that as the release takes place the thumb and left hand are not touching the ball. The legs are extended the right arm is medially rotated, and the forearm and hand are pronated. The greater the extent of these actions, the greater the possibility for attaining greater velocity at release. Immediately after release, the velocity will decrease because of the pull of gravity and because of air resistance.

This type of pass may be thrown while the player is in the air, when less distance is required. The turn to face the court would be initiated before leaving the floor in the jump.

Shooting

One of the most difficult and perhaps the most important skill in basketball is shooting. It takes years of practice for the action to become automatic. As in other aspects of the games, the players shouldn't have to think with the higher brain mechanisms while in the act of shooting. The shooting should be done intuitively. Changes in shooting style are difficult to perfect for the older player. A motion learned as a youngster even though it may be considered incorrect (and corrected to a degree later) will be reverted to often under stress. "Bad habits die hard."

Shooting is a type of specialized throwing action in which the ball is usually propelled upward toward an elevated, fixed target. Wooden (p. 71) calls the throw "a pass to the basket." The throw at the basket is released quickly but with much less force than in a throw for distance or high velocity. However, from a mechanical point of view, some of the principles involved in most throwing action are present in basketball shooting.

Cousy distinguishes between sighting and aiming. To many, this would be only a study in semantics. However, in support of Cousy's concept, the shooter first attempts to focus on locating the target, the basket, by sighting, to determine how far and how high the opponent guarding will attempt to jump up in the air to block the shot. All such necessary calculations are accomplished before the ball is released or projected toward the basket. Thus, sighting is an act of locating, focusing, and determining a target out in space. Aiming involves deciding on a specific target, such as the front rim of the basket, a spot on the backboard (glass), or the center of the basket. A type of training procedure involved in this process of aiming is mental imagery. Mental imagery enables a basketball player to prepare for shooting a ball at the goal by just reflecting on the image of the action.

Furthermore, the muscles performing the act of shooting have memory in a sense. If a shooting action is successful and satisfying, this action is recorded and later fed back to the shooter. At a later moment, the muscles again are called upon to contract (flex and extend) and communicate to the shooter if a degree of duplication has been accomplished. The player calls this having a "feel" (kinesthesis) for what was achieved.

A player usually has only a few tenths or hundreds of a second to make decisions on range, angle, and velocity. The path of the ball is parabolic in nature. This means the ball will be elevated gradually in the first part of the parabolic path. A shot blocker must recognize this path.

The word "flip" is used sometimes to describe shots which utilize fast hand action as well as softness of the throw. A quick release is essential. Brancazio (p. 308) mentions that in basketball the shooter is launching "the projectile (ball) up an incline."

In modern-day basketball, the dominant hand is the last hand to be in contact with the ball as it is released toward the basket. Additionally, it has been found that in shots of the past, such as the underhand shot, two-hand set shot, and the two-hand jump shot, the right hand and fingers of that hand (for right-hand shooters) were the last to give impetus to the ball before it was released. This action has been observed in re-inacted slow motion film. So it is with the one-hand set, the jump shot, the hook shot, the underhand layup, the scoop shot, the push one-hand layup, etc. There is a similar pattern found in each, and the relationship to each other and to the past styles is remarkable.

Cooper and Siedentop have mentioned certain shooting principles:

1. "Good shooters should always aim at a specific target." The target area might be the front of the rim of the basket, the back of the rim, the open area within the basket, or a spot on

the board (glass). In the past, the good shooter often used the backboard as a target at distance 20 feet from the basket and to the side of it or at an angle to the basket. There was greater friction with the spinning ball against the wood backboard than against a glass backboard. Accuracy was high at this distances for the wooden backboard. That is not true to the same extent with glass backboard. Close-to-the-basket shots, such as a la-yup, and even close-in hook shots, however, will usually re-bound off the glass board into the basket if thrown to the correct spot.

2. "Good shooters should maintain constant eye focus on the tar-get until the ball is released." Some shooters raise their eyes to observe the flight of the ball toward the basket just prior to releasing the balls. This eye, and consequently head and even torso movement, raises the center of gravity of the player and changes the flight path of the ball. This may cause enough of a deviation in the flight path of the ball to cause it to miss the basket.

3. "The ball should be wiggled, if possible, just before the release is begun in order to have good touch in shooting." This action activates the nerve endings in the fingers and the propriocep-tors in a joint so an acute awareness of the ball and its position in the hands is communicated to the player. Some would call this a "feel" for the ball.

4. "The shooter should not hold the body in a fixed position for a long time before releasing the ball (especially the arms and hands)." It has been found that to remain in a state of readi-ness, to perform a gross body action, to more than 1.7 seconds causes the body to lose some of its fluid, smooth muscular co-ordination and efficiency of movement.

5. "The ball should be delivered with a reverse spin in most in-stances." In order for the ball to rebound effectively away from the glass or other type of backboard as well as the rim of the basket, reverse spin should be imparted. Due to the spin, fric-tion is created, which causes the ball to lose some of its speed, and rebound more softly and relatively higher than if there were no spin. The action of the ball under these conditions makes it easier to rebound defensively and to tip in offen-sively. In addition, because of the softness and higher bounce, the ball may strike the goal or backboard and still go into the basket.

6. "The better the shooter, the more intense is the concentration on the act of shooting." The good shooter is one who is pre-pared to shoot at the basket when within range and partially free from a defender. The great shooter-passer is one who is able to change from a shooter to passer or the reverse within fractions of a second. Such a player is rare since the body is being called upon to change movement patterns rapidly and

as intuitively as possible. If the player has to "cerebrate," that is, think before acting, the opportunity to shoot or pass may be lost.

7. "Shooting is characterized by slight and almost imperceptable medial rotation at the shoulder, by extension at the elbow, forearm pronation, and by flexion at the wrist." A clear understanding of the extent of these actions is necessary.

Shooting in modern-day basketball rarely takes place farther than 20 feet from the basket. Therefore, the less pronounced the limbs' actions are, the more accurate the toss and the slower the ball velocity in flight. The legs are slightly flexed and the forearm and hand actions are less pronounced. The release is slightly out in front of the body so the actions mentioned above are seen to a far lesser extent than those seen in a baseball pitcher. Although the actions are the same they are not performed to the same extent.

Jumpshot. The most universally executed shot is the jump shot. It began as a two-hand jump, but it was actually a one-hand shot as the dominant hand was the last to touch the ball as it was being released. It is generally believed that Cooper (one of the authors) and Roberts were the first to use the jumpshot (late 1920's). A discussion of the jump shot (Gates and Holt) follows:

1. More successful shooters demonstrated a greater angle at the shoulder at the point of releasing the basketball (lateral view).
2. More successful shooters used a smaller elbow angle at the start of the shot than the poorer shooters.
3. A greater backspin during flight was associated with the high performance shooters.
4. The successful shooters demonstrated a closer alignment of the upper arm with the vertical at release than the lower percentage shooters.

Cousy (p. 46) reminds the readers that the jump shot can be executed from "a standing position, off a dribble and after a cut is made and the ball is received." While the mechanics of delivery are the same in each instance, the mechanics for preparing for the shot prior to the launching of the shot are different.

Many authorities believe that a one-step method is the best to use in an approach to executing the jump shot from a dribble, receiving a pass while stationary, or while moving and receiving a pass. The front foot is planted, then the trail foot joins it. The jump is accomplished by flexing the knees and pushing against the floor with the feet (action-reaction). The body position in shooting the jump shot is facing the basket. Students of shooting call this position "squaring up" to the basket with the feet parallel in the air.

This "squared-up" position (right shoulder slightly in front of the left shoulder) is the one assumed by all performers in throwing and striking as the object is being thrown or struck. The basketball jump shooter's position is comparable to the final position of all throwing action. But Gates and Holt found that the best shooters were slightly less "squared" to the basket than the poorer players. The dominant eye focusing on the basket causes the head to be turned so that this eye is the one sighting on the basket.

Depending on what is desired by the shooter, the legs may be flexed or extended while in the air. A quick, not very high, jump may be necessary in order to fool the defensive player. Prior to takeoff, the feet should be six to ten inches apart and under the center of gravity.

There has been discussion on the question of balance in the air. Players are said to drift in the air as they shoot. An off-center jump is initiated as the player is still on the floor. A tilt of the head, a movement of the shoulders, and a change of the center of gravity will change the direction of the flight of the ball. While in the air the player may move one or more body parts, for example, arms, head, or legs to cause this unbalance, but the path of the center of gravity is not changed.

It is necessary to keep the head, shoulders, and trunk (torso) over the feet. As the push against the floor takes place, the floor pushes back and this force should be through the feet and center of gravity in order to be in balance.

Students of the shooting phase of basketball believe that the position of the elbow and hand are the keys to successful shooting. The starting position of the elbow is not as important as the release position. It is believed that the elbow of the shooting arm should be pointed toward the basket as the ball is released. Lehmann says that the elbow should be kept within the plane of the body, not lateral to the body.

The hand position in gripping the ball for the shot is generally thought to be one where most of the ball rests on the fingers. Some modern players' hands, however, are so large that the ball, out of necessity, needs to be resting slightly on the palm of the shooting hand. As a rule, a true palm shooter is an unsuccessful shooter. Sharman believes the thumb and the index finger of the shooting hand should form a V and should be in line with the shoulder of the shooting arm. (See Fig. 19-5.) The correct position and two incorrect positions are shown. Visualizing the line of force, can you explain why the two incorrect positions are likely to result in an unsuccessful shot at the basket? Do Sharman and Lehmann agree? At what point in the jump shot is the ball released? Strength of the shooter, distance from the basket, and position and size of the defender are among the variables that help determine the release points. Most writers, such as Brancazio, Hess, Martin and Macaulay, favor shooting at the peak of the jump.

Shooting occurs at the peak of the jump because at this position the upward momentum and the force of gravity are neutralized. It is easier to perform an action under these circumstances. It may be necessary to shoot quickly with only a slight jump to outmaneuver a tall

GRIP

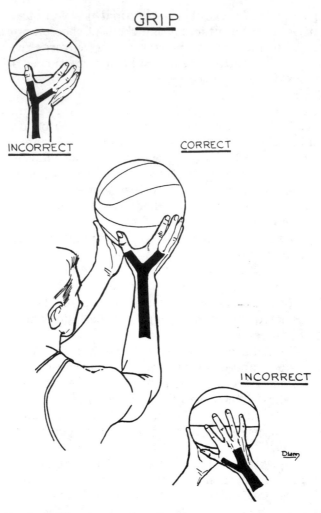

INCORRECT

CORRECT

INCORRECT

Fig. 19-5. *Hand positions in shooting. Two incorrect grips are depicted and the correct grip is Y position such that the ball is well balanced between the thumb and fingers with the distal phalanges holding the ball. The fingers are spread in a comfortable position for maximum control of ball and subsequent shooting accuracy. (From Sharman, by permission)*

defender. To shoot on the way down also confuses a defender. A shooter who is a long distance from the basket (35 feet or more) may release the ball on the way up.

The follow-through in jump shooting is a continuation of the shooting procedure. It prevents the shooter from stopping the shooting action too soon, and, thus, making a jerky motion. It makes the shooting rhythm natural and smooth in transference of action from one component part to another. Flexion of the hand and forward movement of the arm can be seen in Fig. 19-6.

More and more shots will be taken at the basket when the offen-

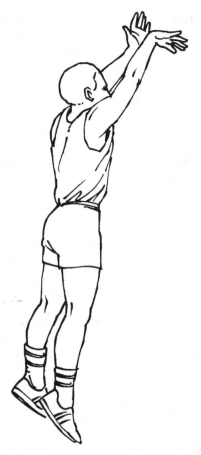

Fig. 19-6. *The one-hand jump shot includes a follow through of the hand and arm after release. There also is a response of the non-shooting arm. Describe the actions after release of the ball of this basketball shooter.*

sive player is running, jumping, and shooting on the move. The player will be trying to propel the ball toward the basket before the defense is ready. At release, the shooter must have control over the speed of movement and the angle of projection.

Balance on the floor and in the the air has been discussed by students of basketball. It is generally believed that the best shooters are balanced when they shoot. From the on-the-floor position, it is easy to visualize balance being maintained. An unbalanced position in the air is often initiated by a push of the feet when they are not under the center of gravity. Misalignment of the head and shoulders with the rest of the body may also cause an imbalance to occur.

A variety of other shots, such as the one-hand set, the hook, front layup, scoop, reverse layup, free throw, and even the dunk have some of the same mechanical elements as the jump shot. These include target area selection, pronation of forearm and hand, maintenance of head and shoulder level, eye focus on the target, and follow-through. Even the fade-away jump shot involves most of the mechanics mentioned in this discussion, with the exception that the center of gravity moves to the rear, however, the actions in the air are similar to the regular jump shot.

It is believed that in the future the in-the-air shots will be performed with the ball held above and behind the head, as in a jump shot, while facing the basket. The hook shot will be combined with a jump shot by the inside players. It will be a half hook. These positions of the ball will prevent the defenders from blocking the shot.

Foul Shooting. Foul shooting is similar to one-hand jump shooting and to the set jump shot, in that this 15-foot shot involves a balanced stance, usually with the feet parallel and shoulder-width apart. The foul shooter's head remains stationary. There is medial rotation at the shoulder and pronation of the forearm and hand. The elbow faces the basket at release and the body of the shooter is "squared up" to the basket. Hudson found that women performers were characterized by a high point of release, a well-balanced weight distribution and minimal trunk inclination. Also, the better players had a higher angle of projection (62 degrees) and greater projection velocity.

The following principles of performance in foul shooting are from Cooper and Siedentop:

1. The player should dry the fingertips.
2. The feet are placed in a stride position close to the foul line, the right foot is in advance of the left (right-handed shooter). The toes of the right foot should be pointing inward and the toes of the left slightly outward. The head is kept down to observe correct foot placement; the ball is kept just overhead or close to waist to avoid creating tension in the arms.
3. The ball is moved so that the same grip is used in one-hand set shooting. The ball rests on the fingers, not in the palm of the hand. The ball is loosely placed in the hands to establish the sense of feel and either the ball is shaken with the hands by moving at the wrists or the ball is bounced on the floor once or twice. Such movements release tension.
4. The player now takes a deep breath. This helps relax the shooter and also prevents the chest area from moving while shooting, which would interfere with accuracy. The shooter looks up at the goal, and focuses attention on shooting just over the rim (a target point must be selected). The head is held up and the back kept straight.
5. The legs are slightly bent, the ball is brought back and down, the hand is flexed, and the ball is released. The hand and finger action is executed as the ball is released and then the follow-through is done rhythmically. There is a dip in the knees, then the legs are extended vertically. There should be

no break in rhythm after the eyes are focused on the basket. The arms and the body follow-through are pointed directly toward the basket.

6. The ball should be released with a slight backspin which will make it easier to catch on the rebound and may cause it to go into the basket from the board or back rim. It has been estimated that a correctly delivered shot will make several revolutions before reaching the goal.

7. The ball must be tossed softly in harmony with the rhythm of the entire body.

8. The eyes should not follow the ball in flight, but should be fixed on the target. However, if a player can concentrate on the target until after the ball is released from the hands, the accuracy of the shot is not affected if the ball is followed visually in flight.

9. The shooter should be sure not to step toward the basket too soon. This can be prevented by keeping at lease one foot firmly on the floor until the ball is released.

10. Producing the least amounts of extraneous movements possible aids in the accuracy of the shot. A rhythmic, smooth movement assures that a soft, accurate shot is accomplished.

Angle of incidence and angle of basket reflection are the striking and rebounding angles of an object (ball) contacting a surface (backboard or floor). If the two objects come in contact with one another and if the impact is perpendicular, there is no friction because friction is parallel to the interacting surfaces. If the impact is not perpendicular to the floor, then the force of friction changes the rebound angle so that the parallel component of the rebound is reduced. If there is any spin on the ball, this modification is a bit more complicated.

The angle of incidence is equal to the angle of reflection only when the ball is thrown against the backboard in a near-perpendicular line, such as is sometimes done by a high-jumping player near the basket from a position in front of the basket. The ball will rebound directly forward, and gravity will bring it down onto the court. However, if the ball impacts the backboard at an angle (oblique angle of incidence), the angle of incidence will be different from the angle of reflection because the vertical velocity is affected by the coefficient of restitution and the horizontal velocity is affected by friction. (See Figure 19-7.)

Usually, the change in the angle of reflection makes it easier to rebound or tip in the rebounding ball. This is particularly true with the common high angle of reflection of a shot with a soft backward spin. Incidentally, a ball thrown from one side of the basket which misses the basket but strikes high on the backboard will rebound to the opposite side more than 50% of the time. Players know this and try to station themselves in the best position to catch the rebound.

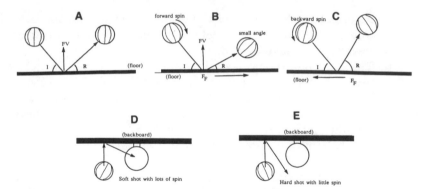

Fig. 19-7. *Angles of incidence and rebound of a basketball as measured from the rebounding surface. A, Non-spinning ball, rebound angle (R) from floor or backboard will be slightly less than incidence angle (I) because elasticity coefficient is less than 1.0. B, Forward spinning ball against the floor (or inward spinning ball against the backboard) will result in reduced angle of rebound because of friction of spin causing increased tangential speed (Vt). C, Backward spinning ball will result in an increased angle of rebound. D, low velocity shots with high velocity spins have a high percentage of rebounding into the basket. E, high velocity shots with low velocity spins have a low percentage of rebounding into the basket. Complex spins, such as a backspin/sidespin combination, is more difficult to diagram. The ratio of the two spinning frequencies or the resultant direction of spin will need to be diligently measured.*

MINI-LAB LEARNING EXPERIENCES

1. Duplicate the situations depicted in Fig. 19-7. Use lay-up or close-to-the-basket shots and try to predict the rebound of the ball. Experiment with different movements and types of spin, different placements on the backboard, and different types of backboards.
2. List other sports in which these principles are applicable. Name an activity in which precision in achieving correct angles of incidence and reflection determines success of the action.

The trajectory of the basketball is predictable. It is the path of an object (ball or person) moving in space. For example, a ball thrown into the air will rapidly move upward until its velocity is zero. If an object lands at the same height that it has been released, the velocity at release and the velocity at (immediately prior to) landing will be identical. During shooting, the basketball follows a curved path, parabolic in nature. The horizontal and vertical displacement are dependent on the angle and speed at takeoff. In the case of a basketball launched toward the basket, the speed and angle of release will determine the distance the ball will travel. A basketball player, desiring to shoot the ball at a higher angle than usual, may have a slower speed of release and a decrease in distance. However, a low angle of release means the ball is traveling too fast to ordinarily score a basket. A small player driving toward the basket and confronted by a taller player will change the angle of release to a higher one to avoid the shot being blocked. Such a player is close enough to the basket that distance is of no concern, angle of release and softness of shot being the important factors.

It must be kept in mind that, given a constant velocity, as the angle of release is increased in degrees, the object will increase in displacement, up to a release angle of approximately 42–43 degrees. In other words, in mathematical terms, a theoretical angle to use when throwing for a distance is approximately 43 degrees from a player in a set position. With a constant speed, any release angle above or below that theoretical angle should result in diminished distance. In basketball, a ball released with controlled speed from a height of 7 feet probably should be released at a 46 to 55 degree angle except when very near or above the basket where a release angle up to nearly 90 degrees can be used. This principle is true because maximum distance is not usually the object in shooting a basketball, and the landing target is 3 feet above the 7 foot release height. Hudson found the proper angle of release in a free throw may be as high as 62 degrees.

From a theoretical point of view only, the ball that is descending vertically into the basket has the best opportunity to go through the basket and to score a goal for a player. A slam dunk, where the ball is elevated directly above the basket, is the easiest position from which to score. It obviously favors the taller and/or the high jumping player. The farther the distance the ball is launched away from the basket, the more "arch" (angle of release) is necessary for the best descent toward the basket. The shooter is usually within 15–20 feet of the basket or closer and the ball may be released near or above the level of the basket height. In such situations, if the angle of release 46–62 degrees, the ball may not enter the basket. If the shooter pushes the ball too vertically to get more height in the shot, horizontal release speed imparted to the ball is reduced. The result is a "short" shot or one not released under control with the proper touch and perhaps not propelled in the desired direction. Too flat a shot (low projectile angle) often results in lack of success and long rebounds.

Jumping

Jumping is the act of projecting the body upward by means of the force produced by the foot (feet), pushing against the floor and the floor pushing back. The amount of "G" is often three or four times greater than body weight.

A person jumping either forward or backward in space will go up vertically but travel horizontally, too. The vertical impulse at floor takeoff contact will determine the height of the jump (force × time). The angle of takeoff is also a factor in determining the horizontal distance from takeoff to landing. Most jump shooters try to jump as nearly vertical as possible.

The preliminary movements prior to jumping into the air involve:

1. The required takeoff speed.
2. The angle of projection, which depends on the desired outcome.
3. The force exerted against the floor and the amount of time the force is applied. Force × time equals impulse. The greater the impulse, the higher the jump. Most top jumpers exert a maximum force in a minimum time. What they lose in time, they gain in force production.

The basketball player is confronted with decisions on which determine the type and style of jumping. Thus, a small and quick player may wish to gain some height quickly in order to offset the very high jumping ability of an opponent. Therefore, the small, quick player maneuver for an advantageous position, such as close to and under the basket, and to be off the floor before the taller and perhaps higher jumper has created the force against the floor that would propel the body upward.

A player who cannot jump high makes it a point to correctly judge the rebound angle or path flight of the ball and to attempt to be inside the opponent under the basket area for a rebound. Low jumping height and slow feet still may be offset by quick hands and effective body position under the basket.

It is known that increased takeoff velocity will result in a longer and/or higher jump. The basketball player may not wish to jump as high as possible because of the defensive player's height, location on the court, the position of all the other players and the distance the ball is from the basket. The jumper defensive or offensive, takes a reading on many situations and factors, and by virtue of many experiences, intuitively responds on how to jump. A shooter may decide not to drive and jump because of a congestion of players. A fade-away shooter may want a displacement to the rear at takeoff in order to elude the defensive player, but this requires greater force in shooting the ball and an adjustment to maintain balance. A defensive player may wait and jump to try and steal the ball or not jump at all, but to steal the ball if the rebounder brings the ball down and in toward the body. Many rebounders will spread their legs to block out the opponents as they jump for the ball.

While airborne, the use of one arm up and the other moved forcefully downward causes the raised arm to move higher. This is termed "diagonal and spiral movement" of the trunk and elevated arm. As much as 6 inches is added to arm-hand reach. Even if the off arm isn't forcefully moved downward, as much as 3 to 4 inches in height will be gained by the use of a one-hand reach rather than the two-hand.

There are several types of jumps that a basketball player may use, however, the emphasis here will be placed on the vertical jump. From a standing position, the feet should be placed apart approximately equal to the width of hip sockets (10–12 in). The angle at the knee should be approximately 115 degrees for maximum lift. An explosive movement will increase the height of the jump.

The swing of the arms, first downward to add force to the floor push, and then upward for position to catch or bat the ball away is used. A shooter brings the ball downward by flexion of the arms and then elevates it to shoot. It has been shown that with the feet against the floor, the downward movement of the arms first adds force that later helps in the upward movement. Then the upward movement of the arms raises the center of gravity of the player still higher within the body.

The reports of 44 to 48 inches vertical leaps from a standing position with feet parallel seem to be grossly exaggerated. A vertical jump is measured by the difference in the standing hand reach and height of the hand reach in the vertical jump without a "crowhop" or a run being permitted. The highest height recorded for an entire basketball conference was 29 inches. (See Table 19-1)

A jump preceded by a run can cause the player to jump higher. A run, however, introduces other factors into the jump. The most notable is the conversion of horizontal velocity into vertical lift. The runner-jumper attains a certain velocity toward the basket in preparation for a shot. The run must be fast enough to attempt to outdistance the defense, yet the player must be under control. If the player

Table 19-1. *Frequency distribution of vertical jump abilities of 24 skilled basketball players starting from a stationary position.*

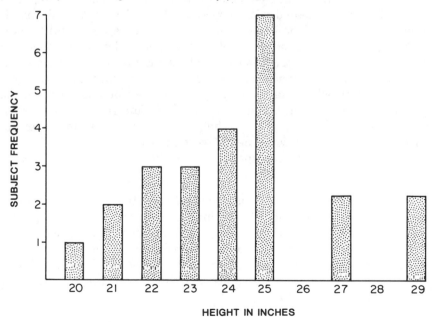

is running too fast, it will be impossible to jump off the floor in an effective manner.

The tendency will be for the jumper's center of gravity to move forward as the jumper-shooter goes into the air. The jump should be as vertical as possible to gain height and to avoid jumping into defensive players. Some control of the center of gravity and the parabolic flight path must be made. The parabola or the path of the center of gravity must be a high elevated one, not a long low one. There is also a rotational component present in run-jump situations. This rotational aspect is overcome by moving the torso backward and attempting to jump as nearly vertical as possible. The jump shooter's takeoff and landing angles are similar, about 160 degrees.

The layup shot usually involves a run and a jump toward the basket. This action is best accomplished more as a high jump than as a long jump. The takeoff angle is 165 degrees. The jumper-shooter travels horizontally in the air $1^{1}/_{2}$ feet. The path of the center of gravity is shown as a parabola.

In the driving layup situation the takeoff is by one foot with a minimum of reduction in momentum. The penultimate (next to last) stride should be longer and lower than the final stride to direct the jumper upward. The player going up for a layup must jump more up than out and shoot quickly if guarded.

Guarding

Defense is a team concept, as well as an individual concept. The most exacting so-called individual defense is that played in a player-to-player style. One player is accountable for one opponent. Zone defense can be individual to a degree, but is less precise, less demanding, and not as clearly delineated with respect to individual responsibility. It is not as easy in a zone-style defense to pinpoint accountability as it is in a player-to-player style. A delineated space is being defended and different opponents enter this space. Since the mechanics of action in a player-to-player are more easily recognized and definable, this discussion is limited primarily to player-to-player defense, known as, guarding. Even though the style of play can be a zone, press, a combination of player-to-player, or a helping type of player-to-player defense, all involve individual defensive maneuvers.

Cooper and Siedentop (pp. 107–108) have listed the following principles of individual defense:

1. "Playing good defense in a competitive situation is more (often) a matter of attitude, desire, and concentration than it is proper execution of skills." Perhaps this statement has some truth in it, yet the mastery of defensive skills are essential.
2. "The main purpose of individual defense is to contain the player who has the ball and to prevent the player and the offensive team from scoring."

3. "Individual defense can be aided by the use of mechanically sound stance."
4. "Variations in defensive stance used may depend upon the immediate situation and the planned team strategy." It is possible to assume a defensive stance in which the offensive player is overplayed to one side, forcing certain responses from the offensive team.
5. "The use of proper eye focus and concentration is essential to a good defensive player."
6. "The manner in which the first defensive stride (step) is taken as the offensive player moves and the angle of pursuit used are fundamental to displaying good defensive play."
7. "The footwork used by the defensive player should be continuously altered by the needs of the situation."

It is believed that the movement skills used in defensive play are not difficult to execute, yet some players are slow in reacting to clues given by the offensive player. It may take such slow-reacting players several years to learn to play individual defense intuitively.

If a basketball player who has played inside positions (forwards or centers) is shifted to a guard position, the footwork and actions are now different, especially with respect to the defensive distance which must be traveled both forward and backward. It becomes more difficult to keep up with an opposing player who now moves a much greater distance. There are some players who are quite capable defensively when they move forward or laterally but who have difficulty moving backward when trying to guard a cutting player. This problem is mainly due to the fact that they are unable to move their feet and shift their center of gravity quickly enough in the rear direction to counteract the drive of the offensive players. Furthermore, when they are moving sideward or forward, they step in the desired direction with the center of gravity projected in that direction. To slide or step in a backward direction, unless the center of gravity is also shifted quickly backward, leaves them vulnerable to a drive toward them. They are in a sense polarized.

The stance of a defensive player out on the court is at best "liable to attack." It is a compromise between being balanced and stable, and being unstable enough to move quickly in any direction. It becomes a guessing game between the defensive player and the offensive player. To limit the offensive possibilities, the defensive player may try to cause the offensive player to move in a path less desirable or make a move too soon.

If an opponent has dribbled, it is expected the player will pass, fake or shoot. If the defensive player moves the hand close to the ball, the offensive player will be forced to turn and may make a mistake. Some offensives are geared to take place beginning with defense, waiting until the offensive team makes a mistake. Thus, defense players take stances that do not immobilize them to an extent that movement is hampered. They are geared to take chances.

Cooper and Siedentop (pp. 108–109) state, "The stance must be a stable one so that a slight reaction (counteraction) by the defensive player to a false (or fake) move by the offensive player will not throw the defensive player off balance. Increased stability (balance or equilibrium) is achieved by widening the base of support and lowering the center of gravity. Stability can be considered in direct proportion to the vertical and horizontal distance the center of gravity is from the base of support (feet). The feet (often in a stride position) are usually spread a distance just beyond the width of the shoulders (or even more, depending on the speed of the offensive player). The defensive player may assume a wide enough base in a stride position to stop a speedster. The legs are flexed to an angle at the knee between 90–120 degrees.

Cooper and Seidentop also have said, "If the defender increases the angle of flexion, thus lowering farther the center of gravity, the defender would gain additional stability but at the expense of mobility. Also, the increased low position makes the player unable to raise the center of gravity and the body, including the arms, fast enough to defend against a jump shooter."

Other principles of guarding are:

1. The guarding position is characterized as similar to sitting in a chair. Weight is equally distributed between the feet.
2. Each type of guarding stance has its advantage. For example, a parallel foot stance is best to use in guarding lateral movements. The stride stance is best to use against a cutting player because the center of gravity is more toward the rear. The fencer's stance with the rear foot turned sideward gives the defensive player an opportunity for quick forward movement since the player is able to push with greater force against the floor (action of the feet and reaction from floor) but is not too adaptable to use against lateral or backward movements. The stride position of the feet is the best all-around stance.
3. A defensive player should not leave the floor to block a shot until the offensive player is fully committed to jumping and shooting or passing. A player in the air cannot alter the flight pattern until returning to the floor. The defensive player is almost helpless while in the air. To leave the floor is usually a mistake unless done at the very last second. Some coaches won't permit their player to jump into the air to block a shot.
4. The defensive player focuses the eyes on the offensive player's belt-buckle area (which is approximately the center of gravity). This is especially true when the offensive player is a cutter or driver.
5. The arms of the defensive player are placed where best to counter a pass, shot, or dribble. This means that one hand might

be held high to protect against a shot or high pass and one low to counter a dribble or low pass. Zone players should keep both arms extended overhead to help close open gaps in defense.

In case of a non-cutter, both hands might be held high, and against a dribbler-cutter and passer both hands might be kept very low.

Each change in arm positions changes the position of the center of gravity and has its advantages and disadvantages. The ability to move the hands through the full range of arm movement without unduly altering the position of the center of gravity is also essential to guarding mechanics.

6. It is possible for a defensive player to "close the gap" and be very close to the offensive player. This may be disconcerting, especially if the defensive player shifts so the favorite driving path is closed and only an alternative direction is available. For example, over-shifting of the upper body, but not the feet, may cause the offense to respond favorably for the defense, that is, move toward the sidelines. Thus, it is evident that defense should be considered in terms of the total body rather than just the position of the feet and arms. This is done by over-playing one way and leaving the alternative open for easy movement.

A defensive player has to be careful not to shift the feet, particularly in a forward direction, just as the offensive player starts a drive for the basket. Recovery cannot be accomplished until the movement of the shifting of the foot (feet) is completed. This would be too late to stop the drive. If a foot is raised into the air only a few centimeters off the floor in the so-called slide, the center of gravity of the defensive player is so far forward that, until the foot is firmly planted on the floor again, no movement can be made by the player to correct the mistake. Even a lean of the body in one direction (which is a shift of the center of gravity) in response to a fake may leave the opposite side open for a move by the offensive player.

The position of the trunk is held essentially upright in a defensive stance. In this position, the defensive player is able to quickly lean the body (shift the center of gravity) in any desired direction. It is also possible to anticipate the direction the offensive player will move and be mentally moved before the actual movement takes place.

In the past, there has been much discussion about the defensive player always using the slide step rather than a crossover step when moving on defense. This is a true statement when the defensive player is moving laterally a short distance. However, if an offensive player cuts quickly for the basket, the only way the defensive player can hope to stay with the offensive player is with the use of a crossover step and to run the shorter distance to the basket. This is especially true if a "back-door" situation is taking place. In any situation that involves moving a large distance the crossover step is faster than the slide step. However, when using the crossover step, recovery in the opposite direction is difficult because the center of gravity is projected quite far in the one direction. It may then be best to use the slide step in short quick counter movements. The closer to the floor the step is made, the less the center of gravity is raised and the less likely it is that the offensive player can drive by the defensive player.

The defensive player also has to be alert to offset a screen being set by one of the offensive players. This involves having a teammate notify the involved defensive player. This latter player should be able to "feel" an offensive player coming up or across the floor to screen. Continually shifting the body to fight through a screen is a necessary prerequisite for a skilled defensive player.

Guarding a player without the ball means the defensive player may retreat to a certain distance from the defensive player out on the court. Nevertheless, the defensive player must know the location of the ball and if possible, keep it in view at all times. This is done by constantly moving the body so the ball is seen peripherally. The defensive player focuses the eyes (looks out of the corner of the eyes) on an object somewhat distant such as a spot on the floor. Since objects are seen quicker with peripheral, rather than with direct vision, this is an asset. The ball can be seen, yet the player being guarded can also be seen. If one is to sacrifice seeing one thing, it would be seeing the location of the ball, not the offensive player. Yet, in the zone style the location of the ball is usually the number-one priority.

The hand to use when attempting to knock the ball out of the hands of the offensive player is normally the lead hand, not the trail hand. To move the trail hand forward toward the ball causes the body to move a greater distance in one direction, so the defensive player may be out of position if the ball is missed. In fact, in most instances, a foul will be called. The movement of the hand should be up, not down, as it moves to knock the ball loose.

Guarding inside players is normally easier since the inside offensive players cover less distance. Many of the principles previously mentioned should be utilized. If the offensive player's back is to the basket, the defensive player guarding from behind should concentrate on a point on the body near the belt line (center of gravity). If the offensive player's belt line, from the rear, starts to move up when in possession of the ball, then it is possible shooting at the basket may take place. The defensive player must be prepared for this eventuality. It should be kept in mind that the offensive player cannot move without taking the belt line along.

Guarding a much taller inside player means the defensive player must slide from one side to the other in line with the ball to prevent the taller player from receiving a pass. Playing behind such a player can be difficult because of the height differential. Help from teammates may be necessary. Sometimes two or three players sink back toward the taller player to prevent the taller player from receiving the ball.

The defensive player covering the inside player has the added responsibility of screening out the inside player so rebounding the ball cannot take place. A quick turn inside or a turn around pivot into the path of the offensive rebounder should prevent an easy tip in or offensive rebound. If an inside player moves out on the court, then the principles of guarding are the same as previously presented. If an outside offensive player moves to the basket for a rebound, the defensive player first retreats and screens with a pivot as mentioned for a defensive inside player. If the offensive player comes in full contact with the defensive player, deceleration takes place and it is difficult for the offensive player to rebound.

MINI-LAB LEARNING EXPERIENCES

Dribbling

1. Count the number of dribbles made by the left hand and by the right hand in 30 seconds. Observe and estimate the action of the fingers, hand, forearm, arm, and body.
2. Dribble behind the back and between the legs, alternating these actions for 30 seconds. Evaluate the performance, especially as changes occur with fatigue.
3. Observe videotapes of basketball players dribbling in the game situation. Analyze their movements.

Passing

Using a videotape (or real life observations) of a top passer, describe the planes and axes of the different passes.

Shooting

1. View a videotape of six top shooters, varying in anthropometric characteristics. Describe their shooting kinematics.
2. Observe the head and eye positions of successful shooters. Draw conclusions.
3. Observe the angle of release of a shot at the basket by a teammate. Ask your teammate to deliberately change the angle of release. Observe the results. Discuss the results.

Jumping

1. Through use of videotape or actual movements on the court, observe the jumping angles of defensive and offensive rebounders. If using video, measure the angles with freeze-framing of video images. Discuss the differences.
2. Describe the single and double jump action of shooters. How is each accomplished?
3. How can injuries be prevented in jumping actions? During a game, observe the ways in which players are, or could be, hurt in jumping situations.

---

1. Ask a basketball player to demonstrate the speed of a crossover step by moving ten steps as rapidly as possible. Time this movement, and then time a shuffle step also traversing ten steps as rapidly as possible. Compare and explain the results.
2. Using a videotape count the number of shuffle-step situations occurring in a given game as compared to the number of cross-over steps.
3. Try to analyze why one method of guarding is more effective than another. Check with basketball coaches and players to determine the methods used by them (or refer to guarding section in this chapter).

FIELD HOCKEY

Field hockey is a game involving linear and curvilinear motion. Performance also includes changing direction while running, and maneuvering and striking a field hockey ball with a flat, one-sided, curved shaft. (See Fig. 19-8) Men and women participate in the sport at all age levels throughout the world. Women in the USA have reached a high level of participation, finishing third in the world at the 1984 Los Angeles Olympics.

In the linear running aspect of the game, the performers must learn to use the same mechanics as do sprinters, with the exception that the performer runs under control, at about 80% maximum speed. This control is necessary because it enables the player to change direction, using maximum agility in response to movements of other players and the ball.

Curvilinear motion is incorporated as the ball carrier maneuvers the ball in the dribbling action. The curved running feature, which

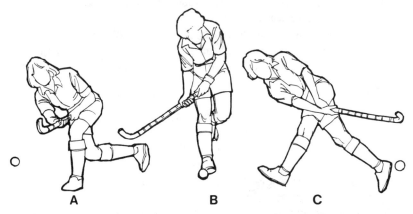

Fig. 19-8. *Note the differences in balance and positioning of the body parts in the execution of the following field hockey strokes: A, the push pass; B, the drive; and C, the drive on the run.*

occurs frequently, involves moving the body's center of gravity laterally toward the inside portion of the curve and then accelerating after "setting" into the curve.

All these movements are made while the player is carrying or maneuvering a field hockey stick. The additional weight of the stick, combined with its length and one-sided design (right-handed only), requires the player to have strength and considerable skill in manipulating (wielding) the stick effectively.

The striking aspects are identical with those mentioned previously in other striking actions. The curved stick increases the length of the lever arm, increasing the possibility that greater ball velocity can be developed than would be possible with a straight stick.

Skills that must be mastered for effective and efficient play include achieving maximum ball velocity, and being able, to deliver the ball at a variety of angles, and receive a ball coming in at a variety of speeds. (See sections on throwing and catching.) Patterns of movement include pushing and pulling as well as sequential joint action, using the underarm and sidearm patterns.

Klatt studied the temporal and kinematic characteristics of a successful penalty corner. Components include a hit-out, reception, and shot on goal. On the hit-out, a drive or push stroke is executed in approximately one second. She found that the average speed of the hit-out of the elite athlete was 15.42 m/sec (50.57 ft/sec) for women, whereas men executed the hit-out at 16.52 m/sec (54.19 ft/sec). The hit-out involves a high-velocity action, as long a traversed distance as possible, and a ball path that will enable the ball to be received and shot for goal with as large an angle open to the goal mouth as possible. Female Olympic players received the ball in .56 seconds and executed a shot on goal with an average velocity of 25.39 m/sec (83.30 ft/sec); the male Olympians executed the reception in .54 seconds and recorded an average velocity of 28.58 m/sec (93.75 ft/sec) for the shot on goal. Klatt used three-dimensional cinematography and computer simulation to determine the following optimum action to be executed by offensive and defensive performers in the hit-out:

1. Develop a consistent speed and angle on the hit-out; the direction should be such that the ball is received directly in front of the goal mouth.
2. Have the receiver sprint into the circle to receive the ball, decreasing the time of the hit-out and increasing the angle open to the goal.
3. Designate a "corner team" of three players; the corner team must practice the drive or push out, have consistent location of reception, and timing and direction of the shot on goal. Practice needs to be independent of the whole team as well as with it.
4. Position the defensive team so that no one crosses the visual path of the goalkeeper on the defensive rush.

5. Have the goalkeeper move in direct line with the point of reception, moving out from the goal to decrease the opening to the goal mouth.

During the 1984 Olympics in Los Angeles, the male as well as female goalkeepers used a slide tackle with success to defend against the penalty corner situation. Total distance traveled by the goalkeeper from the time of the hit-out through the time of reception was 6.23 meters (20.45 ft) for the females and 11.31 meters (37.10 ft), for the males. A horizontal position in the direction of the goal mouth was determined to be best to defend against an immediate shot on goal.

The penalty corner continues to remain a great offensive and defensive strategy "game." Ten years ago, the offense had the advantage on the corner. At the 1984 Olympics, the offense and defense were equalized with the use of the slide tackle by the goalkeepers.

MINI-LAB LEARNING EXPERIENCES

Use a stationary ball on the ground or batting tee and attempt to:

1. Contact the ball at the center of percussion. Include a variety of surfaces, i.e., floor, turf, and grass. Then contact the ball off center, and observe the translatory motion that results.
2. Run carrying the hockey stick for 50 feet. Repeat without the stick. Repeat dribbling a field hockey ball. Run executing an air dribble. Time all runs and compare results.
3. Determine the distance a goalie can reach with the stick, with and without movement of the feet in relation to coverage of the entrance to the goal. Hint: draw a triangle with the apex at the center of the goal.
4. Try a flick (aerial) shot and a shot on the ground. Note the difference in the distance attained, especially in deep grass. Hint: friction may cause the difference.
5. Measure the dimensions of a field hockey stick and an ice hockey stick. Particularly note differences in length, blade portion, and curvature. Strike a hockey puck with the field hockey stick and strike a hockey ball with the ice hockey stick. Experiment with different sticks: goalkeeper sticks, floorhockey sticks, and weighted sticks. How do these sticks influence techniques, strategy and general game play?
6. Discuss the effects or potential effects of the following upon the game of field hockey.
   a. crowned synthetic turf playing field
   b. metal hockey sticks
   c. flat synthetic turf playing field
   d. changes in hockey stick weights: heavier, lighter, built up on back side of blade

VOLLEYBALL

Volleyball was transformed from an easy, recreational, fun game during the late 1950's and early 1960's to that of a complex, highly competitive game known as "power volleyball." This change caused the top players to develop high-level ability in striking, passing, jumping, and landing skills.

Some basic concepts that are involved in the game are:

1. The various movements involved in the game must be understood since player positions are specialized based upon which movements the player can best execute.
2. Specificity of training must be recognized. A performer may be effective in one sport, but will need to perfect volleyball skills.
3. The better the feedback, the better the learning of motor skills.
4. Perhaps one of the most difficult skills in volleyball is spiking, since the performer must become airborne in an effort to exert maximum force on another airborne object, the ball. Often, otherwise perfected technique results in unsuccessful performance because of timing errors and inaccurate position to the ball.

The physical laws and principles that are involved in the various movements in striking, stopping an object, and passing, etc., apply in the game of volleyball. These will be discussed throughout this section. One of the most important concepts, the effect of impact on the ball or floor and these on the body, is determined by several factors:

1. The magnitude of the force can be reduced by prolonging the period of energy absorption.
2. The duration of the impact, if of high intensity, can be tolerated for only a brief period of time.
3. Spreading the forces over a large part of the body reduces the severity of the force.
4. A part of the body, such as the forearm, is best able to resist an impact if the focus of force is applied gently at first, and then gradually increased.
5. A joint struck when it is at the extreme range of motion causes the joint to be moved beyond the normal range. Thus, not only the force of the blow, but the position of the body parts at the joint receiving the blow, determine the effect of the force.

Serving

All three basic patterns (underhand, overhand, and sidearm) of striking or projecting a ball can be used in executing the volleyball service. Although many players have been able to produce considerable spin using the underhand and sidearm services, the overhand service is the most effective type of service. The best type of service occurs when the ball travels with the fastest possible speed and flattest trajectory, thereby forcing the receiver to respond in the shortest possible amount of time. Because of the law of gravitation—that is, all objects fall at the same rate—the overhand service will have the shortest air time and cause the receiver to make decisions and move more quickly than if either of the other two services were used. In addition, the lever systems and muscles utilized during the overhand service have the potential to create the greatest horizontal speed. Thus, the ball will be descending at a faster rate and a more horizontal angle, which is more difficult to receive than the sidearm and underhand services. For example, if the served ball is descending at a 30-degree angle, the arms of the receiver would need to be more vertical than horizontal. In terms of perception, this position is more difficult, and attentuation, by moving the arms in the same direction as in the incoming ball, is also more difficult.

In volleyball, the most widely used types of serves are the overhand floater, overhand topspin, roundhouse floater, and roundhouse topspin. The topspin serve is sometimes referred to as a drive or power serve. Accuracy as well as speed of travel are important considerations in serving. A taller player will have an advantage in serving because of increased linear velocity resulting from a longer system of levers. Additionally, the ball can be contacted at a decreased angle of projection, which increases the margin for error from an accuracy perspective, and thus it is advantageous in serving the ball to the specific target area. Another factor influencing a lower projection angle and a decreased time of flight is a fast arm swing. Beginning players often cannot generate the desired arm swing speed and, as a result, have to project the ball at a higher angle. Opponents, then, have more time to position themselves for the service reception. Since serving is a sequential striking skill (Fig. 19-9), immature and ineffective patterns often appear as a pushlike pattern with simultaneous segmental rotations occurring. In introducing overhand serving, it may be easier for the beginning server (6th or 7th grader) to learn a roundhouse pattern since it is possible to achieve a longer lever action and produce more force on the ball with this pattern. It is a suitable choice of serve style especially if the server is unable to develop an effective sequential pattern such as is required in the traditional style of the overhead serve.

In any style, it is important to hit with an optimally extended (not fully extended or locked) arm to increase linear velocity. It is also important to contact the ball in front of the body and to take a step or to shift the weight forward, thus transferring the momentum of the body to the ball at time of contact. By hitting approximately 6–12 inches in front of the body, the server can see the intended target area and the opponents' reception alignment.

The float serve, equivalent to the knuckleball pitch in baseball, is an aerodynamic "wonder" and is often the serve style of preference

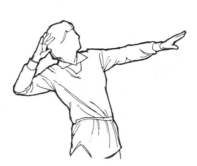

Fig. 19-9. *The overhand float service requires sequential segmental rotation with precise ball contact for successful force production and absence of spin on the ball. Note again the similarities to the basic overarm pattern, including the non-striking arm and shoulder girdle force couple.*

because of the simplicity of the technique. It requires a lower projection angle and velocity than topspin serve styles because the ball is not dropping due to spin. Its unpredictable flight path can make it a difficult serve to receive and often requires the receiver to make last-minute positional adjustments because of a sudden flight path deviation. Flight deviation may occur in a float serve as a result of the orientation of the seams and valve relative to the airflow. The non-symmetrical surface of a volleyball gives rise to the turbulence and lower pressure zones that tend to shift around on the ball as it travels. Lift forces are produced at different areas, producing movements of the ball. Often players are instructed to position the air valve toward the opponent in order to induce greater movement on the ball. However, researchers have failed to validate this concept.

Since the ball is not perfectly symmetric with respect to weight, this type of flight will not maintain a parabolic curvature or a predictable modification because of spin, but will "wobble" or "float." The flight path depends on the ball's center of gravity, which may be to the right or left or the geometric center of the ball, or above or below it. A volleyball is relatively light in mass with a large, nonstreamlined profile and is usually out-of-round. In addition, it has patterned but irregular seams and an air valve. For the player to execute the float serve correctly, the ball must be struck through its center of mass so that rotation is not induced. The wrist should be kept extended (180 degrees) at contact to minimize hitting the ball off center whereas in a topspin serve, wrist flexion is important in producing an off-center hit.

Another style of serving that is gaining popularity is the jump serve. This was initially used in the 1976 Montreal Olympic Games by several of the men's teams. It was commonly used in the 1984 Olympic Games. Although this is a difficult serving style to master, the server can "spike" from the baseline at a higher velocity than is normally achieved in other patterns. It has a relatively short time of flight and often is hit with excessive topspin, which causes it to drop markedly during flight. Frequently this results in an ace serve because the opponents do not make the necessary reception adjustments in time. Another factor that makes this service such an effective offensive weapon is that the server can actually be making ball contact from within the court, as long as the jump is initiated from behind the baseline. Two or three running steps may be taken to build up momentum for increased jump height. The coordinated action of trunk and shoulder rotation increases the range and speed of the sequential striking actions employed in serving.

Spiking

The spike may be sub-divided into the following phases for analysis: (1) approach, (2) takeoff, (3) body preparation during airborne phase, (4) contact, (5) follow-through, and (6) landing.

(1) **Approach.** For a regular high set, the spiker starts 8–12 feet from the net and takes a two- or three-step approach which develops horizontal momentum. This horizontal momentum is converted to vertical momentum at takeoff to achieve jump height. In hitting from the side positions, the spiker should approach from outside the sideline in order to keep the ball in front of the hitting arm and to maximize the hitting area. Most hitters use a step-close or pre-jump approach and both are considered to be equally effective. On the plant step just prior to takeoff, the body is positioned at approximately 45 degrees to the net when hitting strong side (left front) and middle (center front). This positions the hitting arm away from the ball, in addition to partially hiding the hitting arm from the opponent. The spiker can rotate through a large range of motion before contact, thereby generating a high hitting velocity.

(2) **Takeoff.** A forceful extension at the hips, knees, and ankles occurs as the spiker takes off from both feet. On quick sets, a one-foot takeoff is often used since jumping height is not as crucial. Quickness in getting to the set is a priority in hitting a front or back one-set. The one-foot takeoff enables the hitter to pivot and position behind the ball more effectively when running the various fast play patterns. A vigorous upward arm swing evokes additional force for takeoff propulsion. Estimations of arm swing contributions have been as much as 15% of the height of the jump. Spiking requires coordinating the jump and armswing in order to contact the moving ball in front of the body with an optimally extended contact arm.

(3) **Body Preparation During Airborne Phase.** Once airborne, the spiker executes counter-rotation patterns on the backswing

(forearm flexed, upper arm outwardly rotated, and hand hyperextended), which reduces the moment of inertia and increases the speed of rotation away from the ball prior to contact. The trunk is hyperextended, the hips and shoulders are rotated, and the striking arm is cocked, which increases the distance over which velocity is developed. The non-striking arm is extended upward.

(4) **Contact.** At contact, the body rotates and the left arm and shoulder drop quickly as the right arm moves toward the ball, with the elbow leading the motion. The striking shoulder elevates (left shoulder drops so right shoulder can get higher) to maximize a high ball contact point. The trunk pikes (flexes), thus increasing momentum of the body. The more sequential the action of the trunk, upper arm, forearm, and hand, the more force produced. The ball should be contacted in front of the body and with the arm optimally extended to maximize hitting velocity and to achieve the appropriate hitting angle (Fig. 19-10). The distance through which the hand is accelerated is increased by inward rotation of the upper arm, forearm pronation and hand flexion. "Snapping the wrist" (hand flexion) results in topspin being imparted to the ball as the hand wraps around the ball at contact producing an above-center eccentric force. Topspin results in a low pressure zone developing on the bottom of the ball, which causes the ball to drop more rapidly in flight and increase the chances of it staying in the court without compromising ball velocity.

(5) **Follow-through.** The follow-through of the spiking arm should be performed in a way that prevents violating the playing rules (e.g., hitting the net), losing linear velocity at contact by decelerating prior to contact, and preventing injury caused by the abrupt stopping of a fast-moving hitting arm which requires high-stopping forces.

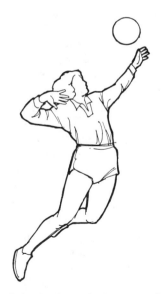

Fig. 19-10. *Position of the body and upper arm for a successful spike.*

(6) Landing. Landing should be on both feet to increase the area over which landing forces act. Flexion occurs in the hips, knees, and ankles which increases the time and distance over which force is absorbed.

Volleyball Injuries and Prevention

Load is recognized as a critical factor in the occurrence of pain and injury in volleyball. Whereas most moves in volleyball occur without the ball, the highest loading occurs during landing movements associated with high intensity jumps at the net which are involved with spiking and blocking. A player may jump and land as many as 100 times per hour of play, and many of these landings occur on one foot. Many volleyball injuries occur in the lower extremity and back usually as a result of landing on another player's foot. A sprained ankle can result from the unstable position of the ankle that occurs when the body is airborne. The relaxed foot tends to supinate, which is a most unstable position, and landing with the foot in this position makes it vulnerable to injury.

Stacoff, Kaelin, and Stuessi (1987) report that impact forces in landing range from 1000 to 2000 N under the forefoot and from 1000 to 6500 N under the heel. The elastic limit of the cartilage is reached at approximately 5000 N. This limit was exceeded in almost 10% of the jumps analyzed in their study. Clearly shoes, surface, conditioning and landing techniques should be scrutinized carefully. In volleyball competition as recently as 10–15 years ago, players preferred a thin-soled shoe that provided little cushioning and force absorption. Modern shoes can reduce landing forces by up to 30%. If a player, however, has weak ankles, the increased leverage provided by a thicker sole may cause the ankle to be more susceptible to sprains. If a player is suffering from jumper's knee, the extra cushioning provided by a thicker sole will minimize landing forces and is recommended. Athletes with ankle problems should train the peroneal muscles, wear thin-soled shoes and use external devices such as high-topped shoes, ankle braces and taping. Athletes with knee problems should wear thicker soled shoes, develop the calf muscles, and work on improved landing technique.

In preventing injuries associated with floor skills such as diving and rolling, several factors should be considered. In diving, split chins resulting from "bottoming out" (i.e. all body parts impacting the floor at the same time) in the dive can often be prevented through proper flexibility exercises in the neck and spine. In fact, certain players should not be taught to dive unless they have an adequate level of upper body strength and flexibility in the neck and spine which will allow the player to safely position the head off the floor when impact occurs.

Other factors often overlooked are the floor surface on which the dive is being executed and the jersey material and type and placement of the number on the player's jersey. Many of the synthetic surfaces impede the sliding of the player's body across the surface which results in high level of forces being concentrated in certain areas of the player's body; namely the chin, neck, and chest. If a player is wearing a jersey with a plastic number or logo which further increases the level of friction, the sliding action of the player during the floor move may be slowed, which decreases force absorption in the dive and increases stopping forces. More than one diver has had his/her chin stitched up as a result of sudden stopping action caused by a shirt number or rough textured floor or even a dirty, sticky floor. Additionally, proper technique must be emphasized in teaching floor skills. The worst scenario may involve a broken neck if the diver is unskilled and the dive is initiated from too high a position and too large an angle to the floor, negating proper dissipation of landing forces.

Jumping and Jump-Training in Volleyball

In the sport of volleyball, jumping depends not only on correct technique and leg strength but also on the ability to correctly load the muscles during the set-up phase. This phase begins when one foot hits the floor at the end of the approach and terminates when the legs reach maximum flexion. During negative work involved in the set-up phase, a certain quantity of elastic energy can be stored in the elastic elements in series which are found in the tendons and muscles. The energy stored during this eccentrically-controlled work phase may be re-utilized during the following concentric phase to improve jumping performance. A rapid lengthening of a muscle just prior to contraction will result in a stronger contraction. This phenomenon is believed to be a result of the stretching of muscle spindles involving a myotatic reflex which results in increased frequency of motor unit discharge, stimulation of other receptors and an increased number of activated motor units. Other factors influencing the set-up phase include the velocity of the stretch and the time between the eccentric and concentric phases.

For more than two decades, volleyball players have experimented with depth jumping (drop jumps or rebound jumps) as part of their jump training regime. Depth jumping is a plyometric exercise designed to enhance the stretch-shortening cycle to increase elastic potential of leg extensor muscles. Depth jumping involves dropping from a specified height and immediately rebounding (jumping) off the surface, which is often a mat. Different drop heights have been utilized, ranging from .3 m which is recommended for first-year depth jumpers, to 1.10 m, which has been reported for training of elite athletes. Most researchers support the fact that depth jumping increases jump height, but fail to support that depth jumping is superior to other types of jump training. Bosco et al. (1981) were able to demonstrate that after 18 months of special plyometric training, 8 volleyball players on the Finnish National team increased the elastic potential and stretch load tolerance of leg extensor muscles. Jensen and Russell (1986) report that depth jumping may be useful for teaching the regulation of muscle stiffness. They characterize optimum jump performance by high stretch velocities and short transitions between eccentric and concentric phases.

Based upon research, Colvin et al. (1984) of the 1984 men's Olympic volleyball team suggests that optimum jumping technique is characterized by a forceful arm swing, a decisive blocking action with the arms (designed to transfer momentum developed in the arm swing to the body) and simultaneous extension at the hips, knees and ankles during the extension phases. The lesser skilled jumpers tended to extend at the knees and hips earlier than did the more skilled jumpers. Time of support during the jump ranged from .26 s to .38 s.

Setting

Frequently the setter in volleyball is compared to the quarterback in football—the "brains" of the outfit. Accuracy, speed of delivery and deception are all necessary ingredients of good setting. Setting technique involves a push-like pattern, requiring simultaneous segmental rotations. As in other pushing patterns, the involved segments are aligned behind the object to be projected to allow for a flattening of the arc of the ball flight and greater accuracy. Finger action during the absorption phase involves stretching of the flexor muscles as a result of ball impact. This recoil action aids in ball projection.

In a study by Ridgway and Wilkerson (1986) of front setting and back setting, the investigators found that over 50% of the setters did not exhibit simultaneous extension of the legs and arms. The arms had begun movement toward the ball prior to leg extension. In high levels of quick, fast-paced play, frequently the setter has little opportunity to position in such a way that allows the use of the legs. As a result, the setter has an arm-dominated pattern (Fig. 19-11). Quick sets such as the one-set or two-set are characterized by a greater ball absorption phase in the setter's hands and a slower projection velocity. The time of ball contact in the hands ranges from .054 s for low set to .072 s for a high outside front set to .086 s for a high back set. The volleyball official has a difficult task in judging the legality of a set because of two obvious factors: (1) the ball actually does comes to rest in the setter's hands as it changes direction of motion during the absorption and propulsion phases, and (2) the setting technique whether it be a high set or a quick set often occurs in less than .01 s. An official must not be too quick to make a judgment regarding an illegal hit because the setter appears to be poorly positioned for executing the set. Judging how long the ball rests in the hands in beyond the scope of this text.

Forearm Pass

Passing may well be the least glamorous of all volleyball techniques. Every offensive player, however, begins with a pass. Some of

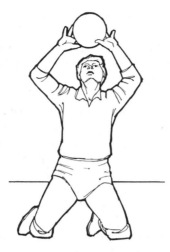

Fig. 19-11. *The setter must develop enough strength in hands, arms, and fingers to pass the ball without the use of the legs. Strong legs are required to position the body for the best angle for passing. In this situation the lower legs support the body.*

the variables influencing forearm passing success are the varying ball speeds, angles, and unpredictable flight paths associated with float serves and block deflections. In order to meet one of the goals of today's game, that of isolating hitters against only one blocker, passing must be quick, accurate, and consistent. The position of the setter should be such that there is a choice of several quick play-sets rather than a single choice through a double block.

Contour and size of contact area will influence both the consistency of execution of the skill and the likelihood of injury to the body. "The greater the surface area, the less force per square centimeter" is a principle that can be applied to this skill. Injury is not likely to occur to hands; however, forearms do become bruised because the ball impacts against the flesh surrounding the radius and ulna. If there is insufficient adipose tissue or muscle, the deformation caused by the impact will force the small blood vessels against these bones, causing hematoma. Long-sleeved shirts are often worn to protect the forearms from bruises.

Receiving a Spike or Service in Volleyball

Served balls and spiked balls usually are received by means of an underhand hit termed a "forearm pass." In these situations, the volleyball has greater speeds, and, therefore, more kinetic energy and momentum, than in any other situation occurring in the volleyball game. Thus, the volleyball player uses the forearms as rebounding surfaces, rather than using the hands with the active flexion of the fingers (overhand passing technique). The speed and angle of the incoming spike and serve and the distance the ball must be passed will

TEAM SPORTS   **613**

determine whether the receiver will attentuate (absorb) the force or will apply force to the ball.

The first goal of the passer receiving a spiked or served ball is to establish a stable base of support. This base is best taken with the feet shoulder distance apart with one foot slightly ahead of the other with the weight on the balls and insides of the feet. When it is not possible to play the ball off the midline of the body, a step with a pivot to the side will be used to position the arms toward the path of the ball. Since spiked balls have a primarily downward flight, there is no need to widen the base of support in the anteroposterior direction to any great extent. Even in the case of served balls, the trajectory is apt to be 30 to 60 degrees with the horizontal. Thus, the horizontal momentum will be less than one-half that of a well-hit volleyball spike traveling 120 kmph (74 mph).

The type of contact and the surfaces of contact will determine the amount of rebound velocity of the ball. Any forward motion of the arms will apply a force to the ball and thus impart additional velocity to it. If the arms are stationary at contact, the amount of tension and the amount of fleshy tissue will determine the amount of attentuation of the force of the ball. For example, a ball dropped from a height of approximtely 7 m will rebound almost 2 m after impact on a wooden floor, whereas the ball will rebound 1 m (half that distance) if the impact is made on a maximally tensed, bony, tendinous surface such as the forearm. If, however, little effort is made to tense the arms, the rebound will be greatly reduced, to as little as, or less than 20 cm. If the shoulders are pulled back and the hips thrust forward, greater force absorption will occur in response to hard-hit balls. Thus, it is important both to develop kinesthetic awareness of the amount of tension in the arms, including the shoulder stabilization tension, and to be able to estimate the speed and angle of the incoming ball.

The flatness of the contact area is paramount for consistency in directing the ball. Theoretically, the anterior surface of the wrist and heel of the hand are best because of their flatness and large surface area. There is the problem of stabilizing the two hands so that the forearms act as one unit. Normally it is not recommended that the hands or the heels of the hands be used for contact on the forearm pass. The contact should be above the wrist and below the elbow, on the fleshy portion of the forearm, although some passers do clasp the hands together and use the radial surfaces of the forearms as the contact site.

The positioning of the rebounding surfaces for the desired angle of rebound is done primarily by means of shoulder flexion. The angle of the arms with respect to the trajectory of the ball determines, in part, the angle of rebound. For example, if the ball enters at a 90-degree angle to the arms, it will rebound at a nearly 90-degree angle. Angles of rebound and incidence are often dissimilar in volleyball, since balls have spin and are impacted with moving arms. This statement is based on Newton's third law and the coefficients of friction and elasticity. As the ball rebounds, the speed can be vectorally added to show the influence of spin, elasticity, and friction. Knowing the incoming speed and angle of the ball, a person can predict the speed and angle of the rebound. Frequently, teams running fast offenses want low-trajectory passes to shorten the time it takes to run an offensive play. This decreases the time the defense has to set up against the attack. To accomplish this fast, low-arc pass, the passer has the arms pointing toward the floor and the back held straight. Projection angles of 30 to 50 degress are not uncommon, but, since the time of flight has been reduced, low passes require greater setter mobility.

Ridgway and Hamilton (1987) profiled low-skilled and high-skilled passers. The low-skilled passers were junior high and junior varsity players and their passing patterns were characterized by: (1) overswinging at the shoulders; (2) short ball contact time, which decreased force absorption of the ball; (3) contacting the ball too close to the thumbs and wrists, thus decreasing force absorption, and (4) passing too high (71 degress vs. 63 degrees), which apprently resulted from an erect head and upright trunk posture. Due to gravitational acceleration, high passes have a greater descent velocity, which makes it difficult for the setter to set. The setter must focus too high above the court, which interferes with the peripheral vision used in locating the hitters and opponents. High passes also have a longer flight time, which gives the opponents more time to set up their defense.

Blocking

Blocking the ball is done to prevent the opposing team member from making a successful hit over the net; reducing the force on a spiked ball; forcing the opposing attacker to hit the ball toward the defense; or taking away the favorite shots of the opposing hitter. There may be one, two or sometimes three blockers at the net. One blocker's action will be described here.

The blocker is positioned close to the net so that the plane of the net may be penetrated in blocking the ball. In preparing for the jump to block the hit, the blocker places the feet approximately hip width with legs flexed. The arms are first moved to bring force against the feet and then moved upward to aid in summation of the forces in the upward vertical jump to increase the height of the reach of the arms.

The arms of the blocker are elevated vertically and then the hands are flexed and moved forward above and across the net. The blocker's hands reach across the net to prevent the ball from coming down on the blocker's side. This arm movement takes away a larger portion of the hitting area of the court than if the hands are just above the net. (See Fig. 19-12).

The blocker jumps after the hitter jumps in order to time the block and to keep the ball from rebounding from the hands and going out-of-bounds. The blocker actually delays the jump for the block until the hitter is near the apex of the jump.

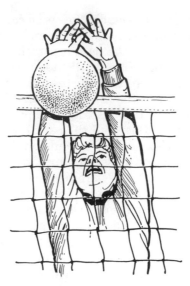

Fig. 19-12. *Blocking requires not only precise timing, but the appropriate positioning of the hands. This player has extended the upper body to its maximum after a forceful jump. The hands then reach forward toward the net fully extended to contact as much of the ball as possible.*

Since new ways of placing the hands during a block may arise, the main concept is to maximize hand area so a block can be successful. The wrists and hands should be firm at ball contact so injury to the finger joints will not occur.

EFFECTS OF FATIGUE ON TECHNIQUE

A major goal of the volleyball player is the replication of performance: the ability to continue successful execution of skills throughout the practice or competition. As fatigue occurs, various performance variables are affected, which may result in a poorer performance, pain, or injury. Stress fractures are thought to be a result of fatigued muscles. According to this hypothesis, there is decreased elastic energy storage in the muscles and the forces generated in jump landings and other strenuous moves are transmitted to the bone and joints instead of being neutralized by the surrounding musculature. Depth jumping is particularly stressful if improper jumping technique or inadequate strength exists in the leg extensor muscles controlling the impact of landing.

Sardinha and Zebas (1986) studied the effects of perceived fatigue on selected spike performance variables. They concluded that perceived fatigue alters spike efficiency. Their subjects spiked the ball at a lower position and at a slower velocity and committed a greater number of timing errors when fatigue was perceived to have occurred. The velocities of the hand and forearm decreased giving the blockers

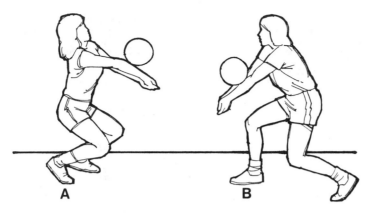

Fig. 19-13. *Examples of two volleyball players prepared to receive and pass the volleyball using a forearm bump type pass. Describe the differences and problems with the low skilled technique (A) compared to the higher skilled passer (B).*

and defensive players more reaction and movement time. In addition, vertical velocity at takeoff decreased and inaccurate positioning to the ball increased.

MINI-LAB LEARNING EXPERIENCES

Study the low-skilled and high-skilled execution of a forearm pass. Discuss observable differences in technique and how these differences influence passing performance (Fig. 19-13).

REFERENCES

Allsen, P. E. and Ruffner, W. (1969). Relationship between the type of pass and the loss of the ball in basketball, *Athletic Journal* 49, September, p, 94, pp. 105–107.

Bosco, C., Komi, P., Pulli, M., Pettera, C. and Montonev, H. (1981). Considerations of the training of the elastic potential of the human skeletal muscle. *Volleyball, IFVB Official Magazine,* No. 2:22–30.

Brancazio, P. J. (1984) *Sports science physical laws and optimum performance,* New York: Simon and Schuster.

Coleman, J. E. and Liskewych, F. N. (1974). *Pictoral Analysis of Power Volleyball.* Creative Hollywood Sports Books. CA.

Colvin, W., Beal, D. and Zier, D. (1984). A kinetic analysis of the vertical jump with arm swing. Paper presented at the 2nd International Symposium of Biomechanics in Sports. Colorado Springs, CO.

Cooper, J. M., and Siedentop, D. (1969). *The theory and science of basketball,* Philadelphia: Lea and Febiger.

Cooper, J. M. (1987). *Basketball: Player Movement Skills,* Indianapolis: Benchmark Press.

Cousy, B. and Powers, F. (1970). *Basketball concepts and techniques,* Boston: Allyn and Bacon, Inc.

Jensen, J. and Russell, P. (1986). Depth jumping and the volleyball spike. In J. Terauds, B. Gowitzke, and L. Holt (Eds.), *Biomechanics in Sports IIV & IV.* Del Mar, CA: Academic Publishers.

Klatt, L. A. (1977). Kinematic and temporal characteristics of a successful penalty corner in women's field hockey, doctoral dissertation, Indiana University.

Ridgway, M. and Hamilton, N. (1987). The kinematics of forearm passing in low skilled and high skilled volleyball players. *Biomechanics In Sports V.* Del Mar, CA. Academic Publishers (in press).

Ridgway, M. and Wilkerson, J. (1986). A kinetic analysis of the front set and back set in volleyball. In J. Terauds, B. Gowitzke, and L. Holt (Eds.), *Biomechanics in Sports III & IV.* Del Mar, CA: Academic Publishers.

Sardinha, L. and Zebas, C. (1986). The effect of perceived fatigue on volleyballspike skill performance. In J. Terauds, B. Gowitzke, and L. Holt (Eds.), *Biomechanics in Sports III & IV* (pp. 249–257). Del Mar, CA: Academic Publishers.

Stacoff, A., Kaelin, X. and Stuessi, E. (1986). Foot-movement, load and injury in volleyball. In J. Terauds, B. Gowitzke and L. Holt (Eds.), *Biomechanics in Sports III & IV* (pp. 258–262). Del Mar, CA: Academic Publishers.

Wooden, J. R. (1980). *Practical modern basketball, 2nd edition,* New York: Wiley and Sons.

20
Combatives

SCENARIO I

The smoke rises like solid grey beams in the hot light. All attention is focused on the two men in the small canvas square below, their bodies slick with sweat, faces distorted with mouthpieces, hands taped and gloved into shapeless weapons. What protection do they have from the blows of the opponent? Will conditioning and fast reflexes save them? How much force can a punch produce? How will the opponent minimize these forces?

What part will friction play? Who designed the shoes the way they are and why? Could they be better? What about the surface of the ring and the interface between the shoe-foot-ring surface? What are the ideal frictional values and what are the real ones?

SCENARIO II

In total silence, the two figures play each other up and down the narrow copper strip. Opponents, yet moving as partners, as though dancing an adagio in white. Each looks for a concentration break, one movement a little too large, and three feet of steel move forward at dazzling speed to find the open target with the tiny point. How fast is the attack? What is the time span between the decision to act and the act itself? Is speed more important than deception? The defense, how fast is it? Is it reflexive? How much force do fencers impart to the target? What is the line of force? Does it vary? Do skilled fencers produce and use forces differently than less skilled fencers?

The questions never stop. Each answer provides a small piece of information which gives the next curious person a starting place. We know so little; we need to know so much more. Some of what we know may not even be true. We can be statistically positive; but we can never be sure; We must always remember to doubt. But the doubt must be informed,; otherwise, it lapses into opinion.

How can we support the statements we make? Since the combatives can all be broken down into the basic movements of kicking, striking, pushing and pulling, we can apply certain principles of mechanics to the questions we wish to answer. What are these principles? Certainly the Newtonian principles of SF = ma, impulse-momentum and work (kinetic energy) will apply. In defenses, such as blocks and parries, the principles of stability and force absorption can be guides in answering questions.

KARATE

Karate is the art of hand and foot fighting. The stances in karate are patterned after animal stances. The two basic stances are the horse stance and the cat stance. The wide lateral position of the horse stance provides great stability, whereas the one-footed cat stance is ideal for mobility. Common attacks include punching and kicking. In karate, three basic concepts govern the effectiveness of attack and defense. These concepts are:

1. Center of gravity;
2. Base of support;
3. Force production and absorption.

These concepts will now be discussed more entirely.

Concept of Center of Gravity

The center of gravity is an imaginary reference point around which the weight of the body is evenly distributed. The location of this point varies with the body type of the individual, and the activity in which the person is engaged. An individual can change the position of the center of gravity simply by changing the position of one or more body segments. In some cases, the center of gravity can be located outside the body itself. But no matter where the center of gravity is, the body weight will always be divided equally on all sides of it.

A person's stability is closely related to the position of the center of gravity. Since the center of gravity can be changed at will, it follows that stability can be changed at will. For a karateka, this principle is vital. When delivering a blow with great force, the karateka needs to be stable. In fact, the reason that the karate punch is so powerful is that it is delivered from a position of great stability. Conversely, to move fast, the karaketa must be in an unstable position.

What factors govern the stability or instability of the body?

Concept of the Base of Support

The base of support refers to the area which supports the body. Part of the base of support may be outside the body. For example, when standing with the feet apart, the base of support includes the area between the feet. For stability, the larger the base of support, the more stable the position.

Stability and center of gravity are closely related. The lower the center of gravity, the more stable the stance. The converse is also true. Additionally, the center of gravity must fall within the bounds of the base of support for equilibrium to exist. The body will be most stable when the center of gravity is directly over the base of support.

Stability and instability must also be considered anthropomorphically. Although a larger, heavier person will be more stable, a ligher, smaller one may move more quickly.

The center of gravity also plays a part in the speed of motion. The karateka strives to keep the center of gravity at the same height when stepping forward to deliver a punch. By maintaining the center of gravity in a direct line, the karateka shortens the movement time to the target and because the movement occurs in a straight line, extraneous movement is eliminated and the karateka can move with incredible speed (Fig. 20-1).

Concept of Force

Unless force is applied, motion cannot occur or cease. A body in equilibrium remains that way until force is applied to cause movement (Newton's first law). In the body, force is produced by muscle action.

In order for large amounts of force to be developed and transmitted to the target, a karateka takes advantage of various principles relating to force production and absorption. For example, a skilled performer in any sport takes advantage of what is called "summation of forces." This means that the muscles contract in order, so that the force of each muscle group is added to the force of the succeeding muscle group. This summation produces a final force much greater than would occur if less muscle groups were utilized, or if the muscle groups were coordinated improperly. In a skilled performer, the strongest muscle group usually contracts first and the weakest group last. The

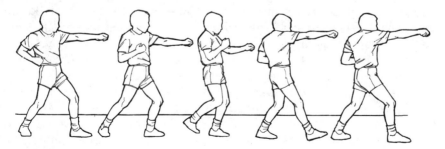

Fig. 20-1. *The forward step is executed without raising the center of gravity of the body. The body moves directly forward in a linear, horizontal displacement. Note the adjustments that must be made with the legs in order to execute the most effective forward step.*

COMBATIVES   **621**

trick learned by all skilled performers, however, is to have the succeeding group of muscles contract at the precise moment that the preceeding group has caused a body part to reach its maximum velocity.

In karate, correct summation of forces is readily seen in any skilled punch or kick. This is part of the reason why karate punches and kicks impart such great force to the target. Another important factor in martial arts is that of the amount of time the force is applied.

The longer the time during which a force is applied, the greater will be the force. Additionally, the longer the distance over which a force is applied, the greater the resultant force. The karetka must carefully balance the amount of force imparted versus the time taken to impart it. If the distance through which the force is applied is shortened, greater speed will be achieved, but less force will be generated. In a tournament where contact is minimal, force is a negligible factor and the performer strives for speed. When defending oneself in a street situation, however, the karetka, may strive for maximum force to disable an attacker. This principle can be further demonstrated by reviewing the basic leverage principles; i.e., a short lever moves faster than a long lever, but a long lever develops more force and more kinetic energy (which could be applied to the target) than a short one.

The principles of collision and of receiving impact forces can be applied to the impact of the punch and kick. To increase the time of impact the performer thinks of punching or kicking "through the target." This enables the performer to maintain the necessary velocity and prevent premature deceleration. In addition, the muscles are tensed at contact, which produces less deformation of the striking limb, less recoil from the joints, and therefore reduces the force absorbed by the striker. Additionally, the wrist or ankle will be firm and in alignment with the striking limb, and form a rigid bar at impact. The entire body is held rigid, with the rear foot and leg extended to act as a brace to counteract the collision.

Finally, to intensify the force imparted to the target, the kareteka will endeavor to strike the smallest part of the target, i.e., employ the principle $P = F/A$. Two persons who impart equal force (F) into a target may strike with quite unequal pressure (P) if they strike an area (A) differing in size. This principle is one which makes the force delivered by a kick or blow in karate so powerful. The karetka strives to strike the smallest area possible with the greatest amount of force possible. This can be achieved in two ways: (1) by decreasing the contact area of the striking part, and (2) by decreasing the area of the body part struck. For example, the hand strike is made with the side of the hand rather than the palm, and the punch is delivered with two knuckles of the fist making contact, rather than all four. The lateral edge of the foot is used in kicking, rather than the sole of the foot. Furthermore, the target struck is a vulnerable area, such as the bridge of the nose or knee.

To deliver more power, the body should act as a system of rigid levers, rather than "collapsible" levers. In reality, however, the hand and foot are not rigid; they deform on contact with the target. Additionally, the skin, the muscles and tendons deform to absorb some of the force of impact, thereby protecting the body part from injury.

Now to address some of the questions which were raised at the beginning of this chapter—how fast does the kareteka move and what magnitude of forces can a skilled performer develop?

The hand of the kareteka can exert a force in excess of 3,000 N (675 pounds). A force of 670 N is required to break wood, and force of 3,100 N is required to break concrete. Additionally, to break wood, the hand must reach a velocity of 6.1 meters per second, and to break concrete, a velocity of 10.6 meters a second must be achieved. Hand velocity in a skilled kareteka has been measured as high as 14 meters per second. The hand also needs 12.3 joules of energy to break wood and 37.1 joules to break concrete. (A joule is the amount of energy required to displace 1 newton a distance of one meter. Thus a joule is a unit of work as well (newton-meter).

Finally, trauma to the part of the body used in striking and kicking causes either injury or anatomic changes resulting from adaptation to trauma. Hypertrophy of the two knuckles used in striking with the fist frequently occurs as one of these adaptations.

FENCING

Fencing is unique in many ways. It involves no ball, but does involve a long striking implement (foil, epee, or sabre). This implement is not swung, but used as an extension of the arm. A sport of body propulsion, it involves neither running, jumping, or kicking, yet the body is propelled rapidly forward and backward during the course of the bout. Speed is very important, and the line of action should be direct to the target as previously explained in the karate section.

The basic stance in fencing has little similarity to other sports, except certain positions in the martial arts. In the basic stance, the feet are at right angles to each other, with the lead foot facing the opponent.

This stance provides both lateral and sagittal stability. The width of the feet is such that the center of gravity may be lowered for stability and increased flexion at the knee is possible in order to execute a forceful lunge. In addition, the knees should be above the feet to reduce the moments of force and stress at the knee joints. The feet should also be spread a distance that provides optimum mobility.

The method of delivering the attack in fencing, and in some cases the attack itself, is termed the lunge. The force produced in the lunge is obtained through extension of the rear leg and movement of the lead leg and rear arm. The more directly horizontal this force can be directed, the faster and more effective will be the lunge. Note in Fig. 20-2 the differences in peak forces of the rear leg during the lunge of

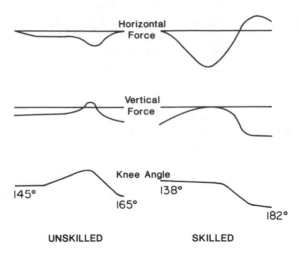

Fig. 20-2. *Force-time histories and angular displacement of the rear leg during an unskilled and skilled fencing lunge. The body weight is depicted as a horizontal line. The skilled fencer extends the lower leg immediately from the flexed support position. What does the unskilled fencer do? The skilled fencer develops greater horizontal momentum as evidenced by the large impulse (area under the horizontal force-time curve). The unskilled fencer exerts a vertical force that exceeds the body weight.*

a skilled performer and that of an unskilled performer. The unskilled performer did not extend the rear leg completely until after landing, and vertical forces were greater than horizontal ones. In addition, the vertical impulses were greater than the horizontal impulses. The skilled performer developed 355 N of peak force and five times more impulse in the horizontal direction than did the unskilled fencer. The skilled fencer showed no vertical force greater than body weight.

Further research concerning horizontal work and power in the lunge was carried out on fencers of university varsity caliber. The amount of work done was calculated using the formula work = force × distance of application. Body weight represented force. Duration of horizontal force production was divided into work to determine power produced. In the lunge, power ranged from 1988 watts to 2105 watts, and work done ranged from 1196 joules to 1256 joules.

Electromyographic and electrogoniometric data on both correctly and incorrectly performed lunging are depicted in Fig. 20-3. Note the differences in muscle action potentials with respect to position of the knee. Such data not only can assist a fencer in determining performance faults but can be used to determine which muscles are vulnerable when performance is incorrect.

High-speed photography is also valuable to the movement analyst in noting the movement of the muscle itself. For example, the movement of the triceps surae (the gastrocnemius and soleus considered together) during a fencing lunge can be seen in Fig. 20-4. Is the muscle more susceptible to tearing in image C of this figure?

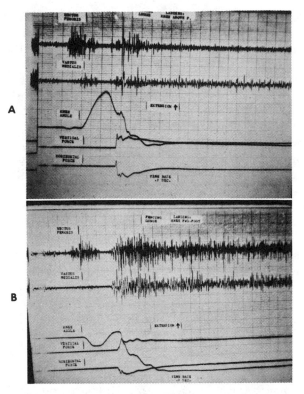

Fig. 20-3. *Comparison of electromyographic and electrogoniometric recordings as a function of the position of the knee during landing after two fencing lunges. A, Knee is above base of support (foot) at end of lunge and muscular activity is low in the rectus femoris and vastus lateralis muscles. B, Knee is outside base of support at end of lunge and muscular activity is high in both muscles. Why is this so?*

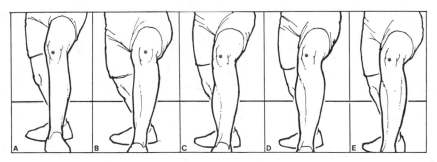

Fig. 20-4. *High speed cinematography captures human tissue phenomena unseen through normal visual observations. The two heads of the gastrocnemius muscle displace from their vertical shank alignment to wrap around the shank at the instant of contact during a fencing lunge. This can also be seen during lunges used in other sports situations, such as in racquetball. The five sequences depicted occurred in 0.025 seconds (camera was operating at 200 frames per second.)*

COMBATIVES   **625**

Further analyses of elite performers in the lunge were carried out on 3 male members of the 1984 Olympic team. The duration of their lunges, from start to finish, ranged from 250 to 600 milliseconds, and were fastest when they responded to conditions which simulated actual bout. The velocity of the fencers varied from a low of 1.2 meters per second to 4 meters per second, with the greatest velocity again being recorded in the bout simulating condition.

Acceleration in the attack is important since varying speeds are difficult for the opponent to judge and defend against. To determine acceleration, hip translation was investigated. In elite performers, acceleration did occur in the lunge, but it occurred in different phases of the lunge with each performer. Hip translation and lower extremity displacement during a lunge by one of the elite fencers is depicted in Fig. 20-5.

In fencing, to be elite is to be individual, within certain technically prescribed parameters. These individual differences may be due to anatomical factors, age, weapon fenced, or other variables.

More research is needed in fencing, and fencing is conducive to study since many of the gross moves are uniplanar and the fencers maintain a definite spatial relationship to one another.

BOXING

Boxing has been practiced both as a sport and for defense since prehistoric times. Although professional boxing has waxed and waned in popularity, amateur boxing still enjoys a high number of participants. Whereas the boxer is one of the fittest of athletes, some object

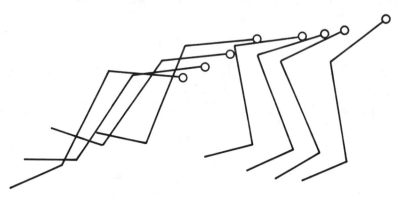

Fig. 20-5. *Line segment tracings of thigh, shank, and foot of lead leg executing a fencing lunge. The thigh moves from a downward inclination to a horizontal position. The shank initially is inclined forward and passes through the vertical during midlunge and then is inclined backward at landing. The foot begins in plantar flexion, dorsiflexes and again plantar flexes. Place a piece of transparent paper over this figure and plot the movement of the hip, knee, ankle and toe. How are the patterns similar and how are they different from each other? Given the goal of exection of as fast and forward a lunge as possible, what changes should be made in the segmental displacements of this lunge?*

to boxing on moral grounds. Since the object of boxing is to incapacitate the opponent, boxing can, by its very nature, cause injury. Boxers have much in common with karatekas in that they must impart and withstand forces and must move with precision and speed.

The boxer, however, imparts a large amount of momentum to the entire mass of the opponent, whereas the karateka focuses power on one small body area.

Additionally, boxing involves the extraneous movements of bobbing, weaving, and ducking, either to avoid punches or set up the opponent. The boxer must carry the center of gravity higher than either the judo or karate participant, because boxing is more mobile than either of these sports. Additionally, the boxer does not always deliver power in a straight line, but often moves the hands in a circular type of motion to the target, as, for example, when delivering a roundhouse punch.

For the boxer, the problems of generating and absorbing force are of prime importance. From a position less stable than that of the judo or karate performer, the boxer must generate force and absorb it, not once but many times over. How does the boxer deal with these problems?

First, the boxer develops a great deal of musculature, and the larger the muscle, the more strength available which can be used to generate power or to absorb the force of repeated blows. The boxer is also able to take advantage of the summation of forces principle. Primarily, however, the amateur boxer especially counts on repeated impacts to "wear the opponent down." Herein lies the basic problem concerning boxing. Although boxing actually ranks only 10th or 11th as a sport which causes serious injury, repeated impacts cause trauma which may not become apparent for a number of years.

When a boxer sustains a blow to the head, the head is accelerated backwards. The brain, which is suspended in a cerebrospinal fluid inside the skull, will move the same way. The two main areas of the brain, gray and white matter, are accelerated, too, but at different rates. This difference in rate leads to shearing forces between the gray and white matter. Thus, some nerve cells can be damaged, and others can die, never to be replaced. Additionally, in the collision of the brain with the skull, both the front and back of the brain can be damaged. The common manifestation of this type of injury is the individual who appears to be in a stupor or drunk. Loss of memory as well as loss of functional ability may occur.

A primary concern related to these symptoms is that the boxer could suffer a ruptured blood vessel in the brain. The bleeding which could occur from this rupture could lead to pressure on the brain, which could ultimately cause death. Such intracranial bleeding is thought by some authorities to be due to prolonged battering. Because of this possibility, amateur bouts are usually restricted in length to three rounds. Professional boxers, however, are often required to fight fifteen rounds (McLatchie).

COMBATIVES 627

When studying boxing, the question always arises as to the amount of force which can be generated by a punch, the amount of force necessary to cause body damage, and the force absorption characteristics of the boxing gloves and headgear. The Wayne State tolerance curve (WSTC) has been used to establish that forces sufficient to cause head accelerations of 80 g (784 n) of approximately 8 msec. duration are of knockout proportions (Smith and Hamil). A force of about 1100 N is required to break a mandible.

Studies were conducted on subjects punching a bag with no gloves, with karate gloves, and with boxing gloves. The boxing gloves imparted more momentum to the bag than did the bare fist, and the karate glove imparted momentum similar to the bare-fisted condition. Peak forces transmitted to the target were also higher with the boxing glove than with the karate glove. For this reason, the boxing glove would tend to cause more damage to hard tissue, such as bone and cartilage. Additionally, boxing gloves lose much of their force-absorption characteristics after the first few impacts. Boxing gloves tested by Therrien (1981) lost as much as 50% of their force-absorption capability after only a few impacts. This is quite a serious liability, considering that a boxer may use one set of gloves for a number of fights. There were also large variations in force absorption characteristics between boxing gloves of the same pair.

Finally, researchers suggest that neither boxing nor karate gloves offer much protection after the first few blows. Even-low skilled punchers could deliver blows of concussive force while wearing either type of glove.

JUDO

Judo is a sport of high impact and torsional forces. The main goal of judo is to break your opponent's balance while keeping yours. While timing and correct execution of technique are essential in judo, so is an understanding of torque and the center of the gravity. It is by moving the opponent's center of gravity outside the base of support that a judoka can unbalance and ultimately throw the opponent.

Breaking and Keeping Balance

Balance may be upset in eight conventional directions: forward, backward, right, left, and in the four corners. Force-application patterns used to produce this loss in equilibrium consists of (1) push, (2) pull, (3) push followed by a release, (4) pull followed by a release, (5) push-pull (force couple), (6) pull-push (force couple), and (7) combinations of all the above. Combinations of push-pull and pull-push always produce rotations of the opponent's body about its longitudinal axis.

The defensive position is taken with the center of gravity lowered by flexion at the knees. The feet are more than hip width apart, and they are at right angles to each other to provide both lateral and anteroposterior stability. This stance is similar to the fencer's stance, but in judo the torso is facing the opponent.

As the judoka face each other in this defensive stance, they grasp one another's lapel and sleeve. The material is held with the third and fourth fingers while the other fingers and thumb exert little pressure. This grip can be changed easily to achieve better leverage. Grasping the lapel causes any force by fingers or hand to control the midline of the opponent's body, whereas the grasping of the sleeve causes a moment of force to be applied to the torso.

Since the judoka must always be prepared for an attack, locomotion in made with short, quick steps of a sliding nature, with a lowered center of gravity. These movements provide maximum stability and promote maintenance of balance during the locomotion itself. The weight is often maintained over the leading foot so that the rear foot can be quickly used for sweeping and other attacks.

Preparation for a throw consists of interplay between the opponents in which they search for the timing and position to unbalance each other. For example, after some pushing and pulling and sliding of the feet, the opponent may push. A counteraction may be pulling against this opponent with greater force than of the push. This action may unbalance the opponent.

Since they are rotational, judo throwing techniques rely on the development of torque to make them efficient.

The Concept of Torque

Torque is simply rotational force. To calculate a torque, it is necessary to know two factors: (1) The force acting to cause rotation and, (2) the lever arm (moment arm) between this force and the pivot point (fulcrum). The magnitude of these two factors are multiplied together to calculate torque. In judo especially, after the opponent is unbalanced, some torques are cuased by the force of gravity.

Classifying Judo Techniques

Because there are so many types of throws and moves in judo, biomechanists and students of judo have long looked for a way to classify judo throwing techniques (which are called Mage Waza). Dr. Kano, the founder of judo, established the Kodokan classification, which is still used today in judo establishments the world over. The classification is based on the tori's (thrower) body movements. Another classification is based on the movements of the uke (person being thrown).

Dr. Kano further suggested that the judo throw is subdivided into three parts: (1) preparatory movements intended to unbalance the uke's body, (2) the final unbalancing, and (3) the execution of the throwing movement.

Looking for a better way to classify judo movements biomechanically, Sacripanti suggested that all the movements in judo could be divided into categories. The first category included all techniques in which the tori employed a force couple. These techniques would include leg sweeps and pushing and pulling the uke's body simultaneously. The second category included all techniques in which the tori primarily used principles of leverage. This would include all throws which occured as a result of turning the uke's body around a pivot point (fulcrum).

This method of classification enables researchers to utilize two sets of easily understood principles to analyze the majority of judo throws. All that is necessary is to decide the category in which the throw belongs. To illustrate the usefulness of this system, 2 judo moves, the hip throw (seoi nage) and the major outer reaping throw (o soto gari), will be analyzed. After reading the analysis, you determine the category to which each throw belongs.

Basic Principles Applied to Seoi Nage (Hip Throw)

See Fig. 20-6 for a general description of the throw, termed seoi nage, in which the tori rotates in front of the uke. The tori drops low and then moves diagonally upward as the uke is pulled into the circle of the tori's hip. As contact is made, the uke is already off-balance, and the throw is executed. The following principles govern this throw:

1. Maintain a low center of gravity.
2. Take short preparation steps to maintain equilibrium.
3. Place the center of gravity below the level of the opponent's center of gravity.
4. Move continuously and in a circular fashion.
5. Unbalance the opponent.
6. Draw the opponent sideward, rather than moving toward the opponent.
7. Throw in the direction of the opponent's movement. Bring the opponent's body over you in a curved path, caused by unbalancing the uke's body, and keep the hip firmly under that of the opponent.

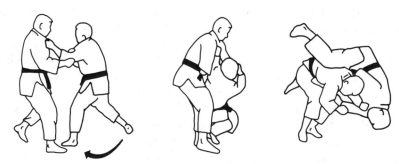

Fig. 20-6. *Note the use of both linear and rotary movements to position the center of gravity of the uke in a favorable position to execute the seoinage judo throw.*

Step 5, unbalancing the opponent is accomplished in two ways. First, by pulling the opponent toward you and to the right, your opponent's center of gravity is moved outside the base of support. As this occurs, the gravitational pull on the opponent's body creates a torque (t1) which alone could cause a fall. As explained previously, torque is the product of force multiplied by the lever arm. In this case, the force is the uke's weight, and the lever arm is the amount he is unbalanced. The more unbalanced the uke is, the greater the lever arm. Seio nage is typically done to one side of the body, as it is much easier to unbalance an opponent to the side than to the front. Why is this so? Because in pulling sideways the uke's center of gravity only needs to be displaced a short distance before it is no longer within the base of support. If the tori pulls the uke directly forward, the uke will not be unbalanced because a simple shift of body weight over the front foot can be executed. The tori would then become engaged in a strength contest with the uke, which would negate the idea behind judo.

As the tori turns and brings the unbalanced uke over the hip (tori's fulcrum), a second torque (t2) is applied, which causes the uke to roll over the tori's hip.

The hip throw, then, uses the first torque to unbalance the opponent and the second torque, caused by the tori's pull and pivot turn, to execute the throw.

In the o soto gari (Fig. 20-7), the object is to force your opponent to fall on one side of the body. In order to keep from injuring your opponent, it is wise to always hold the opponent firmly and gradually lower the opponent to land in a side fall position. The o soto gari begins when the opponent, as a result of preliminary pulling and pushing, steps back on one foot (left foot). Since the uke is already going backward, the tori steps to the side and pulls down on the uke's uniform. This pull is in the direction the uke is already going, so there is no resistance to the move. The pull also bends uke's body backward, causing an unbalancing because the center of gravity has been moved

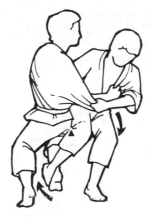

Fig. 20-7. *O soto gari, a judo throw consisting of the force couple (⌢) at the arm and foot and the fulcrum (▲) at the upper thigh/hip.*

away from the base of support. An initial torque has now been established, again caused by the uke's own weight. The tori takes advantage of this initial unbalancing by stepping behind the uke with the right foot and placing it behind the uke's right foot. The tori then sweeps the right hip and leg to the rear as rapidly as possible. This removes the rest of the uke's base of support, and there is nowhere for the uke to go but down. The two torques which have been created have caused the uke to rotate around a fulcrum on the tori's leg. The tori completes the throw by pulling down on the uke's uniform while simultaneously sweeping the uke's legs off the ground.

Now, you be the judge. In which category or categories do these two throws belong? Be sure to base your answer on mechanical principles.

Breaking the Fall

Since all throws involve a landing, the basic techniques described in Chapter 14 are applicable. The hand slap is unique to judo. Although the slap does not absorb a great deal of force, it is useful in placing the rest of the body, especially the trunk, in the most advantageous landing position. The goal of the landing is to absorb the force over the greatest possible body area and for the longest amount of time. If the landing will be a rolling type, the back is curved and the head is flexed to produce a low resistance to rolling.

Sports Medicine Problems

Nage Waza are typically performed toward one side. Thus a judoka may become overdeveloped on one side of the body. Since judo is basically a unilateral sport, except at high competitive levels, scoliosis, which is due to shortening of muscles on one side of spinal column, may result unless there is concomitant development of general body strength.

Another sports medicine problem caused by the force production and by the timing of the throw to coincide with the ideal position of the opponent's gravitational line is that of elbow injury. This injury is similar to "baseball pitcher's elbow," "tennis elbow," and other conditions caused by stress on the elbow.

MINI-LAB LEARNING EXPERIENCES

1. Observing maximum safety precautions, try to seio nage, (a) using a tall tori and short uke, and (b) using a short tori and tall uke. Why was the short tori more successful than the tall tori? How could the tall tori modify the technique to be more effective for his/her particular body type

2. Obtain an old pair of boxing gloves. Open one and observe the type and condition of the padding. Where is it all con-

---

centrated? What effect would this have on the boxer? On the body of the opponent? What material(s) do you think would make better padding? How would you modify the glove to make it safer for the wearer? For the boxer being hit?

3. Select a skill which interests you from any one of the sports in this chapter. Analyze the mechanics of the skill, using free body diagrams, force vectors, and/or any other principles of mechanics applicable to the skill.

4. From a mechanical viewpoint, which of the sports or activities in this chapter would you recommend for (a) young children, (b) elderly persons, (c) differently abled persons, and (d) developmentally delayed persons?

5. Explore the use of leverage in the following ways: (a) Grasp a person's arm in the following three positions and attempt to turn the person: (1) near the shoulder, (2) below the elbow, (3) at the wrist. (b) Name the levers involved and the relative success of each; explain why success differs for the three situations.

6. Observe a karate class practicing punches and kicks. Describe the position of the center of gravity and how it changes during the execution of the skills. Can you notice a difference in the mechanics employed by less and more skilled participants? If so, try to describe the differences. Do you think the skills could be taught more effectively if correct mechanics were explained and stressed, rather than the "imitate the leader" type of learning?

7. Which of the described combatives is most similar to wrestling? Observe a wrestline match and identify the basic principles involved in the skills.

REFERENCES

Adams, S., Adrian, A. and Bayliss, M. (eds.): (1987) *Catastrophic Injuries in Sports Avoidance Strategies*, Indianapolis: Benchmark Press.

Adrian, M., and Klinger, A.: (1977) A Biomechanical Analysis of the Fencing Lunge, *Swordmaster*, July.

Basmajian, J. V.: (1957) New Views of Muscular Tone and Relaxation, *Can. Med. Assoc. J.* 77:293.

Basmajian, J. V.: (1984) *Muscles Alive: Their Functions as Revealed by Electromyography*, ed. 2. Baltimore: The Williams & Wilkins Co.

Feld, M. S., McNair, R. E., and Wilk, S. R.: (1979) The Physics of Karate, *Sci. Am.* 240

Klinger, A., and Adrian, M.: (1985) Effect of Pre-Lunge Conditions on Performance of Elite Male Fencers, *Proceedings of ISBS Biomechanics in Sports, II*, Terauds and Barham (Eds.). Del Mar, CA: Academic Publishers.

Klinger, A., and Adrian, M.: (1987) Power Output as a Function of Fencing Technique, *International Series on Biomechanics*. vol. 6B. Human Kinetics Publishing Co., Champaign, Illinois.

Klinger, A. K.: (1977) Teaching mechanical principles through self-defense, In Dillman, C. J., and Sears, R. G. editors: *Proceedings, Kinesiology: a National Conference on Teaching*. Urbana: University of Illinois.

Kodokan: (1968) *Kodokan Judo*, Tokyo: Kodansha.

McLatchie, G. R.: (1981) "Injuries in Combat Sports," In *Sports Fitness and Sports Injury*, Reilly, T. (Ed.) London: Faber & Faber.

Sacripanti, A.: (1987) Biomedical Classification of Judo Throwing Technique. Unpublished paper presented at International Society of Biomechanics in Sports Symposium, July.

Schroeder, C. and Wallace, B.: (1982) *Karate, Basic Concepts and Skills*. Reading, Mass: Addison Wesley Publishing Co.

Smith, P. and Hamil, J.: (1985) Karate and Boxing Glove Impact as Functions of Velocity, *Proceedings of the ISBS Biomechanics in Sports, II*, Terauds and Barham, (eds.) Del Mar, CA: Academic Publishers.

Walker, J.: (1980) The Amateur Scientist: In Judo and Aikido Application of the Physics of Forces makes the Weak Equal to the Strong. *Scientific American.* 243:150–161, July.

Walker, J.: Karate strikes, *American Journal of Physics* **43**(10).

Westbrook and Ratti: (1980) *Aikido and the dynamic sphere: an illustrated introduction*, Rutland, VA: Charles and Tuttle Co.

21A
Aquatic Activities

As previously stated movement of human beings and animals on land is made possible by the relatively rigid surfaces on which the living body exerts a force and by the coefficient of friction between the surfaces. This frictional element produces a resistance to movement. Friction is a result of the normal force causing an equal and opposite reactive force, which results in deformation on the land surface. The air constitutes a nonrigid substance that normally produces a negligible resistance to movement of the body parts. Forces exerted by the human being or animal against the air are virtually ineffective. The air moves away from the body part; it does not become deformed or compressed to any significant extent. Water constitutes an environment that is less rigid (less compressible) than land, but is more rigid (more compressible) than air. As with land surfaces and air at different altitudes and temperatures, not all water is alike. For example, saltwater, cold water, hot water, oil-saturated lake water, fast-flowing river water, and choppy, windswept water all change the aquatic environment slightly for the person attempting to use the water. These uses of a physical nature can be grouped into floating activities, therapeutic exercises, swimming, surfboarding, and all types of small-craft activities.

RELATIONSHIPS OF BODY AND WATER WEIGHTS

If the human body, either stationary or moving, is supported by water, the mechanical problems the human being encounters differ from those encountered when it is supported by a more rigid surface and also when it is surrounded by air. When the body is supported by the ground or a floor, those surfaces are usually more than strong enough to resist the weight of the body and any additional force applied by moving body segments. When the supporting surface is water, this surface is unable to support the body; it gives way, and the body sinks, wholly or partially. It will sink until the weight of the displaced water equals the weight of the body. Before the latter is completely

635

immersed, the body will float. The first recognition of this weight relationship is attributed to Archimedes (287-212 B.C.), who said, "A body immersed in a fluid is buoyed up by a force equal to the weight of the displaced fluid." This concept is known as Archimedes' Principle.

The weight of a body compared to that of an equal amount of water is known as the specific gravity of the body:

$$\text{Specific Gravity} = \frac{\text{Weight of body}}{\text{Weight of equal amount of water}}$$

Human bodies differ in specific gravity: those with greater proportions of bone and muscle will be heavier. However, all are close to a specific gravity of 1, some being slightly less than 1 and some slightly more than 1.

The specific gravity of a given body can be determined by various methods. If the body is a regular geometric solid, its dimensions can be measured and its volume calculated. If the volume is known, the body weight can be compared to the weight of an equal volume of water.

If the body is irregular in shape, it can be submerged to determine the weight of the water that is displaces. If the body sinks, its weight can be determined while the body is completely submerged. The loss of weight when it is submerged is the weight of the displaced water.

$$\text{Specific gravity} = \frac{\text{Body Weight}}{\text{Loss of Weight in water}}$$

If the body does not sink or does not sink readily, additional weight may be attached to it to ensure complete submersion. The submerged weight of the attached mass should be determined. The loss of body weight in the water will be the total weight of the submerged body and attached mass minus the weight of the mass under water. The formula just given for bodies that sink readily can be applied to determine specific gravity.

In measuring 27 college women, Rork and Hellebrandt found that, after full inspiration, the mean specific gravity was 0.9812, ranging from 0.9635 to 1.0614; when the lungs were deflated, the average was 1.0177. Only 5 subjects had a specific gravity of less than 1 on full expiration. According to these authors, their findings compare favorably with those reported by previous investigators. It is to be expected that, in general, the specific gravity of women will be less than that of men, and that of children will be less than that of adults, especially at ages when the trunk is a greater proportion of the total body mass.

Since the specific gravity of most nonpowered small craft (rowboats, canoes, kayaks, sailboats) is less than 1, these objects will float upright or when capsized. Because of the relative size of these objects, the volume of water displaced is high compared to their weights. Some small craft have air chambers, or float spaces, to provide or enhance their floating ability.

FLOATING POSITION IN WATER

Persons whose specific gravity is less than 1 will float with some part of the body above the surface of the water. The position of the body as it floats will depend on the relationship of the center of gravity of the body to the center of weight of the displaced water. In most individuals, the lower limbs will sink because they are heavier than the water that they displace. However, the chest, which displaces water weighing more than this portion of the body, will float. The lungs assist in flotation by causing a balloonlike effect. The center of weight of the water displaced by the total body will therefore be nearer the head than is the center of gravity of the body. As the lower limbs sink, the spine will be arched, and the center of gravity will move toward a vertical line passing through the center of weight of the displaced water. When these two centers are in the same vertical line, the downward rotation of the lower limbs will cease.

Since in the adult the center of gravity is farther from the head than is the center of weight of the water, any changes in relative position of body segments that move the center of gravity closer to the head will bring the centers closer together. Raising the arms overhead in line with the trunk would do so, as would flexing the legs. For floating, the head, as well as all other body segments, should be resting in the water. The center of buoyancy of a body is also a factor in flotation.

Since muscle is heavier than fat, clearly a heavily muscled person will sink lower in the water than will a fatter person of the same size. This difference in body composition determines the extent of immersion in the water.

Knowledge of the relative position of the center of buoyancy in the body is helpful in teaching persons to float (Fig. 21A-1). Since most persons float in other than in a horizontal position, the legs and hips will descend into the water when a prone or supine floating position is assumed. Moreover, the descent of these body parts produces a rotation about the center of buoyancy, as well as a downward movement. Consequently, the momentum created will cause the head of the individual to submerge, and any hopes, of floating is soon dissipated.

A reverse momentum, creating a pleasant feeling rather than fear, occurs when a person begins the floating experience from a vertical position. The buoyancy force causes the legs to rise toward the horizontal position until the position of equilibrium occurs. Since the body motion is opposite the direction of gravity, the movement will stop at the point of equilibrium. This is not the case for the body descending from a horizontal position toward the diagonal floating position.

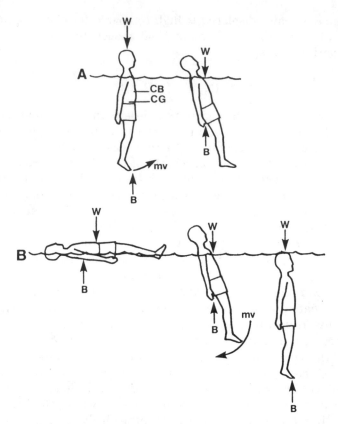

Fig. 21A-1. *Relationship of center of gravity (CG) of body and center of buoyancy (CB) of body and floating ability. A, Buoyancy force (B) and weight force (W) create momentum (mv) to rotate body to floating position, which is the position of vertical alignment of the two centers. B, When the body that does not float horizontally begins in the horizontal position the momentum rotates the body into the water. The body tends to pass through the balancing (floating) point because of the momentum. This causes the body to submerge and assume a floating position with total body under water.*

With respect to synchronized swimming, including stunts, the performer who floats horizontally has the advantage with respect to efficiency over the person who floats at a diagonal. For the horizontal floater, few or no sculling movements would be required to maintain the floating position. An action such as raising one leg above water, as in the ballet leg stunt in which the leg is perpendicular and completely above the water, requires a force only equal to the weight of the leg. The person who does not float horizontally is already using muscle effort to maintain the body position at the surface of the water. Additional force will be required to support the leg out of the water. Likewise, all the slow, propulsive strokes displaying exaggerated arm movements above the water level are more easily performed by the floaters.

FORCES ACTING DURING LOCOMOTION IN WATER

Resisting Forces

As the body moves through water, its progress is resisted by this medium. Karpovich stated that, as investigations on plane and ship models have shown, this resistance consists mainly of three factors: skin resistance, eddy resistance, and wave-making, or frontal, resistance. The opposing force of frontal resistance is the greatest of these. In addition, it has been found that a looser-fitting suit offers more resistance than does a tighter-fitting suit. In observing the drag, Karpovich found less resistance in the prone position than in gliding on the back. This finding has been disputed by some. Counsilman found that the prone position offers less resistance than does the side position, and that, if the body is rolled by an external force, the resistance increases and is still greater with a self-rolling position. However, all top swimmers utilizing either of the crawl strokes roll their bodies to some extent. There evidently are advantages to the roll that are greater than those lost through resistance. Among them are the following: (1) The arm is closer to the midline of the body rather than to the side and consequently its pull is more effective; (2) the recovery of the arm is facilitated; and (3) the breathing position is improved.

Form, or frontal, resistance during swimming changes continuously as both the velocity and the body position change.

In observing the effect of the speed of the body on resistance, Alley found that when the body is in the prone position, resistance increases up to approximately 0.6 m/sec (2 ft/sec). At speeds between 0.6 and 1.5 m/sec (2 and 5 ft/sec), the lower limbs are lifted toward the body line. This action, of course, decreases the resistance. When the speed reaches 1.8 m/sec (6 ft/sec), a noticeable bow wave adds to the resistance. These observations were made while dragging the body through the water without changing limb positions. Resistance values during these towing conditions ranged from 1.0 N to 2.5 N at approximately 1 m/sec.

During the glide phase of swimming, the resistance is termed passive and remains relatively constant. Active resistance, however, occurs during the remainder of the swimming cycle and varies as the position of the body changes with an application of force by the swimmer. Rennie and associates measured active resistance as 2.3 to 5.0 N at 0.9 m/sec for women swimmers. Thus, twice as much resistance may be expected during the act of swimming than during gliding.

One of the more commonly investigated cross-sectional characteristics (and therefore an indirect measurement of form resistance) is the breast stroke kick and its variations. For example, differences in the spread of the feet vary from 30 cm in the preparation phase of the whip kick to 180 cm in the preparation phase of the breaststroke kick. The frontal area changes almost fourfold between glide and preparation in the latter kick. In addition, the duration of the preparation phase is longer for the breaststroke kick than for the whip kick.

Alteveer recorded the minute changes in speed during swimming and found that the sidestroke, elementary backstroke, and breast stroke showed a loss in speed of greater than 50% during the recovery phase. This loss was attributed to the increase in frontal area during that phase. The crawl strokes and dolphin stroke showed less than 15% reduction.

Since active drag is one and one-half to two times that of passive drag, researchers have attempted to determine the effect of anthropometric characteristics on active drag. None of the correlations were greater than 0.46, an indication that anthropometric characteristics are not the primary factor in the production of active drag, but that swimming technique is more important.

Many practices have been utilized by swimmers and coaches to reduce frictional (surface) resistance, including shaving the body, oiling the body, and changing the material of the swimsuit. An exceptionally hairy man was able to reduce towing resistance by approximately 1% after having shaved. Woolen suits have been discarded because of their absorption of water and the consequent increase of resistance. Nylon and other artificial fibers have provided suits that prevent water absorption, but there are no other measurable differences among styles or materials.

Tethered swimming, swimming in a water treadmill, swimming with hand paddles, drag suits, or other resistance devices all have been utilized by coaches to increase the work required of the swimmer. Since force characteristics change in these situations compared with free swimming, one may assume that the mechanical characteristics of the stroke itself may change. For example, when the swimmer is tethered, the water is churned up, and the same water is being engaged with each stroke, causing turbulence. This turbulence causes the water particles to move in a haphazard fashion, increasing the resistance but varying it in an unknown amount from one stroke to the next. Thus the application of force by the swimmer will not be the same for each stroke.

Maglischo (1985) studied what effects using surgical tubing (stretch cords) as a means of sprint assisted and sprint resistive training had on stroke mechanics. With the tubing attached to a wall and to a waist belt on the other end, the person would swim away from the wall. This resulted in increased resistance (spring resistive). Shortly after this trial, the individual swam to the original starting position, trying to move as fast, or faster, than the recoiling tubing (sprint assistive). He found a definite change in stroke mechanics, but no conclusive results pertaining to the improvement or lack of improvement during the pull pattern.

Nelson attached a resistance training device to the waist of women being towed in the prone position (Fig. 21A-2). The average resistance during towing with the device was 90% greater than during towing

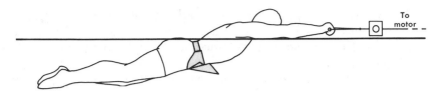

Fig. 21A-2. *Resistance device captures water inside pocket. Towing speed decreases or greater force is required for motor to tow person at the same speed. The resistance is measurable and is analogous to the drag force of the swimmer in the glide position. This technique, or a modification thereof, can be used to test persons with other devices and in different body positions.*

without the device, as recorded by strain gages. One group of swimmers trained with the device, and one group trained without the device. The following conclusions were drawn:

1. The resistance while a swimmer is wearing the device will vary among subjects because of the size of the sagittal-thorax area, which is the primary cause of turbulent flow into and around the device.
2. Wearing the device will drop the lower half of the body, thus causing a change in the body orientation. This change could prevent the swimmer from practicing the specific movements of stroking needed to train effectively.
3. The evidence suggests that swimmers who continue to use the device believe that it is beneficial in spite of perceived problems with specificity of training.

PROPULSIVE PRINCIPLES COMMON TO ALL STROKES

Improving swimming speed by application of biomechanical principles has been of interest to both the researcher and coach at all levels of performance. Because of the complexity of the many variables involved, the primary concern becomes one of separating which factors are most important, and which are less important.

Counsilman (1977) identified six factors that are common to all competitive strokes:

1. All strokes have some type of elliptical pull pattern; i.e., the swimmer should never pull on a straight line (Barthels & Adrian, 1975; Hay, 1978; Maglischo, 1982; Rackman, 1975).
2. In all strokes, the pull pattern occurs with what is called a high-elbow position (Colwin, 1965; Maglischo, 1982).
3. All strokes begin the pull pattern with the arms extended (straight), then they begin to flex, and continue to flex until the maximum forearm flexion occurs just over halfway through the pull pattern. At this point, the arms begin to extend again for the completion of the pull pattern; i.e., an extend-flex-extend (straight-bent-straight) arm relationship exists.

AQUATIC ACTIVITIES   **641**

4. All strokes have a maximum angle at the elbow of 90 degrees, except the breaststroke, which has a maximum of 120 degrees. This flexion should take place just over halfway through the pull pattern.
5. The pitch of the hands is important during the entry, pull pattern and exit.
   a) During the entry, the hands should enter the water in a manner that will eliminate any entrapment of air, causing a decrease in the efficiency of the pull pattern (Maglischo, 1982). This is accomplished by entering with the thumb and index finger first on the crawl and butterfly, and with the little finger first on the backstroke.
   b) During the pull pattern, the hands should be pitched in a manner to optimize the lift and drag forces (Barthles 1979; Hay, 1978; Maglischo, 1982; Schleihauf, 1978).
   c) The hands should be pitched on the exit to allow for a smooth transition from the pull pattern to the recovery. The hands should exit the water as if being taken out of the pocket on the crawl and butterfly stroke. During the backstroke, the hand should exit the water with the thumb first (Maglischo 1982).
6. The most important principle is one of hand acceleration. All strokes are performed with a hand-speed pattern that begins relatively slowly and progresses to a speed of 21.0 ft/sec in world-class swimmers at the end of the pull (Counsilman and Wasilak 1981).

PROPULSIVE FORCES

Any study of propulsive forces in swimming should focus upon the hydrodynamic forces acting on the hand. To convince oneself that movement of the hand provides the dominant force in swimming, one need only attempt to swim with a clenched fist. "The reduction in surface area of some 50 percent will produce a disproportionate decrease in swimming propulsion. This is because propulsion in swimming is largely dependent upon the shape and orientation of a broad, flat, propelling surface" (Schleihauf, 1978, p. 2).

The arms are generally regarded as the prime source of forward propulsion, but opinions differ concerning the exact magnitude of the contribution. Karpovich (1935) determined experimentally the speeds that a group of crawl swimmers could develop using the arms alone, the legs alone, and the arms and legs together. He concluded that skilled crawl swimmers derive about 70% of their forward speed from their arms and 30% from their legs. Armbruster, Allen, and Billingsley (1970), however, stated, "The arms provide about 85% of the total power of the sprint crawl stroke" (p. 53). Counsilman (1968) goes still further with his statement:

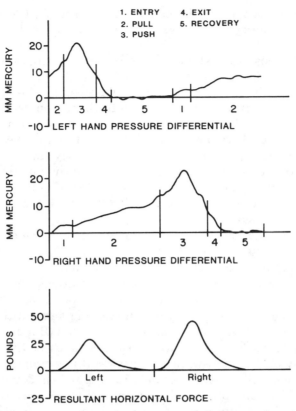

Fig. 21A-3. *Resultant horizontal force and palmar-dorsal pressure differential recordings during crawl stroke swimming. Note the differences between the right and left hands. (Courtesy J. Scheuchenzuber, Doctoral dissertation, Kinetic and Kinematic Characteristics in the Performance of Tethered and Non-tethered Swimming of the Front Crawl Stroke. Indiana University, Bloomington.)*

The arm stroke in the crawl is the main source of propulsion and, in the case of most swimmers, the only source of propulsion. This is because the forward force of the kick is less than the forward force of the arms. (p. 25)

Counsilman (1968) also compared the situation to that of a car with four-wheel drive where the front wheels (the swimming arms) turn at 30 mph and the rear wheels (the swimming legs) turn at 20 mph. In this situation, on a dry road, the rear wheels would actually slow the car to about 25 mph. In swimming, the retarding drag created by the kick is minimized by the water, which allows the legs to slip forward to a certain point. But at racing speeds there is still a retarding drag created by the legs. Counsilman (1968) found at speeds greater than 5.0 ft/sec (1.5 m/s) the kick of the swimmer did not contribute anything to the speed at which he was being towed, and in some instances, actually created and increased drag as a result of the kick. Regardless of the exact amount of total propulsion for which the legs are responsible (whether 5%, 10%, or 15%), the researchers agree that on the crawl stroke, the hand pull is the dominant force in propulsion.

The forearms are of slightly more importance than the legs. Consilman (1968), with his research on the "high elbow position" (an arm position where the humerus medially rotates to get the elbow higher than the hand), verifies the existence of forearm propulsion. However, the insignificance of the forearms can be seen by referring back to the first example where the swimmer swam with a clenched fist. When swimming with a fist, one proceeds very slowly, and only a small amount of the total propulsion is attributed to the forearms. At slow speeds, both the legs and fists contribute to the minimum motion created. Therefore, the arms, and specifically, the hands dominate in swimming propulsion.

Studies on the importance of the magnitude of the application of force in swimming are plentiful (Counsilman 1955, 1977; Goldfuss & Nelson 1971; Scheuchenzubur, 1974; Schleihauf, 1974). A major breakthrough came in stroke mechanics when Counsilman (1971) discovered that world-class swimmers use "lift" (an application of Bernouli's principle), as well as "drag," in creating forward thrust. Since then, research of others have supported this claim (Barthels & Adrian 1974; Hay, 1978; Schleihauf, 1974). During much of the arm movement of any of the four swimming strokes, the swimmer is actually sculling through the water (Barthels 1979; Barthels & Adrian 1975). In addition, drag also plays an important role since it is a combination of these two forces that a world-class swimmer uses to achieve maximum forward thrust (Barthels, 1979; Counsilman, 1977; Schleihauf, 1978). "Poor swimmers rely on drag, while good swimmers rely on lift force for propulsion" (Counsilman and Wasilak, 1981, p. 1). The old idea that to swim forward one should push the water straight back is now known to be inefficient and is a principle utilized only by poor swimmers.

The hand movement of any world-class swimmer is three dimensional: it moves up and down in the vertical plane; forward and backward in the horizontal plane; and laterally, inward, and outward from the midline of the body (Counsilman, 1977; Barthels, 1979; Maglischo, 1982). The pull pattern of all strokes is elliptical. Following an elliptical pathway (with the lateral movements being especially important) permits the hand to develop lift. In order to push the water backward at an angle, Schleihauf (1974) commented: "The propellor is the most efficient means of propulsion in water currently known" (p. 90). To obtain lift, therefore, the hand must be pitched in much the same manner as the blades of an airplane or boat propeller. Consequently, the term "sculling" is the most correct term to describe hand movements of the swimming pull.

Recommendations for the optimum angle of attack have varied. The flow pattern becomes confusing when the direction of flow is considered across the ulnar, radial, distal and proximal sides of the hand.

Schleihauf (1979) has found the optimum angle of lift for swimming propulsion to be between 37 and 40 degrees, relative to the principal plane where the movement of the hand takes place. Maglischo (1982) suggested the optimum angle of lift for the hand to fall somewhere between 20 and 50 degrees.

The hand's position and orientation is constantly changing to maintain the desired pitch. When observing underwater movies of such "natural" swimmers as Tracy Caulkins, Mary Meager, Mark Spitz, Alex Baumann, and Rowdy Gaines, one can see that they do perform these precise changes (Counsilman and Wasilak, 1981).

Another important reason why the elliptical pull pattern is efficient is that it allows the hand to encounter still water, that is, water without turbulence (Counsilman, 1977; Maglischo, 1982). Maximum efficiency is achieved when the hand does not push the same water back continuously, but can find still water. Counsilman (1971) stated:

> The greater efficiency in water is achieved by moving a large amount of water a short distance than by moving a small amount of water a great distance. Perhaps the ability to find still water constitutes one aspect of that nebulous quality that coaches call having a good feel for the water (p. 3).

A quality that may be of equal, or even greater importance, than this "feel for the water" is the manner in which this force is applied in terms of its variance. Scheuchenzuber (1974) used an apparatus that measured the force generated by the arm pull by detecting the pressure differential between the palmar and dorsal surfaces of the hand. The results are presented in Fig. 21A-3.

As shown in the two upper graphs, there were two power surges in the crawl stroke that occur during each arm pull. Counsilman and Wasilak (1981) gave further support for that concept with the following statement:

> In any physical activity that involves overcoming inertia and developing acceleration, such as putting the shot, throwing a ball, running, and possibly swimming, there should be a force that begins at a relatively low level, and is progressively applied throughout the movement. The force should progressively increase until the peak force is achieved when the shot or ball leaves the hand, the foot leaves the ground, or the hand finishes the pull. This is the ideal application of force, but it may not often occur due to muscular weakness, changing mechanical advantage, or other factors (p. 3).

Studying acceleration patterns in physical activities has been neglected. Counsilman and Wasilak (1981) believed:

> The ability to accelerate is one of the most important variables in nearly all athletic events. In throwing a baseball, the hand of

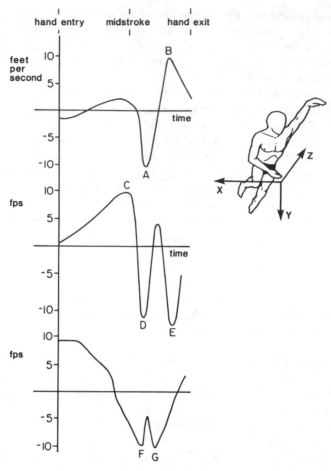

Fig. 21A-4. *Hand velocity curves of Mark Spitz during crawl swimming. A, Medial and lateral velocities; B, Upward and downward velocities; C, Forward and Backward velocities. The ranges in all cases are + or − ten feet per second. Visualize the direction and velocities at the points labeled A through G. (Modified from R. Schleihauf, A Biomechanical Analysis of Freestyle Aquatic Skill. Swimming Technique, 11, p. 93.)*

a fastball pitcher can accelerate from a few feet per second to over 90 miles per hour (660 ft/sec) in a little over one tenth of a second. In a good crawl sprinter, the hand accelerates from zero feet per second to 20 feet per second in less than 4/10ths of a second (p. 3).

The study of hand-velocity patterns can become very complex when they are expressed in either one, two, or three dimensions. The hand-velocity pattern can also be expressed in relation to the hand relative to still water, or in relation to the hand movement relative to the body. They can also be expressed in terms of acceleration curves. There are, in fact, several ways in which hand-speed can be represented. (Counsilman and Wasilak, 1981).

Both Schleihauf (1974) and Counsilman (1977, 1980a) have mentioned the importance of hand acceleration during the pull. Schleihauf (1974) presented hand-velocity patterns of Mark Spitz as shown in Fig. 21A-4. These patterns depict the hand-velocity patterns in their relationships to still water and not the body.

Presenting the hand-velocity patterns relative to still water makes it difficult for the swimmer to grasp the concepts. Counsilman (1980a) has found that swimmers cannot easily orient this thinking and coordination, with respect to hand movement and acceleration in still water. Hand-velocity data in several modes may be informative and interesting to the researcher but confusing to the swimmer, or anyone contemplating the material for the first time. In discussions with competitive swimmers, Counsilman and Wasilak (1981) concluded that average swimmers relate their hand movement to their bodies.

Counsilman and Wasilak (1981) analyzed hand-speed patterns relative to the body in all four strokes, and found that all world-class swimmers began the pull pattern with a relatively low level of force

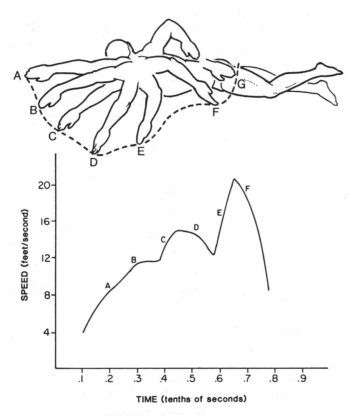

Fig. 21A-5. *Hand speed of Rowdy Gaines (world-class swimmer) relative to his body during the crawl stroke. The maximum hand speed was greater than 21 ft./sec. (approximately 6.5 m/sec) occurring toward the end of the pulling phase which was nearly 0.7 seconds in duration. (Courtesy of J. Counsilman and J. Wasilak)*

and increased the magnitude continuously until the maximum forward thrust created by the hand reached its peak near the end of the pull. This can be seen from the four graphs of world-class swimmers in Fig. 21A-5 through 21A-8.

Rowdy Gaines in the crawl stroke reached a peak hand-speed of over 21.0 ft/sec (6.4 m/s) at the end of the pull. The total time involved in performing the propulsive phase of the stroke is slightly over 0.5 of a second (Counsilman and Wasilak, 1981).

Jim Haliburton also reached a peak hand speed in the butterfly of 1.80 ft/sec (5.4 m/s) at the end of the pull. The total time of the propulsive phase was just over 0.5 of a second (Counsilman and Wasilak, 1981).

Alex Baumann's hand-speed curve of the backstroke is the only representation of a swimmer not swimming at a maximum effort. It was included to show that world-class swimmers tend to have similar hand-speed patterns even at moderate speeds, the basic difference being in the time it takes to complete the pull—in this case, 0.8 of a second compared to 0.5 of a second, when the swimmer is swimming at maximum effort (Counsilman and Wasilak, 1981).

Nobutaka Taguchi's hand speed during the breast stroke is bi-

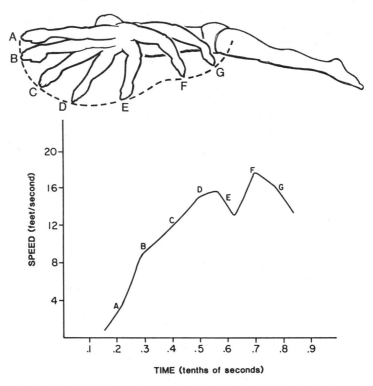

Fig. 21A-6. *Hand speed of Jim Halliburton (world-class swimmer) relative to his body during the butterfly stroke. The maximum hand speed was 18 ft/sec (5.5 m/sec) occurring toward the end of the pulling phase which was nearly 0.7 seconds in duration (Courtesy of J. Counsilman and J. Wasilak).*

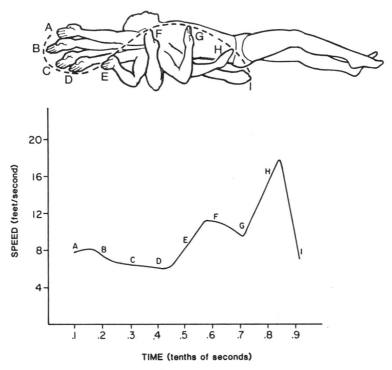

Fig. 21A-7. *Hand speed of Alex Baumann (world-class swimmer) relative to his body during swimming the backstroke at a moderate speed. At this speed his maximum hand speed was approximately 18 ft/sec (5.5 m/sec). His pattern was similar for faster speeds but the pulling time was shorter. (Courtesy of J. Counsilman and J. Wasilak)*

modal in nature, but in many respects is similar to that of other strokes. The dip in the hand-speed between points C and D, (Fig. 21A-8) occurs when the hand changes direction of the pull from outward to the inward scull. The entire propulsive phase of the stroke takes less than four-tenths of a second. The maximum speed is achieved on the inward sculling action of the hands from D to E (Counsilman and Wasilak, 1981).

It was found that to achieve this variance in force, there was a constant increase in hand speed during the arm pull of all competitive strokes. There was one exception to this increase in variance when the hand decelerated and there was a corresponding dip in the hand-speed curve.

Counsilman and Wasilak (1981) believed:

That in all but the breaststroke pull, even during the period of time when the hands are decelerating, there can be an increase in the magnitude of the forward thrust. This is possible, apparently, because the main source of propulsion at this point in the stroke is derived from lift (as the hands are sculling) inward laterally (p. 9).

AQUATIC ACTIVITIES

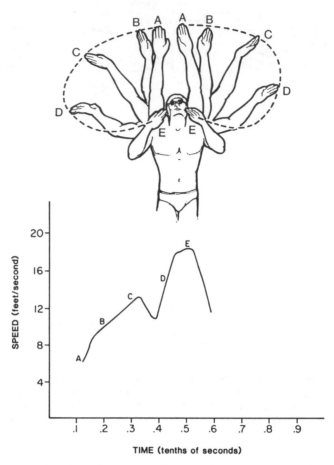

Fig. 21A-8. *Hand speed of Nobutaka Taguchi (world-class swimmer) relative to his body during the breast stroke. The maximum hand speed was nearly 8 ft/ sec (5.5 m/sec) occurring on the inward sculling action (D to E) near the end of the pulling phase which was less than 0.5 seconds in duration. Refer to previous three figures and compare the hand speed patterns for these other swimming strokes, bearing in mind that these are individual patterns and not all swimmers will produce identical patterns or force magnitudes.*

Counsilman (1980), in comparing hand-speed patterns of poor swimmers and world-class swimmers, found several obvious differences:

> The poor swimmers take longer to complete their underwater arm pull. The average time for the poor swimmers was 1.05 seconds, while the average time for the world-class swimmers was only 0.7 seconds. The average top hand speed of the swimmers at the swimming speed used in the study was 7.3 feet/second or 4.99 miles per hour, while that of the world-class swimmers was 17.4 feet/second or 11.91 miles per hour. The poor swimmers believed they maintained the same muscular effort throughout the arm

pull, while the world-class swimmers thought their effort increased as the pull progressed. The latter, however, did have trouble verbalizing the exact manner in which this effort increased (p. 7).

If the poor swimmers did maintain the same muscular effort throughout the entire pull, the increase in speed, even though not of the magnitude of that of the world-class swimmers, could be explained in terms of the mechanical advantage of the muscles as the pull progressed.

If this were true, it would seem that for a swimmer to simulate the hand-speed patterns of world-class swimmers, it would be necessary, either consciously or unconsciously, to increase the force exerted by the pulling muscles. In other words, "The swimmer could not rely entirely on the increased force created by the mechanical advantage by the changing position of the arm" (Counsilman 1980, p. 9).

In summary, the hand-speed patterns of world-class swimmers have obvious similarities in all four competitive strokes. The peak hand speeds of the world-class swimmers studied were between 18.0 ft/sec to 21.0 ft/sec (5.4m/s–6.4m/s). It can be seen that the hand should exert a force on the water that begins at a relatively low level and is increased in magnitude continuously, until the maximum forward thrust created by the hand reaches its peak near the end of the pull (Counsilman and Wasilak, 1981).

MINI-LAB LEARNING EXPERIENCES

Experiment with the relationship of stroke frequency, stroke distance, and speed of swimming.

A. Ask swimmers to swim at the following cadences. Count the number of strokes, and record the time taken to swim a prescribed distance (i.e., 30 feet):
1. 60, 80, 100, and 120 strokes per minute.
2. Calculate distance traveled per stroke and speed of swimming.
3. Plot the relationships of stroke rate, distance per stroke and speed of swimming, and compare the data with that of Craig and Prendergast.
B. Repeat procedure A with running, race walking, or other cyclic forms of locomotion and compare results with those of swimming.

REFERENCES

Armbruster, D., Allen, R., Billingsley, H. (1973) *Swimming and Diving,* St. Louis: C. V. Mosby.
Adrian, M. J., Singh, M. and Karpovich, P. M. (1966) Energy cost of leg kick, armstroke, and whole crawl stroke, *J. Appl. Physiol.* 21:1763–1766.
Alley, L. E. (1952) An analysis of water resistance and propulsion in swimming the crawl stroke, *Res. Q.* 23:253.

Alteveer, M. (1976) Minute changes in speed during execution of several strokes, master's thesis, Springfield College.

Barthels, K. (1976) Re-evaluation of swimming movements based upon research. In Adrian, M. and Bramne, J., editors: *Research: women in sport, vol. 3,* Washington, DC: American Association for Health, Physical Education, and Recreation.

Barthels, K. (1979) The mechanism for body propulsion in swimming. In *Swimming III.* Terauds, J. Bedington, W. (Eds), Baltimore: University Park Press.

Barthels, K., Adrian, M. (1975) Three-dimensional spatial patterns of skilled butterfly swimmers. In *Swimming II.* LeWillie, L., Clarys, J. (Eds), Brussels: Universitie Libre de Bruxelles.

Clarys, J. P. and LeWillie, L. (1975) *Swimming, II.* International Series on Sport Science, Baltimore: University Park Press.

Colwin, C. (1969) *Cecil Colwin on Swimming.* London: Pelham Books.

Counsilman, J. E. (1955) Forces in two types of crawl stroke, *Res. Q.* 26:127–139.

Counsilman, J. E. (1968) *The Science of Swimming.* Englewood Cliffs: Prentice Hall.

Counsilman, J. E. (1980) *The application of Bernoulli's principle to human propulsion in water,* Bloomington, IN: Indiana University Publications.

Counsilman, J. E., Wasilad, J. (1981) Hand speed and hand acceleration patterns in swimming strokes. Unpublished paper presented at American Coaches Association, Chicago.

Cureton, T. K. (1930) Mechanics and kinesiology of the crawl flutter kick, *Res. Q.* 1:87.

Goldfuss, A., Nelson, R. (1971) A temporal and force analysis of the crawl arm stroke during tethered swimming. In *Proceedings of the First International Symposium on Biomechanics on Swimming, Waterpolo, and Diving.* Brussels: Universite Libre de Bruxelles.

Hollander, P., Huijing, P., de Groot, G. (1983) *Biomechanics and Medicine in Swimming.* Champaign, IL: Human Kinetics Publishers Inc.

Karpovich, P. V. (1933) Water resistance in swimming, *Res. Q.* 4:21.

Maglischo, E. (1982) *Swimming Faster.* Palo Alto, CA: Mayfield Publishing.

Maglischo, E., Maglischo, C. (1985) The effects of sprint assisted and sprint resistive training on stroke mechanics. *The Journal Swimming Research* 1.

Nelson, L. J. (1976) Drag and performance analysis of a resistance device in swimming, thesis, Washington State University.

Rackham, G. (1975) An analysis of arm propulsion inswiming. In *Swimming II,* LeWille, L, Clarys, J. (Eds.), Brussels: Universite Libre de Bruxelles.

Rennie, D. W., Pendergast, D. R., and DiPrampero, P. E. (1975) Energetics of swimming in man. In Clarys, J. P. and Lewillie, L., editors: *Swimming, vol. 2,* Baltimore: University Park Press.

Ringer, L., Adrian, M. (1969) "An electrogoniometric study of the wrist and elbow in the crawl arm stroke." *Res. Q.* 40:353.

Rork, R. and Hellebrandt, F. A. (1937) The floating ability of college women, *Res. Q.* 8:19.

Scheuchenzuber, H. J., Jr. (1974) Kinetic and kinematic characteristics in the performance of tethered and nontethered swimming of the front crawl arm stroke, doctoral dissertation, Indiana University, August.

Schliehauf, R. E. (1979) A hydrodynamic analysis of swimming propulsion. In Terauds, J. and Bedingfield, E. W., editors: *Swimming, vol. 3,* Baltimore: University Park Press.

Scott, S. (1969) Factors influencing whip-kick performance, thesis, Washington State University.

Ungerechts, B. E., Wilke, K. and Reischle, K. (1988) *Swimming Science V,* Champaign, IL: Human Kinetics.

Wasilak, J. (1988) Unpublished dissertation, Indiana University, Bloomington.

Wood, T. C. (1979) A fluid dynamics analysis of the propulsive potential of the hand and forearm in swimming. In Terauds, J. and Bedingfield, E. W., editors: *Swimming, vol. 3,* Baltimore: University Park Press.

21B

Gliding with Rolling and Sliding Blades

Which devices are used by human beings to glide for short or long periods of time? What will we see as devices in the future? Maybe you'll invent one of these future devices. Gliding has always been exciting and dangerous, a combination which renders it appealing. In some countries, skiing is a daily method of transportation. Although the term skiing originally meant to glide on snow by means of a pair of slender boards of wood known as skis, the definition has changed with the advent of new materials, single water skis, roller blades, and dry-land skis. In addition, one might consider surfboarding and skateboarding to be forms of skiing, since each resembles the single-ski technique of waterskiing. Since both skateboards and the dry-land skis use a form of roller, there is a need for a clear delineation between types of gliding. For ease in biomechanical analysis, those forms of locomotion which utilize some type of device to produce a gliding motion may be placed into the following two categories: sliding friction devices and rolling friction devices. Examples of locomotion with sliding devices include downhill skiing, cross-country skiing, waterskiing, surfboarding, and ice-skating (including ice hockey). Rolling friction devices can be sub-divided into (1) devices that roll as a result of a gliding of the body and (2) devices that roll because of the turning of pedals by the person. Examples of locomotion in which the body glides on roller devices include roller skating, skateboarding, and dry-land cross-county skiing. Examples of rolling friction devices in which pedals are used include unicycles, bicycles, tricycles, wheelchairs, and other human-powered machines.

Since skating, skiing, and cycling skills are not taught nationwide in the public school curriculum, and few participants have been able to enjoy a financially rewarding professional career in these sports, there has been a sparsity of biomechanical literature with respect to most gliding activities. The water, snow, and ice media have not always proved to be convenient places for conducting research. With the advent of controlled wave-making surfing areas, artificial snow, indoor ski hills, and indoor ice rinks, however, data collection on these media is not only easier but can be standardized. An increase in research concerning the biomechanics of winter sports and cycling has occurred because of the interest in understanding and improving international sports performances. For example, skiers have been filmed, force transducers have been attached to the skis, and electrodes for electromyographic recordings and electrogoniometers for angular displacement recordings have been attached to their bodies. Most of the researchers utilize telemetry equipment, cinematography, or videography. The equipment and environment are equally important in the biomechanical analysis of the human gliding constraints. Thus the information in this chapter will include such topics as fitting the bicycle to the person and the effects of powder snow and icy snow.

BASIC PRINCIPLES

1. A step/stroke will produce momentum (gliding of the body) proportional to the impulse (SFt = mv) produced. The greater the force-time product, the longer will be the glide, and the fewer the strokes (steps) that will be necessary to traverse a predetermined distance.
2. Maximizing the step/stroke-frequency is dependent upon optimum timing of the next step/stroke prior to losses in speed. This is similar to loss of momentum in gliding action during swimming.
3. Since the base of support is narrower (i.e. skates) or is longer (i.e. skis), equilibrium may be more difficult to maintain. Changes of direction require precise timing in shifting the position of the center of gravity.
4. When executing turns, the greater the arc, that is, the longer the radius of the turn, the greater will be the tangential velocity. This creates problems when executing this turn on a slope.
5. In order to change direction, stop, or start, there must be a change in friction and reaction forces.
6. Waxing changes the surface friction and will facilitate maneuvers on water skis and snow skis. Snow does not pack under the waxed ski but will turn to water and maintain a more laminar flow across the ski bottoms.
7. With every change in body position (or body parts), there is a change in the center of gravity and gravitational line and thus the reactive forces between the ground and the tire or ski will change.

8. The body position influences the form and surface area drag and thus will increase or decrease the velocity of the person.

9. Use of rolling and gliding devices in natural environments results in unexpected changes in the coefficient of friction. For example, snow changing to slush may cause the greater friction and stop the momentum of the ski, catapulting the skier in a forward rotational movement. Likewise, pedaling the bicycle too fast may cause tires to spin on wet pavement and therefore prevent the bicycle from rolling forward.

10. Tactile and kinesthetic sensations may not be recognized as readily when using gliding and rolling devices.

CYCLING

Bicycling

Startling changes occurred in both the bicycle and the riding attire of competitive cyclists at the 1984 Olympic games. Spectators saw aerodynamic helmets, skin-tight clothing, and disc wheels. Truly, the equipment influenced the cycling performances at these Games. Bicycling will never be the same! In addition, there has been a more scientific interfacing of the cyclist to the bicycle. In recent years, for example, numerous studies have been conducted with respect to best saddle height, best pedaling rate, best trunk position, and most effective use of toe clips. Guidelines for the average cyclist have been proposed and published using data from performances of elite cyclists. These guidelines should not be considered as standards, since elite cyclists may have different styles based upon habits, physical characteristics, and other factors. In addition, the pedaling rate, bicycle model, trunk position of rider, and saddle height will vary depending upon the distance of the race, the type of terrain, and the goal of the ride. The biomechanical analyses of these cycling factors are described in the following sections.

Pedaling Position

Movements of the legs during bicycling cause the pedals to move a gear that turns the wheels of the bicycle. The bicyclist varies the handlebar and seat-post (saddle-post) positions to obtain the most effective position for force production and for decreased surface resistance of the trunk. These two effects are accomplished by adjusting the seat post so that it is equal to a near extension at the knee when the leg is in the "down position" (pedal at the lowest point in the circle). A quantitative measure of this saddle height is 107% to 109% of the height of the symphysis pubis from the floor. It has been suggested that the saddle height of 109% is conducive to greater power output, and therefore useful for sprint racing. The height of 107% is better for minimum energy expenditure and for long races. These, of course, are general guidelines only and must be evaluated for each individual. Analysis of actual performance speeds, energy required (fatigue level), and comfort, as well as trial-and-error, will make it possible to determine the optimum saddle height for a given individual. The handlebars are placed in a position to enable the body to lean forward, reducing the hip angle in flexion, which allows the use of the powerful gluteus maximus muscle during cycling. Researchers have shown that there is greater electrical activity in the hip extensors when the cyclist is in this low, crouching position (termed the racing position) than when the cyclist is in the upright-trunk position. That a cyclist is able to exert more force in the racing position than in the upright position has also been substantiated by research in which strain gauges were utilized to measure the forces exerted on the pedals by the feet of the cyclist.

If the cyclist is not cycling in hilly terrain or is not attempting to achieve speed, the upright body position may be the preferred trunk posture. This might be especially true for older persons, persons with kyphosis, or persons who wish to isometrically contract the abdominal muscles while cycling, thereby improving strength in these muscles as a concomitant value. The upright position may also be advocated for persons who have excessive tension in shoulder, neck, and upper back because of habitual work or sport postures. Conversely, the person with low-back pain may prefer the flexed-trunk position to relieve stress to the lumbar region (Fig. 21B-1).

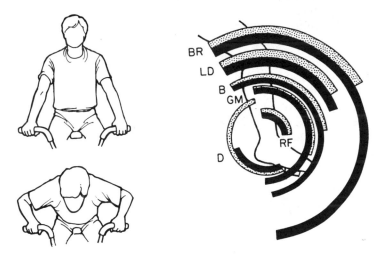

Fig. 21B-1. *Postures and surface areas related to erect and racing cycling positions. The erect position is also a high handlebar position and the racing position is a low handlebar position. The erect position may be likened to sitting in a chair without a backrest. With implications does this have for the muscles of the trunk and the pressure on the spine? How does the reaction forces acting at the hands affect these trunk and spine forces? Note the differences in six muscle contributions during these two riding positions. Although intensities are not known, there is more involvement of these muscles during riding using the high handlebar position (the erect trunk). Is it any wonder the racer uses the flexed trunk position?*

Clips

To increase the speed of cycling, competitors use toe clips. These clips help maintain the foot position on the pedal and enable the leg muscles to apply force during the upward movement of the pedal, as well as during the downward movement. Researchers, however, have shown clips to be more important for effective pushing and stability of foot than actually applying a pulling force.

Air Resistance (Drag)

Although the rolling resistance of bicycle tires can range from one third of a pound to more than 2 $\frac{1}{2}$ pounds, and bicycles can have relative drag forces that differ eightfold, the greatest significant drag component is that of the rider. The human body accounts for 70% of the wind resistance acting on the rider/cycle system while the bicycle accounts for the remaining 30%. The amount of the surface area encountered by the air can be decreased with a lowering of body position. The racing position decreases the frontal area exposed to the air, thus causing lowered frontal air resistance (drag).

MINI-LAB LEARNING EXPERIENCES

Measure the differences in surface area by tracing the shadow of a cyclist in the upright and racing position. Use a photo flood light and paper taped to a wall if indoors; use the sun outdoors. At least 20% greater drag exists in the upright position than in the racing position. In terms of power, the drag force multiplied by the velocity cubed is a reasonable estimation of the amount of power required for cycling.

Calculations can be made placing a cyclist in an instrumented wind tunnel. Values that have been derived with a skier in a wind tunnel are as follows:

The velocity was 8 m/sec; the drag force, in the upright position was 2 N; and the drag force in the racing position 1.5 N. The power output needed to maintain this velocity would be 1024 Nm/sec in the upright position, compared with 768 Nm/sec in the racing position.

Based upon your surface area measurements, would you expect the changes in drag to be greater or less for the bicyclist than the skier?

Another 10% reduction in drag force can be achieved when in a hill-descent position (greater crouch). The greatest reduction in drag, however, can be achieved during drafting. Drafting is the act of riding closely behind another cyclist in order to ride in the artificial tailwind of the other rider. If the drafter has the front wheel within 0.2 m of the rear wheel of the lead rider, wind drag can be reduced 44%. At a 2.0 m wheel gap, the reduction in wind drag is still an appreciable 27%. Implications for such advantages in wind drag relate to pursuit racing; racing times can be reduced and increased speed of the group of cyclists occurs, as the cyclists change "the lead." Only the lead cyclist must work hard; the others can "take a rest." In team competitions, the cyclists will deliberately travel closely behind each other so that only the lead cyclist encounters air resistance relative to the speed of cycling. The other cyclists travel in the wake or draft or each other. This is analogous to traveling in a vacuum.

Cycle Frequency and Speed

Gregor and Rugg have summarized the research findings related to cadences for optimum efficiency during bicycling and they indicate that seven factors influence this cadence. These factors are: type of bicycle used, rider's position, use of toe clips and cleated shoes, speed of riding, gear ratio, physical condition of rider, and rider's perception of exertion. Thus it is obvious that optimum cadence is an individual matter. Data from populations of elite cyclists and recreational cyclists can be used to estimate the range in which a cyclist might most efficiently function. Most studies of noncyclists, recreational cyclists, or persons using a bicycle ergometer preferred pedaling rates between 33 and 80 rpms as their optimum rates. Cadences outside this range were less efficient, since low-pedaling rates require longer durations of contraction (therefore greater energy is required) and high-pedaling rates require ability to produce greater force and power. Elite cyclists prefer cadences of 72 and 102 rpms. Recommended pedaling rates, based upon research of Habert et al. in 1981, are as follows: long-term endurance—80–100 rpm, minimum sprint cadence—110 rpm. The highest reported cadence of a cyclist in their study was 160 rpm.

The Bicycle

The adjustment the cyclist can make in body position as a result of saddle and handlebar positioning, as well as the cycle design itself, influences the level of efficiency of the cyclist. The circular sprocket design of the cycle is not efficient; it has two locations at which the cyclist has difficulty in maintaining force and therefore momentum against the pedals. The beginning cyclist will have several problems. For example, the feet will slip from the pedal, causing the pedals to stop and the cycle to decrease in speed. The results will be a problem in equilibrium if the cycle is one- or two-wheeled. The beginner must be taught to extend the leg through the down position, which is one of the two problem spots. This action of one leg will help the other leg through the second site of inefficient force application, which is the pedal-up position. At this spot, the angles of the segments of the leg are such that leg extension is difficult to initiate. Many researchers are investigating elliptical and other types of sprocket design in order to improve efficiency and/or power.

Friction and Balance

The coefficient of friction between the tires, the supporting surface, and the weight of the cycle will determine how easily the cycle can be accelerated. Low friction and lightweight cycles are the goals for racing. At some point, however, and depending on the skill of the cyclist, lateral stability will become a consideration. If the cyclist has difficulty in balancing a bicycle, a wider-track tire may be required. The three-wheeled cycle used for teaching children to ride has also become popular with older persons who have problems in equilibrium or who wish to use the cycle as a vehicle to carry parcels. This type of vehicle is helpful for persons with neurological problems or strength deficits.

As with walking and running, the speed of locomotion via cyclic rpms is influenced by the power capabilities and efficiency of the performer. Mechanical efficiency varies with speed. There is an optimum speed that will require minimum muscle force to keep the pedals rotating. This muscular force is assisted in the down phase by the weight of the leg. Speeds faster and slower than this optimum speed will require greater muscle force to propel the cycle. To allow for increased speed with minimal muscle force, a series of gear ratios have been built into bicycles. A change in gear ratio will cause the cyclist to pedal several revolutions while transversing only a short distance, thereby sacrificing movement efficiency for a gain in force efficiency. Using the tenth gear of a ten-speed bicycle increases the movement distance of pedaling to ten times that of a first gear to traverse the same distance on the ground. Thus improved efficiency for different types of terrain and different goals is possible with a bicycle with multiple gears.

Pedal Force

Several researchers have instrumented the bicycle pedal and calculated the actual forces exerted by the cyclists upon the pedal. The amount of wasted force and impeding (negative) forces, as well as the positive (effective propelling) forces were identified. The pattern of these forces can be used as criteria for evaluating the skill level of the cyclist, according to Cavanaugh and Sanderson. Pedal force patterns of elite cyclists appear in Fig. 21B-2. Positive and negative impulses are shown in fifteen degree sectors of the crank revolution. During the third and fourth segments from TDC (60–120 degrees) more than half of the total propulsive impulse is applied. Slight negative impulse is noted in the 8th to 11th sectors. In this figure, unused and negative effective forces are diagramed to serve as a criterion diagram for assisting the cyclist in modifying force application. The

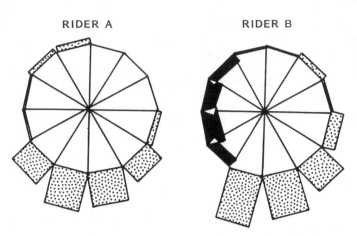

Integral of Unused Positive Force

Integral of Negative Force

RIDER A   RIDER B

Fig. 21B-2. *These pedal force patterns can be used to compare cyclists with respect to effectiveness of application, that is, the amount of effective negative force application and the amount of unused (ineffective) positive force application. Which is the more effective rider? At which areas of the pedal cycle are the riders most effective?*

unused force near the BDC position needs to be reduced. Such pattern analysis is valuable for analyzing left and right symmetry as well, since most riders show different force patterns with their two legs. If large discrepancies are identified, they should be alleviated so that performances can be improved.

Modeling for Safety and Effective Performance

The functions of the human leg during cycling can be modeled as a three-link mechanical system of rigid levers rotating about axes. An example of modeling the thigh, shank, and foot diagrammed with the major muscles as a two-dimensional model appears as Fig. 21B-3. Since the bicycle imposes constraints upon the leg, the movement is almost totally predetermined. Thus, by means of a computer, any saddle height, handlebar position, and anthropometry body configurations, i.e. thigh-shank-foot length, can be modeled and the pedaling action simulated.

The leg then is modeled to move in a circular path. The angle at each joint changes in order to effectively push the pedal with the foot. The vector for the pushing force would be tangential to the circle.

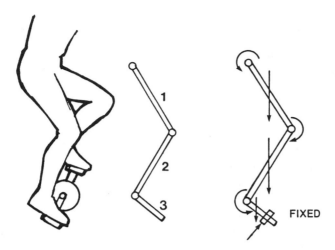

Fig. 21B-3. *Planar model of the leg during cycling using a 3 segment link system. Note that the metatarsal joint has not been modeled; it is considered rigid or of no consequence since the ball of the foot rests on the pedal. Start at the foot and analyze the forces and moments acting on the foot and ankle. Next study the shank, noting the effect of the moment at the ankle upon the shank. Do the same for the thigh and hip. What effect would a faster pedal rate (increases the angular movements of the body segments) have upon joint moments?*

Ranges of motion at the three joints would be approximately 42 degrees at the hip, 73 degrees at the knee, and 25 degrees at the ankle for an average leg. Moments of forces, and force acting at the joints, including muscle forces, can be predicted at selected speeds and gear-ratios if the forces at the pedal are known. For example, the moment at the ankle would be equal to the force at the pedal times the distance from the ankle times the angular acceleration of the foot (provided there is some) times the moment of inertia of the foot. This moment of force at the foot is countered by an equal and opposite moment created by the muscles. A three-dimensional model is useful to determine frontal deviation of the leg and therefore predict stress to the foot or knee soft tissues, such as medial collateral ligaments. The three joints are now assumed to be pin type, rather than the hinge type of the two-dimensional model.

Anatomical characteristics such as bowleggedness, knock-knees, forefoot and rear foot valgus and varus, can be investigated using this model. Muscle forces are used to maintain straight leg alignment. The movement out or in from the straight line of action is considered to be an undesirable deviation, and, if detected, needs to be corrected. Any deviation from this straight line places the force line outside the mid-joint position, thus creating greater stress at these sites. Orthopedic bicycle pedals to allow for anatomical anomalies and correct foot alignment have been developed.

SKATING

Skating requires and builds leg strength and calf and thigh muscles; the quadriceps developing nearly the same amount of strength as the hamstrings. In addition, the pushing-off action of skating work the gluteal muscles. Skating is less traumatizing to the joints than running, and can be used to improve balance and coordination to strengthen the ankles and leg bones and to improve aerobic capacity. Different types of skating techniques are used in different skating events, such as free style (jumps, spins, fancy footwork), figure skating, ice dancing, speed skating, and power skating used in ice hockey. (When skating fast around an ice rink, you are working against centrifugal force.)

Although skating can be considered a form of stepping, its mechanics differ in several ways from those of walking. In ice-skating, the differences are caused by two aspects of the situation: (1) the base of support is much smaller (the width of the skate blade compared to that of the shoe or foot) and (2) the supporting surface offers little resistance to a horizontal push (ice compared to ground or floor). In roller skating, the base is wider, but the lack of friction between the rollers and the supporting surface is comparable to that in ice skating. The major adjustment to this low coefficient of friction for the skater is to always keep the center of gravity over the supporting foot. The center of gravity cannot be allowed to fall ahead, since backward rotational movement and slippage of the foot will result, and balance is likely to be lost.

The muscles involved in skating are the leg extensor muscles, the abdominal muscles, and the arm/shoulder flexor muscles. The leg extensor muscles used in skating are: the gastrocnemius and soleus muscles acting at the ankle joint, the quadriceps femoris muscle group acting at the knee joint, and the gluteus maximus and upper hamstring muscles acting at the hip joint (for pushing the leg back). The hip joint flexor muscles (the rectus femoris, the pectineus, and the illiopsoas) are used to lift the leg and to place the foot on the ice for the forward glide. A strong midsection (the abdominals and the erector spinae) is needed in order to keep the body in the desirable body position (either erect or flexed trunk) and to be able to transfer the force of the arms and legs in order to propel the body forward. A person can skate faster when the legs and trunk are flexed. To facilitate shoulder action and full range of motion of the arms, the following upper body muscles are used: the anterior deltoid, the pectoralis major and minor, the serratus anterior and the trapezius.

Beginning skaters have trouble with balance. Windmilling the arms backward assists in regaining balance, by rotating the lower body backward, which compensates for the forward rotation of the upper body.

Speed skaters use certain techniques to reduce drag, for example, having the upper body flexed almost parallel to the ice to reduce the frontal area, keeping one arm tucked behind the back to reduce the drag, and swinging the other arm to maintain balance. They also wear tight-fitting clothes to keep their body surface smooth.

Power Skating

Power skating is taught especially for use in ice hockey and speed skating. Power skating requires mastering the use of the inside and outside edges of the skate blade and obtaining maximum leg power with minimum work and extraneous motion. Force applied correctly in a short period of time translates into power, which, in turn, is an important component of speed. The power-skating stride segments are divided into the areas of (a) the wind-up, (b) the release, (c) the follow-through, and (d) the return.

The wind-up is the preparation phase of the stride and prepares the skater to push, by digging the blade edge into the ice and pressing the body weight down over the blade edge (coiling). The thrusting leg will provide great power if the edge is digging into the ice at an optimum angle (approximately 45 degrees) ankle roll, and if the leg is strongly flexed to approximately 45 degrees at the knee. The feet are positioned in a "V" formation—toes apart, heels together. For an explosive start, both heels are lifted from the ice so only the front one-third of the inside edges of the blades are touching the ice, and the upper body is angled forward with the legs flexed. The skater actually tries to fall forward while maintaining the body position. For explosiveness, there is no glide phase. Using the blade edges correctly in the wind-up prepares for rapid acceleration.

The release phase is the actual leg thrust in which power is applied. The thrusting leg must drive against the blade edge and must reach to full extension. The legs push (uncoil) quickly to get maximum speed. The thrusting leg pushes on a side and back diagonal. The toe of the thrusting leg points outward (not down) at the finish of the push and very close to the ice surface. The support leg is flexed. Driving hard with the thrusting leg and reaching with the knees achieves power and distance with each stride. The main power of the thrust is provided by the thigh muscles. Rapid leg turnover is essential to an explosive start.

The return is a critical determinant of effectiveness of both the forward stride and the explosive start. The outstretched leg must return quickly, staying close to the ice surface and keeping the toes and knee pointed outward. Keeping the foot close to the ice surface helps keep the center of gravity low so speed will not decrease, and progress can be made in a straight line, which is more effective for speed. Keeping a strong "knee bend" the gliding foot will momentarily meet the returning foot in a "V" position as it sets down on the ice to become the gliding foot. Every push must start with the feet centered under the body.

In a study concerning acceleration in skating, it was found to be more important to place the foot directly underneath rather than in front of the body to aid in the next propulsive phase. This rapid striding pattern generates velocity. Getting a full extension at the knee during the push-off resulted in the ability to cover a greater distance in less time. Also, rapid strides rather than long strides facilitates quickness in skating starts. A higher stride rate, which is greatly related to acceleration and skate time, is also accompanied by a large propulsive angle. The glide phase of the skating stride denotes a deceleration in the horizontal direction; therefore, for a quick start, very little gliding is used. To optimize the magnitude and the direction of propulsion, a low angle of forward body lean, approximately 42 degrees, is desirable.

In ice racing, one of two foot positions is commonly used as the skater is waiting at the starting line for the starting signal. In one, the skates are placed shoulder width apart, one ahead of the other and both at an approximate angle of 40 degrees with the starting line. In the other, the front skate is pointed forward at 90 degrees to the starting line, and the rear skate approaches a parallel position with the starting line. Skaters who use the second position believe that it saves a fraction of a second in the start, since the foot need not be lifted and turned to take the first step.

At the starting signal, the center of gravity is lowered by increasing flexion at the knee and hip. The weight is shifted to the rear foot so that the forward one can be lifted slightly for the first step. With this step, there is extension at the rear knee and hip. For a brief time, the center of gravity falls ahead of the supporting foot; this is possible because the angle of the skate resists the backward push of gravity and the extension continues until the rear limb is straight and inclined approximately 45 degrees from the horizontal. After a short step, the front foot has in the meantime been placed on the ice and angled, as was the rear foot. The rear foot now steps. This type of stepping continues for three or four strides, each stride increasing in length over the previous one. During the beginning strides, the arms move as they do in running, in opposition to the lower-limb movements.

After the starting strides, the weight is carried over the front foot. As the rear foot pushes, it does not affect equilibrium. As the push from the ice is applied to the body a low center of gravity is advantageous. After the push, as the supporting foot glides, the rear foot is brought forward; as it passes the gliding foot, it takes the weight of the body. The push will have a sideward, as well as backward, component. The former component should be minimized by placing the skate, as it takes the weight, in a forward direction and close to the other foot as it begins the glide.

The Skating Stride. Ice skating is biphasic, with each stride consisting of alternate periods of single support and double support. In speed skating, the period of single support is the glide phase and propulsion occurs during the double-support phase. In a hockey start, as in power skating, propulsion occurs during the single support. Because of the resistive forces of drag and friction, the body will tend to accelerate when a propulsive force is being applied and will decelerate during the glide phase. In a study by Marino and Weese, it was revealed that the ice-skating stride consists of two functional phases: (a) glide during the single support, (b) propulsion during single and double support, beginning halfway through the single-support phase and lasting through the end of the double-support phase. In the technique of the skating stride, a long single-support time is related to relatively slow skating time and with a low rate of acceleration. A high stride rate was commensurate with fast skating time and a high rate of acceleration.

The mechanics of the skating action change somewhat with respect to the length of the race. Filmstrips were prepared in 1962 by Freisinger, the 1964 Olympic team coach. He showed that in the 500-meter race the trunk is slightly above the horizontal, whereas in the longer races it is horizontal. Additionally, in the short-distance race, alternating flexion and extension of the spine is seen. At the end of the push, one limb is well back of the gliding foot, and the trunk is fully extended. At this instance trunk and limb balance each other over the supporting limb like two ends of a teeterboard.

Marino investigated the factors that determine high acceleration rates obtained in the ice-skating start. Although the regression equation for the relationship between technique variables and acceleration showed a multiple correlation of only 0.78, the following factors were identified as forming the ideal skating start pattern: High stride rate, significant forward lean, low takeoff angle, and placement of the recovery foot directly under the body at the end of the single-support phase.

The form (shape) of the body influences the magnitude of drag in a similar fashion to that of bicycling. The surface area encountering the air will create resistance that the skater must overcome with muscle force.

Stopping

There are many different techniques for stopping in skating. All of the different stopping positions consist of leaning the body backward and digging (sliding) the blades into the ice causing an increase in friction.

Spinning, Turning, and Twisting in Skating

The moment of inertia is the smallest about the horizontal axis and can be increased by extending the arms or legs or by flexing at the waist. A skater spins faster if the arms and legs are close and tight to the body. Positions of arms and legs, i.e., planting the foot out to the side to provide an effective push-off for turning, and swinging the arms horizontally in the direction of the turn/twist, provide torques needed to initiate spins. Raising the arms overhead will increase the rate of spin. Unfolding the arms or a leg to the side while spinning will bring about a deceleration.

MINI-LAB LEARNING EXPERIENCES

Estimate the differences in surface area drag as follows:

Place a flood light (any bright light with a wide area of dispersement) behind a person standing several feet in front of a wall. Estimate the surface area of the shadow on the wall of the person as varying skating positions are taken (actual measurements can be taken if paper is taped to the wall and the shadow traced.) Another method is to videotape or photograph the shadows, and measure the projected image.

Figure Skating

Basic Fig. skating is the utilization of medial and lateral and inside and outside edges of the skates. The inside edge is always toward the center of the curve and may be the medial or lateral edge depending upon the situation. Skating in a curved path involves one medial and lateral edge, whereas fixing the skates in one position requires both medial edges or a flat blade (no edging).

The toe of the skate is used to create friction, and thus a change in direction and/or reduction in speed. Detailed exploration of edging and changes in friction are included in the skiing section.

Roller Skating

Although research does not exist concerning roller skating skills, the information given with respect to ice-skating can be used as a basic foundation for the analysis and improvement of roller skating skills.

Skiing

Skiing is a form of locomotion within a relatively frictionless environment. In many ways, then, it is similar to roller skating, ice-skating and water-skiing, in which the gear attached to the feet slides, or rolls, along the supporting surface. Therefore, skiing becomes a sport in which it is paramount that the skier control the direction and magnitude of the sliding of the skis. This control (or regulation) of the slide is a matter of balance and steering.

Effect of Steepness of Slope on Movement

What is the optimum slope angle for executing skiing techniques? Is one slope best for all skill levels? Once again, an understanding of the movement situation may be acquired by means of a free body diagram in which all the forces are identified. Before motion begins, there are two major forces acting: body weight (gravity) and friction. Additionally, there are two forces that react to body weight and friction (termed reaction forces). These forces with respect to zero slope (level ground) are depicted in Fig. 21B-4. Notice that there is no propulsive force because gravity acts at right angles to the ground. Therefore, the skier would have to exert an additional force—for example, pole plant and push—to initiate movement. Friction is equal to the coefficient of friction times the normal force. The normal force in this case of zero slope is equal to body weight.

Definition alterations in force occur with the introduction of an incline or slope (Fig. 21B-5). As the slope increases, the normal force is now that component of the body weight which is perpendicular to the slope. Since the normal force decreases, the force of friction also decreases. Movement is therefore facilitated and will occur with less

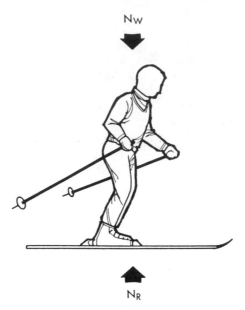

Fig. 21B-4. *Contourogram of natural gliding posture of skier. Free body diagram of forces applied when slope is level and skier is stationary. (Nw, Normal force of body weight; Nr, normal reaction force.)*

resistance or opposition than on a level surface. In addition, there is a component of body weight acting parallel to the slope. This component is termed the propulsive force because it causes the skier to be accelerated down the slope. This propulsive force increases in direct proportion to the increase in the slope. A skier, then, will have an acceleration in direct relationship to the slope of the hill. The analysis of skiing is another example of the necessity for resolving one force vector into pertinent components, in this case with respect to the slope of the hill.

The optimum slope for skiing will vary with the individual and the techniques to be performed. There must be a propulsive force to

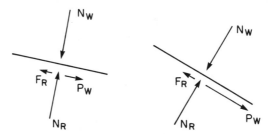

Fig. 21B-5. *Free body diagram representing magnitude and types of forces acting on a skier under two different inclinations of the ski slope. (Nw, Normal force; Fr, friction force; Pw, propulsive force; Nr, reaction force.) Some portion of the body weight vector (not shown) constitutes the normal force and the other portion is in the propulsive force. Calculate these portions knowing that the slopes are 10 degrees and 20 degrees respectively.*

668   *THE BIOMECHANICS OF HUMAN MOVEMENT*

cause motion, but this force must not be so great that the body accelerates so rapidly that the person panics or does not have time to react and execute desired techniques. A slope that is too gentle is less dangerous, although equally difficult in terms of performance, than a slope that is too steep.

Concomitantly, one cannot disregard the type of snow and the surface of the skis. The interaction of these two materials produces a coefficient of friction that affects movement on a slope. An excellent treatise on this subject has been published as a result of the Winter Olympics in Sapporo, Japan, and the concern for maximizing the snow conditions for that event. The advent of indoor areas, artificial snow machines, and other advanced technology could result in ideal conditions for enhancing performance of both the beginning and the competitive skier.

Too often the environment is ignored by the analyst of animal and human movement. Snow skiing, waterskiing, and surfboarding are excellent examples of activities in which the environment plays a dominant role in the success of the performer. Throughout this book an effort has been made to show the importance of the environment in mechanical and anatomic considerations. Truly the best performer is in harmony with the environment.

Balance

Persons are more stable on skis over packed snow than on shoes having the same type of surface as skis, since the base of support of skis is three to six times longer than that of shoes. This greater stability on skis is primarily in the anteroposterior direction, which is an asset when a skier is sliding down a steep slope. Keeping the skis apart, about hip width, will provide greater lateral stability than placing the skis together. This wide position, called wide tracking, places the hips directly above the knees and the knees directly above the feet, thus ensuring that there will be equal weight on both skis and that the line of gravity of the skier will be midway between the skis when the skier is going down the fall line (line of the slope that is the most direct). The weight of the body is distributed on the whole of both feet, the skis are flat, and the body is in a "natural position." This position places the center of gravity of the body lower than does the erect standing posture, thus increasing stability of the body. The term "natural position" means that the body segments are slightly flexed and thus able to respond easily to bumps and other changes in the terrain or the changes in the snow. This semiflexed position of the legs allows further flexion and also extension. The body faces squarely in the direction of travel, and it is in a state of differential relaxation; that is, only a minimal number of essential muscles are contracting, and these muscles are contracting minimally.

Turning on skis, walking on level ground, stepping around, and climbing the slope all necessitate transference of the line of gravity from between the skis to a position over one ski. The shift of body weight should involve as little modification as possible in the trunk, arm, or leg positions, since the shift is a lateral shift of the total body. Fundamental to being able to achieve skill in skiing is the ability to change the body weight line (line of gravity) from one ski to the other, and from one ski to both skis. The achievement of this ability, known as dynamic balance, can be fostered by placing the skier in situations that require combinations of single and double balance conditions. Thus dynamic balance may be practiced in such situations as stepping out (walking) at the end of a straight run (descent down the fall line), deliberately lifting one ski and then the other while in a straight run, and executing two steps to the side and back again during a straight run.

Steering

Steering refers to turning or changing direction of the slide of the skis. Since a turn requires greater movement of the tail of the ski than of the ski tip, the sliding action of a turn is also called skidding. Short skis, or the graduated ski-length method (GLM) will provide greater success in learning the technique of skidding than will long skis. The reason is that longer skis will have a greater radius and greater arc of turn for the same angle of turn. There also is more time to commit errors, and greater centrifugal force is developed when long skis are used than when short skis are used.

Regardless of what length ski is used, the wedge, or V position, is recommended to facilitate turning. This position presets each ski at an angle to the fall line, thus creating a turning angle. Shifting the weight from the center of the V to one ski will cause the skier to execute a turn in the direction of the ski tip. A series of turns can be executed by alternately shifting body weight from a position above one ski to above the other ski. The speed and magnitude of the turn are dependent on the slope, snow, duration of single ski support, and edging, that is, tilting the ski so that one edge penetrates the snow while the other edge is elevated.

Edging and Moments of Force

When skis are in the traverse position (across the slope), they will tend to slide down the fall line if they are flat. The cause is the effect of gravity, which translates the skis as a unit. The speed of the slide will be directly related to the steepness of the slope and inversely related to the amount of friction between the ski and the snow. The friction is affected by such factors as the type and temperature of the snow and the type of wax used. In addition, the direction and speed of the slide can be regulated by the position of the line of gravity of the skier with respect to the ski length and to the amount of edging of the skis. If the skis are flat and the body weight is shifted forward, this places the line of gravity forward in relation to the balance point of the skis and creates a moment of force, causing the tips to rotate downward. By the same reasoning, if the skis are flat and the skier leans backward, the tails will rotate downward. In both instances, the results are caused by the creation of a moment of force. An analogy could be made to loading one end of a teeterboard with more weight than the other end. The weighted end rotates downward and the lighter end goes upward. (See Fig. 21B-6.)

The introduction of ski edging, however, creates a reactive force than can be greater than the moment of force produced by body weight. Thus edging the skis while leaning backward increases the friction on the tails, which prevents their rotation and causes the tips of the skis to rotate downward. Forward lean with ski edging causes the tails to rotate downward. (See Fig. 21B-7). Thus it is evident that the skilled skier has learned to create the precise moment of force required for a turn by regulating the amount of edging and shifting the line of gravity in the anteroposterior plane of the body.

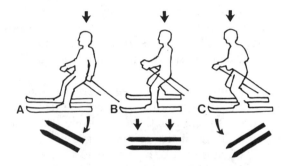

Fig. 21B-6. *Effect of shift of body weight upon flat skis set across the ski slope. A, Backward shift causes ski tails to slide down slope faster than tips producing a clockwise rotation; B, Balanced position causes skis to slide down slope in a parallel position; C, Forward shift causes ski tips to slide down slope faster than tails producing a counterclockwise rotation. The change in friction is the primary factor explaining these movements.*

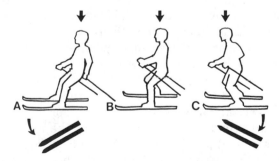

Fig. 21B-7. *Effect of shift of body weight upon edged skis set across the ski slope. A, Backward shift causes ski tips to slide faster; B, Balanced position prevents sliding; C, Forward shift causes ski tails to slide faster. The change in reaction force is the primary factor explaining these movements or lack of movement.*

ROLLING AND SLIDING BLADES   **671**

Methods of Initiating Turns

The three major methods for initiating a turn, that is, shifting the weight and rotating the skis, are (1) rotation of body parts, (2) use of the external environment, and (3) unweighting. The anatomical, mechanical, and environmental considerations for each will be presented. There usually is more than one biomechanically correct way of performing a skill. There probably, however, is one optimum way for a given set of constraints (environment included).

Rotation of Body Parts. Almost any body part can be used to initiate a turn. Rotations at the shoulder, spinal column, hip, knee, and ankle are executed in a direction counter to the turn and then in the direction of the desired turn. These actions are similar to the preparation, coiling, or backswing of many throwing movements. Each rotation can be forceful enough and can be in the correct direction to cause turning. Knee steering (rotation at the knee) has two advantages over all the other rotations: 1) The knee is at an equal distance between the center of gravity of the body and the ski. Thus the rotation at the knee is easy to control and does not displace the line of gravity excessively. 2) The knee is an important joint in the balance phases of walking. Therefore, the use of the knee for locomotion is familar.

Likewise, rotation of the feet (heel thrust or foot steering) is an effective means of producing a turn because the feet are used in walking. Although closer to the ski than the knee, the foot has the disadvantage of being far from the center of gravity of the body. In addition, the range of motion at the ankle is limited, as is the force. Some persons, therefore, have difficulty in performing the heel thrust technique. The heel thrust, however, is useful in deep-powder snow and advanced turns and usually is combined with the method of unweighting.

Arm and trunk rotations, initiated by movements at the shoulder, hip and spinal column, will cause the skis to turn if the action is forceful enough. This necessity for force, acceleration, and large motions is a source of "overturning" and loss of control. Why is loss of control apt to be more prevalent with this method than the others? When the trunk is moved, approximately half the body weight is being moved. Usually the line of gravity is displaced a greater distance than necessary, thus causing the turn to be greater than 90 degrees and inhibiting the second turn or causing a straight run backwards.

Use of External Environment. A bump, or mogul, may be used to effectively initiate a turn. The ski tips or the area under the feet can be used as a pivot point as the terrain elevates tips, tails, or both from the snow. Change in body lean or the use of knee steering or heel thrusts can produce the pivot. Release of the edges of the skis may be the only action necessary to have an effective turn on a mogul.

The use of one or both poles may produce a turn. The friction between the ski and the snow may be decreased by transfering some of the body weight to the pole, or it may be eliminated altogether by transfering all of the body weight to two poles. The initial pole plant is nearly vertical but downhill from the position of the feet, so that the most effective reaction forces can be attained.

Underweighting. There are two types of unweighting: up-unweighting and down-unweighting. Each has its use; although many beginning skiers find up-unweighting to be a more familiar or natural movement. In both cases the principle underlying the method is that the acceleration of the body mass can create a force that reduces the normal force, thus decreasing the reaction of the skis with the snow and decreasing the resistance to turning.

$$F = ma + BW$$

If the acceleration is fast enough, the person can completely unweight, that is, have zero force between the snow and skis. This can occur without the skier becoming airborne. Acceleration of body mass is an outcome of rapid flexion or extension at the knee. The hips, trunk, and arms maintain their position of the line of gravity. The unweighting method makes it possible to turn with the skis in the wide-tracking (parallel) position.

$$F = Bw - ma = 0$$

The up-unweighting technique consists of an acceleration of the body due to leg extension. There is an initial overweighting followed by an unweighting as the legs reach the extended position (Fig. 21B-8). The turn must be executed in the latter part of the upward movement of the body, when the friction is least. This fact, and the fact that, in general, upward movements are thought to be lifting, or unweighting, movements, probably are the reasons that beginners more easily learn to turn with this method than with the down-unweighting method.

The down-unweighting technique (Fig. 21B-8) creates an unweighting in the initial part of the movement. Therefore the turn must be executed in the early part of the downward movement. If the turn is attempted later, as in up-unweighting, the reaction force is greater than body weight, and friction has increased proportionately, causing great difficulty and possibly producing no success in turning. Timing, or fast reaction time, is the key factor to success with this technique. Since the down-unweighting technique utilizes gravity and has the potential for attaining greater acceleration than is possible with unweighting, down-unweighting can be a more effective and efficient turning technique.

General Concepts. Turns may be executed from the wedge, stem (one ski in partial wedge position), and parallel positions. The method of turn is dependent on the steepness of the slope, the type of snow, the radius of turn desired, the speed of turn, and the skill of the skier.

ROLLING AND SLIDING BLADES 673

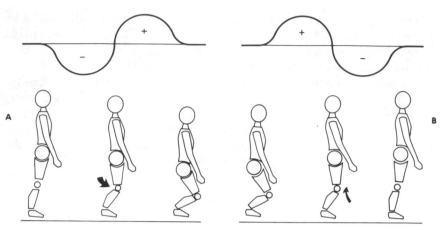

Fig. 21B-8. *Effect of fast flexion movements (down-unweighting in skiing) and fast extension movements (up-unweighting in skiing) upon ground reaction forces. These force-time histories were obtained from a force platform recording system. The horizontal line is the body weight line, also termed the body weight reference, and extends as a time continuum. The + depicts the positive impulse produced by the duration and magnitues of forces greater than body weight. The − depicts the negative impulse produced by forces less than body weight. A, Negative and positive impulses occurred in that order during flexion at the ankle, knee, and hip. B, Positive and negative impulses occurred in that order during extension at the ankle, knee, and hip. Since A represents down-unweighting and B represents up-unweighting it is readily apparent that the down-unweighting style of skiing turn must be initiated earlier than the up-unweighting style.*

Wedges and stems provide a slowing-down capability useful on steep slopes or difficult terrain. Edging, whether in parallel position or not, will reduce the skier's speed.

Human beings tend to be asymmetric, that is, they perform a turn more succcessfully in one direction than in the other. Leg dominance with respect to balance usually determines the preferred turning direction. Turns are easier to perform when the skier is going fast and is close to the fall line. However, the acceleration rate and ultimate speed that can be tolerated by both the skier's leg muscles and mind will determine the skier's need to check speed by stemming, edging, or deviating from the fall line. The larger the radius of rotation of the turn, the greater the speed and centrifugal force created—and, therefore, the more difficult it will be for the skier to remain in control of the turn. The major danger is that the skier will be unable to turn from the fall line to complete the turn started by a traverse. The reason is that centrigual forces causes the skier to "fly off at a tangent," that is, to continue in the tangential velocity at the midpoint of the turn, which is the fall line position (Fig. 21B-9). Large-radius turns on steep slopes should not be attempted by beginning skiers because they will not be able to adjust their speed appropriately and soon enough.

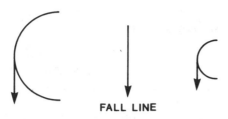

FALL LINE

Fig. 21B-9. *The tangential velocity of a skier is dependent upon the radii of the turn all other conditions being kept constant. As the radius of the turn increases the magnitude of the tangential velocity in the direction of the fall line (direct line down) the slope increases.*

SURFBOARDING

Balance, or attaining a position or a series of positions of equilibrium on the surfboard, is the first skill in acquiring surfboarding expertise. Practice in still water and in a towing situation before beginning small-wave surfboarding will allow the person to realize similarities between the principles of equilibrium specified for walking, running, standing, and other land locomotion patterns and those utilized in surfboarding.

A low center of gravity produces greater equilibrium. A change in vertical position of the center of gravity should be made without horizontal displacement when moving from the kneeling position to the standing position. The line of gravity is kept near the midpoint of the base of support to provide the greatest distance for adjustments. The feet are positioned slightly more than hip width apart to provide control of the front and rear of the board without excess movement of the feet. The feet are set in a forward and backward stride position to provide control of the hydroplaning of the board. Lateral stability is achieved by a lateral spread of the feet approximately hip width apart. When riding the crest of a wave that elevates the surfboarder and the board, the surfboarder will lower the center of gravity by assuming a semi-squatting position.

Depending on the weight of the surfboarder and the length, width, weight, and design of the board, the position of the surfboarder will be forward or in back of an average position. This average position, the riding position, is closer to the rear of the board than to the front of the board. It is the position that allows the surfboarder to keep the "nose" of the board above water, which produces a hydroplaning effect comparable to that of the skis in powder snow. Any displacement of the tips of the skis or nose of the surfboard below the surface level causes the snow or water to act as additional drag and will stop or decrease the motion of the tips while the body and remainder of skis or board continue to move and are rotated upward. This action plunges the ski tips or board nose deeper and causes the person to fall or capsize.

ROLLING AND SLIDING BLADES 675

To keep the correct degree of hydroplaning, walking on the board is necessary as the velocity and height of the wave diminish. The board must be positioned to ride the wave and not to prevent the leading edge (nose or side) from plunging under water. Once the surfboard is positioned correctly, the surfboarder glides just as on snow skis. A turn is executed according to the basic principles of motion in a curved path.

The feet are placed with the rear foot at right angles to the line of the board, while the leading foot remains in the direction of the board. This stance resembles the fencing stance. To execute a turn, the person counterrotates toward the rear of the surfboard and then, using hip, knee, and foot steering as described in the section on snow skiing, rotates in the direction of the tip of the board. Once set, the surfboarder adjusts balance with body lean and rotation while maintaining contact with both feet, especially the ball of the rear foot.

Basic biomechanical principles may be more important to the surfboarder than to athletes on land, since the former must shift body weight in response to a moving environment that is also the base of support. The water and waves are a constantly changing medium that would be difficult to understand without formulating some general principles about motion and forces. The waves are not repetitive; each is different in height, direction, and place of occurrence. The surfboarder must "read" the waves and adjust the position of the surfboard by shifting the line of gravity right, left, forward, or backward, depending on the crest and direction of the wave with respect to the surfboard. In addition, the environment represents a four-surface frictional environment. The coefficient of friction between the feet and the surfboard and the coefficient of friction between the surfboard and the water may be two very different values. This difference, as well as the newness of the skill, often causes beginning surfboarders to experience muscle aches and "cramps" resulting from excessive tension in the muscles of the lower extremities, especially the feet.

SKATEBOARDING

Surfboarding and skateboarding appear to have several similarities, but there are also several major differences. The balancing techniques and shifting of weight front, back, right, and left are similar. When a performer is executing a turn, both activities utilize the same type of body position, the "C" shape. See Fig. 2-6. This position also is commonly used in snow skiing and waterskiing. The major differences between surfboarding and skateboarding are the greater speeds achieved by skateboarders and the static environment of the ground used for skateboarding. Speeds of 100 kmph have been recorded for skateboarding competitors. Such speeds allow a person to skate around the inside of a cylinder, becoming upside down during the mid-point of the loop. At such speeds, the potential for serious injury exists if the person loses control and falls. Elbow and knee pads, wrist and hand protection, and helmets are some of the devices necessary to the safety of skateboard competitors. Should the body weight shift quickly to one or two wheels, causing a proportionately greater friction on these wheels than on the other wheels, turns can occur. If the friction is too great, these wheels will be prevented from rotating and will "lock," thus causing the person to be catapulted from the skateboard at the velocity achieved before the wheels stopped. This is another instance in which the safety of the performer is dependent not only on performance but on equipment as well.

BOBSLED

The sport of bobsled is the only sliding event in which the athletes travel downhill in a seated position. Two- and four-person teams ride in a large sled down a banked track which is usually close to one mile in length. The sled can weigh anywhere from 300 to 500 pounds (not counting the weight of the athletes) and can reach speeds in excess of 90 mph. In some of the sharper turns on the course, the athletes may experience forces up to five times that of their body weight. The average amount of time required by a bobsled team to complete a one mile run is one minute, which means that the average speed of the slide is 60 mph.

The bobsled is made of steel with fiberglass cowling to provide an aerodynamic form. It is articulated in the middle such that the rear of the sled can rotate slightly on the long axis relative to the front of the sled. There are four blades beneath the sled, and the front blades pivot slightly, providing the driver with the ability to steer the sled. The rear blades are fixed. Steering is accomplished by pulling on one of two handles connected to either side of the front "axle" by means of an aircraft cable. Braking is accomplished in much the same way as it is on a child's race car buggy. The designated sledder (brakeman) pulls up on the handle of a lever, which has a row of shark-like teeth on the opposite end. The teeth simply bite into the ice to slow the sled.

The brakeman pushes the sled via push-bars which protrude from the rear of the sled. These bars are part of the steel framework and do not change position throughout the run. The driver (and passengers in the four-person event) pushes on a single bar which protrudes from the side of the sled and then retracts into the cowling once the driver is in the sled. Retracting this bar insures that no objects protrude from the sled and that the aerodynamic properties are maintained.

The sledders are able to push the sled on ice because of a unique type of shoe which they wear. The front half of the sole of this shoe looks very similar to the nylon portion of a velcro surface. There are hundreds of long thin spikes which enable the sledders to run on ice almost as well as on concrete. The remainder of the uniform consists of a skin-tight suit which may have several layers of padding underneath. In addition, the sledders wear a helmet which is very similar in nature to a motorcycle helmet.

In order to insure fair competition between sledders, each sled is required to have its blades below a specified temperature (dependent upon outdoor temperature) at the time of the start. Warm blades provide an unfair advantage via a decrease in blade/ice friction, and their detection results in the elimination of that sled from competition. This condition also applies to all other sliding events.

The event starts when the athletes push the sled through a starting gate. In the two-person event, (Fig. 21B-10), the brakeman pushes the sled from behind while the driver pushes from the side. In the four-person event, the driver is joined on the sides by two passengers. As in other sliding events such as luge, the start in bobsled is one of the major determinants of performance and must be perfectly executed. Because of the large mass of the sled, bobsled athletes must be large, strong, and fast. In addition, they need to coordinate their efforts with other team members.

The athletes push the sled until they approach their maximum sprinting speed. At this point, they board the sled and assume a low-profile position. The driver then has the responsibility of guiding the sled down the track, keeping it off the walls and as low as possible on the turns. The event ends when the sled crosses the finish gate. The sledders are in tremendous danger if the driver loses control of

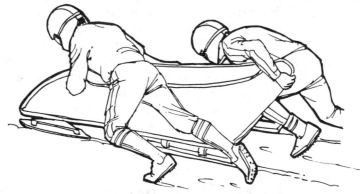

Fig. 21B-10. *A world-class driver and brakeman perform a start in the 2-man bobsled event. The brakeman is behind the sled and the driver is on the side. Measure the angles of each leg thrust in support of one aspect of their skill in starting. Note the aerodynamically designed bobsled and headgear. (Courtesy of James Richards)*

THE BIOMECHANICS OF HUMAN MOVEMENT

the sled and it overturns. When this happens, the sledders may end up rolling around a narrow channel of ice with a 500-pound sled at speeds greater than 60 mph. Broken bones and severe lacerations (from the ice) are not uncommon during this type of occurrence.

Research in the sport of bobsled is focused in two primary areas: sled design and start technique. Scientists in the areas of engineering and biomechanics are currently trying to surpass old competition records by applying the latest technologies to this event.

The sled design efforts currently underway focus on four areas. These are: (1) reducing the longitudinal friction of the blades, (2) increasing the steering capabilities, (3) safety, and (4) reducing the wind resistance of the sled and riders. Researchers are performing extensive wind-tunnel tests in order to accomplish the latter goal. Major design changes are being made to the cowl (the covering over the front of the sled), the push bars, and the blade housings in order to minimize friction from the wind.

Biomechanists are working with instrumented sleds in an effort to measure and optimize forces exerted on the sled by the athletes during the starts. As with most other sports, success in the starts has been found to be heavily dependent upon technique and upon the coordination of efforts between team members. And, although the start represents a very simple mechanical problem (producing a maximum acceleration on a constant mass), the large mass of the sled and the fact that the performance is on ice dictates that the forces exerted during the start have to be precisely directed and controlled. (See Fig. 21B-11.)

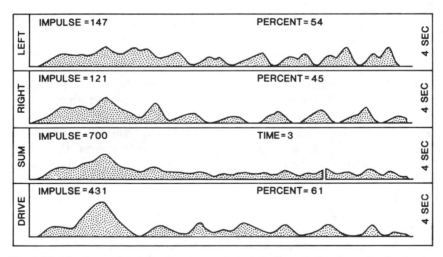

Fig. 21B-11. *A graph of the forces produced on the starting bars by the brakeman (left and right upper graphs), the driver (bottom graph), and the sum of both (graph above the driver's graph). The percent value in the driver's graph represents 61% of the team impulse, whereas it is more typical among world-class teams that the brakeman exerts that amount. The symmetry of the right and left force production of the brakeman can be evaluated. (Courtesy of James Richards)*

LUGE

The sport of luge involves a sledder maneuvering down a channel of ice characterized by extremely sharp turns and high arching banks. The event consists of both, one- and two-person teams for men, and single-sledder events for women. The sledder travels through a frozen maze while lying on his/her back on top of a 50-pound sled, which may reach speeds of greater than 60 miles per hour at various points throughout the run. The object of the sport is simple: travel the entire track, from top to bottom, in as short a time as possible.

There are several factors involved in accomplishing this objective. First, the sledder must have an effective start. This provides the sledder with a high initial velocity on the track which, when all other factors are accounted for, results in a fast finish time. Second, the sledder must minimize wind resistance while riding the sled by adopting and maintaining an efficient sliding position. Third, the sledder must have a "clean" run; that is, no part of the body should touch the ice at any time. In addition, the sledder must stay low in the turns, as this has the effect of shortening the track. A sledder who stays low in the turns will have a shorter distance to ride than a sledder who takes the turns high. Finally, the sledder must have equipment which is technologically competitive with the rest of the world. The sled should have an efficient aerodynamic design and offer minimum resistance to the ice surface. In addition, it must also have very controllable and predictable steering qualities. The uniform which the sledder wears must provide some degree of protection while at the same time offering a minimum amount of wind resistance to the rider. This is currently a skin-tight glossy Lycra suit with booties and a low-profile helmet with a visor.

The sled itself consists of a semi-rigid framework which encompasses two steel blades and a fiberglass pod on which the sledder lies. The overall structure resembles a high-tech version of an old recreational sled, except that it is much heavier and aerodynamically designed. The blades mounted on the sled are slight convex, such that only a few inches of the blade are in contact with the ice at any time. This design allows the sledder to steer the sled by "bending" the frame. For example, if the sledder pushes down on the sled simultaneously with his/her right shoulder and left leg, the sled will steer to the right. Pressing with the left shoulder and right leg will subsequently result in steering the sled to the left.

All of the equipment components of luge must be optimized in order for the sledder to achieve competitive results. The aerodynamic properties of the sled and sledder as well as the frictional properties of the sled play an extremely important role in the success of the sledder. In addition, the steering properties of the sled, governed by the flexibility of the frame and the design of the blades, must fit the style of the sledder in order to insure a clean run and a fast time on the track.

The human element in luge is the additional obvious factor which accounts for a sledder's success or failure. The sledder in the sport of luge must perform three primary tasks. These are: (1) produce a maximum starting velocity, (2) accurately steer the sled down the track, and (3) maintain an efficient aerodynamic profile throughout the entire run down the track. Of these three tasks, the generation of a maximum starting velocity may be the most difficult for many sledders to perform.

The luge start is performed with the sledder in a seated position on the sled, facing the run and positioned between a set of starting bars. The starting bars are large handles attached to the track which allow the sledder to overcome his/her inertia by pulling and then pushing out of the starting gate. The race does not start when the sledder leaves the starting bars but rather several meters later; therefore, the sledder is already moving when the timing of the race begins. The object is to enter the first timing photocell with as high a speed as possible and to maintain a maximum speed throughout the course. Because of this, the speed reached at the start plays a major role in determining how fast the sledder can complete the rest of the run.

Based upon research performed on the luge start, the start consists of two separate phases: a pull phase and a push phase. (See Fig. 21B-12.) The pull phase is the power phase and accounts for approximately 75% of the impulse (and thus velocity) generated at the start. The push phase, as well as the transition into the push phase (from the pull), accounts for the remaining 25% of the starting impulse. In addition, researchers indicated that the start, despite its simplistic appearance, is extremely technique-dependent. Carefully designed technique changes employed by several members of the United States National Luge team accounted for as much as a 20% increase in starting velocity during the 1986–87 season.

Additional research in the sport of luge centers around the design of the sled and the clothing worn by the sledder. Wind tunnels have been utilized in order to test the aerodynamic qualities of different

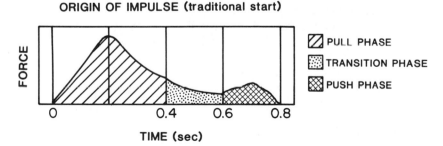

Fig. 21B-12. *A typical force pattern created by a luger on the starting bars. Note that the pull phase has the greatest impulse and is the primary determinant of success of the start. (Courtesy of James Richards)*

ROLLING AND SLIDING BLADES   **681**

sled designs as well as varying styles of helmets and face shields. In addition, wind-tunnel experiments centering around various types of fabric to be worn by the sledders have been conducted.

MINI-LAB LEARNING EXPERIENCES

1. Using a bicycle, skis, skateboard, skates, tobaggan, or other gliding device, in an appropriate environment, perform the following:
   A. Glide in a straight line and experiment with various body positions. Describe the balanced position of the body that appears to be best. State why.
   B. Assume different amounts of lateral lean of the body when gliding in a curved path at three designated speeds: slow, moderate, and fast.
   C. Estimate the amount of lean possible for each of the speeds, and discuss the basic principles involved in the determination of lean.
2. Take a small toy car or truck and attach a weight to the front.
   a. Push the weighted car down an incline.
   b. Describe the path of the car.
3. Repeat step 2, changing the weight from the front to (a) the rear, (b) the right, and (c) the left. Describe what happens to the path of the car for each situation and explain the reason or reasons.
4. Study Fig. 21B-13 and explain the following:
   a. The forces acting on the skier;
   b. The relationship of radius of the turn and the magnitude of these forces acting on the skier;
   c. The magnitude of the displacement of the center of gravity outside the base of support with respect to speed and radius of turn.
5. Apply the information in this chapter to the following sports:
   1. Cross Country Skiing
      a. differences with respect to walking
      b. differences with respect to slope
   2. Ski Jumping
      a. determine the velocity at takeoff.
      b. compare differences in drag with respect to different body configurations
6. Ski Jumping
   a. Determine the velocity at takeoff.
   b. Compare differences in drag with respect to different body configurations.

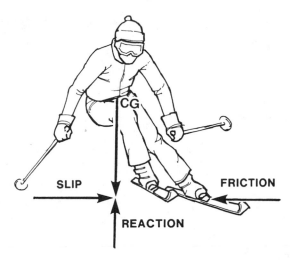

Fig. 21B-13. *A down hill skier on a giant slalom course. Note the force vectors superimposed as a free-body diagram of the kinetics to be considered at this instant in time. (Courtesy Sports Information Office Washington State University)*

REFERENCES

Brancazio, P. (1984) *Sport Science*, New York: Simon & Schuster.
Burke, E. (1984) *The Science of Cycling*, Champaign, IL: Human Kinetics.
Emmert, W. (1984) The Slap Shot, *National Strength and Conditioning Journal*, Apr–May, 4.
Faria, I., Cavanagh, P. (1978) *The physiology and biomechanics of cycling.* New York: John Wiley and Sons.
Hahn, M. R. (1980) A kinematic analysis of selected body segments during the start in luge, unpublished masters thesis, University of Illinois at Urbana-Champaign.
Howe, J. (1987) *Skiing Mechanics*, Laporte, CO: Poudre Press.
Leonardi, L. M., DalMonte, A., Faina, M., and Rabazzi, E. (1982) Quantitative and qualitative measurement of the force exerted on a bobsled in the push-off phase. First results, Proceedings, XXII World Congress of Sports Medicine, Vienna.
Marino, W. (1983) "Selected Mechanical Factors Associated with Acceleration in Ice Skating", *Research Quarterly for Exercise and Sport*, Vol. 54(3), Sept.
Marino, G. W. & Weese, R. G. (1979) Systematic Analysis of the Ice Skating Stride, *Science in Skiing, Skating, & Hockey*, J. Terauds, Ed., Del Mar, CA: Academic Publishers.
Official American Ski Technique (1966) Professional Ski Instructors of America, Inc., Salt Lake City.
Paul, J. C. (1986) Progress in bobsled technology. *The Bobsledder*, 3(1), fall.
Richards, J., Tyler, J., Walter, J., Lapham, E., and Higgs, C. (1986) An analysis of forces involved in the 2-man bobsled start, *The Bobsledder* 3(1) fall.
Rogowski, P. and Wala. (1978) *The sport of luge*, Baltimore: University Press, Inc.
Society of Ski Sciences: Scientific study of skiing in Japan (1972) Tokyo: Hitachi, Ltd.
Stamm, L. & Reilly, R.: Powerskating, *American Hockey*, Summer 1986, Fall 1986, Winter 1986.
Terauds, J., Gros, H. (Eds.) (1979) *Science of skiing, skating, and hockey*, DelMar, Ca: Academic Publishers.

21C
Gymnastics and Diving

Why place these two in the same chapter? Both gymnasts and divers appear to defy the restrictions of bipedal locomotion. With courage and daring they catapult themselves into the air, executing complex rotational movements of the total body. Single, double and triple somersaults, combined with twists of varying degrees are not only performed at all International competitions, but throughout the nations' gymnastics clubs and school teams. Somersaults and diving are a part of the entertainment industry—acrobatics are performed at the circus, dinner club, and carnival. In addition, competition occurs in such activities as board skating, acrobatic skiing, trampolining, rebound tumbling, and gymnastics.

These stunts can be initiated by applying force from a land surface, either by the feet or the hands, or from an arm-supported position involving swinging, mounting, and dismounting from gymnastics equipment. Correct execution of these stunts is dependent upon achieving adequate air time to complete the aerial stunts and on the ability to generate angular momentum and to regulate changes in angular velocity and changes in direction throughout the swinging and rotary activities.

The planar arm-supported and aerial movements are relatively easy to analyze, as was noted in other airborne activities, but the activities that consist of movements in two or more planes are very difficult to analyze. These complex activities may be analyzed by separating each rotary component and defining the basic mechanical principles and anatomic considerations involved in each component. The combination, however, must also be investigated, since a person who can perform one rotation such as a twist, as well as another type of rotation such as a somersault, may not be able to perform a twisting somersault.

BASIC PRINCIPLES RELATING TO AIRBORNE
AND ARM-SUPPORTED ACTIVITIES

Some of the basic principles that can be applied to rotary aerial stunts and arm-supported swinging activities are as follows:

1. Rotation can be produced only by an eccentric force; that is, the force must create a moment about the center of gravity of the body and must not be directed through the center of gravity of the body.
2. The moment of force must be optimized. This requires that the person cope with the desired rotation and the speed of rotation without being disoriented.
3. Sufficient vertical height must be produced to facilitate the aerial skill. The required height can be mathematically calculated by using the equation of falling bodies:

$$S = 1/2at^2$$

with t equal to rotary time of desired number of rotations.
4. While the person is airborne and during swinging, the principle of conservation of angular momentum will determine the speed of rotation with respect to changes in body position.
5. Movements while the performer is airborne will not change the flight of the center of gravity of the body, but they will create reaction forces within the body, causing movements of body segments that may or may not be desirable.
6. The time of execution of a movement will determine success or failure, or it may necessitate modification of the movement before it can be completed. For example, if the projection of the body is executed too early, the result will be insufficient height, greater horizontal velocity, and greater rotary velocity than if the force for the body projection occurred at the biomechanically correct instant in time.
7. Movements of body parts, including hand-position changes, are easiest to perform at zero velocity during the swinging movements.
8. Producing rotations simultaneously in two of the principal planes is a complex phenomenon.

For example, twist requires a horizontal moment of force, whereas the somersault requires a vertical moment of force. Thus, when a person attempts to generate both moments of force, the result often is insufficient vertical force, since effort was required to produce the twist. Therefore, the twist may occur, but the complete somersault might fail. In addition, the correct timing of each movement may be difficult to achieve. A simple one-rotation movement allows the person to concentrate on the time of initiation of that rotation. Initiating a second rotation approximately at the same instant as a rotation in another plane is a task of greater difficulty, although some persons have more difficulty than others. In addition, a movement requiring rotation in two planes changes the body's orientation in space compared with that of a single rotation. Various reflex responses and possible disorientation may interfere with the performance.

Reflex Patterns

Because the body is placed in upside-down positions and in other orientations to earth, and because the position of the head with respect to the trunk deviates from a straight line, many swinging, suspended, and airborne activities are often facilitated or inhibited by the labyrinthine righting reflexes and the tonic neck reflexes. The head will reflexively orient itself to the upright position in headstands, handstands, somersaults, cartwheels, and upward swings. This change in the position of the head for the purpose of righting the body often interferes with the maintenance of a stable support position, since the action of the head may move the line of gravity outside the base of support.

The head movement also will elicit a response from the body based on the tonic neck reflex. For example, an extension of the head, such as the act of "throwing the head backward" for initiation of a backward somersault, will elicit the tonic neck reflex, in which body parts respond reflexively to movement of the head as determined by tension in the muscles crossing the neck. Extension of the head causes both flexion of the legs and extension of the arms. These actions facilitate the backward somersault by decreasing the moment of inertia and the radius of rotation. This same reflex acts to flex the arms and extend the legs when the head is flexed. This time the reflex interferes with the execution of the movement pattern—the front somersault.

Trampoline and Diving Skills

Gaining Height. Gaining height is essential in diving and trampoline skills to provide time for the desired movements of body segments while the body is airborne. The more complex the movements, the greater must be the height. Since the force of projection is derived mainly from the rebounding net or board, these surfaces must be depressed as much as possible when great height is desired. Depression is achieved by several means.

First, the performer approaches the net (trampoline bed) or board from a projection. In running dives, this is the hurdle that precedes the final landing on the board. On the trampoline, the performer uses repeated bounces. When the height of the bounce and the resulting depressions of the net were measured, the data shown in Table 21C-1 were obtained from a film of a highly skilled performer. The relationship of depression to height of drop is not linear. Smaller gains are obtained as the height is increased, since the depression is determined by the tension in its springs, which is nonlinear.

GYMNASTICS AND DIVING   **687**

Table 21C-1. *Comparison of first, second, and third bounce heights and resultant depression on the trampoline. Note that the trampoline appears to have reached its maximum depression on the second bounce.*

	Height	Resulting net depression
First bounce	0.53 m (21 in)	0.51 m (20 in)
Second bounce	1.14 m (45 in)	0.76 m (30 in)
Third bounce	1.50 m (60 in)	0.78 m (31 in)

Second, the center of gravity of the body should be directly over the feet as the contact is made, so that the direction of the landing force is kept directly downward.

Third, there is no "give" by the performer as the feet contact the net or board. Ordinarily, the jar of landing is decreased by flexion at the ankles, knees, and hips. In dives and on the trampoline, the depressing surface takes over the task of eliminating the jolt, and landing is made with full foot contact and with flexed ankles, knees, and hips held firmly as the feet land. The arms are extended downward and just back of the hips on landing. The relationship of these flexed positions should be such that the center of gravity is over the feet.

Fourth, as the surface depresses, the flexed joints extend, pushing the net or board downward, beyond the depth that it would reach were the landing the only force acting on it. On the trampoline, the ankle reaches an angle of 90 degrees; the extension at the hips and knees bring the legs, thighs, and trunk into a straight line. The arms, at the same time, are swung forward and upward and add to the downward force. In dives, the lower legs are not fully extended; they reserve some of their power for the projection.

When great height is desired, the trampoline performer takes repeated bounces; the diver can use only one landing, and for those dives which require longer time in the air, a high diving board is used.

Projectial Direction. From the low point of depression the performer rides upward on the rebounding surface. During this time the center of gravity develops a velocity equal to that of the net or board. At the departure point, this velocity is increased by extension at the ankle and some further arm flexion, and in dives, by the remaining amount of possible lower leg extension. The direction of the center of gravity during flight is determined by the position of the center of gravity in relation to the feet at the final thrust. The diver must have some forward lean to enter the water a short distance from the board. The position of the entry will depend on the lean. Beginning divers are likely to lean too far forward as they attempt a straight front dive; they concentrate on clearing the board rather than on gaining height. Consequently, as they enter the water, their bodies approach a horizontal, rather than a vertical, line. Since the center of gravity follows a parabolic curve, the time of flight from takeoff until the hips enter the water is a measure of the height attained. Block has suggested that the beginner be given a distance goal of 1.5 to 2.4 m (5 to 8 ft) from the board as the desirable entry, and that the diver attempt to develop a projection that would have a minimal time of 1.1 seconds. Such projections would mean that the center of gravity would have an inclination of 22 to 30 degrees beyond the perpendicular at takeoff and a velocity of 3.9 to 4.2 m/sec (9.13 to 14 ft/sec). These goals were found, experimentally, to be within the capacity of beginning college women divers. Groves found that with an expert male diver the lean for various dives ranged from 20 to 34 degrees at takeoff and that the height reached by the center of gravity ranged from 0.73 to 1.4 m (2.4 to 4.6 ft).

On the trampoline, no forward component of velocity is needed, and the center of gravity can be in a line that is perpendicular to the final thrust. In bounces to gain height, this will be done to convert the rebounding force as much as possible into an upward projection.

Rotations and Twists in Flight. As the performer leaves the net or board, the position of the center of gravity also influences the body rotations in the sagittal or transverse planes or both. The amount of lean depends on the amount of rotation desired during flight. The performer riding upward on the rebounding surface has the desired body rotations in mind and makes adjustments to place the center of gravity in the needed relationship to the final thrust. In Fig. 21C-1 are shown line tracings of the takeoffs of an expert performer planning to execute forward and backward somersaults during flight. In the forward movement, the center of gravity has been carried ahead of the toes by hip and shoulder flexion. The thrust will start the rotation in a counterclockwise direction. For the backward movement,

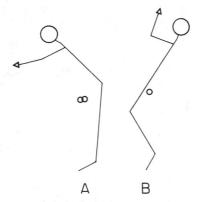

A B

Fig. 21C-1. *Takeoff position, from trampoline, of highly skilled college man executing a forward somersault (A) and a backward somersault (B). Position of the center of gravity (O) with respect to the base of support is a major determining factor for production of total body rotation. At this instant in time, and for each condition, where is the line of gravity?*

GYMNASTICS AND DIVING   **689**

knee flexion has carried the center of gravity back of the toes, and rotation in a clockwise direction will be started. Once the body is in flight, joint actions will add to the speed of rotation of the segments.

Reuschlein measured on film the rotation of body parts of an expert performer executing a forward somersault in the pike position. The degrees of rotation in space of the trunk and the lower limbs and the changes in the hip angle were measured. Rotation was produced by creating a moment of force before becoming airborne. The trunk, slightly above the horizontal at the beginning of flight, rotated counterclockwise until it reached the 12-o'clock position—more than 270 degrees—whereas the lower limbs, starting near the 6-o'clock position, rotated more than 360 degrees counterclockwise. In the first 0.284 second, the trunk rotated 110 degrees and the limbs 61 degrees. Trunk movement was facilitated by gravitational force, while the lower limbs opposed gravity. In the next 0.521 second, the limbs rotated faster than the trunk. Thus, to speak of the angular velocity of the total body may not always be valid, since positioning of the limbs and changes in the angles at the joints cause independent segmental angular velocities different from the total body rotation.

If greater speed of rotation is desired, the body will assume a tuck position to shorten the length of the moment arms. While the body is in midair, the speed of rotation will be decreased by extending the limbs and the trunk, as is done in preparation for landing or entering a body of water.

A diver does not require as much trunk flexion as the trampolinist, because the diver's flight will always have some horizontal velocity. The diver can use full body lean to displace the center of gravity of the body in front of or behind the base of support. For the reverse and inward dives the body position appears similar to that of the trampolinist. Swain studied dives performed at an Association for Intercollegiate Athletics for Women (AIAW) national diving championship and discovered a relationship between type of dive (number of rotations) and body position at takeoff (see Fig. 21C-2). The more rotations, the greater the lean. The lean was unique to each classification. Prior to reading the legend under Fig. 21C-2, study the illustration and identify the direction of the somersaulting action that is being initiated.

State the principle (concept) utilized in identifying the resultant somersaulting actions.

What are the characteristics of a successful diver? Prior to and after the 1984 Olympics, Miller and Munro (1985) studied in detail the temporal, joint positions, and linear and angular momentum characteristics of diving performances of Greg Louganis (gold medalist). No twisting dives were analyzed. Probably the two most important contributors to Greg's success were his vertical velocity at the beginning (4-4$\frac{1}{2}$ m/sec) and end of takeoff (5-6 m/sec). Greg consistently had greater vertical velocity than other competitors. Stick figures (line-

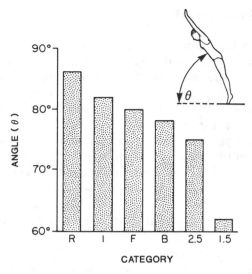

Fig. 21C-2. *Relationship of body lean to type of dive. R, Reverse layout; I, inward layout; F, front layout; B, back layout; 2¹/₂ somersault back layout; 1¹/₂ somersault front pike. Although these precise values may not be true for all divers, the trend (ranking) should be the same. For example, the diver's height will influence angle of body lean prior to takeoff. What other factors will influence body lean?*

segment tracings) from cinema films of preliminary and final performances were compared. Greg's segmental tracings were consistently different from other competitors. There were greater ranges of motion at the knee, hip, and shoulder joints during takeoff. Graphical portrayal of angular momentum of the trunk and head, of the upper extremities, and of the lower extremities from one trial to another of this diver were nearly identical.

The angular momentum was calculated by estimating the body segment mass, centers of gravity, and moments of inertia (based upon values and procedures in literature and Greg's body weight) and utilizing the kinematic data derived from the analysis of cinemia films of Greg's performances. Total body angular momentum was the sum of the local body segment contribution (its moment of inertia x its angular velocity) and the remote body segment contribution (its linear momentum x the moment arm from the center of gravity of the body). The local body segment contribution was found to be small (7-21%), with the trunk (because of its large mass) accounting for at least 4/5th of the resultant total body momentum, except in the case of the reverse dives.

The total body angular momentum is achieved during the recoil of the board. Greg used almost the same amount of contact time on the board regardless of the type of dive being performed. Angular momentum was positively correlated with the number of somersaults achieved.

Rotary Capabilities of Human Body

The human body can rotate about the three principle axes: vertical, frontal-horizontal, and sagittal-horizontal. These rotations are termed (1) pitch, which is about the frontal-horizontal axis as in a front somersault; (2) yaw, which is about the sagittal-horizontal axis as in a cartwheel; and (3) roll, which is about the vertical axis as in twists. In addition, the body may rotate about any diagonal axis or about more than one axis. In certain movements, it is possible for a person who is rotating about one of the horizontal axes to lean the body to one side and be able to twist about the vertical axis. By redistributing the body mass, the performer may change the direction of the main axis, which may give rise to a conical motion about the axis of momentum and cause the performer to rotate about more than one axis at the same time.

Usually, angular momentum is produced while the performer is on a supporting surface, whether a foot support or arm support. Thus rotations are begun before the person terminates contact with the supporting surface. Even in twisting movements, the body shifts the line of gravity from between the feet or hands and toward one of the supports before the instant of takeoff. When the performer is in the air, the arms or lower limbs or both are moved to accentuate the twist.

Ramey and others have shown that the human body cannot execute even one complete rotation of the body in the pitch or yaw planes if no angular momentum exists at the time of takeoff. The reason is the principle of the conservation of momentum, which states that momentum cannot be created or destroyed once the body is airborne and no external forces or couples are acting on the body. Stated another way, the law of interaction functions in airborne situations, produces a counterrotation of one body part whenever a rotation is produced with another body part. For example, the front pike dive will result in a leg entry, as shown in Fig. 21C-3A, if the upper body flexes after the diver becomes airborne and the total body has no angular momentum. The lower body will rise to meet the upper body because of the law of interaction. Contrast this with Fig. 21C-3B, in which angular momentum exists before the upper body flexes. The lower body reaction still causes the upper body parts to approach each other, but the pitch rotation places the body in a more favorable angle for head-first entry into the water.

The "biomechanically ideal" method of assuming the extended inverted position at water entry is to use minimum acceleration of the legs when extension at the hip is executed. The equal and opposite reaction, therefore, will also be small and can be counteracted by muscle force at the hip joint. Should the leg extension be one of moderate to great acceleration, thus creating a high velocity, the upper body reaction will be pronounced. The back will most likely arch, and the head and arms will rise. Persons with weak abdominal muscles will

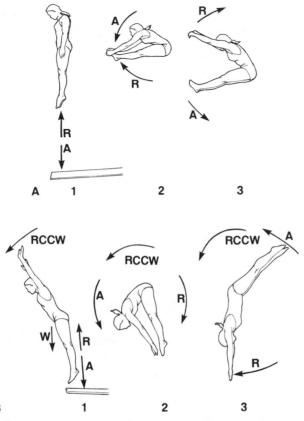

Fig. 21C-3. *Effects of rotation and action-reaction as a person is airborne. A, Vertical takeoff result in foot first entry and no total body rotation despite efforts of the diver to execute a pike somersault (A2). B, Total body rotation in sagittal plane is produced by eccentric action (A1). (A, Action; R, Reaction; RCCW total body reaction moment; W, Weight.)*

experience pain in the lumbar region of the spine and have an uncontrolled landing.

Although pitch and the rarely used yaw, rotations cannot be initiated successfully while the diver is airborne, twisting movements can be and are initiated at that time. This is possible because the rotation is about the longitudinal axis of the body. The body parts may be redistributed about this axis to produce favorable moment-of-inertia ratios with respect to the law of interaction. The easiest way to understand this concept is to visualize the twist as it is initiated from a pike position, with the upper body inverted and the legs horizontal, as shown in Fig. 21C-4. As the arms are moved to cause the upper body to twist, the opposite reaction in the legs will be one of low velocity, and therefore low displacement and counter twist, because of the high moment-of-inertia ratio. The legs have a long moment arm and a small twist in the horizontal plane, in contrast to the

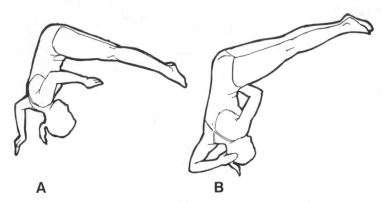

Fig. 21C-4. *Twisting is possible to initiate after diver leaves the board; diver is airborne. In this example, the twist is executed from the pike position. This upper body twist creates only a small amount of reaction movement since the moment of inertia of the legs is great compared to rest of the body.*

short moment arm of the horizontal twist by the upper body. The arms and trunk will move at a greater velocity and have a larger angular displacement because their moment of inertia is small compared to that of the legs. This example not only provides an understanding of the biomechanical principles but illustrates how important it is for the performer to execute movements at precisely the most optimum point in time within a movement pattern.

Twisting movements can be executed in a variety of ways. Individual differences may account for one performer's method in comparison with another, or the particular stunt may influence selection of the method of initiating the twist. Many gymnasts use what is termed a high arm throw, whereas the low arm throw is more common to divers. Thayer studied these two types of arm actions used in diving. She concluded that the high arm action is biomechanically better because the velocity is in the direction of the twist, and in addition, the line of direction of the possible muscles involved and the moments of inertia appear to be more effective during that action than during the low arm action. More research, however, should be conducted with different populations and with respect to twisting movements in general.

MINI-LAB LEARNING EXPERIENCES

One of the best examples of conservation of angular momentum is achieved by standing on a freely rotating board (such as a twister board) or a chair (swivel type) and changing the moment arms of the upper extremities while spinning. Use the experimentation in Chapter 5.

1. Spin a person who is standing on a freely rotating surface.
2. Have the person begin with the hands at the sides (anatomic position).

3. After the spin has started, ask the person to abduct the arms to the horizontal position. Note the decrease in angular speed.
4. Now spin the person, beginning with arms in the abducted position and adduct the arms during the spin. Note the increase in angular speed.
5. Add weights to the hands and repeat steps 1 to 4.
6. Other examples of the conservation of angular momentum can be observed in sports. One of the easiest and safest ways to experience the increase in angular speed is with the forward roll. Since the person is not airborne, there is little danger if the person fails to achieve high angular speeds. In fact, less speed is safer than developing too much speed. Thus one can experience the trade-off that occurs between the momement of inertia and angular speed (velocity). Estimates of differences in moments of inertia of body parts among persons and between one person's body parts may be made by estimating differences in angular velocities by means of time or radian measurements.

George (1980) identified four basic principles that differentiate between skilled and unskilled performers in gymnastic movement. These are as follows:

1. Amplitude—The gymnast should strive to increase appropriate internal and external amplitude. External amplitude is dependent upon the power (velocity—force product) of the propulsive actions of the skill. Usually the lesser skilled gymnasts do not maximize their potential because of ineffective and reduced speed. Internal amplitude is dependent upon range of motion utilized in the execution of the skill. Thus, the greater the velocities and ranges of motion, the greater the ability to perform complex stunts and to complete the stunts in "good form." Note the differences in amplitude of the two performers depicted in Fig. 21C-5.

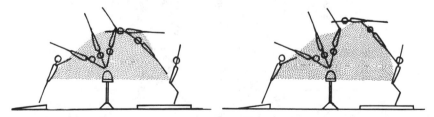

Fig. 21C-5. *Comparison of amplitudes of two performances. Note how the stunt itself dictates amplitude. The amplitude pattern of each stunt can then be used as a criterion for success (both in technical execution and quality). (Modified from G. George,* Biomechanics of Women's Gymnastics, *Prentice-Hall)*

GYMNASTICS AND DIVING   **695**

2. Segmentation—Skill proficiency is inversely related to the number of segmental body parts used in a particular stunt. Another way to state this is that skill proficiency reduces extraneous independent body segment actions. Thus, symmetry of motion, both legs moving identically and the body moving as a unit, can be observed in the performance in Fig. 21C-6A more so than in Fig. 21C-6B. The latter has not applied the segmentation principle.

3. Closure—Closure is the achievement of the body shape alteration within each phase of the stunt. For example, the pike position, the tuck position, and the layout positions are precisely achieved. The attainment of the precise shape is desirable both for aesthetic and mechanical reasons.

4. Peaking—This is also referred to as the timing principle. The performer utilizes principles of momentum and direction of forces to change the body shape at the most advantageous instant. Common examples of correct peaking occur in swing-to-vertical lifts on parallel bars, rings, and uneven parallel bars at which the lift occurs prior to swinging through the vertical. Other examples are peaking from lay-out to tuck somersaults. The tuck must be delayed (properly timed) in order to achieve sufficient angular velocity for a high quality performance.

Using the principles of this chapter analyze the actions of the stunts depicted in figures 21C-9, 21C-10, and 21C-11. Indicate why one is more biomechanically executed than the other.

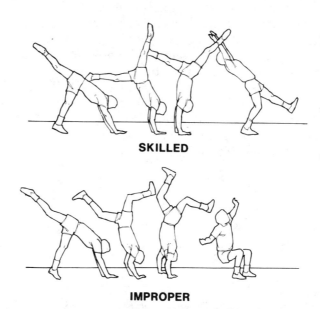

SKILLED

IMPROPER

Fig. 21C-6. *Segmentation. Each body segment creates a line of force and balance. Different stunts consist of different level of segmentation. Improperly performed stunt differs from skilled performance on segmentation.*

A. (1) Observe a dive forward roll.
  (2) Describe the angular velocity during different phases of the roll.
  (3) Estimate the radius of rotation (length of lever).
B. Ask the performer to execute the roll in the following ways:
  (1) Tuck as soon as possible and maintain tuck throughout the roll.
  (2) Extend the legs and maintain this extension until upside down and then tuck rapidly.
  (3) Extend legs and assume a pike position as soon as possible; assume the tuck position when upside down.
C. (1) Observe the rolls performed in step B.
  (2) Evaluate whether or not the performer executed the task.
  (3) Assess the performances as in step A.

ARM-SUPPORTED SKILLS

Mechanics of Arm-Supported Skills

In many gymnastic skills, the body is supported by the hands as it is rotated in a vertical or horizontal plane around the support. In the vertical plane as the body rotates downward, gravitational force aids; as the body rotates upward, gravity resists the movement. Therefore, on the downswing, the skilled performer will move the body's center of gravity as far as possible from the center of rotation; this is done by full extension at the hip and shoulder girdle depression. On the upswing, the center of gravity will be moved toward the center of rotation by flexion at the hip and shoulder girdle elevation. In skills in which the body is rotated in the horizontal plane, the body segment actions will be those that tend to keep the center of gravity directly over the supporting base.

Simple Underswing

The simple underswing (swinging back and forth) is a preliminary movement that is used in preparation for the execution of more advanced moves. The hands provide the point of support and the center of rotation. To develop a simple underswing the legs should flex (at the hip) on the upswing (forward and backward), thereby shortening the radius of rotation (with the result that the center of rotation moves closer to the center of support). The performer, by elevating the shoulder girdle when the body is directly under the point of support, may also help increase the angular velocity. In gymnastic terms, this is known as hollowing the chest. As the body starts downward at the end of the swing, the velocity can be increased by leg extension (at the hip) and shoulder girdle elevation.

Giant Swing

The giant swing may be done both backward and forward. On the upward swing the radius of rotation is shortened by flexion at the hips and by shoulder girdle elevation. Actually, the hollowing of the chest has the effect of causing a slight flexion, as well as depression of the shoulders. (If the arms were flexed, the radius of movement would be shortened much more; however, in topflight gymnastic competition the flexing of the arms is considered poor form.) All these actions bring the center of gravity closer to the center of support (shortening the radius) and in turn accelerate the upward angular velocity. As the center of gravity moves over the center of support (the hands), the grip has been moved upward, and the performer momentarily pushes the body up to a handstand position. On the downswing, the body is fully extended. The extension is made just before the body reaches the high vertical position to gain the full effect of gravity and to develop the greatest possible velocity in preparation for the next upward swing. (See Fig. 21C-7 and 21C-8.)

The following are kinetic findings reported by Valliere on performers executing the backward giant swing on the still rings:

1. A decline in force was exerted during the descent phase.
2. A sudden increase of force coincided with the greatest shoulder joint velocity.

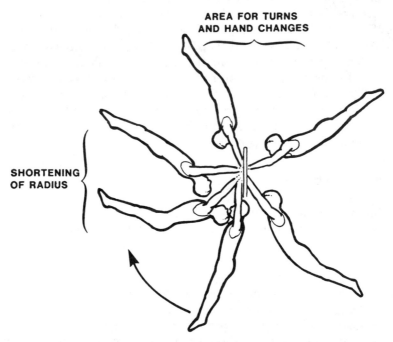

Fig. 21C-7. *The back giant swing on the high bar has commonalities with giant swings on parallel and uneven parallel bars, the rings, and the front giant swing. Note the area of longest radius of rotation (body extension), the area of shortening of the radius, and the area in which hand changes and turning can occur.*

THE BIOMECHANICS OF HUMAN MOVEMENT

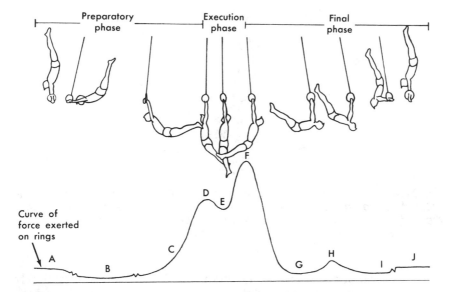

Fig. 21C-8. *Kinetic and kinematic diagram of backward giant swing executed on still rings. Special strain gage transducers within the supporting cable structures of the rings were used to obtain the force-time curve. Selected points on the force-time curve were synchronized with corresponding body positions traced from movie film. (From Valliere, A. Kinetic and kinematic analysis of the backward giant swing on the still rings in gymnastics, Doctoral dissertation, Indiana University, 1973)*

3. A drop in force coincided with the whiplike action of the legs, occurring at the bottom of the swing.
4. A sharp increase in force moving to a maximum coincided with the upward lift of the body in the ascent phase. (See Fig. 21C-8 for a view of this special apparatus; and the force-time curve.)

MINI-LAB LEARNING EXPERIENCES

Refer to Chapter 6 (Work-Kinetic Energy) and estimate changes in velocity, work, and energy of gymnasts performing giant swings. Use video tapes, films, tracings.

Stunts on Parallel Bars

In the swing from the support position (Fig. 21C-9) on the parallel bars, much of the skill depends on adjustments made to keep the body's center of gravity over (or near) the supporting hands. Note that in the supine position the arms are tilted to the left and the legs are flexed; both adjustments move the body mass toward the vertical plane of the hands. In the prone position, flexion at the elbow occurs, this is a reversed muscle action that moves the upper arm and with it the

GYMNASTICS AND DIVING   **699**

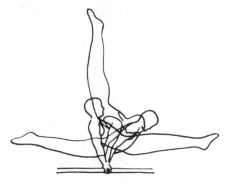

Fig. 21C-9. *Swing from support position on parallel bars into a hand stand. Note the shift of the shoulders about the hands. The arms flex at the elbows when the body is in the prone position. This would be an example of incorrect segmentation and judges would deduct a fraction of a point.*

upper portion of the trunk to the right to balance the lower limbs. In the final position, extension of the spine and backward rotation of the pelvis have moved the lower limbs close to the support to balance the head and shoulder girdle. As the arms moved to the right on the downswing, the effect of gravitational force was increased by increasing the distance between the hands and the center of gravity. As the flexion occurs at the elbow on the first part of the upward swing, the moment arm was shortened to make better use of the momentum developed on the downward swing.

Stunts on Uneven Parallel Bars

The same principle involved in swinging activities on the high bar and on parallel bars apply to swinging on the uneven parallel bars. In addition, however, the transfer of a body swinging on one bar to the other bar increases both the complexity and the possibilities of stunts that can be performed. The lower bar of the uneven parallel bars also may be an obstacle to the execution of stunts that normally are routine on a high bar. For example, women are performing the giant swing of the high bar on the top bar of the uneven parallel bars. The downswing essentially is the same as in the high bar performance, but the upswing necessitates a piking and an upward extension of the body, which is by far more difficult than the upswing on the high bar.

One of the most important mechanical principles is that of continuity of angular momentum, that is, the maintenance of the rotary momentum for the execution of a series of stunts, especially those which involve transference from one bar to the other.

The cast-off from the high bar to a back hip circle on the low bar is one of the more common stunts, and it is one that shows the applications of swing and moment of inertia. The swing is begun by a clockwise rotation of the lower body to overcome inertia, produce a

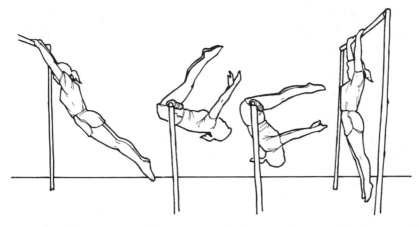

Fig. 21C-10. *Cast-off from high bar to back circle on low bar of uneven parallel bars. Note periods of long radii and short radii, as well as movements with gravity and opposing gravity.*

forceful counterclockwise rotation, and thus acquire the greatest height for the starting point of the swing (Fig. 21C-10). The body is extended, with chest hollowed to provide the longest lever possible for the downswing. As the center of gravity reaches a point below the bar, the body arches slightly and causes the legs to move behind the trunk. As the trunk leads, the lever length is decreased somewhat and angular velocity increases. This facilitates the piking action necessary to execute the back hip circle around the low bar. The piking action increases the angular velocity considerably and, when perfectly timed, will cause the axis of rotation of the body to coincide with that of the lower bar axis. The body will rotate around the lower bar with a minimum of pressure between the bar and the body. In essence, this back hip circle is similar to the back pike somersault dismount from a high bar. The only difference is that the bar contains the horizontal velocity and maintains a fixed axis of rotation about the bar. The performer then grasps the lower bar with her hands and increases the moment of inertia by extending into the front support position.

MUSCLE FUNCTION

The amount of muscular activity in selected shoulder muscles during four stunts on the uneven parallel bars has been studied by Landa. She used surface electrodes to record the action potentials from the pectoralis major, three heads of the deltoids, the biceps brachii, the superior and inferior heads of the trapezius, and the latissimus dorsi. Muscle activity was positively related to increases in swing amplitude, which also meant that it was related to swing velocity. Both the stationary hang into a squat on the low bar and the jump-catch swing into a squat on the low bar showed less activity than did the cast-off into a pike around the low bar and the cast-off into a back

GYMNASTICS AND DIVING   **701**

hip circle on the low bar. The latissimus dorsi contributed a greater amount of electrical activity with respect to potential than any of the other muscles. Landa concluded that strength improvement exercises in the shoulder and upper back, especially for the latissimus dorsi, are vital for performers on the uneven parallel bars.

Oglesby also investigated muscle activity in women gymnasts. She studied the upper, middle, and lower portions of the rectus abdominus muscle to determine their magnitude and time of activity in the kip and single-leg shoot-through on the uneven parallel bars, as well as in three floor exercise stunts and two balance beam stunts. She found that the muscle, especially the lower portion, performed a major function in the execution of five of the seven stunts. Since each stunt showed a unique pattern of electrical activity, Oglesby suggested that exercises which simulate the stunts should be used for abdominal strength training.

Flyaway

The flyaway is a type of dismount that usually follows a giant swing. The performer first does a giant swing and then prepares for the flyaway by increasing speed. The radius of rotation is shortened as the body passes over the bar. This is done by flexing at the hips and depressing the shoulder girdle. (The arms could be flexed, but this is considered poor form.) The back is then arched (by extension) just before coming directly under the bar on the downswing. This arching helps shorten the radius as the body rises in the upswing and aids in accelerating the angular velocity. As the body rises above the horizontal, the arch is continued with the head held well backward (upper back and head extension) and the legs and arms (slightly) fixed (Fig. 21C-11). The reaction from the bent bar gives added upward velocity to the performer. Centrifugal force pulls the body away from the bar, as the hands are released.

Action on Still (Stationary) Rings

The two basic principles for successful performance are to shorten the moment arm (radius of swing, length of arms) for efficiency of energy and balance and to utilize continuity of motion throughout the routine, again for efficiency, but also for success. The movement of the preceding stunt is necessary to perform the next stunt in the routines.

Back Uprise to a Handstand on Rings. To execute the back uprise to a handstand on the still rings (Fig. 21C-12A), the performer swings the body to and fro by alternate flexion and extension at the hips to gain momentum, and on the downswing, the radius (the distance from the hands to the toes) is lengthened. The center of gravity is kept under the point of suspension of the cables. On the upswing, the radius is shortened by arching the back and in-locating the shoulders, that is, internally rotating the humeral head in the glenoid fossa.

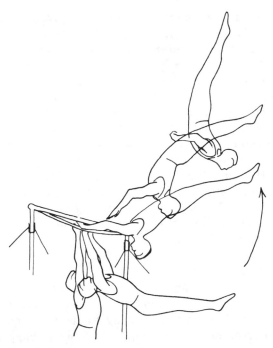

Fig. 21C-11. *Flyaway (layout) from back giant swing on high bar. Head appears to extend too early, thus reducing maximum lift of body from the bar. The action of the arms after pushoff also is not appropriate to optimum performance since the arms remains slightly flexed.*

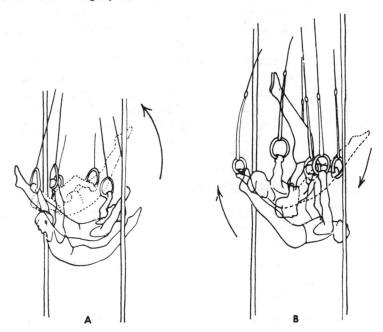

A   B

Fig. 21C-12. *Movements on the still rings have high potential for injury to the shoulders, especially dislocations. Note the movements of the body about the shoulders in the back uprise to handstand (A) and the shoot to handstand (B).*

(This helps overcome the force of gravity and gives the performer accelerated upward angular velocity.) The body is moved forward, placing the center of rotation nearer to the point of support (hands), which is kept behind an extended line from the shoulders. The center of gravity is still kept under the point of suspension of the cables and rings. As the point of support moves under the point of suspension of the rings, the center of gravity moves upward and inward at the same rate. The performer pulls the body up by forceful scapular abduction and arm extension and then pushes upward to a handstand in continuous motion as the rotary swing diminishes. This is accomplished by flexing at the hips and abducting the scapulae.

Since the rings should be as stationary as possible while the exercises are being performed, the performer should attempt to stop or prevent movement of the cables. Usually swing occurs when the performer fails to keep the center of gravity under the point of support and along the rope suspension line. When the swinging begins, it is difficult to stop, and thereafter all movements on the rings are difficult to execute. Developing a certain amount of swing is inevitable during the course of a competitive routine, and the accomplished gymnast learns to "kill," or stop, the swing in some movements and use it to advantage in others. Usually one of two things happens: the swing continues to increase (most commonly) or may be controlled or partially dissipated. Movement of the center of gravity of the body against the direction of the swing may help control or stop it.

Cross-hang Position on the Rings. The cross-hang position, known as the iron cross, is an exercise of simple joint action requiring tremendous strength because the supports (the hands) are not directly above the body's center of gravity but rather at arm's distance from it horizontally. To maintain the arm position, the shoulder adductors must contract forcefully. The elbow and wrist joints must be stabilized; however, the muscular effort for maintaining the positions of these joints is not great if the shoulder position is held. From this position, upper trunk rotation takes place to either the right or the left.

MINI-LAB LEARNING EXPERIENCES

What advantage does the short-armed person have compared with the long-armed person performing on the rings? Refer to information in Chapter 4.

Side Horse Activities

The movements on the side horse are normally those of pendulumlike swinging, rotary movements, and variations of these two.

A type of pendulum-like swinging is observed in the execution of simple leg cuts and scissor actions (Fig. 21C-13). The points of sus-

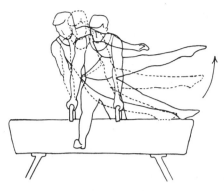

Fig. 21C-13. *Pendulum swing in scissors action on side horse. Note shift of shoulders during regrasping.*

pension of the pendulum are the shoulder joints. The radius is short-ened as the performer moves the center of gravity nearer to the base of support on the upswing and is lengthened on the downswing to increase angular velocity. This is accomplished by flexing at the hip, accompanied by flexion and lateral rotation of the trunk. On the up-swing, the top thigh is abducted. The resistance arm of the lever (dis-tance from the point of support to the center of gravity of the com-bined mass of the trunk and lower limbs) is also shortened on the upswing and lengthened on the downswing. As the upswing dimin-ishes until the velocity is zero (the upward velocity and the pull of gravity nullifying one another), the performer flexes at the hip, flexes and laterally rotates the trunk, and executes leg crosses and scissor-like actions.

When high double-leg circles are executed, the center of gravity must be kept over the center of rotation and base of support during most of the move. The body rotates about the center of support by means of lateral trunk flexion, with the shoulders held more or less at the same elevation (Fig. 21C-14). The shortening of the radius and raising of the center of gravity during the movement allow the return swing to be made more easily. Takemoto and Hamaido liken this ac-

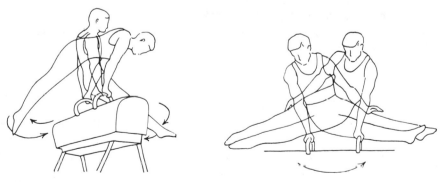

Fig. 21C-14. *High double leg circles on side horse. Is the circle symmetrical with respect to the different right and left circles?*

GYMNASTICS AND DIVING

tion to the spinning of a top. No pause (or slowing down) may occur while the action takes place, or the performer will fall off the apparatus.

Balance Beam

The gymnastic event executed on the balance beam is one in which the woman performer is called on to do many acrobatic stunts while maintaining balance. The duration of the movements on the beam is restricted to not less than 1 minute 15 seconds and not more than 1 minute 35 seconds.

To counteract toppling in one direction, the gymnast rotates her arms and sometimes the non-supporting leg in the direction of unbalance to cause the rest of the body to move in the opposite direction, thus counteracting the overbalance.

It is evident that this event, in which a mounted beam of narrow width constitutes a performance area where dance steps, turns, jumps, leaps, and gymnastic twists are executed, calls for great skill involving principles of equilibrium. The placement of the body's center of gravity must be directly over the feet so that the performer is able to stay on the beam after executing a move. During the execution of the stunt, the center of gravity must move in the direction of movement so that the movement flows as progress is made back and forth on the beam (Wilkerson).

Beginning and novice performers view the width of the beam as a requirement for precision of execution, but view the height of the beam fearfully. Thus, analyses of movements on the balance beam should include direct or indirect measurement of muscle activity. Tension in extraneous muscles is a primary cause of unsuccessful or unskilled performances. If the actions can be performed on a painted line on the floor, why can't they be performed on the beam. This is a perfect example of the necessity of analyzing the psychological environment in order to interpret the biomechanics of performance.

MINI-LAB LEARNING EXPERIENCES

Observe, videotape, or record EMG from arm and trunk muscles, or otherwise record three skipping patterns with the following constraints:

1. Skip forward on the floor.
2. Skip forward along a line 4″ wide.
3. skip forward on a 4″ × 4″ × 6' board set on the floor.
4. Skip forward on the 4" × 4″ × 6' board elevated from the floor.

Record results in the form of a table or graph. Discuss results. Does the skip change? How? Estimate planes of movement, ROM, and sequencing of movement.

Vaulting

Vaulting may be thought of as consisting of two jumps, one from the feet and one from the hands. Therefore, many of the principles described in the chapter on jumping can be applied to the skill of vaulting. Since the goals of vaulting and jumping differ, however, some differences are evident. Since the distance allowed for the approach in vaulting is less than 8 m, vaulters do not attain maximum running speeds before takeoff. Average speeds of skilled vaulters immediately before contact with the takeoff boards have been reported as being 6.09–7.9 m/sec. The difference between male and female United States elite junior vaulters was approximately one foot per second (1985 data obtained by Sands and Cheetham). The runup speed for the Yamashita vault performed by the gold medalist Nelli Kim in 1976 was measured as 7.64 m/s as compared with the runup for the full-twisting Tsukahara vault (7.4 m/sec.). The fastest speeds of runup have been found in performances of the 1984 Olympic male finalists in which the speeds ranged from 7.6 m/s to 7.99 m/s.

Investigations have been conducted of the changes in speed during the runup. Theoretically, the speed increases until the hurdle is taken. The following results, however, were obtained from the final four steps of elite juniors: increase in speed from fourth last step to third last step, lesser increase in speed from third to second last step, and slight decrease in speed from second last to last step.

Little or no speed is lost during board contact, because of the rebound capabilities of the board as well as the vaulter's ability to apply force during the contact phase. Less skilled vaulters are not able to maintain their speed and show decreases of 1 or 2 m/sec during this phase. In addition, skilled vaulters can develop the required vertical and angular speeds, while maintaining the majority of the horizontal speed.

The speed of the approach is a major determinant of flight speed. The faster the approach speed, the greater the possibility of a more skilled performance. The correlation between the peak velocity of the runup and number of steps and the score awarded was .953 for nine vaults by elite juniors. There is no doubt that gymnasts should utilize a long approach to achieve a fast runup.

Dynamic control of the approach speed is the next determinant of skilled performance, since the takeoff determines the angle and speed of the preflight (airborne phase between takeoff from the board and contact with the horse), just as the direction of the initial contact with the horse will influence the effectiveness of the postflight (from leaving the horse to landing on the mat). The preflight velocity of skilled vaulters is greater than that of less skilled vaulters.

The runup also produces the momentum to achieve as high and as long a trajectory as possible during the flight between the horse and landing (postflight and stance) while performing somersaults and twisting actions. Dainis has shown that a decrease of 7% in the runup speed will cause a decrease of 13% in the postflight distance. In addition, a decrease of 7% in the vertical speed results in a decrease of 25% in the postflight distance.

Researchers on the handspring vault showed that vaulters contact the takeoff board at an angle producing 75% horizontal force and 25% vertical force. Their takeoff velocity shows approximately equal horizontal and vertical components, a significant change in direction.

As with other forms of jumping, a compromise must be made between magnitude of force and magnitude of time during the takeoff phase. Skilled vaulters have a relatively short contact time, both on the board and on the horse. Contact times on the takeoff board are about 0.1 second (100 msec) but will vary with respect to type of vault, type of board, and vaulter. Contact times on the horse for handspring vaults of 10 advanced female gymnasts ranged from 130 msec to 295 msec. This vault was characterized by a takeoff from the horse before the body passed the vertical. Less skilled vaults were characterized by takeoffs after the body passed the vertical position on the horse (Daniels).

Basic Principles of Vaulting:

1. Attain an approach speed that is as fast as possible without loss of dynamic equilibrium.
2. Learn to obtain maximum mechanical energy from the takeoff board. Penney has shown that skilled vaulters adapted to the rebounding surface, but some vaulters exceeded the limits of the Reuter board, formerly used extensively for vaulting competitions.
3. Determine the angle of the preflight which will result in the best body position and the least amount of inhibiting or detrimental reaction force at contact with the horse.
4. Apply force during contact with the horse to attain adequate velocity for the postflight.

MINI-LAB LEARNING EXPERIENCES

1. Set up a series of photocell timing devices and record the speed of runup of vaulters at intervals of 1 meter. If photocells are not available, videotape the runup, and record the time to execute each step of the runup. Plot the results on a graph using step numbers for the x axis and time for the y axis. Assume equal length of steps. A digital time code on videotape and single frame advance capabilities on the playback unit are necessary. An alternate approach is to use an audiocassette recorder and record the sound of the steps. Estimate cadence or changes in time intervals. Qualitative assessment of positive and negative acceleration is probably all that is feasible in this case.

2. Observe and measure (during the performance or with a postperformance evaluation of a videotape) the distance of preflight and postflight.
   Compare these distances with respect to type of vault and score awarded for performance.

Anthropometric Considerations

An anatomic consideration of importance to successful performance in gymnastics, especially with respect to the uneven parallel bars, is the length of the body. It is essential that the levels of the two bars and the distance between the two bars be adjusted precisely to the length, therefore, the swinging distance, of the body of each performer. Beginners, who strike the bar and possess little thigh mass, may find padding useful and necessary during the learning stages of movements such as back hip circles after swinging movements from the high bar. Improper timing will cause impact trauma to the body rather than a "wrapping of the body around the bar."

As with most sports in which equipment is essential to the performances, biomechanists working with a team of researchers and coaches are attempting to investigate the precise influence of equipment upon gymnastics performance and to redesign gymnastics equipment. In the past, persons of all possible anthropometric characteristics were unable to perform satisfactorily in all gymnastics events. For example, the uneven parallel bars were built to accommodate the typical short stature female gymnast. A tall woman was unable to swing from the high bar without her feet striking the ground. Today, the uneven bars have been modified and are more adjustable to different-sized individuals. The size of the rings, and hand contact points on the pommel horse, high bar, parallel bars, and uneven parallel bars are not always suited to the size of a person's hand. Gripping may be comprised. Use of hand grips compensates for gripsize, as well as strength. An analysis of performance, thus must include an evaluation of anatomical characteristics of the performer and its influence upon performance.

Biomechanics and Safety

In the same way that body alignment is the key to biomechanically sound standing posture, body alignment is the key to gymnastics activities. The handstand and the bar-hang are considered the foundation for practicing the straight line body alignment. The arms, trunk, neck, and legs are in a straight line, and the shoulders are depressed.

Low back pain is a common complaint among gymnasts. Repeated and excessive arching of the lumbar spine is a typical posture in the routines of gymnasts. If such a posture occurs during dismounting from a piece of gymnastics apparatus, trauma from the impact forces is apt to occur. Since gymnastic activities are replete with landing

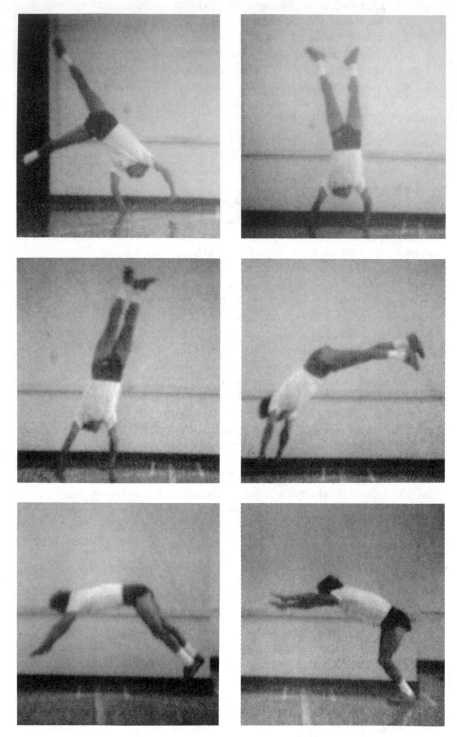

Fig. 21C-15. *Round-off Cartwheel.*

710

activities, special landing mats have been constructed that are appropriate for each piece of apparatus.

What are the risks of trauma to the joints of the body in gymnastics and how would you estimate them?

Step 1. Hypothesize that the greater the landing forces, the greater the risk of injury. This is based upon the stress-strain relationship which, in review, can be stated as follows: As stress is increased, the strain increases. Thus, a body will deform positively with increased force applied to it until it fractures.

Step 2. Review literature to determine impact values and tools used to obtain these values. Too and Adrian found values of 5–6 BW

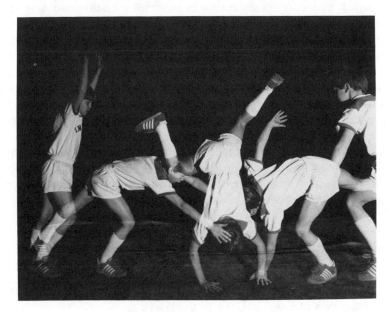

Fig. 21C-16. *Cartwheel.*

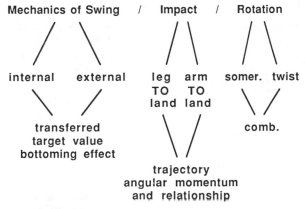

Fig. 21C-17. *A model schematic for analyzing gymnastics performances. Performances can be categorized into swing, impact, and total body rotation.*

GYMNASTICS AND DIVING   **711**

(5 to 6 times body weight) during landings from a vaulting box .85 meters high. A change in the surface mat resulted in a difference of almost 20% BW with an increase in mat thickness. Mat 1 was 1 cm thick with a coefficient of restitution of .78 (as calculated from the rebound height of a dropped ball). The second mat was 5 cm thick with a coefficient of restitution of .58.

A comparison was made of those gymnasts landing with a flat trunk (no increased curvature at the lumbar spine) and those with an arched trunk (increased curvature at the lumbar spine). Mean vertical impact forces were 5.47 BW flat trunk response and 6.62 BW arched trunk response.

Step 3. Select subjects (persons who follow standard test directions) who will perform different types of landings. Measure the vertical ground reaction forces. A force platform or other force transducer can be used. If neither is available, an animal, truck, or other floor scale with a range of zero-to-one thousand pounds could be used. For relative estimation (ranking of different conditions), a sand landing pit could be used. Measurement of the depth of foot penetration for each condition could be recorded and ranked. The deeper the penetration, the greater the impact force.

Step 4. Observe, videotape, or film the kinematics of the subjects as they perform landings from different heights.

Step 5. Based upon your data derive one or more principles with respect to impact force and body segment motion.

MINI-LAB LEARNING EXPERIENCES

Study, measure and describe the performances of Figs. 21C-15 and 21C-16. Use the model in Fig. 21C-17 to categorize the performances of Figs. 21C-15 and 21C-16

REFERENCES

Daniels, A. (1979) Cinematographic analysis of the handspring vault, *Res. Q.* 50:3
Darda, B.: Springboard diving. *Encyclopedia of Physical Education,* Cureton, T. K. Cureton, editor, 1986, pp. 460–463.
George, G. (1980) *Biomechanics of women's gymnastics,* Englewood Cliffs, NJ: Prentice-Hall.
Hay, J., editor: *Starting, stroking and turning, a compilation of research on the biomechanics of swimming,* Iowa City, IA: 1983–86, University of Iowa.
Hay, J., Wilson, B., Dapena, J., Woodworth, G. (1977). A computational technique to determine the angular momentum of a human body. *Journal of Biomechanics,* 10:269–277.
Landa, J. (1973) Shoulder muscle activity during selected skills on the uneven parallel bars, Unpublished thesis, Washington State University, Pullman.
Oglesby, B. (1969) An electromyographic study of the rectus abdominus muscle during selected gymnastic stunts. Unpublished thesis, Washington State University, Pullman.
Miller, D. I. and Munro, C. F.: Greg Louganis' springboard takeoff: II linear and angular momentum considerations, *IJSB,* 1(4):288–307, Nov., 1985.
Miller, D. I. and Nissinen, M. A.: Critical examination of ground reaction force in the running forward somersault, *IJSB* 3(3):189–206, August, 1987.
Prassas, S., Terauds, J. (1987) Gaylord II: A qualitative assessment. In *Biomechanics in Sports III & IV,* Terauds, J., Gowitzke, B., Holt, L. (Eds), Del Mar, CA: Academic Publishers.
Rackham, G. (1975) *Diving Complete.* London: Faber and Faber.

Reuschlein, P. (1962) An analysis of the forward somersault in the pike position. Unpublished paper, University of Wisconsin.

Sands, B. and Cheetham, P.: Velocity of the vault run, *Technique* 6(3):10–14, October, 1986.

Stroup, F. Bushnell, D. (1969) Rotation, translation, and trajectory in springboard diving. *Res. Q.* 40:812–817.

Swain, R. (1979) A comparison between coaching cues and the execution of that dive. Unpublished paper, Washington State University.

Too, D., Adrian, M. (1987) Relationship of lumbar curvature and landing surface to ground reaction forces during gymnastic landing. In *Biomechanics in Sports III & IV*, Terauds, J., Gowitzke, Holt, L (Eds.), Del Mar, CA: Academic Publishers.

Valliere, A. (1973) Kinetic and kinematic analysis of the backward giant swing on the still rings in gymnastics. Unpublished dissertation, Indiana University, Bloomington.

Part V   *Biomechanics for Better Understanding and Self-Improvement*

Now and in the Future

22
The Future

We don't know whether you'll read this chapter first or last, but we do know that once you begin it, you won't be able to stop.

Lean back in your water-warmed flexible glass recliner chair, designed to fit your particular anatomy, and flick the switch that slides back the solar panels to reveal your skylight. Watch Skylab wink its way across the night sky. Your house robot appears at the side of your chair, bringing you a drink which your computer has designed. It contains the precise amount of vitamins and minerals you need to replenish those you've used during the day. Fantastic, you say? Not nearly as fantastic as the things which already exist in everyday use which were unheard of 10 years ago.

In the past 50 years, television networks have been created and now every home in the U.S. has an average of two television sets. Jet planes and commercial airplanes speed us around the world. Satellites monitor weather, defense, and communications. Overall, the omnipotent computer keeps track of the massive data collected every moment of the day.

We live in an age of creativity and excitement that surpasses even the Renaissance. Never before has the human race faced the challenges it faces today. Knowledge is expanding at an exponential rate. The sophisticated experiments in today's "high tech" labs will be carried out tomorrow by graduate college students, and in a few years by undergraduates.

Some of the most exciting research will occur in the field of biomechanics. Biomechanists, combining with biomedical personnel, anatomists, and ergonomic specialists, will form high-powered research teams and consortiums, linked by computer, and will solve movement problems and create equipment undreamed of at this time.

Let us look, for example, at the future in clinical and orthopaedic biomechanics.

717

NEW CLINICAL DEVICES

An understanding of factors influencing safe and effective movement is the foundation for prevention or reduction of trauma to the human body. Devices have been instrumented to alert the wearer to dangerous conditions. For example, a force transducer shaped as an insole and fitting inside a shoe (see Fig. 22-1), has been connected to an activation box that beeps when a prescribed vertical load is exceeded. This device has been used to assist osteoporotic, diabetic, and other afflicted persons who must prevent excess impact forces during the landing phase of walking. Recently a more sophisticated device (pressure relief and asymmetry monitor) has been designed to monitor the sitting behavior of wheelchair users, as they sit in their chairs. Excessive and long-term pressure during sitting often results in trauma to the soft tissues of the body. The most common effects are ulcers, blisters, and circulatory restrictions. Monitoring the magnitude of pressures, the pressure patterns, and the shifting of pressures and pressure patterns results in information that can be used to prevent excessive pressures and long-duration pressures. We predict that computer-interaction with the seated person will be available soon. Imagine this, the person would receive signals (both auditory and tactile) to shift weight-bearing areas or unload the buttocks.

Musculoskeletal scanning machines have been developed for assessments of musculoskeletal abnormalities. One such device is depicted in Fig. 22-2. This is a total body scanner from which three-dimensional graphics are generated. Postural evaluations, including scoliosis screening and potentially high stresses to body areas, can be performed in the clinic or on-site, since the scanner is a portable unit.

One of the fastest-growing areas in rehabilitative biomechanics is that of screening of back patients and evaluations of risk of back

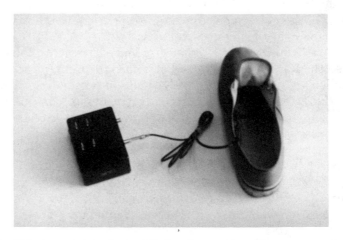

Fig. 22-1. *This force insole fits inside the shoe and can be connected to a dual microprocessor circuit that will send an audible signal any instant that predetermined threshold force is exceeded.*

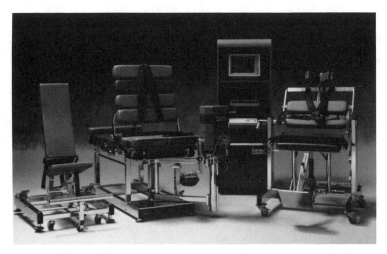

Fig. 22-2. *Musculoskeletal scanning machine. (Courtesy of Universal Gym Equipment, Inc.)*

injury. Several new devices have been developed to record dynamic strength, power, muscular work capacity, range of motion, and to simulate actual job tasks. See Fig. 22-3 for one example.

Can you create a use for this machine (or redesign this machine) in another area of human movement? Why not in sports, music, or activities of daily living?

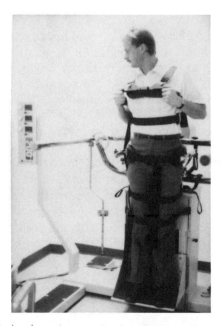

Fig. 22-3. *Isokinetic back and upper body assessment machine. Range of motion and dynamic strength throughout the range can be assessed in three dimensional space.*

THE FUTURE   **719**

HOW WILL EXERCISE BE PRESCRIBED AND PERFORMED IN THE 21ST CENTURY?

Overwhelmingly, the new exercise machines include digital display which monitor performance. We predict that, in the 21st century, exercise centers will not only use these high tech programmable machines, but also use computers to evaluate and individualize exercise prescriptions. Unfortunately, these prescriptions could be based upon inadequate knowledge and, therefore, may be dangerous to the user. Machines can be built to record any type of movement or force data and can manipulate and compare treatment protocols and control the operation of the machine, based upon feedback mechanisms. All these, however, are not valid if the parameters of the exerciser are not known or are calculated incorrectly. Too much assumed data, generic data, cadaver data, or otherwise normative data are the basis for the algorithms in today's powerful software interfaced with the exercise machines of today's technology. Collaborative efforts of life science researchers, engineers, and kinesiologists must be escalated if the customizing of fitness machines is to produce the desired benefits to individual exercisers.

DESIGNER SPORTS EQUIPMENT

It is evident that customization of sports equipment has become important to sporting goods manufacturers and the elite athlete and will become more and more so in the future. For example, have you heard of the robotic golfer? This is a robot programmed to produce the ideal biomechanical golf swing. Although one golfer was found who could reproduce this swing, we know that there is more than one biomechanically ideal-golf swing. The anthropometric characteristics and club characteristics influence the characteristics of the swing. Two writers in SOMA have modeled the anthropometric characteristics of men and women and predicted the length of club that will result in the most effective golf performance.

Some of the greatest technological changes have influenced the sport of tennis. In fact, as Wendland has written: "Tennis racquets enter the space age" (High Technology, April 1986). New materials for the frame and the strings, new shapes of racquet heads, new stringing patterns, and adjustable mechanisms are the common changes that have been developed to produce lighter and more durable racquets with greater damping of vibrations. In addition, each racquet can be evaluated with respect to its rebound, vibration, and duration of ball contact time on the racquet. How is this possible? This is possible through computer-aided design technology (CAD, CAM, CAEDS, etc.). This is the same technology used in the design of automobiles, airplanes, and racing vehicles. Finite element analysis is utilized to theoretically slice the racquet and calculate stresses on each slice to determine the deformation of racquet and strings. Subsequently, the vibrations caused by prescribed impacts of the ball on the string are calculated. Such complex analylsis (virtually impossible without a computer) accrues complex data for design of racquets. We now know, for example, that there actually are three "sweet spots" in the strings:

1) The well-known 'sweet spot' representing the center of percussion at which the shock to the human hand is minimized. This spot is usually closer to the handle than in the middle of the stringing pattern.
2) The sweet spot at which racquet vibrations are minimized. This is the node of the various natural frequencies and harmonic frequencies of the racquet and usually is farther from the handle than the middle of the string pattern.
3) The power sweet spot at which maximum rebound power is transmitted to the ball. This sweet spot is closest to the handle. Examples of the sweet spots of several racquets are depicted in Fig. 22-4.

Future technologists will need to design racquets with the power and center of percussion sweet spots coincidental.

The amount of time the ball remains on the strings determines the amount of spin. Players can adjust the tension in the strings to suit their stroke and optimize spin production. Unfortunately, such adjustments are selected by the player based upon what feels and appears to be the best. In the future, it might be possible to quantitatively assess racquet-player effectiveness and maximize the applications of this technology in programmable tennis racquets.

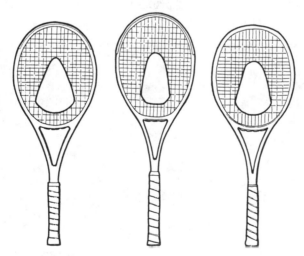

Fig. 22-4. *Note the varying sites and areas of sweet spots on different tennis racquets.*

THE FUTURE

SHOE TECHNOLOGY

Aerobic, running, and walking shoes are now a part of everyday life. But what about new technologies—the marching shoe, the fiber optic shoe, and the NASA shoe?

The advent of the marching shoe follows the trend to design specific shoes for specific purposes. Theoretically, human performance can be maximized if the shoe-surface interface is optimized. Traction, friction, and resiliancy are factors considered in the design of the shoe. Pragmatically, where does this trend lead? What will a person do if a "general" shoe must be worn one day? How many shoes must one own and pack for a day's activities? What are the similarities and differences among the movements performed in work, sports and daily living? More research must be conducted, and the existing research must be analyzed to avoid decision-making on the basis of non-interpreted or mis-interpreted data.

The latest in walking shoes is based upon cushioning mechanisms used in footwear on the moon. The midsoles consist of interlocking coil fibers that contract when the foot strikes the ground, generating a flow of energy the length of the sole and terminating in a potential upward force. The shoes act as a spring, much as the widely publicized Harvard University track surface acted as a spring to runners. One new spring-loaded system patent is depicted in Fig. 22-5.

Do you want to monitor the ground reaction forces continuously when you walk? By means of fiber optics, these forces can be measured with negligible increase in weight. The potential use of fiber optics for clinical assessment, biomechanical modeling, lower limb prosthetic design, evaluation of podiatric orthotics, and general research, such as investigation of neurological and circulatory problems, is beyond a single person's comprehension. We may finally, through fiber optics, solve the problem of how to measure shearing forces during continuous walking.

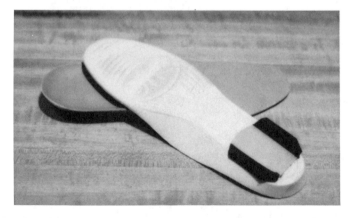

Fig. 22-5. *A stainless steel spring loaded heel designed shoe. Return of energy to the person to produce more efficient locomotion is the 1988 design trend of the athletic footwear industry.*

OUR ENVIRONMENT IN THE NEXT DECADE

Did you realize that some sports equipment have basic designs (or lack of design) created a century ago and that many of our home and garden tools are based upon archaic designs from the time of the Industrial Revolution? These earlier designs did not consider the heterogeneity of the population and the optimization of productivity.

A number of design changes today are based upon a vast amount of information. For example, the avid golfer can take a telescopic putter on business trips and putt in the hotel room. The putter extends from less that 12″ to a regulation length putter.

We can also go back to the stone age and use a reconstructed putter. (See Fig. 22-6). This putter can be used as effectively as most traditional golf putters on sale at sporting goods stores or golf shops.

Some changes in equipment might be detrimental to safe play. For example, if one ball rebounds faster than another, there may be inadequate response time for the player to avoid being struck. Either rules of play must be changed, protective equipment worn, or the equipment declared illegal.

Sports equipment for youth, for women, and for the elite have been developed. The game of basketball has three official sizes: youth size, women's size, and men's size. Also, women play with a softball that is larger than a baseball, but smaller than 12″ circumference. The purpose of these changes was to enable all players to be able to handle the ball equally well. Thus, hand sizes were taken into consideration when designing the ball size. What other equipment requires modification because of mis-matching of anthropometry and size of equipment?

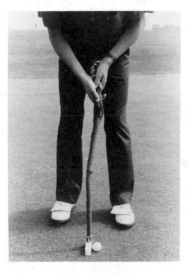

Fig. 22-6. *Golf putting can be performed successfully with this newly designed putter. We must weave historical information and experience into our design of high technology for human movement analysis.*

Designer Bats

House has reviewed and tested the state of the art with respect to softball bats. We are reprinting some of her material, presented at the 1987 National Convention of the American Alliance for Health, Physical Eduction, Recreation and Dance to introduce you to the process of design and evaluation (originally published through that association in 1988). Descriptions of some of the designer bats are as follows:

Nineteen bats, consisting of five normal and 13 designer bats, were measured and tested with respect to the following three mechanical characteristics:

1) location of center of gravity,
2) location of center of percussion (sweet spot), and
3) distribution of mass relative to axis of rotation at impact.

These bats were also classified as end-loaded, double-loaded or unloaded bats, based upon manufacturing processes.

The Broadsider three-sided bat advertises a "220% greater sweet spot for the ultimate in power and control." This means that the spot is more than two times greater on a flat surface than on the round surface of the traditional bat. The sweet spot is increased perpendicular to the length of the bat! The expensive graphite bats supposedly increase the sweet spot by 5% due to the nature of graphite.

The Broadsider also claims that it has a "new geometry for line drive power." Placing the flat surface toward the pitcher at contact is supposed to increase the chance of hitting a line drive. The success of this claim depends largely on the rotation of the hitter's wrists and the amount of spin on the ball. Theoretically, it could increase the chance of hitting a line drive.

Have you seen the Tidal Wave II? It contains water and is legal because it is welded closed and cannot be easily altered. The theory is that while waiting for the pitch, the fluid is nearer to the hands, lessening the radius of gyration. Once the bat has begun to rotate, centrifugal force pulls the fluid out to the barrel end to load the end and move the sweet spot to 4.4 inches from the end. The movement of the water makes it easier to initiate the swing and then creates a longer radius to the sweet spot.

The Bombat features "pressurized air, inside the bat," which "enhances a hitter's power and propels a softball farther." The theory is that the increased air pressure inside increases the coefficient of restitution between the bat and the ball.

Several of the bats sport a rough surface around the barrel. Theoretically this may affect batting in two ways. First, the ball tends to stay on the rough surface longer allowing the bat to do more work on the ball—give its force to the ball for a longer distance. Secondly, the rough surface may work like dimples on a golf ball to reduce the turbulent flow behind the swinging bat.

The Whizz bat is designed with numerous small holes through the barrel end. Air is supposed to flow through the bat to reduce form drag. Does it work? It does make a "whizzing" noise as it passes over the catcher's head! The air enters the bat through the holes thereby reducing the air pressure against the front of the bat, but once inside the air may be increasing the pressure against the back wall of the barrel. Perhaps, nothing is gained. It is interesting to note that the Whizz bat had the center of percussion closer to the end of the barrel than any of the other 18 tested bats.

Before you race out to your local sporting goods store and stock up on the heaviest end-loaded bats you can find, you need to understand the influence of the third parameter which we investigated for each of these bats: the distribution of the mass or weight with respect to the axis of rotation.

If you swing a bat first by its handle end and then turn it around and swing it by the barrel-end, you will notice that although the mass of the bat stays the same, it is harder to swing from the handle. This is because more of the mass of the bat (which is in the barrel) is distributed further from the axis of rotation when swinging with the handle. The parameter measured to compare each of the bats is called the radius of gyration. This is a distance that represents where the mass is concentrated with respect to the swing axis at the hands. In practical terms, we are talking about how hard it is to swing the bat or how much resistance the bat has to being swung. In numerical terms, hard and easy function as a square of the radius of gyration. So, if two bats had the same weight and one had a radius of gyration of 4 (weight concentrated closer to the handle) and the other of 8 (weight twice as far from the handle), then the second bat would be four times as hard to swing. If the bat is hard to swing, you will not be able to generate as much velocity—angular or linear—and will not be able to impart as much momentum to the ball.

In checking the results for our bats we find that the radius of gyration from the axis at the index finger of the top hand ranged from 16.28 to 18.39 inches (mean of 17.28 inches) for the end-loaded bats and from 15.46 to 17.79 inches (mean of 16.76 inches) for the unloaded bats. Again, there is overlap but the end-loaded bats on the whole will be harder to swing.

These bats, with others, were compared by means of a weighted ranking system in which each bat was ranked on the three mechanical factors and awarded a summed score as follows:

(1) weight rank times 1 with the heaviest bat ranked first
(2) center of percussion rank times 2 with the location closest to the barrel-end ranked first
(3) radius of gyration rank times 3 with the smallest value ranked first.

This ranking resulted in the following characteristics identified for the top five bats:

(1) All were end-loaded in some way.
(2) Only the top three bats showed desirable characteristics in all areas.
(3) The best bat was double-end-loaded with a large mass, relatively small radius of gyration (k) and a center of percussion relatively far out on the barrel end.
(4) Bats ranked 4 and 5 balanced a favorable center of percussion location with a very unfavorable radius of gyration which means they would be difficult to swing—making it hard to generate bat velocity.

In conclusion: It is clear that some of these bats have features which, from the point of view of mechanics, should enhance a batter's ability to hit the ball farther and/or harder. Manufacturers, however, are producing bats with greater mass distributed to move the sweet-spot toward the barrel end but at the expense of the ability to swing the bat. Manufacturers need to be encouraged to produce bats which will maximize all three characteristics.

EQUIPMENT AND SAFETY

New designs also are being developed to alleviate common sports injuries. (See Fig. 22-7.) The bent-handled bat, tennis racquet, racquet ball racquet, and golf club all have been developed to reduce either carpal-tunnel syndrome (numbness, paralysis of hand due to impediment of tendons, nerve, and/or arteries traversing wrist) or tendinitis at the elbow.

Guidelines to Design:

> know capabilities of the human body,
> understand the performance pattern and the desired pattern,
> determine best tool to optimize pattern, and
> determine optimum pattern for existing tools.

Modeling and Simulation

Some types of modeling and simulations procedures are the basis for the development of expert systems and the ultimate understanding of how we move, what can be done to improve movement, and how to predict risk of trauma to our bodies. Solid 3-D models, wire models, and 2-D models are rapidly being developed (see Fig. 22-8) from a variety of data, kinematic and kinetic. Imaging with magnetic resonance or ultrasound are avenues by which the biomechanics of the inner body can be studied. (See Fig. 22-9.) The synthesis of inner and outer human movement data will be commonplace and necessary if we are to obtain the required large body of knowledge to formulate expert systems.

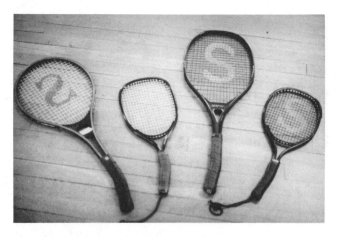

Fig. 22-7. *Bent handled racquets and bats have not been successful despite research supporting their use. Individuals who use these often are confronted with rules against their use, laughter, or inappropriate coaching. Although these may not be the implements of the future, these and other new designs will not be given adequate evaluation if tradition, rules, and other resistances hinder new designs. (Courtesy of Sentra, Chicago.)*

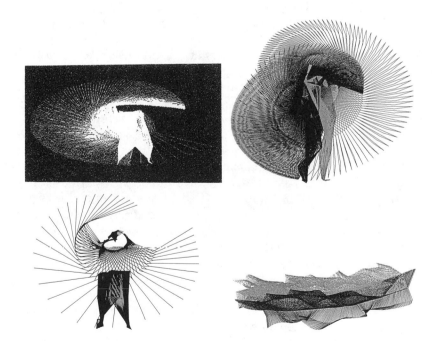

Fig. 22-8. *Computer modeling, simulation, and design is possible in planar, wire and solid 3-D models, and in the 4th and 5th dimensions. Examples related to human movement are depicted as a vision to the future. (Courtesy of Peak Performance Technologies, Inc., Human Analysis Corp., and Ariel Dynamics, Inc.)*

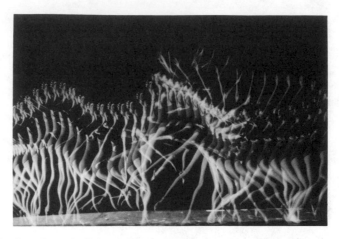

Fig. 22-9. *Imaging of all levels, including holography, thermography, magnetic resonance, and ultrasonic, can be used to more discretely analyze human movement, especially of the internal tissues and organs, and can be used to diagnose with the imaging interfaced computer recognizing the images. Examples are depicted to create ideas for future applications.*

EXPERT SYSTEMS

The next step in the process of maximizing the information gained via human movement analysis is the development of expert systems. Since we are an information society, we collect information, process it to make sense of it, retrieve it to share it, and use it to solve problems. Then we collect data again, add to the body of information, process the information, and continue this cycle over and over. One of the most advanced technological approaches in applying knowledge to the diagnosis of problems is by means of expert systems technology. This technology is commonplace in the field of medicine to diagnose disease states. All knowledge concerning symptoms of diseases, based upon published information and experts in the medical profession, form a computer data base from which the symptoms of a patient can be matched to the appropriate disease filed in the computer. More recently, a "second opinion expert system" has emerged. This expert system serves as a microcomputer-based consultation system and was designed to provide physicians with second opinions in less than one second. The uniqueness of this system is that the physician enters relative-important-ranking of the symptoms. As with all expert systems, this system incorporates inference strategy based upon data existing in the computer. The first step in the process is information gathering. The next step is comparative: normal or abnormal. The abnormalities are then identified with respect to classification, disease state, or other type of profile. Conclusions are then inferred.

No use of an expert system in human movement analysis exists, but we predict that such a use will occur. In the sports world the expert system is being used to analyze game strategy and prediction of probable strategies for success against certain opponents based upon previous game strategies. Expert systems in industry diagnose risk of injury during lifting tasks.

In 1983, Sierig, at the University of Wisconsin, collected data of a limping gait. The orthopedic surgeon needed to excise part of the bone. A computer-generated model of this gait was produced and simulation techniques were used to produce a normal walking and running gait as a result of incremental computer excised bone. Instructions then were given to the orthopedist, who then performed the surgery.

There are several research laboratories in which gait is being performed via artificial muscle activation. Micro-processors are interfaced with a computer preprogrammed to stimulate a biomechanics gait, or preprogrammed to respond to actions of the person, and thus produce the walking pattern.

Highly productive and appealing expert system data bases have been developed in the sports world. One of these is a combination of biomechanical-physiological, developed exclusively in swimming. The other is a biomechanical one exclusively for track and field. Since the concepts and data contained in each approach are valuable for other applications, each is described briefly.

Evaluation Center for Swimmers

This profiling has been one of the most comprehensive internationally publicized programs in the sports world. Each profile card consists of ranked anthropometric, flexibility, strength, and speed parameters. The relationships of motor, time-space, and hydromechanics factors to these parameters also has been investigated.

Altogether (in 1983) 30 time-space, 44 anthropometric, 22 flexibility, 7 strength, 24 swim tests, and 117 derived indices have been used to predict performance. In 1984, the Center organized the European Olympic Solidarity Program Seminar to teach coaches and researchers the procedure for developing and utilizing their evaluative approach and data base. Some of the profile charts and areas of investigation are presented in Fig. 22-10.

TRACK AND FIELD

On-site immediate cinematographic analysis sports movements is happening now, and will be commonplace in the future. International teams of researchers have collected data at the World Junior Championships in Athens in 1986 and subsequent other competitions, and made outputs available between 2 and 24 hours after the end of the competitions. Results included individual performance profiles and comparisons among performances, as well as comparison with the winner. The winner was designated as the model by which individual

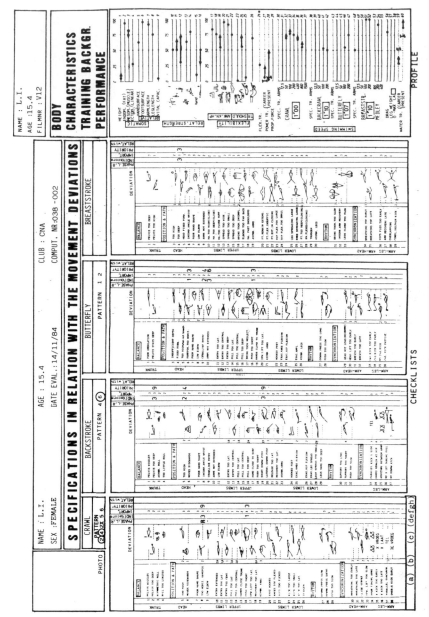

Fig. 22-10. An example of profiling to determine characteristics of swimmers and to predict success in swimming.

730

performances were judged. Selected results are depicted in Fig. 22-11.

If expert systems are to be used, cheaper and easier devices for assessing human movement must be constructed. Videocameras interfaced with user-friendly software and portable free-recording and temporal recording devices are being used in isolated applications. We

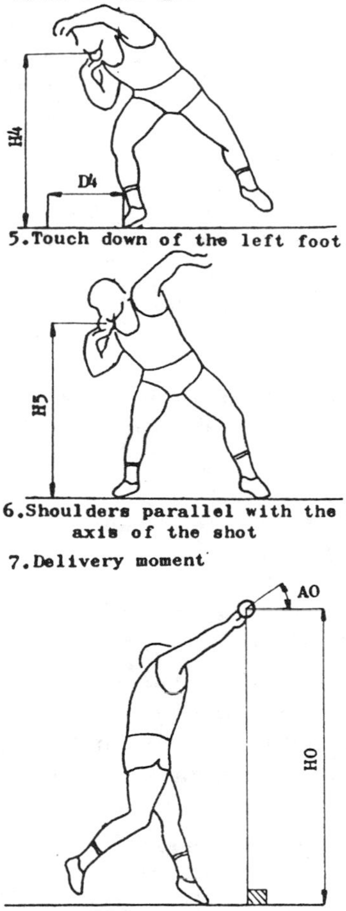

Fig. 22-11. *An example of profiling in track and field activities to enhance performances of the non-champions, as well as the champions.*

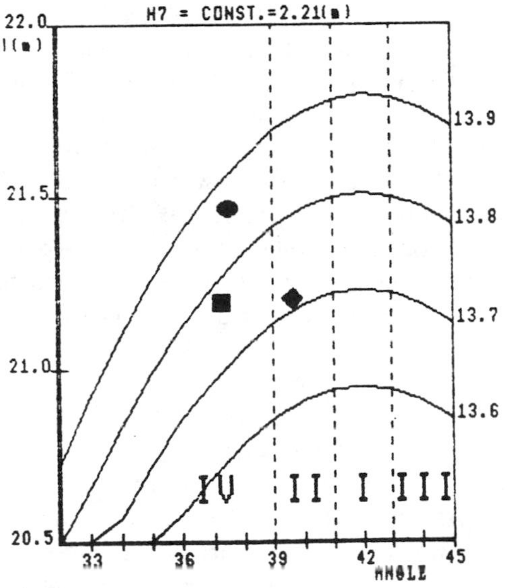

predict that sophisticated assessments (complete with average and elite profiles with which to compare a given group or individual) will be commonplace. Biomechanical expert systems will be merged with expert systems from psychology. Super computers can be utilized. Applications will then be made to learning new skills, matching persons to movement patterns such as a job, sport or musical instrument.

SPACE FLIGHT

Living in space is probably the most exciting thing people can look forward to! What affect will space shuttles and space stations have upon human movement? What happens to the body and life systems as we experience life in zero gravity? What will happen to the body as the mind becomes paramount and all normal reality is suspended? We've already noted the following changes in the astronauts involved in United States space missions and in simulated weightlessness experiments:

1. Loss in body weight.
2. Anatomic and anthropometric changes, such as flexion of upper trunk, flexion of legs, extension of thoracolumbar spine, appearance of a quadruped.
3. Lower body negative pressure; that is, the fluid pressure and volume shifted cephalically, raising the center of gravity of the body and placing stresses on the body.
4. Mineral loss in bones and consequent bone strength loss.
5. Muscle strength decrements, especially in antigravity muscle groups and weight-bearing groups.
6. Reduced work tolerances.
7. Need to relearn simple tasks (indicated to be possible).
8. Disturbances in vestibular function.

Life in outer space necessitates well-designed programs to prevent these changes from occurring. Because of the zero gravity environment and the restricted life-space, innovations will be required. For example, devices were developed such as shoe cleat locking into a grid floor to produce reaction forces so that movements could occur within the spacecraft chamber. Physical exercise programs, new games, sports and ways to perform ADL will need to be developed.

Already we are seeing travel exercise kits for the space age being marketed. Each year new devices, or modifications of old devices, are introduced to the consumer. For example, in 1988, Quik-Fit introduced a Golf Gym kit advertised to develop fitness for golf-specific muscle strengthening and conditioning, and as a power swing workout program. Other sport-specific kits also have been developed (Fig. 22-12). If the trend continues, there will be individualized portable systems for developing movement patterns and fitness for every job, every sport, other leisure activities, and for activities of daily living.

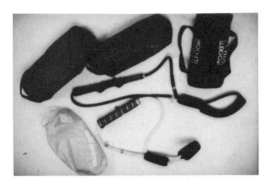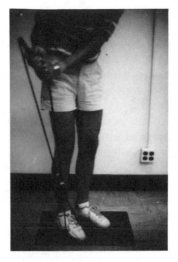

Fig. 22-12. *Specialized exercise-wherever-you-go-kits. Do they work? Analysis of movement patterns performed with the kits should be compared with natural movements. Are there additional benefits obtained with the kits? The time is now to advance human movement performance.*

These would be used in the smallest spaces, such as on a spaceship shuttle, in a train, and in the home and place of work. Coincident with this trend will be development of corporate fitness centers for all employees, not merely the white collar or executive workers. The biomechanics specialist will have a primary role in the directing and setting of these trends.

HUMAN MOVEMENT TOMORROW

During the past decade, Frisbee, walleyball and other new sports and games have created new patterns of movement. Likewise, high technology has been the cause of new ways to perform old jobs and the creation of new jobs. Picture yourself lying prone in a hammock suspended on a wire track as you pick strawberries eight hours a day. Or more sophisticated yet, you direct the picker robot to select the ripe strawberries you are inspecting with a video scanning device. Picture also pressing a few buttons to activate robots to perform all tasks for you. You step onto a platform that carries you to the ocean beach. You select groceries via a video catalog and they are delivered to you. High technology consists of voice activated devices so that fingers need not press buttons.

THE FUTURE

New ways of viewing human movement are beginning to emerge. Three of these emerging perspectives are: 1) control biomechanics, 2) ecological biomechanics, and 3) synergistic biomechanics.

Control biomechanics is a synthesis of traditional biomechanics (time, space, force of human movement and effects of forces upon the human body) and neuromuscular physiology. The end product is a more complete understanding of how optimum movment and force are produced and controlled. At this time the control biomechanists are not concerned with the trauma and safety aspects of biomechanics. Experimental data are collected with respect to movement adaptations to imposed constraints. We see this area of biomechanics as a useful approach to the study of the neurologically impaired person.

Ecological biomechanics is an energy approach to the analysis of goal-directed human behavior. Thus, both psychology and biology are considered as the physical geometry of movement is investigated. This movement lies midway between the highest boundary underlying the theory of relativity—the speed of light and beyond and that of quantum mechanics (movement of particles). Human movement is nonlinear, nonconservative, nonanalytically continuous, and nonholonomic. Because human beings choose to direct, and redirect, their movements according to their goals, the ecological biomechanist perceives space in multiple reference frames and movement in conservative and nonconservative terms. The complexity of this approach requires three-dimensional computer graphics to test the theory. We do not know what concepts and applications will be discovered from this approach.

Synergistic biomechanics is a synthesis of art and science. This implies that the rational and metaphoric, the qualitative and quantitative, and the humanist and reductionist are brought together. Such an integration results in a fuller understanding of movement. The "emergent entity" is greater than the sum of its parts, combining the knowing (feeling and imaging) of the right half of the cortex with the analytical and verbal knowing of the left half of the cortex. In fencing there is a metaphor for how to hold the weapon—like a bird held in the hand, tight enough to keep it from flying and gentle enough to prevent hurting it. Garrett (1986) used computer graphics to produce images of rhythm and flow, and at the same time images with force vectors. The effect is unique and may be the most productive avenue of communication in the area of biomechanics.

Many beginning kinesiology students will soon be able to investigate problems once thought worthy of being studied only by the most sophisticated graduate students. The president of California Polytechnic State University in the early 1960s said that every 10 years the advancement of knowledge has been so rapid that the level of study has moved downward as much as four years in ranking.

Although we are anatomically limited in how we can move, remember the phrase "structure determines function—function determines structure." The human body will change, the devices the human body uses will change, and the environment in which the human body lives will change. Thus the questions of the next decade are unasked and unknown. How then, can be have the answers? Basic concepts concerning what is known must be used to pose the questions of the future and problem-solve for more effective, safer and more rewarding human movement.

Remember, facts are merely items we know; but, facts change and new facts are derived. Human Movement is dynamic. We also must be dynamic and receptive to new concepts.

REFERENCES

Garrett, G. (1986) Synergistic Biomechanics. In *Biomechanics—The 1984 Olympic Scientific Congress Proceedings*, Adrian, M. and Deutsch, H. (Eds.), Eugene, OR: Microform Publications.

International Journal of Sports Biomechanics (1985–1988) Champaign, IL: Human Kinetics Publishers Inc.

Journal of Orthopaedic and Sports Physical Therapy (1979–88) Baltimore, MD: American Physical Therapy Association.

Lipton, L. (1988) Stereoscopic Video. *Advanced Imaging*, Jan. pp. A23–24.

National Strength and Conditioning Association Journal, Lincoln, Nebraska, (1980–1988).

Soma, Engineering for the Human Body, (1986–1988), Baltimore, MD: Williams and Wilkins.

Turvey, M., Kugler, P. (1984). An ecological approach to perception and action. In *Human Motor Actions: Berstein Reassessed*, Whiting, H. (Ed.) Amsterdam: North-Holland Publishing Co.

Winter, D. (1987) Mechanical power in human movement: generation, absorption and transfer. In *Current Research in Sports Biomechanics*, Van Gheluwe, B., Atha, J. (Eds.) *Med. Sport Sci*, vol 25, pp. 34–45. Basel, Karger.

Appendices

Appendix A
International
System of Units

The International System of Units (Système International, or SI) is now the universal system. It is sometimes referred to as the metric system, since distance (meters) is one of the most common items measured. The basic units of measurement for the movement analyst are those measuring time, distance, force, and mass. These form the basis for all the other kinematic and kinetic measures.

Table A-1 lists the SI standard unit and common multiples or fractions for each of the measures together with equivalents from the English system of measurement, the system previously used exclusively in the United States. Table A-2 lists some commonly used units that are derived from mathematical manipulation of the basic units or from a combination of time, force, distance, and mass units.

Table A-1. *SI Units*

SI Unit	English Equivalent
Linear distance	
Meter (m)	3.28 feet (ft)
Millimeter (mm), 0.001 m	0.0394 inches (in)
Centimeter (cm), 0.01 m	0.3937 inches
Kilometers (km), 1000 m	0.621 miles
Angular distance	
Radian (rad)	57.296 degrees (°)
2π rad	360 degrees or 1 revolution
Time	
Minute (min)	Same
Second (sec), $^1/_{60}$ min	Same
Hour (hr), 60 min	Same
Force	
Newton (N)	0.225 pounds (lb)
Kilonewton (kn)	225 pounds
Mass	
Kilogram (kg)*	0.0685 slugs*
Gram (gm), 0.001 kg	0.0000685 slugs

*Note that 1 kg is equal to 1 $Nsec^2/m$; 1 slug is equal to $lb\text{-}sec^2/ft$.

739

Table A-2. *Derived Units*

SI Unit	English Equivalent
Velocity	
Meter per second (m/sec)	3.28 ft/sec or 0.447 mph
Acceleration	
Meter per second per second (m/sec^2)	3.28 ft/sec^2 or 0.447 miles/hr^2
Linear momentum (mV)	
Kilogram-meter per second (kgm/sec)	
(equal to newton-second)	0.225 lb/sec
Impulse (Ft)	
Newton-second (Nsec)	0.225 lb/sec
Moment of force (torque)	
Newton-meter (Nm)	0.738 ft-lb
Work (energy)	
Joules (J) (equal to newton-meter)	0.738 ft-lb
Power	
Watt (W) or newton-meter per second	
(Nm/sec)	0.738 ft-lb/sec
Moment of inertia (I)	
Kilogram-meter^2 (kgm^2)	0.738 slug-ft^2
Angular momentum (I)	
Kilogram-meter^2 · radian per second	
(kgm^2 rad/sec)	0.738 slug-ft^2 rad/sec
Pressure (Pa)	
Pasqual	
Kilopasqual	
Newton per centimeter^2	0.689 lb/in^2

Appendix B
Anatomical Charts

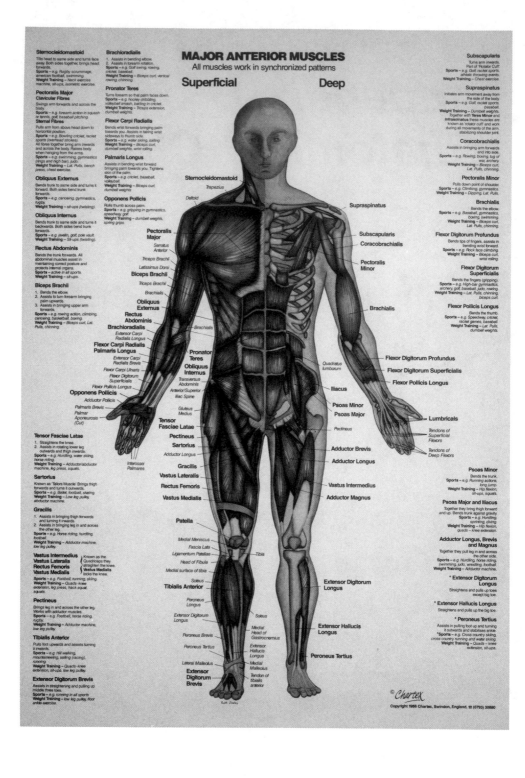

MAJOR ANTERIOR MUSCLES
All muscles work in synchronized patterns

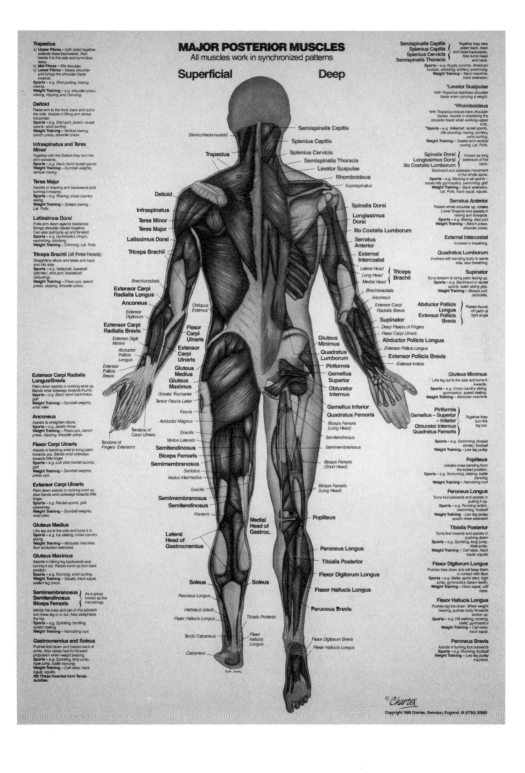

MAJOR POSTERIOR MUSCLES
All muscles work in synchronized patterns

Superficial   **Deep**

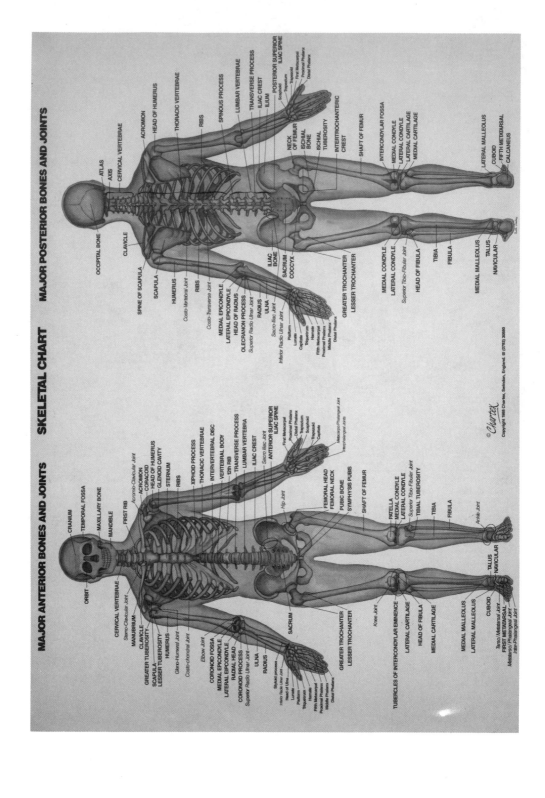

SKELETAL CHART

MAJOR ANTERIOR BONES AND JOINTS

MAJOR POSTERIOR BONES AND JOINTS

Appendix C Trigonometry, Vectors, and Problems

It is possible to solve many force and velocity problems by drawing vector diagrams. However, the degree of accuracy is dependent on the exactness of the drawing and measuring. In addition, this approach is time consuming when compared to the quicker, more accurate method using trigonometry. The word *trigonometry* literally means the *measurement of triangles*. Most problems in motion analysis involve the use of right triangles.

A right triangle is one containing an internal right angle (90 degrees). It should be recalled the *sum of the three internal angles of a triangle always equals 180 degrees*. Also, an *angle less than 90 degrees is called an acute angle* and one *greater than 90 degrees is an obtuse angle*. Two angles are said to be *complementary* if their sum equals 90 degrees. Thus in a right triangle it is apparent that the two acute angles are complementary. (If the sum of two angles equals 180 degrees, they are said to be supplementary.)

To understand the trigonometric functions, one must first be able to identify the parts of a right triangle. The following diagram of a right triangle will be used for the purpose of explanation.

The six component parts of the triangle consist of three angles and three sides. In the diagram below, it should be noted that the longest of the three sides (c) is opposite the right angle (C). This longest side is called the hypotenuse. Since the hypotenuse is always opposite the right angle, it is very easy to identify. The other two sides are called the *legs* of the right triangle. A side may also be referred to as the *side opposite* a particular angle. In the diagram, the side opposite angle A is side a. The side opposite angle B is side b. Ad-

Prepared by Jim Richards, Indiana University, 1979.

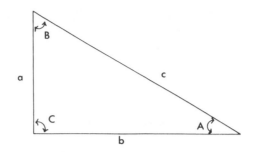

jacent side is a term used to identify the side that, along with the hypotenuse, forms a given angle. Thus the side adjacent to angle A is side b. Likewise, the side adjacent to angle B is side a. It is important to understand that the hypotenuse never changes; which side is opposite or adjacent depends on which angle is being considered.

Of the six trigonometric functions, four will be described here. These functions are based on the relationships between the angles and sides of the triangle.

The *sine* of an angle (pronounced "sign" and abbreviated *sin*) is defined as the ratio of the side opposite to the hypotenuse. Thus the sine of angle A is the length of side a divided by the length of side c, the hypotenuse (sin A = a/c) and the sine of angle B is the length of side b divided by the length of side c (sin B = b/c).

The second trigonometric function is the *cosine (cos)*, defined as the ratio of the side adjacent to the hypotenuse. For angle A the cosine is b/c; for angle B it is a/c.

The *tangent (tan)* is defined as the ratio of the side opposite to the side adjacent. The tangent of angle A is a/b, and the tangent of angle B is b/a.

The *cotangent (cot)* is the ratio of the side adjacent to the side opposite. The cotangent of angle A is b/a; the cotangent of angle B is a/b.

These trigonometric functions have a specific, constant value for any given angle regardless of the size of the triangle. Since the values are constant, they can be compiled in tables such as Table C-1.

Since one angle in a right triangle is fixed, only five parts can vary (three sides and two angles). If either one angle and the length of one side or the lengths of two sides are known, the remaining parts can be calculated. The sides can be used to represent distance, magnitude of force, velocity, or other physical properties (vectors).

EXAMPLE: Assume that the hypotenuse is 6 cm in length and angle A is 40 degrees. Find (1) angle B, (2) side a, and (3) side b.

1. Angle B can be determined very readily since it is complementary to angle A, which is 40 degrees:

$$90 - A = B$$
$$90 - 40 = B$$

2. To find side a, we must select the trigonometric function that involves side a (which is unknown) and side c, the hypotenuse (which is known). The sine of angle A equals side a (opposite) over side c.

$$\sin A = \frac{a}{c}$$

Since c is known to be 6 cm and sin A can be obtained from Table B-1, the only unknown is side a.

$$\sin 40 = \frac{a}{6 \text{ cm}}$$
$$.6428 = \frac{a}{6 \text{ cm}}$$
$$6 \times .6428 = a$$
$$a = 3.86 \text{ cm}$$

3. The same procedure is used to find side b.

The following problems are included as practice exercises. It may be helpful to make a sketch of each triangle to better understand the problem.

1. GIVEN: Hypotenuse = 10 cm; one angle = 30 degrees
   FIND: Both legs (sides) of the triangle
2. GIVEN: One angle = 55 degrees; side opposite = 4 m
   FIND: Hypotenuse and adjacent side
3. GIVEN: Hypotenuse = 4 in; one side = 3 in
   FIND: Both acute angles
4. GIVEN: One leg = 3 m; other leg = 5 m
   FIND: Both acute angles and hypotenuse
5. GIVEN: A ball projected at an angle of 25 degrees with the horizontal; an initial resultant velocity of 10 m/sec (resultant equals hypotenuse)
   FIND: Vertical and horizontal components of the velocity
6. GIVEN: At take-off, long jumper with a forward velocity of 32 ft/sec and a vertical velocity of 12 ft/sec
   FIND: Angle of take-off and resultant velocity

Table C-1. *Trigonometric functions**

Degrees	Sines	Cosines	Tangents	Cotangents	Degrees
0	.0000	1.0000	.0000		90
1	.0175	.9998	.0175	57.290	89
2	.0349	.9994	.0349	28.636	88
3	.0523	.9986	.0524	19.081	87
4	.0698	.9976	.0699	14.301	86
5	.0872	.9962	.0875	11.430	85
6	.1045	.9945	.1051	9.5144	84
7	.1219	.9925	.1228	8.1443	83
8	.1392	.9903	.1405	7.1154	82
9	.1564	.9877	.1584	6.3138	81
10	.1736	.9848	.1763	5.6713	80
11	.1908	9816	.1944	5.1446	79
12	.2079	.9781	.2126	4.7046	78
13	.2250	.9744	.2309	4.3315	77
14	.2419	.9703	.2493	4.0108	76
15	.2588	.9659	.2679	3.7321	75
16	.2756	.9613	.2867	3.4874	74
17	.2924	.9563	.3057	3.2709	73
18	.3090	.9511	.3249	3.0777	72
19	.3256	.9455	.3443	2.9042	71
20	.3420	.9397	.3640	2.7475	70
21	.3584	.9336	.3839	2.6051	69
22	.3746	.9272	.4040	2.4751	68
23	.3907	.9205	.4245	2.3559	67
24	.4067	.9135	.4452	2.2460	66
25	.4226	.9063	.4663	2.1445	65
26	.4384	.8988	.4877	2.0503	64
27	.4540	.8910	.5095	1.9626	63
28	.4695	.8829	.5317	1.8807	62
29	.4848	.8746	.5543	1.8040	61
30	.5000	.8660	.5774	1.7321	60
31	.5150	.8572	.6009	1.6643	59
32	.5299	.8480	.6249	1.6003	58
33	.5446	.8387	.6494	1.5399	57
34	.5592	.8290	.6745	1.4826	56
35	.5736	.8192	.7002	1.4281	55
36	.5878	.8090	.7265	1.3764	54
37	.6018	.7986	.7536	1.3270	53
38	.6157	.7880	.7813	1.2799	52
39	.6293	.7771	.8098	1.2349	51
40	.6428	.7660	.8391	1.1918	50
41	.6561	.7547	.8693	1.1504	49
42	.6691	.7431	.9004	1.1106	48
43	.6820	.7314	.9325	1.0724	47
44	.6947	.7193	.9657	1.0355	46
45	.7071	.7071	1.0000	1.0000	45
Degrees	**Cosines**	**Sines**	**Cotangents**	**Tangents**	**Degrees**

*For angles largers than 45 degrees, be sure to use the headings that appear at the *bottom* of the columns.

748

APPENDICES

PROBLEMS

1. In the following triangle, label the sides (opposite, hypotenuse, and adjacent) with respect to angle a.

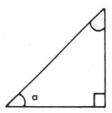

2. In the following triangle, complete the appropriate ratios.
   sin a = _____
   cos a = _____
   tan a = _____

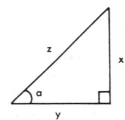

3. Using Table C-1, find the following.
   sin 30°   cos 30°   tan 40°
   sin 60°   cos 60°   tan 60°

4. In the following triangle, find the value of angle a.

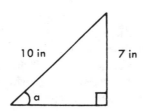

5. If angle a is 20 degrees and side A is 10 inches long, find sides B, and C and angle b.

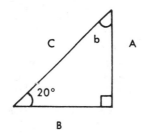

6. Find the two unknown sides and one unknown angle in the following triangle.

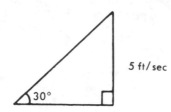

7. A woman walks 8 miles east, turns left, and walks 16 miles north. What is her resultant displacement?
8. The side of a mountain makes a 20-degree angle with the horizontal. If a man walks 1 mile up the mountain, how much has he increased his elevation?
9. A football is kicked with a resultant velocity of 12 m/sec at a 20-degree angle to the ground. What are the horizontal and vertical components of the velocity?
10. Without using trigonometric functions, determine the length of the hypotenuse (also called the resultant side) in the following triangle.

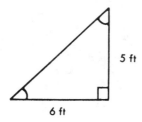

11. A man walks 36 km east and then 10.4 km north. What is his resultant displacement?
12. An automobile travels on a road 50 degrees north of east. If the car goes 17 miles, what are the north and east components of the displacement?
13. The side of a mountain makes a 30-degree angle with the horizontal surface of the earth. If a man walks 2 miles up the mountain side, what is his vertical elevation above the horizontal surface?
14. Find the resultants of the four following vectors:
    a. 100 cm at 0 degrees
    b. 80 cm at 40 degrees
    c. 110 cm at 130 degrees
    d. 160 cm at 210 degrees
15. A runner changes speed from 20 ft/sec to 28 ft/sec in 4 seconds. What is the acceleration? The average velocity? The total distance traveled?

16. A stone is dropped from the top of a vertical cliff. It strikes at the foot of the cliff 3 seconds after it was dropped. How high is the cliff? With what velocity did it strike?

17. If the wheels of an automobile have diameter of 60 cm, how far does the car move when the wheels in contact with the road turn through 9 radians?

18. If a plank 12 ft long of uniform cross-section and density and weighing 120 lb is placed so that 5 ft of it extends over the bank of a creek, how far out on the plank can a boy weighing 75 lb walk without tipping the plank? What is the minimum weight of stone that must be placed on the end on shore to permit the boy to walk to the end over the creek without tipping?

19. A player jumps into the air with both arms extended vertically overhead. Just before the maximum height is reached one arm is forcibly lowered so that the center of gravity is lowered 2 to 4 cm in the body. Do the fingertips of the other hand go higher or lower as a result? How much?

20. If a jumper jumps 2 ft high and takes off at an angle of 20 degrees with the horizontal, how fast is he going forward after the takeoff?

21. If the shot is put at an angle of 42 degrees with the horizontal and with a velocity of 10.8 m/sec in the direction of the put, what will be its upward velocity at the moment of release? What will be its forward velocity? What will be its time of flight from the point of release to the return to the same level at which it was released? How high will the shot go?

22. At the moment of take-off, a broad jumper has a forward velocity of 9 m/sec. Her vertical velocity is 3 m/sec. What is the angle of her takeoff? How high does her center of gravity rise?

23. If the shot were projected horizontally at a speed of 40 ft/sec from a height of 32 ft, how soon would it hit the ground? How far from the starting point would it hit in horizontal distance?

Appendix D
Projectiles

Projection of an object or of oneself is the outcome—the product—of many actions. It is affected by gravity, velocity and angle of projection. The effect of gravity on unsupported objects is the same regardless of the weight of the object (see Fig. D-1). (Metric system would mean a distance of $16.1/3.28 = 4.9$ M.)

The constant acceleration of gravitational force pulls the object downward a distance that equals in feet $16.1\ t^2$, in which t represents the time in seconds during which gravity has been acting on the object. In 1 second an object would be pulled downward 16.1 ft (16.1×1^2); in 0.5 second the distance would be 4.025 ft (16.1×0.5^2). If the velocity and direction imparted by body levers are known, the path of flight can be determined. In Fig. D-1 the horizontal line represents the projection of an object by means of force imparted by the body, a velocity of 80 ft/sec in a horizontal direction. Each dot represents an additional 8 ft in flight and also an additional 0.1 second of time. The effect of gravity at each time interval is represented by the vertical lines. The lower ends of the vertical lines mark the path of flight resulting from the two forces. The path of flight can be determined in like manner whenever the velocity and direction imparted by body force to an object are known.

· · ·

With trigonometric relationships the measures of angles and velocities can be obtained in many ways; those which require the least calculation can be used. As one example the angles of projection might have been determined before the velocities. When the angle is known, another trigonometric value might be used to determine the length of the time to the high point and subtracting from the product, the $16.1\ t^2$ value for this time.

The processes described can be used to determine the position of the projectile at any time in its flight. When the projection has a downward component, the $16.1\ t^2$ value is added, instead of subtracted, in determining the height, and the resulting sum would be subtracted from the starting height.

752

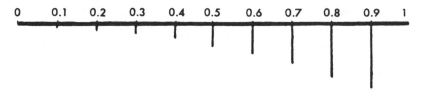

Fig. D-1. *Gravitational effect at each 0.1 second on object projected horizontally at 80 ft. 0.4 in represents 8 ft.*

Knowledge of velocity, angle, and position at any time in flight can be applied to many situations and will enable the instructor to set specific goals for development of skill in a given situation. One illustration is that of developing skill in a tennis serve. Most beginners are likely to direct the ball upward; yet a velocity of 80 to 90 ft/sec can be achieved by the average adult. Suppose that the height at which the ball is impacted is 8 ft and the ball has a velocity of 80 ft/sec. The net is approximately 40 ft from the impact, and the ball would reach it in 0.5 second. The 16.1 t^2 value for this time is 4.025 ft, so that, as the ball reaches the net, it would be 3.975 ft above the ground, thus clearing the net by 0.975 ft. The ball would reach the ground when the 16.1 t^2 value was 8 ft; $8 = 16.1\ t^2$; $t^2 = 8/16.1 = 0.4969$; $t = 0.704$ second. The horizontal distance would be $80 \times 0.704 = 56.32$ ft, which is well within the service court.

Angle, velocity, and ball position have been applied by Mortimer in determining the projection most likely to make a basket from the free throw line when the starting point is 5 ft above the floor. She recommends a velocity of 24 ft/sec and an angle of 58 degrees.

OPTIMAL PROJECTION ANGLE FOR GREATEST DISTANCE

A projection angle of 45 degrees is often recommended as the optimum when the greatest possible distance is desired. This is true only when the vertical distance between the starting point and the end of the flight is zero. Bunn has shown this in discussing the projection of the shot put.

When the vertical distance between the start and the end of flight and the velocity of projection are known, the angle that results in the greatest distance is one in which the following applies:

$$\text{Sine}^2 = \frac{\text{Velocity}^2}{2\,(\text{velocity}^2 - gh)}$$

In this formula, g is 32.2, and h is the vertical distance between the start and end of flight. If the start is higher than the end, h will be a minus quantity.

Bunn gives a table of the distances that the shot put would reach

APPENDICES   753

if projected at angles from 37 through 44 degrees when released at a height of 7 ft at velocities from 20 to 50 ft/sec. If the shot were given a velocity of 30 ft/sec, the determination of the optimal angle would be as follows:

$$\text{Sine}^2 = \frac{30^2}{2[30^2 - (32.2 \times -7)]}$$

In this case the end of the flight is below the starting point, and h has a minus value.

$$\text{Sine}^2 = \frac{900}{2\,(900 + 225.4)}$$
$$\text{Sine}^2 = \frac{900}{2250.8} = 0.39985$$

In this case the sine = 0.6323, which is the value for an angle of 39° 13'. For a 39-degree angle and for a 40-degree angle Bunn's table gives a distance of 34.42 ft, the longest for the angles included in his table.

In jumping for distance the center of gravity is higher at the beginning of light than it is at landing. At the beginning of flight the body is extended, the arms are raised, and in an adult 6 ft tall, the height of the center of gravity can be estimated as 3 plus ft. If the landing is made with the thighs horizontal and some inclination of the legs, it will be assumed for this illustration that the center of gravity is 1.5 ft lower than it was at the beginning of flight. If the velocity of projection is 16 ft/sec, the optimal angle for greatest distance will be one in which the following applies:

$$\text{Sine}^2 = \frac{16^2}{2\,[16^2 - (32.2 \times -1.5)]}$$
$$\text{Sine}^2 = 0.4206$$

In this case, the sine = 0.645. This is the value of an angle of 40°26'.

If the velocity is 12 ft/sec and the other measures remain the same, the optimal angle is 37° 43'. If the positions of the center of gravity are determined at the beginning and end of flight, as they can be from film, the value of h can be more accurately determined. The velocity of the center of gravity can also be determined from these film measures (Chapter 13). In calculating the angle of projection in better-than-average performers, we have found that this angle is less than 45 degrees; this is another example of the body's making necessary adjustments without the person's being aware that it is doing so.

SUMMARY OF CALCULATIONS AND OTHER COMMENTS

For ready reference the calculations discussed here and others that are related and useful are summarized here.

Range is the horizontal distance between the starting and landing point; time means the time in flight.

1. Horizontal velocity = Range ÷ Time.
2. In determining vertical velocity (V. vel.) consideration must be given to the vertical distance (VD) between the starting and the landing point.
   When VD is 0:

   $$V. \text{ vel.} = 16.1 \, t^2 \div \text{Time}$$

3. When the starting point is higher than the landing point:

   $$V. \text{ vel.} = (16.1 \, t^2 - VD) \div \text{Time}$$

   Note that, if $16.1 \, t^2$ is less than VD, the minus quantity indicates that the projection is below the horizontal.

4. When the starting point is lower than the landing point:

   $$V. \text{ vel.} = (16.1 \, t^2 + VD) \div \text{Time}$$

5. For the projection velocity (Proj. vel.):
   a. When the horizontal velocity (Horiz. vel.) and vertical velocity components are known:

   $$(\text{Proj. vel.})^2 = (\text{Horiz. vel.})^2 + (V. \text{ vel.})^2$$

   b. When the angle of projection is known.

   Proj. vel. = V. vel. ÷ Sine, or
   Proj. vel. = Horiz. vel. ÷ Cosine.

6. The angle of projection can be determined by use of trigonometric relationships. For the angle of projection:
   a. Tangent of the angle = V. vel. ÷ Horiz. vel.
   b. Sine of the angle = V. vel. ÷ Proj. vel.
   c. Cosine of the angle = Horiz. vel. ÷ Proj. vel.
7. The high point (h.p.) of the projection can be located by finding first the time to the high point.

   Time to high point = V. vel. ÷ 32.2

8. The distance of the high point above the starting point = (V. vel. × Time to h.p.) -16.1 (time to h.p.)^2
9. The horizontal distance from the starting to the high point = Horiz. vel. × time h.p.

The relationships used in finding the high point can be used to locate the projectile at any time and at any point in flight. For example, a tennis ball was projected from a height of 7 ft and 40 ft from the net at a velocity of 50 ft/sec and at an angle of 10 degrees above the horizontal. Where was the ball when it reached the net? The horizontal and vertical velocity components must be known. They can be found by rearranging the equations in 5b:

V. vel. = Proj. vel. × Sine
Horiz. vel. = Proj. vel × Cosine

For an angle of 10 degrees the sine is 0.173; the cosine is 0.984. In the described tennis situation the numerical values are as follows:

V. vel. = 50 × 0.173, or 8.65 ft/sec
Horiz. Vel. = 50 × 0.984, or 49.2 ft/sec

Following is the time to the net:

40 ÷ 49.2, or 0.81 second

During this time the vertical velocity has moved the ball upward; gravitational force has moved it downward. The combined effect will be as follows:

$(8.65 \times 0.81) - 16.1 (0.81)^2$
7.00 − 10.573, or 3,573 ft

At the time the ball reaches the net, it will be 3.573 lower than the starting point, or 3.427 ft above the ground and 0.427 ft above the net, which is 3 ft in height.

The questions might also arise as to where the ball would be at a given time, such as 0.5 second after the flight began. From the starting point it would travel horizontally as follows:

49.2 × 0.5, or 24.6 ft

Vertically it would travel as follows:

$(8.65 \times 0.5) - 16.1 (0.5)^2$
4.325 − 4.025, or 0.3 ft

In 0.5 second the ball would be 0.3 ft higher than, and 24.6 ft from, the starting point. The spinning ball in flight is affected by the amount and direction of force applied at takeoff and the type and amount of spin (see Figure D-2).

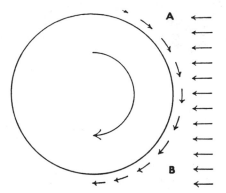

Fig. D-2. *Rapidly spinning ball in flight encounters more resistance at A that at B and in flight will curve toward B.*

Table D-1. *Gravity distance relationship: Given a specific free-fall time, a ball will fall a predetermined distance.**

Time	0.00	0.01	0.02	0.03	0.04	0.05	0.06	0.07	0.08	0.09
0.0	0.000	0.001	0.006	0.014	0.025	0.040	0.057	0.078	0.013	0.13
0.1	0.161	0.194	0.231	0.272	0.315	0.362	0.412	0.465	0.521	0.58
0.2	0.644	0.710	0.779	0.851	0.927	1.006	1.088	1.173	1.262	1.35
0.3	1.449	1.547	1.648	1.745	1.861	1.972	2.086	2.204	2.324	2.44
0.4	2.576	2.706	2.840	2.976	3.116	3.260	3.387	3.556	3.709	3.86
0.5	4.025	4.187	4.353	4.524	4.694	4.870	5.048	5.230	5.416	5.60
0.6	5.796	5.980	6.188	6.290	6.584	6.802	7.014	7.227	7.444	7.66
0.7	7.889	8.116	8.346	8.579	8.816	9.056	9.299	9.545	9.795	10.04
0.8	10.304	10.573	10.825	11.091	11.360	11.632	11.970	12.186	12.468	12.75
0.9	13.041	13.332	13.627	13.925	14.226	14.530	14.838	15.148	15.462	15.77
1.0	16.100	16.432	16.750	17.080	17.414	17.750	18.090	18.433	18.779	19.12
1.1	19.481	19.837	20.196	20.558	20.923	21.292	21.664	22.039	22.417	22.79
1.2	23.184	23.602	23.963	24.357	24.755	25.156	25.560	25.967	26.378	26.79
1.3	27.209	27.629	28.052	28.469	28.899	29.342	29.788	30.208	30.660	31.10
1.4	31.556	32.008	32.464	32.922	33.384	33.850	34.318	34.790	35.265	35.74
1.5	36.225	36.709	37.197	37.688	38.172	38.680	39.180	39.684	40.192	40.70
1.6	41.216	41.732	42.252	42.776	43.307	43.832	44.365	44.901	45.440	45.98
1.7	46.529	47.078	47.630	48.187	48.745	49.306	49.861	50.439	51.011	51.58
1.8	52.164	52.745	53.329	53.917	54.508	55.102	55.660	56.310	56.903	57.51
1.9	58.121	58.734	59.361	59.907	60.593	61.220	61.849	62.482	63.118	63.75
2.0	64.400	65.046	65.644	66.346	67.002	67.960	68.322	68.987	69.206	70.326

t	.00	.01	.02	.03	.04	.05	.06	.07	.08	.09
2.1	71.001	71.679	72.360	73.044	73.732	74.422	75.116	75.813	76.514	77.217
2.2	77.924	78.634	79.347	80.064	80.783	81.566	82.232	82.962	83.694	84.430
2.3	85.169	85.911	86.657	87.405	88.157	88.912	89.671	90.432	91.197	91.965
2.4	92.736	93.510	94.288	95.069	95.854	96.640	97.431	98.224	99.021	99.823
2.5	100.625	101.432	102.341	103.054	103.871	104.690	105.503	106.339	107.168	108.000
2.6	108.836	109.675	110.517	111.362	112.211	113.262	113.917	114.780	115.637	116.502
2.7	117.369	118.240	119.114	119.992	120.872	121.756	122.643	123.534	124.437	125.024
2.8	126.224	127.127	128.034	128.943	129.856	130.772	131.692	132.614	133.540	134.469
2.9	135.401	136.336	137.275	138.217	139.162	140.110	141.062	142.016	142.974	143.936
3.0	144.900	145.868	146.828	147.802	148.790	149.770	150.754	151.781	152.731	153.724
3.1	154.721	155.721	156.724	157.730	158.740	159.752	160.768	161.787	162.810	163.835
3.2	164.864	165.896	166.931	167.970	169.021	170.056	171.104	172.157	173.210	174.268
3.3	175.168	176.393	177.480	178.531	179.605	180.682	181.763	182.846	183.933	185.023
3.4	186.116	187.212	188.312	189.415	190.521	191.630	192.742	193.858	194.977	196.100
3.5	197.125	198.354	199.585	200.620	201.759	202.901	204.045	205.193	206.344	207.498
3.6	208.656	209.817	210.981	212.148	213.319	214.492	215.669	216.849	218.033	219.219
3.7	220.409	221.602	222.798	223.998	225.200	226.406	227.615	228.828	230.043	231.262
3.8	232.484	233.709	234.938	236.169	237.404	238.642	239.884	241.128	242.376	243.627
3.9	244.881	246.138	247.399	248.663	249.930	251.200	252.474	253.750	255.030	256.314
4.0	257.600									

*Distance in feet through which freely falling objects move in a given time, calculated as distance = $\frac{1}{2}gt^2$ (g = 32.2). Conversion to metric system: value in table, divided by 3.28.

Appendix E
Maximum
Moments of Force

Maximum Moments of Force (Torques) Acting At Selected Joints During Various Movement Activities.

	ANKLE		KNEE		HIP		SHOULDER		ELBOW		WRIST	
	Flex.	Exten.	Flex.	Exten.	Flex.	Exten.	Flex.	Exten.	Flex.	Exten.	Flex.	Exten.
Badminton smash	270		39		44		22	17	6	7	2	2
Basketball, vertical jump	300	80	45	75	6	30	6					
Bicycling, 15 mph	3	3	3	40	22	14						
Fencer's lunge, front	275	185	81	130	75	25						
Fencer's lunge, rear	300	290	90	120		63						
Football block		300		240	30	125						
Football punt		300	16	90	75	35						
Golf drive, back arm	200		130				19	9	9	12	5	5
Hammer throw	500	500	300	240	150	200	100	45	90	90	50	90
Head spring					10		33	30	30	24	24	26
Rowing, 36/min.	3		20		3		10	12	9	1	5	1
Swim start		59	11	87	56	26	11	13	5	5		
Tennis serve	150	300	5	95	49	70	27	24	16	14	5	6
Track start	400	400	240	230	60	115						

Measurement is in kg m.

Appendix F
Anthropometric Values

Comparison of 5th, 50th, and 95th Percentile Anthropometric Values of Different Aged Populations.

VARIABLE	AGE	MALE				FEMALE			
		MEAN	5	50	95	MEAN	5	50	95
Weight (kg)	1	9.5	7.8	9.4	11.1	8.9	6.4	8.8	10.6
	6	20.8	15.6	20.7	24.7	19.3	15.2	19.1	23.2
	13	40.7	28.1	39.8	53.4	48.0	35.7	45.9	59.7
	Adult	70.8	55.5	68.6	90.8	60.0	46.6	59.6	74.5
Height (cm)	1	73.5	68.6	72.4	79.8	72.4	67.5	72.7	76.3
	6	133.7	105.4	114.3	120.3	112.8	104.2	113.1	121.5
	13	149.5	137.9	148.3	160.3	155.1	144.0	154.7	164.4
	Adult	174.1	162.8	174.1	185.3	163.0	152.6	162.8	174.1
Sitting height (cm)	1	47.2	44.7	46.3	50.3	46.3	43.0	45.6	50.1
	6	62.4	56.8	62.8	65.8	61.3	56.9	61.2	65.0
	13	76.8	71.5	76.9	82.4	80.0	75.3	80.4	86.2
	Adult	89.3	83.5	89.3	95.4	85.1	79.0	85.2	90.8
Hand length (cm)	1	8.8	8.1	8.7	9.8	8.8	7.4	8.8	9.4
	6	12.6	11.4	12.6	13.6	12.4	11.3	12.3	13.5
	13	15.9	14.3	15.8	17.4	16.8	15.0	16.7	18.4
	Adult	19.0	17.4	19.0	20.6	17.4	16.1	17.4	19.0
Knee height (cm)	1	20.1	18.9	19.9	22.2	19.3	17.1	19.5	21.4
	6	34.1	30.7	34.0	36.8	34.0	30.4	33.8	37.4
	13	47.5	42.1	47.4	55.5	49.0	45.4	49.1	52.3
	Adult	55.1	50.2	55.1	60.2	51.0	46.9	50.9	55.5
Buttocks-foot (cm)	1	35.0	31.6	35.0	37.8	34.1	31.7	33.6	37.0
	6	62.5	57.1	62.7	67.1	63.0	50.9	62.4	69.0
	13	86.9	80.2	86.3	99.0	92.2	83.8	93.1	98.8
	Adult	N/A	N/A	N/A	N/A	N/A	N/A	N/A	N/A
Shoulder breadth (cm)	1	20.7	18.9	20.7	22.5	20.3	18.7	19.9	22.3
	6	27.8	25.2	27.5	30.6	27.3	24.6	27.1	29.8
	13	35.8	32.7	35.7	41.7	37.4	33.5	36.8	41.8
	Adult	45.1	41.2	45.0	49.4	42.1	38.4	42.0	45.7
Lower torso breadth (cm)	1	15.2	13.8	15.0	18.1	14.6	13.1	14.4	16.8
	6	19.6	17.3	19.5	21.9	19.8	17.7	19.7	22.0
	13	26.2	23.8	25.5	30.9	28.7	25.0	28.5	31.5
	Adult	N/A	N/A	N/A	N/A	N/A	N/A	N/A	N/A

INDEX

Isometric exercise, 336
Isotonic exercise, 334

Javelin, throwing, 525–530
Jogging, inadequate equipment for, 436
Joint actions, lower limbs, 286;
  swinging limb, 449–451;
  when running, 448–449, 452–453
Joint stability, 65
Joints, metatarsophalangeal, 57;
  types of, 62–63;
  understanding actions of, 165
Judo, 628–632;
  techniques, classifying, 629;
  throws, movement principles, 630
Jump, distance factors, 471–472
Jumping patterns, older people, 304
Jumping, 467–490;
  basketball, 593–596;
  defined, 467;
  immature patterns, 294;
  types of, 467
Jumps, running, 478–482
Jumpshot, basketball, 586–589

Karate, 620–623
Kicking, 565–574;
  immature patterns, 294;
  joint action in, 109
Kinathropometry, 21, 57
Kinematic, continuum stages, 278;
  factors, pole vaulting, 487;
  link system, 11, 13
Kinematics, 5;
  of projectiles, 151–152
Kinesiology, definition of, 5
Kinetic energy, 159;
  of moving object, 430
Kinetic, factors, pole vaulting, 487–488;
  modeling, 398
Kinetics, walking, 283
Knee action, when running, 445
Knee ligament rehabilitative exercises, 359–361
Knee surgery, effect on gait, 377

Labyrinthine, dysfunction, 303;
  reflex, 180–181
Landing pits, 435
Landing, described, 434–436;
  protective equipment, 435–436
Latissimus Dorsi, adduction of Humerus, 110
Law of inertia, 136
Learning theory, movement patterns, 277
Leg extension, Rectus Femoris, 109;
  standing jumps, 469–471
Leg-length, effect on gait, 379–380
Lever bones, 112
Lever systems, classified, 98;
  elements of, 98–99;
  muscle-bone, 113;
  of humans, 97
Lever, defined, 97;
  elements of, 97–98
Leverage, in artist movement, 408
Levers, bony, function of, 100–101;
  external, 98;

identification of, 98;
  muscle group, 112;
  single muscle, 106
Lifting, 318–319
Limb inclination, supporting, 288–290
Linear momentum, 155–157
Linear motion, 137–138
Linear velocity, 117, 119;
  formula, 120
Locomotion, 311–313;
  described, 10–11
Locomotor patterns, aging, 302;
  development of, 183–186;
  walking, 284
Longitudinal axis, of bone, 102
Longus muscle, 113
Low back pain, in dancers, 410–411;
  pianists, 416
Lower limb adduction, 112
Lower limbs, joint action, 286–287
Luge, 680–682
Lumbar curve, 28

Magnetic resonance imaging, 112, 209
Magnus effect, 537–539
Magnus muscle, 113
Manipulative patterns, 279
Materials handling limits, 392–394
Maturation, of movement pattern, 278
Mechanical considerations, of movement, iden-
  tifying, 272
Mechanical research, in dance, 414
Metatarsophalangeal joints, 57;
  action, 284, 286
Modeling, 726;
  kinetic, 398;
  mathematic, 225–227;
  three-dimensional, 402–403
Moment arm lengths, 122–123
Moment arm, 99
Moment of inertia, 141–142
Moments of force, 399–401;
  effecting skiing, 670–672
Momentum, angular, 157;
  impulse, 153;
  linear, 155–157;
  principles of, 158
Morphology, described, 21
Motion factors, 268
Motion, analysis of, 13;
  concept of, 127;
  described, 9;
  general, 10;
  kinematics of, 5–6;
  laws of, 125–128, 136–138;
  linear, 137–138;
  rotary, 9, 12–13, 138–140;
  spatial characteristics of, 5–6;
  spatial, 9;
  translatory, 9, 11;
  vertical, 136–137
Motor acts, 176–178
Motor control systems, changes, 304
Motor development, children, 279;
  process of, 278;
  inherent, 182–184
Motor skills, stopping moving objects 429–430
Motor units, 171;
  stimulation of, 171–172
Movement analysis models, 264–274

wind instrumentalists, 420;
Potential energy, 159
Power skating, 663–665
Power, definition of, 84
Pressure patterns, foot, 284
Principles of, diving, 686–687;
  gymnastics, 686–687;
  momentum, 158;
  movement, artists, 407;
  movement, biomechanical, 273
Pronated feet, 34, 409–410
Proprioceptors, 173
Propulsive forces, in swimming, 642–652
Prostheses design, 374–375
Prostheses, evaluation of, 375–376
Prosthetics, effect on gait, 370–373
Protective equipment, 436–437
Proximal bone, 100–101
Psychologists, 23–24
Psychometrists, 23

Quadriceps Femoris muscle, 27
Qualitative analysis, 230
Qualitative videography, 240
Quantitative analysis, 230–231
Quantitative video analysis, 240–241

Racewalking, 461–465
Racing dive, 476–478
Racquet sports, 541–557;
  principles, 542–543;
  stroke mechanics, 542–543
Racquets, described, 541–542
Range of motion (ROM), 63–64;
  charts (ROM), 389;
  exercises (ROM), 342–344
Rapid ballistic movement, 93
Rapid tension movement, 93
Reaction, force 103;
  time, 188–189
Receptors, 172–173;
  pacinian, 176;
  skin, 176
Rectus abdominis muscle, 340
Rectus femoris muscle, 117
Reflex acts, development of, 178
Reflex patterns, diving, 687;
  gymnastics, 687
Reflexes, 279;
  labyrinthine, 180–181;
  myotatic, 178–180;
  tonic-neck, 181–182
Rehabilitative biomechanics, defined, 357
Rehabilitative exercises, guidelines, 358–359;
  knee ligament, 359–361
Research tools, dance, 413
Research, defined, 4
Research, electromyography, 191
Resistance arm, 99;
  in a throw, 121
Resistance forces, 98–99
Resistance vector, 99
Reversed muscle action, 284
Rings, in gymnastics, 702
Rising from floor, 317–318
Roller skating, 667
Rope jumping exercise, 346

Rotary motion, 9, 12–13, 138–140
Rotation of axis, 13, 101
Rowing machines, 353–354
Running economy, 457–458
Running foot position, 444–445
Running high jump, 482–484
Running long jump, 478–480
Running, arm action in, 442–443;
  braking force, 445;
  center of gravity, 443;
  curves, 447;
  described, 439;
  efficiency of, 460;
  fatigue effects, 458–459;
  forces affecting, 459;
  grades, 447;
  hip action, 445–446;
  immature patterns, 292–293;
  joint actions, 448–449;
  knee action, 445;
  mechanics of, 440–441;
  older people, 303–304;
  speed, 460;
  terrain, 447;
  track starts, described, 453–456;
  trunk angle, 446

Sagittal plane, 8–9, 13, 186
Sarcolemma, 77
Sarcoplasm, 76–77
Scale method, determining center of gravity, 48
Scoliosis, 34
Segmental method, determining center of gravity, 48–52
Sense organs, of aged, 304–306
Senses, types of, 197
Serving, volleyball, 605–608
Shoe technology, 722
Shooting, basketball, 583–592
Shot put, throwing, 523–525
Shunt muscles, 103–104
Side horse, in gymnastics, 704–706
Sidearm throwing, 501–502
Simulation, 726
Single image photography, 202
Single muscle levers, 106;
  in frontal plane, 110–111
Sinusoidal, center of gravity, 283
Sitting posture, 324–325
Skateboarding, 676–677
Skeletal muscle, 76
Skeletal system, of aged, 305, 307–308
Skeleton, 61–62
Skiing, 667–668;
  balance techniques, 669–670;
  concepts of turns, 673–674;
  effect of terrain, 672–673;
  initiating turns, 672;
  moments of force, 670–672;
  slope angle, 667–669;
  steering, 670;
  underweighting, 673
Skin receptors, 176
Slide manipulation, 414
Soccer, 570–572
Softball batting, 538–540
Soleus muscle, 34
Somatotyping, described, 21

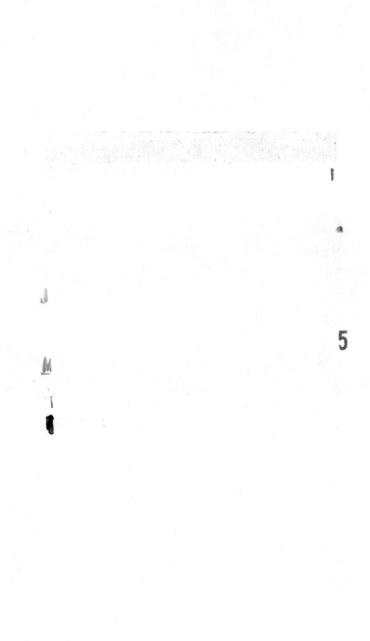